CARDIAC DRUGS

CARDIAC DRUGS

Second Edition

Editors

Kanu Chatterjee MBBS FRCP (London) FRCP (Edin) FCCP FACC MACP

Clinical Professor of Medicine
Kanu and Docey Edwards Chatterjee Chair in
Cardiovascular Medicine
Division of Cardiology
The Carver College of Medicine
University of Iowa
Iowa City, Iowa, USA
Emeritus Professor of Medicine
University of California
San Francisco, California, USA

Eric J Topol MD FACC

Director, Scripps Translational Science Institute
Chief Academic Officer, Scripps Health
Professor of Genomics
The Scripps Research Institute
La Jolla, California, USA

JAYPEE *The Health Sciences Publisher*

New Delhi I London I Philadelphia I Panama

Jaypee Brothers Medical Publishers (P) Ltd

Headquarters
Jaypee Brothers Medical Publishers (P) Ltd
4838/24, Ansari Road, Daryaganj
New Delhi 110 002, India
Phone: +91-11-43574357
Fax: +91-11-43574314
Email: jaypee@jaypeebrothers.com

Overseas Offices

J.P. Medical Ltd
83 Victoria Street, London
SW1H 0HW (UK)
Phone: +44 20 3170 8910
Fax: +44 (0)20 3008 6180
Email: info@jpmedpub.com

Jaypee-Highlights Medical Publishers Inc
City of Knowledge, Bld. 237, Clayton
Panama City, Panama
Phone: +1 507-301-0496
Fax: +1 507-301-0499
Email: cservice@jphmedical.com

Jaypee Medical Inc
The Bourse
111 South Independence Mall East
Suite 835, Philadelphia, PA 19106, USA
Phone: +1 267-519-9789
Email: jpmed.us@gmail.com

Jaypee Brothers Medical Publishers (P) Ltd
17/1-B Babar Road, Block-B, Shaymali
Mohammadpur, Dhaka-1207
Bangladesh
Mobile: +08801912003485
Email: jaypeedhaka@gmail.com

Jaypee Brothers Medical Publishers (P) Ltd
Bhotahity, Kathmandu, Nepal
Phone: +977-9741283608
Email: kathmandu@jaypeebrothers.com

Website: www.jaypeebrothers.com
Website: www.jaypeedigital.com

© 2015, Jaypee Brothers Medical Publishers

Inquiries for bulk sales may be solicited at: jaypee@jaypeebrothers.com

Cardiac Drugs / Editors, Kanu Chatterjee, Eric J Topol

First Edition: 2013
Second Edition: **2015**

ISBN: 978-93-5152-851-7

Printed at: Sanat Printers

Contents

Contributors

EDITORS

Kanu Chatterjee MBBS FRCP (London) FRCP (Edin) FCCP FACC MACP
Clinical Professor of Medicine
Kanu and Docey Edwards Chatterjee Chair in
Cardiovascular Medicine
Division of Cardiology
The Carver College of Medicine
University of Iowa
Iowa City, Iowa, USA
Emeritus Professor of Medicine
University of California
San Francisco, California, USA

Eric J Topol MD FACC
Director, Scripps Translational Science Institute
Chief Academic Officer, Scripps Health
Professor of Genomics
The Scripps Research Institute
La Jolla, California, USA

CONTRIBUTING AUTHORS

Jason A Bartos MD PhD
Cardiology Fellow, Cardiovascular Division
University of Minnesota
Minneapolis, Minnesota, USA

Philip F Binkley MD MPH
Wilson Professor of Medicine and Public Health
Division of Cardiovascular Medicine
Davis Heart and Lung Research Institute
The Ohio State University of Medicine and Public Health
Columbus, Ohio, USA

Prakash Deedwania MD FACC FACP FAHA
Chief of Cardiology Division
VACCHCS/UMC, UCSF Program at Fresno
Fresno, California, USA

Michael E Ernst Pharm D
Professor, Department of Pharmacy Practice and Science
University of Iowa College of Pharmacy
Department of Family Medicine
University of Iowa Carver College of Medicine
University of Iowa Hospital and Clinics
Iowa City, Iowa, USA

Gary S Francis MD
Professor, Cardiovascular Division
University of Minnesota
Minneapolis, Minnesota, USA

Rakesh Gopinathannair MD MA
Assistant Professor, Division of Cardiology
University of Louisville
Director of Cardiac Electrophysiology
University of Louisville Hospital
Louisville, Kentucky, USA

Garrie J Haas MD FACC
Professor, Division of Cardiovascular Medicine
The Ohio State University of Medicine and Public Health
Davis Heart and Lung Research Institute
Columbus, Ohio, USA

Sif Hansdottir MD
Professor of Medicine
Division of Pulmonary and Critical Care
The Carver College of Medicine
University of Iowa Hospitals and Clinics
Iowa City, Iowa, USA

Lee Joseph MD
Fellow in Cardiovascular Diseases
Department of Internal Medicine
University of Iowa
Iowa city, Iowa, USA

Wassef Karrowni MD
Interventional Cardiology
UnityPoint Clinic
Cedar Rapids, Iowa, USA

Suma H Konety MD
Assistant Professor, Cardiovascular Division
University of Minnesota
Minneapolis, Minnesota, USA

Ravinder Kumar MD
Fellow, Division of Cardiovascular Medicine
Department of Internal Medicine
University of Iowa Hospitals and Clinics
Iowa City, Iowa, USA

William J Lawton MD FACP
Associate Professor Emeritus
Division of Nephrology-Hypertension
Department of Internal Medicine
University of Iowa Carver College of Medicine
University of Iowa Hospitals and Clinics
Iowa City, Iowa, USA
Adjunct Associate Professor
Department of Medicine
University of Massachusetts Medical School
Worcester, Massachusetts, USA

Carl V Leier MD
Emeritus Overstreet Professor of Medicine and Pharmacology
Division of Cardiovascular Medicine
Department of Medicine
The Ohio State University College of Medicine
Columbus, Ohio, USA

Brian Olshansky MD FACC FAHA FHRS
Professor, Division of Cardiovascular Medicine
University of Iowa Hospitals and Clinics
Iowa City, Iowa, USA

Krishan V Soni MD MBA
Fellow, Interventional Cardiology
Division of Cardiology
Department of Medicine University of California
San Francisco, California, USA

Sundararajan Srikanth MD
Cardiology Fellow, Department of Medicine
UCSF Program at Fresno
Fresno, California, USA

Thenappan Thenappan MD
Assistant Professor, Division of Cardiovascular Medicine
University of Minnesota
Minneapolis, Minnesota, USA

Byron Vandenberg MD
Associate Professor, Division of Cardiovascular Medicine
Department of Internal Medicine
University of Iowa Hospitals and Clinics
Iowa City, Iowa, USA

Stephen W Waldo MD
Fellow, Division of Cardiology Department of Medicine
University of California
San Francisco, California, USA

Yerem Yeghiazarians MD
Associate Professor, University of California
San Francisco, California, USA

Preface to the Second Edition

Globally, cardiovascular disease is a major cause of morbidity and mortality and the burden of disease is expected to grow even further. Management of cardiovascular disease has been a rapidly evolving field with the ever increasing armamentarium of pharmacological agents for treating these disorders. As new research moves ahead, newer and newer agents with novel mechanisms are being developed. However, this has led to a unique situation where, in many clinical circumstances, the physician faces the dilemma of choosing the most appropriate available drug therapy for the patient. It was our goal to help the care providers identify the best-available drug options when the first edition of 'Cardiac Drugs' was planned.

The first edition was very well appreciated and it is the conviction of the readers that has given us the strength and direction to come out with the second edition in its present shape and form. The chapters have once again been written by experts, amalgamating evidence-based research with years of experience in treating the patients. Like the first edition, this edition is replete with diagrams and illustrations and elaborate tables which help readers understand the concepts clearly and easily. Latest references and guidelines have been incorporated to keep the information current and relevant and some of the chapters have been extensively re-written.

We thank all those who have been associated with us in this exciting journey and once again implore our readers to keep sending in their suggestions and feed back so that we have the opportunity to evolve and live upto their expectations. We thank all the contributors for their efforts and time and for making this book, a reference title, suitable both for clinicians and trainees in cardiovascular medicine.

Kanu Chatterjee
Eric J Topol

Preface to the First Edition

The book *Cardiac Drugs* presents an evidence-based approach towards the pharmacologic agents that are used in various clinical conditions in cardiovascular medicine.

The classes of drugs, such as renin-angiotensin-aldosterone blocking drugs, positive inotropic drugs, diuretics, and anti-hypertensive drugs are discussed in great details with their pharmacokinetics, pharmacodynamics, indications, contra-indications, and doses. Drugs for heart failure, acute coronary syndromes, and pulmonary hypertension are also discussed similarly. Pharmacologic agents, which are in development for various clinical syndromes are also discussed. The unique feature of this book is the detailed discussion on the guidelines of the American College of Cardiology/American Heart Association for the use of pharmacologic agents in various clinical conditions.

Kanu Chatterjee
Eric J Topol

Vasodilators and Neurohormone Modulators

Gary S Francis, Jason A Bartos, Thenappan Thenappan, Suma H Konety

INTRODUCTION OF THE AFTERLOAD REDUCTION CONCEPT

It has long been recognized that impedance to left ventricular (LV) outflow (afterload or increased wall stress during systole) is a critical determinant of cardiac performance.[1-4] This is especially true of patients with impaired LV systolic performance, such as that occurs in systolic heart failure (Fig. 1).[5] Ultimately, the failing heart's ability to respond to increased impedance is diminished. We now know that specific drugs lower aortic impedance, thus, restoring myocardial systolic function to some extent.

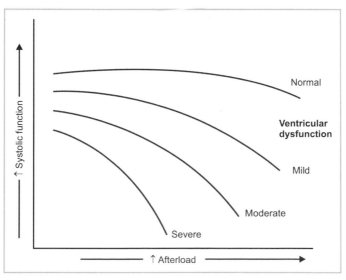

FIG. 1: The relationship between various degrees of left ventricular dysfunction and afterload stress.

The factors that makeup impedance and impair LV ejection of blood in patients with heart failure are multiple, complex, and highly interactive. They include:

● *Peripheral arteriolar vasoconstriction*: This is due to heightened neurohormonal activity including augmentation of the sympathetic nervous system, and intense activation of the renin-angiotensin-aldosterone system (RAAS). There is also release of vasopressin and endothelin, potent peripheral vasoconstrictors.

● Increased LV wall stress during cardiac myocyte shortening—a concept known as "afterload". Afterload is a term that emerged years ago from the study of isolated muscles. It is a laboratory but not a bedside measurement.

● Diminished distensibility of the large vessels such as the aorta and its major branches.

● Reduction in small vessel caliber and compliance.

● Increased blood viscosity and inertia.

Each of these forces can act collectively to impair LV outflow tract flow or cardiac output during contraction and may improve to some extent with vasodilator therapy.

Heightened resistance or impedance to LV ejection is often referred to as "afterload", but the term afterload originates from isolated muscle studies done in the mid-1970s and is not, strictly speaking, appropriately applied to the clinical setting. Afterload is defined as ventricular wall stress during myocyte shortening, and cannot be easily measured in the intact circulation. It is a product of LV cavity size (LaPlace relationship) and systolic arterial pressure and is inversely related to wall thickness or hypertrophy. In clinical practice, systemic vascular resistance (SVR) is a surrogate for afterload that is frequently calculated from right heart catheterization data [SVR = (mean arterial pressure – CVP) × 80/cardiac output], but this calculation is largely an estimate of small peripheral vessel resistance. SVR is, therefore, only a part of the total impedance that affects LV ejection (Table 1). The failing ventricles (both left and right) are exquisitely sensitive to afterload conditions, and it is a logical extension of this concept that drugs that reduce aortic impedance will improve cardiac systolic performance, independent of any effect on myocardial contractility.

TABLE 1: Components of aortic impedance

- Large vessel distensibility
- Small vessel caliber (systemic vascular resistance)
- Small vessel compliance
- Blood viscosity
- Inertia

Vasodilator Drugs and Low Blood Pressure

Patients with moderate-to-severe heart failure often have low blood pressure that is asymptomatic. Low brachial systolic pressure is sometimes perceived by physicians as a contraindication to the use of arteriolar dilator drugs such as nitrates, angiotensin converting enzyme (ACE) inhibitors, angiotensin receptor blockers (ARBs), or carvedilol. However, vasodilator drugs can maintain systolic blood pressure by increasing stroke volume in patients with impaired systolic function. Observations from large clinical trials have challenged the belief that vasodilators are deleterious in patients with low systolic blood pressure.[6-8] Generally speaking, vasodilator drugs should be continued in patients with systolic heart failure and asymptomatic low systolic blood pressure in the range of 80–110 mmHg is not necessarily a contraindication to vasodilator therapy. Severe, symptomatic hypotension can sometimes occur in a volume-depleted patient in response to the first dose of an ACE inhibitor. For example, this might occur following a robust diuresis. Such brisk falls in blood pressure can be treated by leg elevation. Clinicians recognize that symptomatic hypotension is a well described adverse event that can occur when ACE inhibitors or ARBs are used in the context of hypovolemia and an activated RAAS. Symptomatic reduction in systolic blood pressure in response to vasodilators in a euvolemic or volume overloaded patient with severe LV dysfunction is another matter. Such patients are said to be truly intolerant of vasodilators, and symptomatic hypotension in response to drug therapy is a very powerful sign of poor prognosis. Low blood pressure without symptoms is far more common and is usually tolerated by patients using vasodilator drugs.

To avoid symptomatic hypotension when using vaso-dilator drugs to treat heart failure, it is best to begin with the lowest tolerable dose, and then gradually titrate the drugs over several weeks. This requires great patience and frequent contact with the patient. However, the goal is to prevent adverse effects, such as dizziness, light-headedness, syncope, extreme fatigue, and re-admission to the hospital for generalized malaise. It is now a common practice to have highly trained nurses with expertise in heart failure manage such patients soon after hospital discharge (1 week or sooner at our medical center) to carefully proceed with medication titration in a highly monitored setting. In addition to monitoring patient response, serum electrolytes and renal function are frequently assessed. Frequent follow-up soon after hospital discharge with measurement of electrolytes and careful physical examination seems to be an important element in reducing re-hospitalization.

Arterial versus Venous Effects of Vasodilator Drugs in Patients with Systolic Heart Failure

The hemodynamic effects of vasodilator drugs are dependent on the relative effects of the drug on resistance and capacitance vessels. Arterial vasodilators such as hydralazine or amlodipine reduce aortic impedance and thereby increase the velocity of shortening during LV ejection. LV end-systolic volume is thus reduced, and LV ejection fraction increases. With hydralazine, LV end-diastolic volume (i.e., preload) is not acutely altered, so the stroke volume response can be markedly increased.[9] When venodilator drugs such as nitrates are employed in patients with systolic heart failure, blood volume may acutely redistribute into the large capacitance veins, and LV end-diastolic volume or preload is reduced. The reduced LV end-diastolic volume can limit the increase in stroke volume to some extent.[10] With balanced arteriolar-venous vasodilator drugs, such as sodium nitroprusside, a combination of decreased venous pressure (decongestion) and decreased aortic impedance is achieved, which results in improved stroke volume. In patients with severe regurgitant lesions such as mitral or aortic regurgitation, vasodilator drugs also reduce the regurgitant fraction and increase forward cardiac output, thus adding to their beneficial effects. It should be so noted that there are no adequately powered randomized controlled trials with the use of vasodilators in valvular heart disease that support their use to improve long-term outcomes.

The reflex tachycardia observed in normal subjects in response to arterial vasodilators is not seen in patients with advanced systolic heart failure.[11] This is likely due to a reduction in cardiac norepinephrine spillover rate in the setting of heart failure with unloading of the baroreceptors and low pressure mechanoreceptors in response to systemic vasodilation.[12] In fact, the magnitude of the blunted neurohumoral response to nitroprusside infusion in patients with systolic heart failure (i.e., lack of reflex tachycardia) may be a marker of the severity and prognosis of heart failure.[11]

In general, the beneficial response to vasodilator drug therapy is most pronounced in patients with systolic heart failure and a dilated LV. Patients with normal LV cavity size may be more sensitive to changes in preload reduction, and hypotension can occur in response to reduced afterload if the heart is small or there is a relatively reduced preload.

ARTERIOLAR VASODILATORS

Hydralazine

Hydralazine was one of the first drugs used to treat hypertension in the 1950s. Its mechanism of action is still not completely

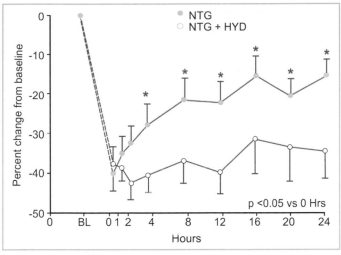

FIG. 2: Nitroglycerin (NTG) alone is associated with the development of early tolerance, whereas the combination of NTG and hydralazine (HYD) 75 mg four times per day is associated with less NTG tolerance. (*: Statistically significant changes)

understood, but it appears to be a direct and potent arteriolar dilator that relaxes the smooth muscles of small resistance vessels. It has essentially no venodilating effects. Hydralazine primarily dilates the renal and peripheral resistant arterioles, and has little effect on coronary or liver blood flow. It may also have antioxidant effects, and can prevent tolerance to nitrates (Fig. 2).

Hydralazine is well-known to cause reflex tachycardia when used in patients without heart failure. For example, in patients with systemic hypertension large doses can produce a reflex tachycardia, edema and may rarely worsen angina. Reflex tachycardia and excess salt and water retention in response to hydralazine is not typically observed in patients with more advanced systolic heart failure because of a blunted baroreceptor response.

Hydralazine can be given orally, where it is rapidly absorbed from the gastrointestinal tract. However, the actual bioavailability is highly variable, and depends on the rate of acetylation by the liver, a genetically determined trait. In the United States, about half of people are fast acetylators and half are slow acetylators. Acetylation activity is not routinely measured in patients. A lupus-like syndrome from hydralazine is more likely to occur in slow acetylators, and this typically wanes when hydralazine is stopped. Fast acetylators may require higher doses of hydralazine. Chronic hydralazine use can cause vitamin B6 deficiency.

The hemodynamic response to chronic oral hydralazine therapy in patients with systolic heart failure is usually characterized by no change in heart rate, a fall in SVR, and about a 50% increase in cardiac output.[13] Most commonly, blood pressure does not change much with hydralazine. Patients with chronic mitral or aortic regurgitation demonstrate a reduction in the regurgitant jet by echo and auscultation, and forward stroke volume is markedly increased. There is no long-term improvement in exercise capacity despite a modest, persistent improvement in ejection fraction. The combination of hydralazine and isosorbide dinitrate ushered in the vasodilator era for the treatment of heart failure in the 1980s (Fig. 3).

Even today we do not know entirely how to properly dose hydralazine for individual patients with advanced heart failure. Because of the high success rate of other vasodilator drugs, such as ACE inhibitors and ARBs, hydralazine has been relegated to second-tier therapy. The one important exception is the safety and efficacy of hydralazine and isosorbide dinitrate in the African-American Heart Failure Trial (A-HeFT) (Fig. 4).[14] In this trial, the fixed combination of hydralazine and isosorbide dinitrate (BiDil) added to standard therapy markedly improved survival and other outcomes among self-identified black patients with systolic heart failure. One rationale for the trial was that isosorbide dinitrate might augment nitric oxide production, and therefore improve endothelial function. Hydralazine may also work as an antioxidant and can reduce nitrate tolerance.[15] The results of the A-HeFT trial have not been robustly translated into clinical practice for a number of reasons. The combination of hydralazine and isosorbide dinitrate today is

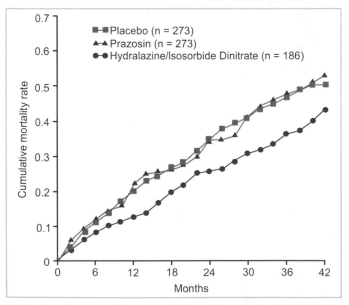

FIG. 3: Mortality curves of patients with heart failure randomized to placebo, prazosin or isosorbide dinitrate/hydralazine in the first Vasodilator Heart Failure Trial (V-HeFT 1); p= 0.046 on the generalized Wilcoxon test, which gives more weight to the treatment differences in the early part of the mortality curves.

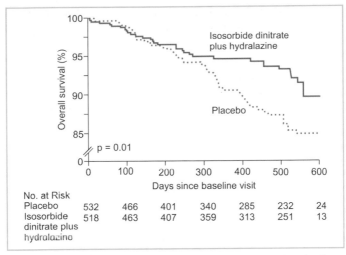

FIG. 4: Mortality curves of African-American patients randomized to placebo or isosorbide dinitrate/hydralazine in addition to standard therapy for heart failure in the African-American Heart Failure Trial (A-HeFT).[14]

generally considered as an add-on therapy, superimposed on more conventional therapy, when patients are demonstrating signs and symptoms of worsening heart failure.

Typically, hydralazine is prescribed along with isosorbide dinitrate to improve cardiac output and reduce pulmonary capillary wedge pressure. The initial hydralazine dose used in A-HeFT was 37.5 mg three times per day and gradually increased to 75 mg three times per day. Isosorbide dinitrate was slowly titrated to a dose of 80 mg three times per day. Doses of hydralazine as high as 1,200 mg/day have been used to treat systolic heart failure, but onset of the lupus syndrome is seen in 15–20% of patients receiving more than 400 mg/day. Fluid retention is also more common when higher doses of hydralazine are used. There is likely a survival advantage associated with long-term hydralazine therapy when taken with isosorbide dinitrate to treat systolic heart failure.

Amlodipine

Amlodipine is a dihydropyridine L-type calcium channel blocking agent that is widely used to treat hypertension and angina. It is a long-acting, potent, arteriolar dilating drug that is well-tolerated. The typical starting dose is 2.5 or 5 mg/day and the target dose for many patients with hypertension is 10 mg/day. Calcium channel drugs are vasodilators and have anti-ischemic effects, so it is logical that they would be investigated in patients with systolic heart failure. The most promising calcium channel blocker to emerge from these studies as potential heart failure therapy was amlodipine. A minor drawback to amlodipine is the frequent development of pedal edema with the higher dose, but this is assumed to be due to benign vasodilation in the small arterioles and venules in the ankles, and not due to heart failure per se. Other non-dihydropyridine calcium channel blockers such as verapamil and diltiazem have negative inotropic properties, may cause cardiac electrical conduction problems, and are not very powerful vasodilators. They have never played a primary role in the treatment of heart failure.

The effect of amlodipine on outcomes in patients with chronic systolic heart failure was evaluated in two PRAISE (Prospective Randomized Amlodipine Survival Evaluation) studies.[16,17] The earlier of the two studies demonstrated that all-cause mortality might be lower in a subset of patients with nonischemic dilated cardiomyopathy treated with amlodipine, though overall, the trial was neutral. The PRAISE II trial was then focused solely in patients with nonischemic dilated cardiomyopathy. In PRAISE II, an overall neutral effect of amlodipine was once again observed. It seems clear that amlodipine is safe to use in patients with systolic heart failure when needed to control hypertension or angina. However, amlodipine is not effective as a life-saving therapy for the treatment of systolic heart failure, despite its powerful vasodilating properties. The observations suggest that vasodilation alone is not enough to provide a mortality benefit. Several other potent vasodilators have failed to improve mortality in patients with heart failure, including prazosin, flosequinan, nesiritide, and synthetic prostacyclin (epoprostenol) or Flolan. Presumably, it is not simple "vasodilation" that provides for the survival benefit, but there should be some neurohumoral modulation property or some other mechanisms beyond simple reduction in afterload.

Oral Nitrates

Nitrates have been widely used to treat angina by physicians for well over 100 years. It is only in the past 25 years that they have been used to treat systolic heart failure. Their favorable effects on angina, systolic heart failure, mitral regurgitation and coronary spasm are now well known. The mechanism of action of nitrates is complex, but these molecules appear to undergo a metabolic biotransformation in vascular smooth muscle, which leads to the formation of nitric oxide or a related S-nitrosothiol. These breakdown products of nitrates stimulate the enzyme guanylate cyclase, leading to the formulation of cyclic guanosine monophosphate (cGMP). cGMP in turn reduces calcium influx, which leads to venous and arterial vasodilation.[18] It is also likely that the vascular endothelium responds to nitrates with the synthesis and release of prostacyclin,[19] thus improving endothelial function. Nitrates primarily cause venodilation, which typically increases venous capacitance and reduces

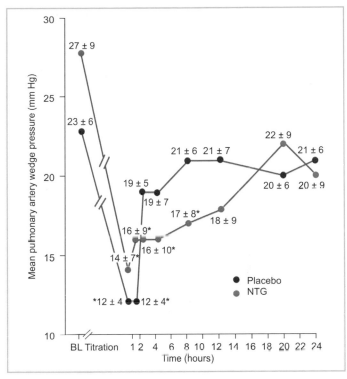

FIG. 5: The data indicate that tolerance can develop to intravenous nitroglycerin (NTG) over 24 hours. There is a brisk initial response to IV NTG manifested by a fall in pulmonary capillary wedge pressure (PCWP) during titration; but during 24 hours of infusion, PCWP increases back toward control in both the NTG and the placebo arms of the study.

preload, thus lowering end diastolic volume, reducing cardiac wall tension and diminishing pulmonary capillary wedge pressure. Dyspnea is relieved. Larger doses lead to arteriolar dilation, further reducing afterload and improving forward flow. LV cavity size diminishes, reducing mitral regurgitation.[20] It is not surprising that oral nitrate therapy has emerged as an important treatment for systolic heart failure. Nitrates are among the few vasodilators that are able to increase exercise tolerance in patients with systolic heart failure.[21,22] However, nitrate tolerance occurs in many patients (Fig. 5), thus casting suspicion on long-term efficiency. This can be offset to some extent by concomitant use of hydralazine.[15]

RENIN-ANGIOTENSIN-ALDOSTERONE SYSTEM BLOCKERS

Angiotensin Converting Enzyme Inhibitors

Angiotensin converting enzyme (ACE) inhibitors were introduced into clinical practice in the 1980s for the treatment

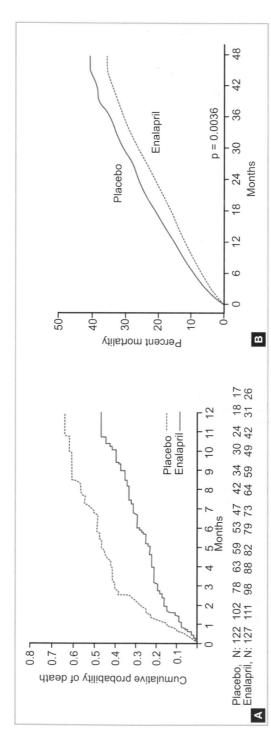

FIGS 6A AND B: In the CONSENSUS Trial, the difference between treatments is even more striking, as the patients likely had more advanced heart failure. Kaplan-Meier survival curves (A) from The CONSENSUS Trial Study Group. Effects of enalapril on mortality in severe congestive heart failure. Results of the Cooperative North Scandinavian Enalapril Survival Study (CONSENSUS).[28]

of hypertension and heart failure. This class of drug therapy has revolutionized the treatment for these two conditions, and has been demonstrated to improve survival in patients with systolic heart failure (Figs 6A and B). The success of ACE inhibitors for the treatment of heart failure was predicated on the observation that the RAAS is activated in chronic systolic heart failure,[23] and this activation contributes importantly to heightened afterload and to the LV remodeling process.

Angiotensinogen is produced in the liver and is converted in the blood by renin to form a small peptide, angiotensin I (Fig. 7). Angiotensin I is then further cleaved to form angiotensin II, a very small peptide, but potent arteriole constrictor. Angiotensin II subserves a host of other biological activities primarily through the angiotensin II receptor, including promotion of volume retention, activation of and sensitization to the sympathetic nervous system, thirst, regulation of salt and water balance, modulation of potassium balance, cardiac myocyte and vascular smooth muscle growth, to name but a few. Its actions are central to the development of acute and chronic systolic heart failure.

Early, overly simplistic thinking was that systolic heart failure was essentially a vasoconstricted state caused by excessive sympathetic nervous system activity and heightened levels of other vasoconstrictor neurohormones, including angiotensin II, arginine vasopressin, (AVP) and endothelin. When it became apparent that ACE inhibitors could block the production of angiotensin II, ACE inhibitors became an attractive candidate for the treatment of patients with hypertension and systolic heart failure. ACE inhibitors would be expected to reduce afterload, and in turn would increase cardiac output and forward flow. Although the initial clinical studies indeed supported this hypothesis,[24] it soon became clear that ACE inhibitors were doing much more than reducing afterload. Long-term clinical improvement was accompanied by reduced LV remodeling and improved patient survival when applied to postmyocardial infarction patients,[25] very similar to the seminal animal work of Pfeffer and colleagues.[26] ACE inhibitors were no longer thought of as simple arteriolar dilators, but were neurohormone modulators that could very favorably alter the natural history of systolic heart failure and improve survival by inhibiting the progression of LV remodeling (Fig. 8).

We now recognize that neurohormonal activation plays a key role in the initiation and progression of heart failure. The RAAS is central to this neurohormonal cascade, as patients with systolic heart failure and high renin levels seemingly derive the most acute benefit from blocking the RAAS.[27] It is now well established that ACE inhibitors slow the progression of heart failure and improve survival in patients with a reduced

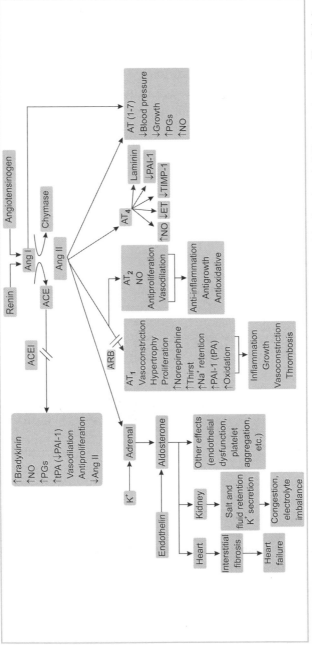

ACE, angiotensin-converting-enzyme; ACEI, angiotensin-converting-enzyme-inhibitor; Ang I, angiotensin I; Ang II, angiotensin II; AT, angiotensin receptor; ET, endothelin; NO, nitric oxide; PAI, plasminogen activator inhibitor; PGs, prostaglandins; TIMP, tissue inhibitor of metalloproteinase; tPA, tissue plasminogen activator.

FIG. 7: The renin-angiotensin-aldosterone system.

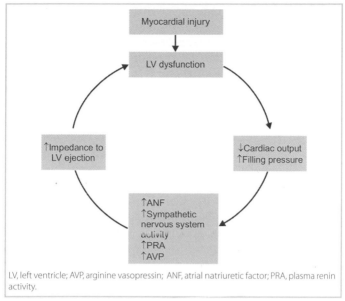

LV, left ventricle; AVP, arginine vasopressin; ANF, atrial natriuretic factor; PRA, plasma renin activity.

FIG. 8: Heart failure is a complex clinical syndrome characterized by extensive neuroendocrine activation. The release of neurohormones appears to be in response to reduced cardiac function and a perceived reduction in effective circulatory volume. It is as if neuroendocrine activity is attempting to protect the blood pressure and maintain circulatory homeostasis. Although this may be adaptive early on, chronic neuroendocrine activation leads to peripheral vasoconstriction, left ventricular remodeling and worsening left ventricular performance, and thus becomes an attractive therapeutic target. Drugs designed to block the exuberant neuroendocrine response, such as ACE inhibitors, have now become the cornerstone of treatment for heart failure.

ejection fraction and congestive heart failure.[28] Much of this improvement is believed to be due to "reverse remodeling". Even patients with a reduced ejection fraction, but few or no heart failure symptoms, derive clinical benefit from ACE inhibitor therapy.[29] The development of symptomatic heart failure is delayed in these patients. The activation of neurohormones (renin, norepinephrine and AVP) appears to occur early in the natural history of the syndrome, before symptoms occur.[30] This observation suggested that early introduction of neurohormonal blocking drugs before symptoms ensue may slow the progression of systolic heart failure or even delay its onset of signs and symptoms.[29] Indeed, today neurohumoral modulating drugs are recommended for patients who demonstrate impaired LV systolic function even in the absence of symptoms. Many investigators observed that the RAAS was markedly activated during decompensated heart failure, but returns to normal once the patient clinically stabilizes, even though severe LV dysfunction may persist.[31] The concept that blocking the RAAS improves patients with systolic heart failure became widely recognized in the 1990s.

In the 1980s, a number of hypotheses and concepts emerged that challenged the long-standing notion that systolic heart failure was fundamentally a mechanical problem. Katz introduced the idea that heart failure may be a disorder of abnormal gene expressional growth response to injury,[32] and many others believed that the myocardial remodeling was at least in part due to activation of neurohormonal systems,[33] which were well known to also be cardiac growth factors when studied in vitro.[34] Alteration of loading conditions due to increased LV chamber size and increased wall stress also undoubtedly led to progressive LV remodeling.[34] Both mechanical and neurohormonal signals regulated the remodeling process, as did altered gene expression. It became clear that the all-important LV remodeling process was largely structural and not functional.[35] Additional data emerged indicating that excessive angiotensin II caused cardiac myocyte necrosis under experimental conditions.[36] Eventually a coherent story emerged suggesting that systolic heart failure was at least in part driven by excessive neurohormonal activation,[37,38] setting up a vicious cycle of worsening heart failure and death (Fig. 8). These neurohormonal systems are likely adaptive in an evolutionary sense,[39] and are not simple biomarkers or epiphenomena. They are known to directly contribute to LV remodeling[40-42] and subsequent patient mortality.[43] The strong notion emerged that pharmacological inhibition of the RAAS (and the sympathetic nervous system) might reduce the progression of LV remodeling,[44-47] and, therefore, such drugs should improve patient survival.[28]

The ACE inhibitors were the first class of drugs to really test the neurohumoral hypothesis (Figs 6A and B). Needless to say, they have now become a standard of care for patients with hypertension, systolic heart failure, acute myocardial infarction and advanced cardiovascular disease. The ACE inhibitor class of drugs reduces afterload, presumably by inhibiting angiotensin II arteriolar constriction reducing sympathetic tone. There is also venodilation with a fall in pulmonary capillary wedge pressure, presumably due to reduction in sympathetic activity to veins and desensitization of venous capacitance vessels to norepinephrine. Angiotensin II does not directly dilate veins, so there is no direct effect of ACE inhibitors on venous capacitance vessels. There is modest improvement in cardiac index with ACE inhibitors, and heart rate may slightly slow. As previously mentioned, if the patient is acutely hyper-reninemic as a consequence of vigorous diuresis, there can be a substantial and prolonged fall in blood pressure with even small doses of ACE inhibition. This is why many physicians prefer to use short-acting ACE inhibitors such as captopril in hospitalized patients with acute systolic heart failure, as patients are less likely to develop prolonged symptomatic hypotension. If symptomatic hypotension ensues, the patient should lie down and the feet should be elevated until these symptoms resolve and the blood pressure improves. Usually a sense of improved well-being is established with the use of ACE inhibitors despite chronically low arterial pressures. Rarely, dysgeusia or loss of taste occurs, sometimes requiring withdrawal of the drug. Rash is uncommon with the smaller doses of ACE inhibitors used today. A dry, non-productive cough occurs in some patients receiving ACE inhibitors, and the drug is discontinued in 5–10% of patients for this reason. The mechanism of the cough is not entirely clear, but is believed to be due to the effects of bradykinin on sensory neurons in the proximal airways.

There is now a long list of ACE inhibitors to choose from (Table 2). They have somewhat dissimilar pharmacodynamics, pharmacokinetics, and rates of elimination. In general, it is best to start with small doses of an ACE inhibitor that has been tested in a large clinical trial and slowly titrates up over days to weeks to a target dose established as safe and effective by use in large clinical trials. It is expected that many patients with advanced systolic heart failure will have about a 20% increase in serum creatinine with ACE inhibitor use. This is usually not reason to discontinue or lower the dose of the ACE inhibitor. However, this class of drug is contraindicated in patients with cardiogenic shock or acute renal failure, and can cause renal insufficiency when used in patients with renal artery stenosis. Occasionally, hyperkalemia can occur requiring alteration of dose or temporary/permanent discontinuation of the ACE inhibitor. Careful, regular follow-up with monitoring of electrolytes, BUN (blood urea nitrogen) and serum creatinine is important in the care of these patients when making decisions about altering the dose of ACE inhibitors. Renal function and serum electrolytes should be checked at about one week following initiation of ACE inhibitor therapy.

Angiotensin Receptor Blockers

Angiotensin receptors of the AT_1 subtype bind angiotensin II with a high structural specificity but limited binding capacity.[48] The remarkable success of ACE inhibitors in the treatment of hypertension, arterial disease, myocardial hypertrophy, heart failure and diabetic renal disease encouraged the exploration of alternative drugs to block the RAAS. It was eventually recognized that ACE inhibitors blocked only one of several pathways that normally increase angiotensin II activity, and that angiotensin II could "escape" from chronic ACE inhibition. ARBs do not demonstrate this "escape" phenomenon. ARBs do not cause cough. They can be used safely in patients who develop angioedema during treatment with an ACE inhibitor. Increased levels of angiotensin II peptides seen with the use of ARBs do not appear to have unexpected off-target effects

TABLE 2: Common drugs used in managing chronic heart failure in the United States

Drug	Trade name	Heart failure indication	Post-myocardial infarction indication	Dosing
Angiotensin-converting enzyme (ACE inhibitors)				
Benazepril	*Lotensin*	No	No	5–40 mg QD
Captopril	Capoten	Yes	No	6.25–150 mg TID
Enalapril	Vasotec	Yes	No	2.5–20 mg BID
Fosinopril	Monopril	Yes	No	10–80 mg QD
Lisinopril	Prinivil, Zestril	Yes	No	5–20 mg QD
Moexipril	*Univasc*	No	No	7.5–60 mg QD
Perindopril	*Aceon*	No	No	2–16 mg QD
Quinapril	Accupril	Yes	No	5–20 mg BID
Ramipril	Altace	Yes	Yes	2.5–20 mg QD
Trandolapril	*Mavik*	No	Yes	1–4 mg QD
Zofenopril	*Bifril*	NA	NA	7.5–60 mg QD
Angiotensin II receptor blockers (ARBs)				
Candesartan	Atacand	Yes	No	8–32 mg QD/BID
Eprosartan	*Teveten*	No	No	400–800 mg QD
Irbesartan	*Avapro*	No	No	150–300 QD
Losartan	*Cozaar*	No	No	50–100 mg QD/BID
Telmisartan	*Telma*	No	No	40–80 QD
Olmesartan	*Benicar*	No	No	20–40 mg QD
Valsartan	Diovan	Yes	No	80–320 mg QD
β-adrenergic receptor antagonists				
Carvedilol	Coreg	Yes	Yes	3.125–25 mg BID
Metoprolol succinate	Toprol XL	Yes	No	25–200 mg QD
Bisoprolol	*Zebeta*	No	No	1.25–10 mg QD
Nebivolol	*Nabilet*	No	No	1.25–10 mg QD
Aldosterone receptor antagonists				
Spironolactone	Aldactone	Yes	No	25–50 mg QD
Eplerenone	Inspra	No	Yes	25–50 mg QD
Others				
Amlodipine	*Norvasc*	No	No	2.5–10 mg QD
Hydralazine-isosorbide dinitrate	BiDil (37.5/20)	Yes	No	1–2 tablets TID
Digoxin	Digitek	Yes	No	0.125–0.25 mg QD

BID, twice daily; QD, once daily; TID, three times daily. Italics indicate drugs that are currently not indicated by the US Food and Drug Administration for treating patients with heart failure).

despite activating AT_2 receptors. First-dose hypotension is not typically seen when ARBs are given to diuretic-treated patients, as often occurs with ACE inhibitors. This is probably because ARBs have a much slower onset of action. Orthostatic hypotension is rare. Rebound hypertension upon withdrawal of ARBs does not appear to be a problem. As with ACE inhibitors, acute renal failure may occur with ARBs if administered to patients with renal artery stenosis or cardiogenic shock. The incidence of renal dysfunction and hyperkalemia is comparable with ARBs and ACE inhibitors.[49] It is now reasonably clear that ACE inhibitors and ARBs should not be used together, as the likelihood of hyperkalemia, hypotension and worsening renal function is greater.[50]

Many randomized controlled trials of ARBs have been performed in patients with chronic systolic heart failure,[51,52] in patients with acute myocardial infarction complicated by heart failure or LV dysfunction,[53] and in patients at high-risk for vascular events.[54] Several important points have emerged from these large trials:

- ARBs and ACE inhibitors appear to have very similar efficacy in these patient groups
- If the patient does not tolerate an ACE inhibitor, an ARB is a suitable substitution
- Although generally more expensive, ARBs are better tolerated than ACE inhibitors
- The combination of an ACE inhibitor and an ARB (dual RAAS blocking effect) is not more effective and is associated with more hypotension, worsening renal function, and hyperkalemia[55]
- Despite earlier favorable reports, ARBs do not appear to prevent recurrent atrial fibrillation.[56]

The dose of ARBs has generally been determined by pharmaceutical generated data and subsequent verification of these doses in large clinical trials (Table 2). Extensive experience with RAAS blockers over the years has led to changes in dose recommendations. For example, the Heart failure Endpoint evaluation of Angiotensin II Antagonist Losartan (HEAAL) trial demonstrated that losartan 150 mg daily reduced the rate of death or admission for heart failure to a greater extent than a dose of 50 mg/day.[57]

Similar to ACE inhibitors, we now have data to suggest that inhibition of the RAAS with ARBs also results in favorable structural and functional changes. Treatment with the ACE inhibitor captopril, the ARB valsartan, or the combination of captopril plus valsartan resulted in similar changes in cardiac volume, ejection fraction and infarct segment length in patients 20 months following acute myocardial infarction.[58] These observations suggest that ARBs are similar to ACE inhibitors with regard to their anti-remodeling properties. Neither ACE inhibitors nor ARBs improve outcomes in patients with heart failure with preserved ejection fraction.[59]

MINERALOCORTICOID (ALDOSTERONE) RECEPTOR BLOCKERS

Aldosterone and Systolic Heart Failure

Aldosterone was structurally identified more than 50 years ago, and was soon after designated a mineralocorticoid due to its salt retaining properties. It also promotes loss of potassium from the kidney, gastrointestinal tract, sweat and salivary glands. It has long been known to play a pathophysiologic role in cardiovascular disease, including congestive heart failure (Fig. 9).[60,61] In addition to its mineralocorticoid properties, which can cause hypokalemia and hypomagnesemia, aldosterone contributes in many ways to the development of heart failure. It likely causes vascular and cardiac remodeling, endothelial dysfunction, inhibits norepinephrine reuptake, and causes baroreceptor dysfunction (Fig. 9). It expands intravascular and extravascular volume. Inhibition of aldosterone is believed to be favorable due to:

- Reduced collagen deposition and possibly anti-remodeling effects
- Blood pressure reduction
- Prevention of hypokalemia and associated arrhythmias
- Modulation of nitric oxide synthesis.

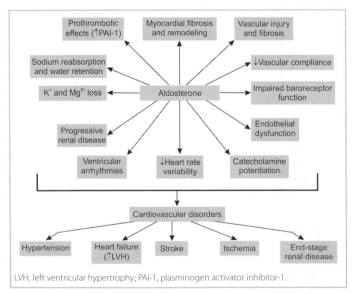

LVH, left ventricular hypertrophy; PAI-1, plasminogen activator inhibitor-1.

FIG. 9: Aldosterone is a mineralocorticoid that has a central role in a host of biological activities. Many of these activities can be excessive due to dysregulation of aldosterone activity, thus contributing to cardiovascular disease.

The major mineralocorticoid in heart failure is cortisol and not aldosterone. Serum aldosterone levels are not consistently elevated in patients with heart failure in the absence of diuretics. Accordingly, it is not aldosterone blockade per se, but mineralocorticoid receptor blockade that is important. Spironolactone and eplerenone are thus mineralocorticoid receptor blockers more than simply aldosterone receptor blockers.

ACE inhibitors were originally believed to chronically suppress angiotensin II in patients with heart failure, a major determinant of aldosterone production by the adrenal glands. This notion probably led to some initial loss of interest in aldosterone receptor inhibitors for the treatment of systolic heart failure. We now know that ACE inhibitors do not suppress angiotensin II long-term, and that there is an aldosterone escape phenomenon. Three landmark studies, the Randomized Aldosterone Evaluation Study (RALES) (Fig. 10),[62] the Eplerenone Post-acute Myocardial Infarction Heart Failure Efficacy and Survival Study (EPHESUS) (Fig. 11)[63] and the Eplerenone in Mild Patients Hospitalization and Survival Study in Heart Failure (EMPHASIS-HF)[64] have remarkably increased the role of aldosterone mineralocorticoid antagonists for the everyday treatment of systolic heart failure. Eplerenone, as compared with placebo, reduced both the risk of death and the risk of hospitalization among patients with systolic heart failure and mild symptoms in the EMPHASIS-HF trial. This finding

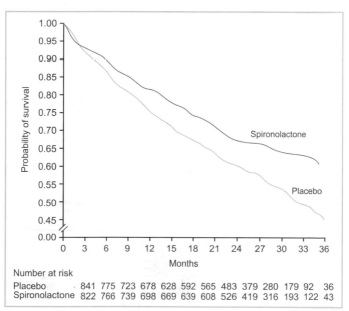

FIG. 10: Survival curves of patients with advanced heart failure randomly allocated to spironolactone or placebo. Most patients were not receiving β-adrenergic blockers. There was a 30% reduction in mortality in patients randomized to spironolactone compared to patients in the placebo group. From the Randomized Aldactone Evaluation Study (RALES).[62]

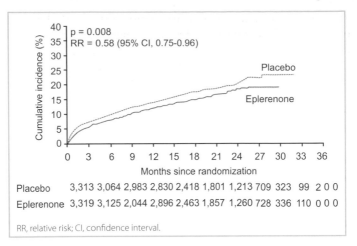

RR, relative risk; CI, confidence interval.

FIG. 11: Kaplan-Meier estimates of the rate of death from any cause in the EPHESUS trial.[63]

is particularly important as it expands the use of mineralo-corticoid antagonists for the New York Heart Association (NYHA) functional class II patients. Spironolactone[62] and eplerenone[63] are now widely used to treat chronic systolic heart failure and postmyocardial infarction heart failure. Despite their greater use today, in the USA it was estimated that less than one-third of eligible patients hospitalized for heart failure received appropriate, guideline-recommended aldosterone antagonist therapy.[65] Some of the reluctance to use aldosterone blockers in patients with systolic heart failure may be justified because of the advanced age of patients, the frequency of chronic renal insufficiency, other common comorbidities such as diabetes mellitus, and the serious threat of hyperkalemia.[66] However, when used according to protocol, hyperkalemia is seemingly not such a major problem. Careful follow-up of patients and frequent measurement of renal function and serum potassium are necessary to ensure safety when using aldosterone receptor blocking drugs.

The RAAS is likely an ancient (~400–600 million years) system that evolved in such a way as to allow them to adapt to salt and volume depletion, as might have occurred during transition from the sea to land eons ago. The notion is that regulation of salt and water retention is adaptive, perhaps by protecting intravascular volume, blood pressure and perfusion to vital organs. We now know that chronic stimulation of the RAAS in patients with heart failure can be maladaptive, and that pharmacologically blocking the RAAS can improve patient survival. Blockade of aldosterone membrane receptors is a widely accepted form of therapy for systolic heart failure. The RALES and EPHESUS studies provide strong evidence that aldosterone mineralocorticoid receptor blockade is effective therapy for patients with heart failure across all degrees of severity. Postmyocardial infarction heart failure is also improved by mineralocorticoid receptor blockers.[63] The role of nuclear aldosterone receptors is less clear, but given the complex array of regulatory properties that angiotensin II and aldosterone demonstrate, including inflammation, collagen synthesis, cytokine production, regulation of nitric oxide and cell adhesion molecules, one has to suspect that the activation of nuclear aldosterone receptors with resultant regulation of selective gene expression is also responsible for many of the biological activities of aldosterone, some of which are seen in systolic heart failure.

Spironolactone and Eplerenone in Chronic Heart Failure

The mechanism of action of spironolactone is complex, as aldosterone mineralocorticoid modulates many features of the heart failure syndrome. Although spironolactone is still used as an antihypertensive agent, it is not considered to be a "vasodilator" in the usual sense. Patients taking spironolactone need to be frequently and carefully monitored (patients in RALES were seen monthly for the first 12 weeks), as hyperkalemia and azotemia can occur with spironolactone,[65] particularly if non-steroidal anti-inflammatory drugs are used concomitantly. Diabetes mellitus, chronic kidney disease, volume depletion, advanced age and use of other potassium sparing agents and non-steroidal anti-inflammatory drugs are all risk factors for the development of hyperkalemia when using RAAS blocking drugs.[61] With careful monitoring, however, serious hyperkalemia is uncommon.[62]

Because of the central importance of aldosterone in the pathophysiology of heart failure, it is not surprising that the aldosterone receptor blocker spironolactone has emerged as an important therapy. Spironolactone is an old drug that was primarily used in large doses to treat ascites, edema and refractory hypertension. Excessive mineralocorticoid, common in patients with heart failure, promotes sodium retention, loss of magnesium and potassium, sympathetic nervous system activation, parasympathetic nervous system inhibition, myocardial and vascular fibrosis, baroreceptor dysfunction, and impaired arterial compliance.[67]

The definitive RALES was published in 1999[62] and clearly demonstrated that spironolactone (25–50 mg/day) added to standard therapy (β-blockers were not yet in widespread use) was safe and reduced mortality by 30% (Fig. 7). Death from progressive heart failure and sudden death were both reduced by spironolactone. The patients who participated in RALES were primarily NYHA class III (70%) and IV (30%).

Eplerenone, a newer, more selective aldosterone mineralocorticoid receptor blocker, causes less gynecomastia and breast tenderness than spironolactone. It is more mineralocorticoid specific than spironolactone. EPHESUS[63] was conducted in patients who experienced a recent acute myocardial infarction with an ejection fraction of 40% or less who had heart failure, or had a history of diabetes mellitus. The patients in EPHESUS were randomly allocated to eplerenone or placebo in addition to standard therapy for acute myocardial infarction. In EPHESUS, eplerenone (average dose 42.6 mg/day) reduced all-cause mortality by 15%, cardiovascular mortality by 17%, and significantly lowered the need for subsequent hospitalization (Fig. 11). Sudden cardiac death was also reduced. As with RALES, serious hyperkalemia was unusual.

The EMPHASIS-HF trial suggests that eplerenone is effective in patients with systolic heart failure and NYHA functional class II symptoms. In EMPHASIS-HF hospitalizations for heart failure and for any cause were also reduced with eplerenone. A serum potassium level exceeding 5.5 mmol/L occurred in 11.8% of patients in the eplerenone group and 7.2% of those in the placebo group (P <0.001). Today, aldosterone mineralocorticoid antagonists are widely used to treat advanced heart failure and selected patients with acute myocardial infarction. However, less than one-third of eligible patients hospitalized for heart failure are receiving guideline-recommended aldosterone receptor blocking drugs.[64] This is perhaps due in part to the need for more frequent and careful follow-up, and the fear of hyperkalemia. There is a perception by some physicians that this class of drugs poses more risk than other RAAS blockers. Nevertheless, aldosterone receptor blockers are effective and safe when properly prescribed and monitored, and their indications are seemingly expanding. There appears to be considerably less reverse remodeling in patients with mild-to-moderate heart failure and LV systolic dysfunction randomly assigned to eplerenone, even though there is a reduction in collagen turnover and a reduction in brain natriuretic peptide (BNP) factor.[68] Despite these surprising neutral effects on reverse remodeling, the results of EMPHASIS-HF trial suggest that patients with mild-to-moderate systolic heart failure still derive a favorable effect on morbidity and mortality from eplerenone.

Recently, the Treatment of Preserved Cardiac Function Heart Failure with an Aldosterone Antagonist (TOPCAT) trial has been completed and published.[69] This was a study aimed at patients with heart failure with a preserved ejection fraction rather than heart failure with a reduced ejection fraction. Overall, there was no improvement in cardiovascular mortality. However, spironolactone was associated with a significant (P = 0.04) reduction in hospitalization (17%). It is unclear how physicians will adopt the results of TOPCAT.

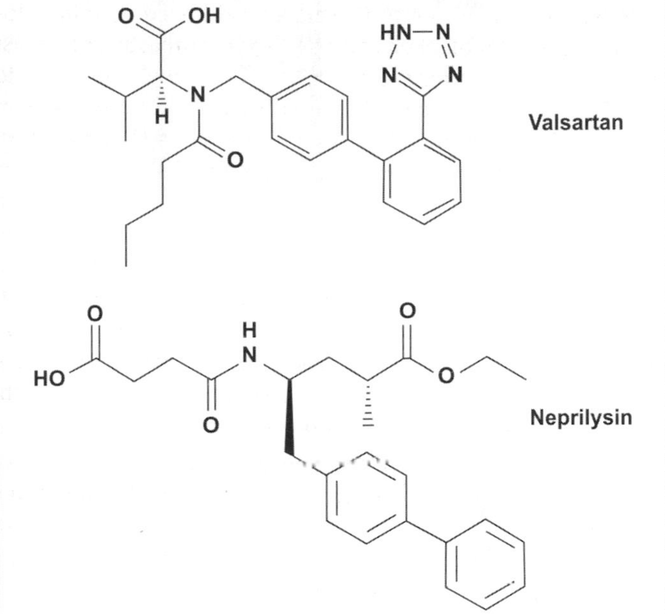

LCZ696: Combination angiotensin II receptor blocker and neutral endopeptidase inhibitor (Novartis).

FIG. 12: Chemical structure of LCZ696.

LCZ696

A new therapy for hypertension and heart failure has been developed by Novartis. LCZ696 is a novel molecule that includes both valsartan and a neprilysin inhibitor. The valsartan moiety of the molecule suppresses the renin-angiotensin system (RAS) while the neprilysin inhibitor reduces the degradation of brain natriuretic peptide (BNP), thereby increasing circulating BNP in plasma (Fig. 12). LCZ696 is taken twice per day. In a recent large clinical trial, 8436 patients with a reduced ejection fraction and NYHA class II to IV symptoms were randomly allocated to LCZ696 at 200 mg twice daily or enalapril at 10 mg twice daily. A favorable effect on survival was observed with LCZ696 relative to enalapril.[70] It is possible that this new form of therapy may emerge as a prominent form of treatment for patients with heart failure and reduced ejection fraction.

PHOSPHODIESTERASE TYPE 5 INHIBITORS

Sildenafil and Tadalafil

Phosphodiesterases are enzymes that hydrolyze the cyclic nucleotides—cGMP and cyclic adenosine monophosphate. At least eleven families of phosphodiesterase isoenzymes have been identified. Phosphodiesterase 5 (PDE 5) degrades cGMP via hydrolysis, thus influencing cGMP's ability to modulate smooth muscle tone,[71] particularly in the venous system of the penile corpus cavernosum and in the pulmonary vasculature. The discovery of sildenafil, a highly selective inhibitor of PDE 5, was initially aimed to be a novel treatment for coronary artery disease. The initial clinical studies in the early 1990s were not promising for this target, but the off-target effect of enhancement of penile erections did not escape the notice of investigators. The use of PDE 5 inhibitors was then redirected toward erectile dysfunction and more recently pulmonary hypertension.

Nitric oxide activates soluble guanylate cyclase, stimulating the production of cGMP. PDE 5 normally hydrolyzes cGMP. Sildenafil inhibits PDE 5, leading to increased cGMP and vasodilation in response to nitric oxide. For years it was known that PDE 5 was not present in normal cardiac myocytes, and the heart itself was not considered an appropriate target. This was challenged by Kass and colleagues[72] who demonstrated that inhibiting PDE 5 in hypertrophied RVs induces a positive inotropic response.[73] In fact, PDE 5 is markedly upregulated in hypertrophied ventricles, and PDE 5 inhibition may lead to regression of RV hypertrophy.[73] PDE 5 has long been known to be highly expressed in lung vasculature, and so it is not surprising that sildenafil is beneficial for the treatment of patients with pulmonary hypertension. As of this writing, it is still not clear if normal cardiac myocytes express PDE 5, but hypertrophied and/or failing myocytes do express it, and PDE 5 inhibition can be clinically helpful in patients with pulmonary hypertension and some element of right ventricular hypertrophy or failing right ventricle.

Sildenafil and tadalafil are both PDE 5 inhibitors that are indicated for use in patients with pulmonary arterial hypertension who have mild to moderately severe symptoms.[74] Preliminary data on sildenafil suggest that its use may also be safe and beneficial in patients with disproportionate pulmonary hypertension and LV dysfunction.[75,76] Sildenafil citrate is prescribed in doses of 20 mg TID and tadalafil is much longer acting and is prescribed in doses of 40 mg/day to control pulmonary hypertension. Hypotension can occur with PDE 5 inhibitors, especially when they are used with nitrates. Visual disturbances and priapism have also been observed with this class of drugs. There is no specific antidote for PDE 5 induced hypotension. Sildenafil and tadalafil are not approved for use in patients with heart failure, but they are being investigated. A small case series (3 patients) has recently implied that a combination of sildenafil and nitrates can be used in patients with heart failure and pulmonary hypertension,[77] though clearly more robust clinical trials are needed. Experimental data indicate that PDE 5 levels are increased in severely failing hearts[78] and that sildenafil reduces myocardial remodeling.[79] Recent data also suggest that PDE 5 is regulated in the LV by oxidative stress.[80] Clearly this story is still unfolding and we have much to learn. Nevertheless, drugs such as sildenafil and tadalafil that selectively restore right ventricular contractility, limit right ventricular hypertrophy and reduce pulmonary artery remodeling are intriguing as potential therapy for right heart failure due to disproportionately increased pulmonary artery pressure. Perhaps PDE 5 inhibitors will also favorably affect left-sided systolic heart failure, particularly if there is associated pulmonary hypertension. More studies are needed, and use of these drugs for the treatment of heart failure remains investigational for now.

Accordingly, the Phosphodiesterase-5 Inhibition to Improve Clinical Status and Exercise Capacity In Heart Failure with Preserved Ejection Fraction (RELAX) trial was designed to test the hypothesis that, compared with placebo, therapy with the PDE-5 inhibitor sildenafil would improve exercise capacity in heart failure with preserved ejection fraction (HFpEF) after 24 weeks of therapy, assessed by the change in peak oxygen consumption.[81] Among these patients with HFpEF, sildenafil did not significantly improve exercise capacity or clinical status relative to placebo. Nevertheless, many experts believe that there still may be a role for phosphodiesterase-5 inhibitors in selected patients with HFpEF and disproportionate pulmonary hypertension.

INTRAVENOUS VASODILATORS

Nitroprusside

Sodium nitroprusside can be dramatic in reversing the deleterious hemodynamics of acute systolic heart failure. Those who have had experienced using the drug in this setting are often astonished how quickly the drug lowers pulmonary capillary wedge pressure (PCWP) and improves cardiac output, leading to prompt and often striking clinic improvement. The drug is usually started as doses of 10 µg/min, and gradually titrated up to no more than 400 µg/min, as needed to control hemodynamic abnormalities and symptoms. Some clinicians give nitroprusside according to body weight, with the typical dose starting at 10–20 µg/kg/min. Our extensive experience with nitroprusside suggests that with low dose infusion rates (<3 µg/kg/min) used for less than 72 hours, toxicity is almost never observed.[82] The systolic blood pressure should not be allowed to be less than 90 mmHg or to a level that includes hypotensive symptoms. Invasive monitoring with a pulmonary artery catheter and an arterial catheter can be useful if the patient has marginal blood pressure. Persistent or severe hypotension will nearly always dissipate as soon as nitroprusside is stopped.

Metabolism and Toxicity of Nitroprusside

Nitroprusside has been used to treat severe heart failure for many years,[83] though the Food and Drug Administration (FDA) has approved it only for severe hypertension and for certain neurosurgical procedures. It must be used carefully by experienced nurses and clinicians. Thiocyanate toxicity can rarely occur, and thiocyanate levels should be monitored, particularly if the patient has received a high dose for a prolonged period of time. Measurement of thiocyanate is a simple, inexpensive colorimetric test, normal levels being less than 10 mg/mL. Metabolic acidosis, anuria, and a prolonged high dose of nitroprusside (>400 μg/min) can predispose to thiocyanate toxicity, prompting measurement of thiocyanate levels. The thiocyanate ion is also readily removed by hemodialysis. When thiocyanate toxicity does occur, the patient may present with confusion, hyperreflexia and convulsions. Occasionally, mild hypoxemia occurs from nitroprusside due to ventilation-perfusion mismatch, but it is usually of little clinical consequence, as cardiac output rises and the delivery of oxygen to tissues increases. Coronary "steal" can occur when nitroprusside is used in the setting of acute myocardial infarction, and it should not be used routinely in this setting.[84,85] If intravenous vasodilator therapy is used for patients with acute myocardial infarction and severe heart failure, intravenous nitroglycerin may be preferred. Nevertheless, nitroprusside has been used successfully in this setting when given in the subacute phase.[84] If nitroprusside is used to treat severe heart failure related to acute myocardial infarction, it should be given later, perhaps 12 hours after admission to the hospital.[85]

Nitroprusside and Severe Heart Failure

Nitroprusside quickly improves hemodynamics and symptoms in patients with severe heart failure.[86] Even patients with hypotension and shock may improve with nitroprusside,[87] as blood pressure may stabilize or even improve with large increases in cardiac output. Patients with severe mitral regurgitations or aortic regurgitation may also demonstrate dramatic clinical improvement with nitroprusside. Patients with severe aortic stenosis and worsening heart failure can be improved with nitroprusside used prior to aortic value replacement,[88] provided they are not hypotensive. It can also be used to stabilize acute heart failure in patients who demonstrate a ruptured interventricular septum following acute myocardial infarction. Recent observational data indicate that in patients hospitalized with advanced, low-output heart failure, those stabilized in the hospital with nitroprusside may have a more favorable long-term clinical outcome.[89]

Intravenous Nitroglycerin

Similar to nitroprusside, intravenous nitroglycerin has an immediate onset and offset of action. The infusion rate is usually initiated at 10–20 µg/min with gradual titration to 200–400 µg/min as needed to control symptoms and improve hemodynamic parameters. It is not approved by the FDA for the treatment of heart failure, but has been widely used for this indication over the past 20 years. Intravenous nitroglycerin is endothelium dependent, and unlike nitroprusside, it has more effect on the venous circulation than on the arterial circulation. However, higher doses of intravenous nitroglycerin have arteriolar dilating properties and may decrease afterload. Therefore, cardiac output may increase and blood pressure can be maintained. PCWP is reduced. Mitral regurgitation improves. There are few data available on the effects of intravenous nitroglycerin on coronary circulation in patients with heart failure. Coronary blood flow appears to improve. This suggests that both the epicardial conductance vessels and the coronary arteriolar resistance vessels are favorably influenced by intravenous nitroglycerin.

Limitations of Intravenous Nitroglycerin in the Treatment of Patients with Heart Failure

Intravenous nitroglycerin causes headaches in about 20% of patients, and when severe, may require cessation of the infusion. Hypotension (10%), nausea and bradycardia occasionally occur. Some patients are relatively resistant to intravenous nitroglycerin and seemingly require very large doses to afford a hemodynamic effect. The reason for this is not particularly clear, but very large doses in excess of 500 µg/min are best avoided. Nitrate tolerance is said to occur when there is a robust initial hemodynamic response, but by 1–2 hours the dose of intravenous nitroglycerin must be increased to establish a continued hemodynamic response. About one-half of patients develop nitrate tolerance, and it cannot be predicted by baseline hemodynamic values (Fig. 5). The mechanism of resistance to intravenous nitroglycerin is not clear, but it is possibly prevented by concomitant use of oral hydralazine (Fig. 2).

Nesiritide

Nesiritide is pure, human BNP synthesized using recombinant DNA techniques. It has the same 32-amino acid sequence as endogenous BNP released from the heart where it is synthesized and stored. When infused intravenously into the circulation of patients with heart failure, the mean terminal elimination half-life of nesiritide is about 18 minutes. Plasma BNP levels increase about three to six-fold with a nesiritide infusion. Human BNP is eliminated from the circulation through complex, multiple mechanisms. Most of the BNP is cleared by c-receptors on cell surfaces, but some is cleared by neutral endopeptidases in renal tubular and vascular cells, and a smaller amount is cleared by renal filtration that is proportional to body weight.

The earliest clinical trial of nesiritide, Vasodilation in the Management of Acute CHF (VMAC), was a comparison study with intravenous nitroglycerin.[90] It demonstrated that nesiritide improved hemodynamic function and self-reported symptoms more effectively than intravenous nitroglycerin or placebo (Figs 13A and B). On this basis, nesiritide was approved by the FDA for heart failure and became widely used. Nesiritide has venous, arterial and coronary vasodilator properties. Cardiac output improves and PCWP is reduced. Hypotension occurs in about 4% of patients, and unlike intravenous nitroglycerin, it can be prolonged (~20 minutes) because of nesiritide's relatively longer half-life. The effects of nesiritide on renal function are variable, but generally only a modest or neutral renal effect is observed, though worsening renal function has been reported.[91,92]

In 2005 Sackner-Bernstein and colleagues reported that nesiritide may be associated with an increased risk of death after treatment for acute decompensated heart failure.[93] At about this time, infusions of nesiritide were also being widely performed in outpatient clinics, and the drug came under severe criticism.[94,95] Ultimately, an outpatient randomized controlled trial of nesiritide vs. placebo was performed which demonstrated that serial outpatient nesiritide infusions did not provide a demonstrable clinical benefit over standard therapy.[96] The drug rapidly fell out of favor.[97] Ultimately, the Acute Study of Clinical Effectiveness of Nesiritide in Decompensated Heart Failure (ASCEND-HF) trial was designed to evaluate the effect of nesiritide, in addition to standard care, on rates of self-reported dyspnea at 6 and 24 hours, re-hospitalization for heart failure or death from any cause at 30 days, and renal dysfunction. The study included more than 7,000 patients and concluded that the IV vasodilator nesiritide did not improve survival or re-hospitalization relative to placebo, but had a small, non-significant effect on dyspnea when used in combination with other therapies. It also did not compromise renal function within a month of its use in acute decompensated heart failure. Therefore, the use of nesiritide for patients with acute decompensated heart failure has further waned over the years, while less expensive intravenous vasodilators continue to be employed.

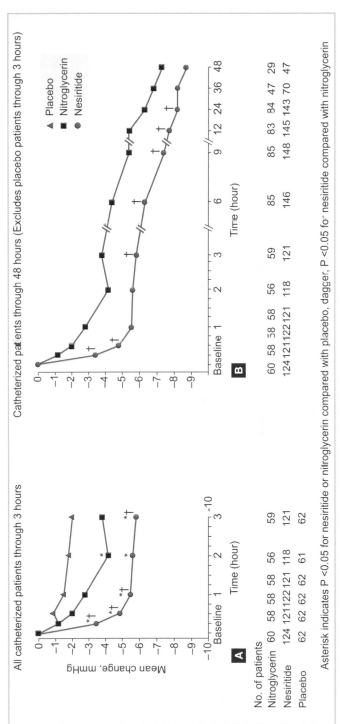

FIGS 13A AND B: Changes in pulmonary capillary wedge pressure from baseline in response to intravenous nitroglycerin, nesiritide and placebo in patients with heart failure.[90]

ORAL β-ADRENERGIC BLOCKING DRUGS

There is a fundamental belief that the biologically powerful adrenergic nervous system compensates for the failing heart by increasing myocyte size (hypertrophy), heart rate and force of contraction (inotropy). The sympathetic nervous system also activates the RAAS, thus conserving intravascular volume and redirecting blood flow to vital organs. However, an overly active sympathetic nervous system has repeatedly been shown to be essentially toxic to myocardial cells in both animals and humans.[98] There have been numerous large randomized trials supporting the concept that blocking the sympathetic nervous system with β-adrenergic blocking drugs in patients with systolic heart failure slows the progression of systolic heart failure and improves patient survival (Fig. 14).

The importance of dysfunctional adrenergic activation in heart failure was first elucidated by work of Braunwald and colleagues at the National Institutes of Health in the 1960s.[99] Since then, there has been an enormous basic and clinical research effort testing the rather counterintuitive concept that blocking the β_1 and β_2-adrenergic receptors will benefit patients with systolic heart failure.[100] It is well known that β-adrenergic receptors downregulate in response to excessive sympathetic drive,[101] presumably in an attempt to protect the cardiac myocyte from overstimulation. Such biological behavior suggests that blocking the receptors pharmacologically may also protect the heart.[102] Moreover, pheochromocytoma (a classic example of long-term hyperadrenergic activity) is well known to express itself as dilated or hypertrophic cardiomyopathy.[103] This provides additional proof of concept that the overly active sympathetic nervous system (SNS) and its dysfunctional status is central to the pathophysiology of heart failure,[104-107] similar to the overly active RAAS.

The first use of β-adrenergic blockers to treat patients with heart failure was the product of a series of carefully written case reports from Göteborg, Sweden.[108-110] This experience was a source of both great excitement and profound skepticism. Eventually, a small clinical trial (Metoprolol in Dilated Cardiomyopathy [MDC]) was launched, but showed only marginal benefit of metoprolol in patients with heart failure.[111] Other clinical trials were performed using bisoprolol (The Cardiac Insufficiency Bisoprolol Study [CIBIS] and CIBIS II)[112,113] and metoprolol succinate (the Metoprolol CR/XL Randomized Intervention Trial in Congestive Heart Failure [MERIT-HF]).[114] Carvedilol, an α1 and non-selective β-adrenergic blocker, was also demonstrated to improve survival in patients with moderate and even very severe heart failure (The Carvedilol Prospective Randomized Cumulative Survival [COPERNICUS] Trial).[115] Some would argue that the α1-adrenergic receptor blockade induced by carvedilol provides an additional

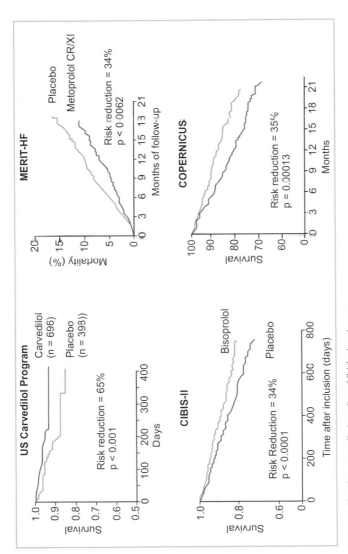

FIG. 14: Placebo-controlled studies of β-blocker therapy.

advantage to standard β-adrenergic blockade,[115-117] but this has remained controversial. Today β-adrenergic blockers are widely used throughout the world to treat patients with systolic heart failure.[118] They are considered "evidence-based" therapy. The suggested initial dose and evidence-based maximal dose are shown in Table 2.

Although it is unusual to see patients with heart failure who are naive to either RAAS inhibitors or β-blockers, occasionally the issue of which class of drug to initiate first arises. Experience indicates that either RAAS blockers (i.e., ACE inhibitor or ARB) or a β-blocker may be initiated first,[119] but that eventually full-doses of both classes of drugs should be attempted. The titration schedule of β-adrenergic drugs should be slow, that is over several weeks. The magnitude of heart rate reduction is significantly associated with the survival benefit of β-blockers in patients with systolic heart failure, whereas the dose of β-blocker is not.[120] There is also a strong correlation between change in heart rate and improvement in LV ejection fraction.[121] It appears as though decreased heart rate, improved LV chamber performance and afterload reduction each contribute to enhanced LV ejection fraction with use of carvedilol.[122]

β-adrenergic blocking drugs are now widely used to treat all stages of heart failure. Some patients admitted to hospital with NYHA class III or IV systolic heart failure may not tolerate β-blockers because of symptomatic hypotension or low cardiac output, but most hospitalized patients with acute heart failure do tolerate these drugs. The continuation of β-blocker therapy in patients hospitalized with acute decompensated systolic heart failure is associated with lower post-discharge mortality risk and improved treatment rates.[123] Withdrawal of β-blocker therapy in the hospital is associated with a higher risk. β-blocker therapy before and during hospitalization for acute systolic heart failure is associated with improved outcomes.[124] In our experience, the most common documented cause of discontinuance of β-blockers in patients with heart failure is failure to restart β-blockers after they have been stopped during hospitalization.[125]

Not all patients with systolic heart failure improve with β-blocking therapy. One possibility is that functional improvement from β-blockers may be related to changes in myocardial contractile protein gene expression,[126] which could vary from patient to patient. Another possibility is that β-blocking drugs are quite different from each other. Metoprolol and bisoprolol are both β-receptor subtype selective (i.e., β_1). Bucindolol, labetalol and carvedilol are each non-selective, and labetalol and carvedilol have α1 blocking properties that produce ancillary vasodilation. Bucindolol, though not generally available, has been intensely studied and has mild vasodilator properties, probably mediated by cGMP.

Additionally, bucindolol has meager "inverse agonism", so there is less negative chronotropism and inotropic effects. Bucindolol can also lower systemic norepinephrine levels substantially in some patients, and therefore has the potential to be a powerful sympatholytic agent. The norepinephrine lowering effects of bucindolol, as well as the clinical response to the drug, are strongly influenced by the pre-synaptic α_2c-adrenergic receptors, which modulate exocytosis and exhibit substantial genetic variation in humans. It is believed that a α_2c-adrenergic receptor polymorphism affects the sympatholytic effects of bucindolol in patients with systolic heart failure.[127] Patients with the α_2c-Del 322-325 polymorphism appear to have a marked increase in the sympatholytic response to bucindolol, and these carriers exhibit no evidence of clinical efficacy when treated with bucindolol. This concept is consistent with observations from other studies that indicate a marked decrease in plasma norepinephrine levels as a consequence of certain drug therapy, such as moxonidine, is associated with increased mortality and more heart failure hospitalizations. This seems also true with regard to the response to bucindolol where carriers of the α_2c-Del 322-325 variant exhibit very low plasma norepinephrine levels during bucindolol use, and a poor response to treatment. The frequency of this genetic variant is ~0.04 in whites and ~0.40 in blacks.

In addition to their favorable effects on LV performance and patient survival, β-adrenergic blockers, like RAAS blockers, slow the progression of LV remodeling. This occurs in patients with heart failure secondary to an acute myocardial infarction and in patients with chronic heart failure from dilated cardiomyopathy. LV end-diastolic volume tends to improve, the LV becomes less spherical and assumes a more natural ellipsoid shape. Mitral regurgitation is ameliorated or improved, and on average the LV ejection fraction goes up by about 5-7 ejection fraction units. In some cases, there is spectacular reverse remodeling, and in other cases this is less apparent or may not be seen at all. Reverse remodeling of the LV is associated with improved survival. We now have three major heart failure therapeutic strategies aimed at producing reverse remodeling: RAAS blocking drugs, cardiac resynchronization therapy (CRT), and β-adrenergic blocking drugs. Of course, coronary revascularization can also improve LV size and performance in selected patients. These therapies have proven to be powerful drivers of improved patient survival.

CONCLUSION

Neurohumoral modulating drugs now have a central role in the treatment of patients with systolic heart failure. This was not the case 35 years ago when only digitalis and diuretics were used.

Annualized mortality has fallen from approximately 20% to less than 10% per year commensurate with the use of RAAS and sympathetic nervous system blocking drugs. Of course, ICDs and CRT have also importantly contributed to this mortality reduction. The total cardiovascular death rate burden has fallen substantially in accordance with the widespread use of these therapies. Although, the incidence of STEMI (ST segment elevation myocardial infarction) has also fallen dramatically, incident systolic heart failure continues to be a major cause of hospitalization. There is now much better treatment for hypertension and hyperlipidemia. Paradoxically, as people live longer, we are now seeing a wave of heart failure in the elderly, the fastest growing segment of our population. The scourge of heart failure has not gone away, but has rather been shifted to people in their 70s, 80s, and 90s. In the end, prevention of heart failure by life-long control of known risk factors and mechanistic enlightenment though additional genomic studies may reduce the burden of heart failures even more, as systolic heart failure is likely a largely preventable disorder.

ACKNOWLEDGMENT

We acknowledge the outstanding help of Marisa Tirimacco in the preparation of this manuscript.

REFERENCES

1. Imperial ES, Levy MN, Zieske H Jr. Outflow resistance as an independent determinant of cardiac performance. Circ Res. 1961;9:1148-55.
2. Sonnenblick EH, Downing SE. Afterload as a primary determinant of ventricular performance. Am J Physiol. 1963;204:604-10.
3. Wilcken DE, Charlier AA, Hoffman JI, et al. Effects of alterations in aortic impedance on the performance of the ventricles. Circ Res. 1964;14:283-93.
4. Ross J Jr, Braunwald E. The Study of left ventricular function in man by increasing resistance to ventricular ejection with angiotensin. Circulation. 1964;29:739-49.
5. Cohn JN. Blood pressure and cardiac performance. Am J Med. 1973;55:351-61.
6. Meredith PA, Ostergren J, Anand I, et al. Clinical outcomes according to baseline blood pressure in patients with a low ejection fraction in the CHARM (Candesartan in Heart Failure: Assessment of Reduction in Mortality and Morbidity) Program. J Am Coll Cardiol. 2008;52:2000-7.
7. Anand IS, Tam SW, Rector TS, et al. Influence of blood pressure on the effectiveness of a fixed-dose combination of isosorbide dinitrate and hydralazine in the African-American Heart Failure Trial. J Am Coll Cardiol. 2007;49:32-9.
8. Rouleau JL, Roecker EB, Tendera M, et al. Influence of pretreatment systolic blood pressure on the effect of carvedilol in patients with severe chronic heart failure: the Carvedilol Prospective Randomized Cumulative Survival (COPERNICUS) study. J Am Coll Cardiol. 2004;43:1423-9.
9. Franciosa JA, Pierpont G, Cohn JN. Hemodynamic improvement after oral hydralazine in left ventricular failure: a comparison with nitroprusside infusion in 16 patients. Ann Intern Med. 1977;86:388-93.
10. Franciosa JA, Blank RC, Cohn JN. Nitrate effects on cardiac output and left ventricular outflow resistance in chronic congestive heart failure. Am J Med. 1978;64:207-13.

11. Olivari MT, Levine TB, Cohn JN. Abnormal neurohumoral response to nitroprusside infusion in congestive heart failure. J Am Coll Cardiol. 1983;2:411-7.

12. Kaye DM, Jennings GL, Dart AM, et al. Differential effect of acute baroreceptor unloading on cardiac and systemic sympathetic tone in congestive heart failure. J Am Coll Cardiol. 1998;31:583-7.

13. Chatterjee K, Parmley WW, Massie B, et al. Oral hydralazine therapy for chronic refractory heart failure. Circulation. 1976;54:879-83.

14. Taylor AL, Ziesche S, Yancy C, et al. Combination of isosorbide dinitrate and hydralazine in blacks with heart failure. N Engl J Med. 2004;351:2049-57.

15. Elkayam U. Nitrates in the treatment of congestive heart failure. Am J Cardiol. 1996;77:41C-51C.

16. Packer M, Carson P, Elkayam U, et al. Effect of amlodipine on the survival of patients with severe chronic heart failure due to a nonischemic cardiomyopathy: Results of the PRAISE-2 study (prospective randomized amlodipine survival evaluation 2). JACC Heart failure. 2013;1:308-14.

17. Packer M, O'Connor CM, Ghali JK, et al. Effect of amlodipine on morbidity and mortality in severe chronic heart failure. Prospective Randomized Amlodipine Survival Evaluation Study Group. N Engl J Med. 1996;335:1107-14.

18. Ignarro LJ, Lippton H, Edwards JC, et al. Mechanism of vascular smooth muscle relaxation by organic nitrates, nitrites, nitroprusside and nitric oxide: evidence for the involvement of S-nitrosothiols as active intermediates. J Pharmacol Exp Ther. 1981;218:739-49.

19. De Caterina R, Dorso CR, Tack-Goldman K, et al. Nitrates and endothelial prostacyclin production: studies in vitro. Circulation. 1985;71:176-82.

20. Franciosa JA, Nordstrom LA, Cohn JN. Nitrate therapy for congestive heart failure. JAMA. 1978;240:443-6.

21. Leier CV, Huss P, Magorien RD, et al. Improved exercise capacity and differing arterial and venous tolerance during chronic isosorbide dinitrate therapy for congestive heart failure. Circulation. 1983;67:817-22.

22. Franciosa JA, Goldsmith SR, Cohn JN. Contrasting immediate and long-term effects of isosorbide dinitrate on exercise capacity in congestive heart failure. Am J Med. 1980;69:559-66.

23. Chatterjee K, Parmley WW. Vasodilator therapy for acute myocardial infarction and chronic congestive heart failure. J Am Coll Cardiol. 1983;1:133-53.

24. A placebo-controlled trial of captopril in refractory chronic congestive heart failure. Captopril Multicenter Research Group. J Am Coll Cardiol. 1983;2:755-63.

25. Pfeffer MA, Braunwald E, Moye LA, et al. Effect of captopril on mortality and morbidity in patients with left ventricular dysfunction after myocardial infarction. Results of the survival and ventricular enlargement trial. The SAVE Investigators. N Engl J Med.1992;327:669-77.

26. Pfeffer JM, Pfeffer MA, Braunwald E. Influence of chronic captopril therapy on the infarcted left ventricle of the rat. Circ Res. 1985;57:84-95.

27. Curtiss C, Cohn JN, Vrobel T, et al. Role of the renin-angiotensin system in the systemic vasoconstriction of chronic congestive heart failure. Circulation. 1978;58:763-70.

28. Effect of enalapril on survival in patients with reduced left ventricular ejection fractions and congestive heart failure. The SOLVD Investigators. N Engl J Med.1991;325:293-302.

29. Effect of enalapril on mortality and the development of heart failure in asymptomatic patients with reduced left ventricular ejection fractions. The SOLVD Investigators. N Engl J Med. 1992;327:685-91.

30. Francis GS, Benedict C, Johnstone DE, et al. Comparison of neuroendocrine activation in patients with left ventricular dysfunction with and without congestive heart failure. A substudy of the Studies of Left Ventricular Dysfunction (SOLVD). Circulation. 1990;82:1724-9.

31. Dzau VJ, Colucci WS, Hollenberg NK, et al. Relation of the renin-angiotensin-aldosterone system to clinical state in congestive heart failure. Circulation. 1981;63:645-51.

32. Katz A. Molecular biology in cardiology, a paradigmatic shift. J Mol Cell Cardiol. 1988;20:12.
33. Packer M. The neurohormonal hypothesis: a theory to explain the mechanism of disease progression in heart failure. J Am Coll Cardiol. 1992;20:248-54.
34. Hill JA, Olson EN. Cardiac plasticity. N Engl J Med. 2008;358:1370-80.
35. McDonald KM, Garr M, Carlyle PF, et al. Relative effects of alpha 1-adrenoceptor blockade, converting enzyme inhibitor therapy, and angiotensin II subtype 1 receptor blockade on ventricular remodeling in the dog. Circulation. 1994;90:3034-46.
36. Tan LB, Jalil JE, Pick R, et al. Cardiac myocyte necrosis induced by angiotensin II. Circ Res. 1991;69:1185-95.
37. Levine TB, Francis GS, Goldsmith SR, et al. Activity of the sympathetic nervous system and renin-angiotensin system assessed by plasma hormone levels and their relation to hemodynamic abnormalities in congestive heart failure. Am J Cardiol. 1982;49:1659-66.
38. Packer M. Neurohormonal interactions and adaptations in congestive heart failure. Circulation. 1988;77:721-30.
39. Harris P. Evolution and the cardiac patient. Cardiovasc Res. 1983;17:313-445.
40. Pfeffer MA, Braunwald E. Ventricular remodeling after myocardial infarction. Experimental observations and clinical implications. Circulation. 1990;81:1161-72.
41. Cohn J. Structural basis for heart failure. Ventricular remodeling and its pharmacological inhibition. Circulation. 1995;91:2504-7.
42. Cohn JN, Ferrari R, Sharpe N. Cardiac remodeling—concepts and clinical implications: a consensus paper from an international forum on cardiac remodeling. Behalf of an International Forum on Cardiac Remodeling. J Am Coll Cardiol. 2000;35:569-82.
43. Packer M, Lee WH, Kessler PD, et al. Role of neurohormonal mechanisms in determining survival in patients with severe chronic heart failure. Circulation. 1987;75:IV80-92.
44. Pfeffer MA, Lamas GA, Vaughan DE, et al. Effect of captopril on progressive ventricular dilatation after anterior myocardial infarction. N Engl J Med. 1988;319:80-6.
45. Konstam MA, Kronenberg MW, Rousseau MF, et al. Effects of the angiotensin converting enzyme inhibitor enalapril on the long-term progression of left ventricular dilatation in patients with asymptomatic systolic dysfunction. SOLVD (Studies of Left Ventricular Dysfunction) Investigators. Circulation. 1993;88:2277-83.
46. Greenberg B, Quinones MA, Koilpillai C, et al. Effects of long-term enalapril therapy on cardiac structure and function in patients with left ventricular dysfunction. Results of the SOLVD echocardiography substudy. Circulation. 1995;91:2573-81.
47. St John Sutton M, Pfeffer MA, Plappert T, et al. Quantitative two-dimensional echocardiographic measurements are major predictors of adverse cardiovascular events after acute myocardial infarction. The protective effects of captopril. Circulation. 1994;89:68-75.
48. Goodfriend TL, Elliott ME, Catt KJ. Angiotensin receptors and their antagonists. The New England journal of medicine. 1996;334:1649-54.
49. Burnier M, Brunner HR. Angiotensin II receptor antagonists. Lancet. 2000;355:637-45.
50. Phillips CO, Kashani A, Ko DK, et al. Adverse effects of combination angiotensin II receptor blockers plus angiotensin-converting enzyme inhibitors for left ventricular dysfunction: a quantitative review of data from randomized clinical trials. Arch Intern Med. 2007;167:1930-6.
51. Cohn JN, Tognoni G, Valsartan Heart Failure Trial I. A randomized trial of the angiotensin-receptor blocker valsartan in chronic heart failure. N Engl J Med. 2001;345:1667-75.
52. Young JB, Dunlap ME, Pfeffer MA, et al. Mortality and morbidity reduction with Candesartan in patients with chronic heart failure and left ventricular systolic dysfunction: results of the CHARM low-left ventricular ejection fraction trials. Circulation. 2004;110:2618-26.

53. Pfeffer MA, McMurray JJ, Velazquez EJ, et al. Valsartan, captopril, or both in myocardial infarction complicated by heart failure, left ventricular dysfunction, or both. N Engl J Med. 2003;349:1893-906.

54. Investigators O. Telmisartan, ramipril, or both in patients at high risk for vascular events. N Engl J Med. 2008;358:1547-59.

55. Messerli FH. The sudden demise of dual renin-angiotensin system blockade or the soft science of the surrogate end point. J Am Coll Cardiol. 2009;53:468-70.

56. GISSI-AF Investigators, Disertori M, Latini R, et al. Valsartan for prevention of recurrent atrial fibrillation. N Engl J Med. 2009;360:1606-17.

57. Konstam MA, Neaton JD, Dickstein K, et al. Effects of high-dose versus low-dose losartan on clinical outcomes in patients with heart failure (HEAAL study): a randomised, double-blind trial. Lancet. 2009;374:1840-8.

58. Solomon SD, Skali H, Anavekar NS, et al. Changes in ventricular size and function in patients treated with valsartan, captopril, or both after myocardial infarction. Circulation. 2005;111:3411-9.

59. Massie BM, Carson PE, McMurray JJ, et al. Irbesartan in patients with heart failure and preserved ejection fraction. N Engl J Med. 2008;359:2456-67.

60. Weber KT. Aldosterone in congestive heart failure. N Engl J Med. 2001;345: 1689-97.

61. Tang WH, Parameswaran AC, Maroo AP, et al. Aldosterone receptor antagonists in the medical management of chronic heart failure. Mayo Clinic proceedings. 2005;80:1623-30.

62. Pitt B, Zannad F, Remme WJ, et al. The effect of spironolactone on morbidity and mortality in patients with severe heart failure. Randomized Aldactone Evaluation Study Investigators. N Engl J Med. 1999;341:709-17.

63. Pitt B, Remme W, Zannad F, et al. Eplerenone, a selective aldosterone blocker, in patients with left ventricular dysfunction after myocardial infarction. N Engl J Med. 2003;348:1309-21.

64. Zannad F, McMurray JJ, Krum H, et al. Eplerenone in patients with systolic heart failure and mild symptoms. N Engl J Med. 2011;364:11-21.

65. Albert NM, Yancy CW, Liang L, et al. Use of aldosterone antagonists in heart failure. JAMA. 2009;302:1658-65.

66. Juurlink DN, Mamdani MM, Lee DS, et al. Rates of hyperkalemia after publication of the Randomized Aldactone Evaluation Study. N Engl J Med. 2004;351:543-51.

67. Weber KT, Villarreal D. Aldosterone and antialdosterone therapy in congestive heart failure. Am J Cardiol. 1993;71:3A-11A.

68. Udelson JE, Feldman AM, Greenberg B, et al. Randomized, double-blind, multicenter, placebo-controlled study evaluating the effect of aldosterone antagonism with eplerenone on ventricular remodeling in patients with mild-to-moderate heart failure and left ventricular systolic dysfunction. Circ Heart fail. 2010;3:347-53.

69. Pitt B, Pfeffer MA, Assmann SF, et al. Spironolactone for heart failure with preserved ejection fraction. N Engl J Med. 2014;370:1383-92.

70. McMurray JJ, Packer M, Desai AS, et al. Angiotensin-neprilysin inhibition versus enalapril in heart failure. N Engl J Med. 2014;371:993-1004.

71. Kumar P, Francis GS, Tang WH. Phosphodiesterase 5 inhibition in heart failure: mechanisms and clinical implications. Nat Rev Cardiol. 2009;6:349-55.

72. Kass DA. Hypertrophied right hearts get two for the price of one: can inhibiting phosphodiesterase type 5 also inhibit phosphodiesterase type 3? Circulation. 2007;116:233-5.

73. Takimoto E, Champion HC, Li M, et al. Chronic inhibition of cyclic GMP phosphodiesterase 5A prevents and reverses cardiac hypertrophy. Nat Med. 2005;11:214-22.

74. Archer SL, Michelakis ED. Phosphodiesterase type 5 inhibitors for pulmonary arterial hypertension. N Engl J Med. 2009;361:1864-71.

75. Semigran MJ. Type 5 phosphodiesterase inhibition: the focus shifts to the heart. Circulation. 2005;112:2589-91.

76. Guazzi M, Samaja M, Arena R, et al. Long-term use of sildenafil in the therapeutic management of heart failure. J Am Coll Cardiol. 2007;50:2136-44.

77. Stehlik J, Movsesian MA. Combined use of PDE5 inhibitors and nitrates in the treatment of pulmonary arterial hypertension in patients with heart failure. J Card Fail. 2009;15:31-4.

78. Pokreisz P, Vandenwijngaert S, Bito V, et al. Ventricular phosphodiesterase-5 expression is increased in patients with advanced heart failure and contributes to adverse ventricular remodeling after myocardial infarction in mice. Circulation. 2009;119:408-16.

79. Nagayama T, Hsu S, Zhang M, et al. Sildenafil stops progressive chamber, cellular, and molecular remodeling and improves calcium handling and function in hearts with pre-existing advanced hypertrophy caused by pressure overload. J Am Coll Cardiol. 2009;53:207-15.

80. Lu Z, Xu X, Hu X, et al. Oxidative stress regulates left ventricular PDE5 expression in the failing heart. Circulation. 2010;121:1474-83.

81. Redfield MM, Chen HH, Borlaug BA, et al. Effect of phosphodiesterase-5 inhibition on exercise capacity and clinical status in heart failure with preserved ejection fraction: a randomized clinical trial. JAMA. 2013;309:1268-77.

82. Cohn JN, Burke LP. Nitroprusside. Ann Intern Med. 1979;91:752-7.

83. Mikulic E, Cohn JN, Franciosa JA. Comparative hemodynamic effects of inotropic and vasodilator drugs in severe heart failure. Circulation. 1977;56:528-33.

84. Franciosa JA, Limas CJ, Guiha NH, et al. Improved left ventricular function during nitroprusside infusion in acute myocardial infarction. Lancet. 1972;1:650-4.

85. Cohn JN, Franciosa JA, Francis GS, et al. Effect of short-term infusion of sodium nitroprusside on mortality rate in acute myocardial infarction complicated by left ventricular failure: results of a Veterans Administration cooperative study. N Engl J Med. 1982;306:1129-35.

86. Guiha NH, Cohn JN, Mikulic E, et al. Treatment of refractory heart failure with infusion of nitroprusside. N Engl J Med. 1974;291:587-92.

87. Cohn JN, Mathew KJ, Franciosa JA, et al. Chronic vasodilator therapy in the management of cardiogenic shock and intractable left ventricular failure. Ann Intern Med. 1974;81:777-80.

88. Khot UN, Novaro GM, Popovic ZB, et al. Nitroprusside in critically ill patients with left ventricular dysfunction and aortic stenosis. N Engl J Med. 2003;348:1756-63.

89. Mullens W, Abrahams Z, Francis GS, et al. Sodium nitroprusside for advanced low-output heart failure. J Am Coll Cardiol. 2008;52:200-7.

90. VMAC. Intravenous nesiritide vs nitroglycerin for treatment of decompensated congestive heart failure: a randomized controlled trial. JAMA. 2002;287:1531-40.

91. Sackner-Bernstein JD, Skopicki HA, Aaronson KD. Risk of worsening renal function with nesiritide in patients with acutely decompensated heart failure. Circulation. 2005;111:1487-91.

92. Teerlink JR, Massie BM. Nesiritide and worsening of renal function: the emperor's new clothes? Circulation. 2005;111:1459-61.

93. Sackner-Bernstein JD, Kowalski M, Fox M, et al. Short-term risk of death after treatment with nesiritide for decompensated heart failure: a pooled analysis of randomized controlled trials. JAMA. 2005;293:1900-5.

94. Topol EJ. Nesiritide - not verified. N Engl J Med. 2005;353:113-6.

95. O'Connor CM, Starling RC, Hernandez AF, et al. Effect of nesiritide in patients with acute decompensated heart failure. N Engl J Med. 2011;365:32-43.

96. Yancy CW, Krum H, Massie BM, et al. Safety and efficacy of outpatient nesiritide in patients with advanced heart failure: results of the Second Follow-Up Serial Infusions of Nesiritide (FUSION II) trial. Circ Heart Fail. 2008;1:9-16.

97. Hauptman PJ, Schnitzler MA, Swindle J, et al. Use of nesiritide before and after publications suggesting drug-related risks in patients with acute decompensated heart failure. JAMA. 2006;296:1877-84.

98. Mann DL, Kent RL, Parsons B, et al. Adrenergic effects on the biology of the adult mammalian cardiocyte. Circulation. 1992;85:790-804.

99. Braunwald E, Chidsey CA, Pool PE, et al. Congestive heart failure. Biochemical and physiological considerations. Combined clinical staff conference at the National Institutes of Health. Ann Intern Med. 1966;64:904-41.

100. Braunwald E, Bristow MR. Congestive heart failure: fifty years of progress. Circulation. 2000;102:IV14-23.

101. Bristow MR, Ginsburg R, Umans V, et al. Beta 1- and beta 2-adrenergic-receptor subpopulations in nonfailing and failing human ventricular myocardium: coupling of both receptor subtypes to muscle contraction and selective beta 1-receptor down-regulation in heart failure. Circ Res. 1986;59:297-309.

102. Eichhorn EJ, Bristow MR. Medical therapy can improve the biological properties of the chronically failing heart. A new era in the treatment of heart failure. Circulation. 1996;94:2285-96.

103. Dalby MC, Burke M, Radley-Smith R, et al. Pheochromocytoma presenting after cardiac transplantation for dilated cardiomyopathy. J Heart Lung Transplant. 2001; 20:773-5.

104. Cohn J. Sympathetic nervous system in heart failure. Circulation. 2002;106:2417-8.

105. Bristow M. Antiadrenergic therapy of chronic heart failure: surprises and now opportunities. Circulation. 2003;107:1100-2.

106. Triposkiadis F, Karayannis G, Giamouzis G, et al. The sympathetic nervous system in heart failure physiology, pathophysiology, and clinical implications. J Am Coll Cardiol. 2009;54:1747-62.

107. Floras JS. Sympathetic nervous system activation in human heart failure: clinical implications of an updated model. J Am Coll Cardiol. 2009;54:375-85.

108. Waagstein F, Hjalmarson A, Varnauskas E, et al. Effect of chronic beta-adrenergic receptor blockade in congestive cardiomyopathy. Br Heart J. 1975;37:1022-36.

109. Swedberg K, Hjalmarson A, Waagstein F, et al. Beneficial effects of long-term beta-blockade in congestive cardiomyopathy. Br Heart J. 1980;44:117-33.

110. Swedberg K, Hjalmarson A, Waagstein F, et al. Adverse effects of beta-blockade withdrawal in patients with congestive cardiomyopathy. Br Heart J. 1980;44:134-42.

111. Waagstein F, Bristow MR, Swedberg K, et al. Beneficial effects of metoprolol in idiopathic dilated cardiomyopathy. Metoprolol in Dilated Cardiomyopathy (MDC) Trial Study Group. Lancet. 1993;342:1441-6.

112. A randomized trial of beta-blockade in heart failure. The Cardiac Insufficiency Bisoprolol Study (CIBIS). CIBIS Investigators and Committees. Circulation. 1994;90: 1765-73.

113. The Cardiac Insufficiency Bisoprolol Study II (CIBIS-II): a randomised trial. Lancet. 1999;353:9-13.

114. Hjalmarson A, Goldstein S, Fagerberg B, et al. Effects of controlled-release metoprolol on total mortality, hospitalizations, and well-being in patients with heart failure: the Metoprolol CR/XL Randomized Intervention Trial in congestive heart failure (MERIT-HF). MERIT-HF Study Group. JAMA. 2000;283:1295-302.

115. Packer M, Fowler MB, Roecker EB, et al. Effect of carvedilol on the morbidity of patients with severe chronic heart failure: results of the carvedilol prospective randomized cumulative survival (COPERNICUS) study. Circulation. 2002;106:2194-9.

116. Poole-Wilson PA, Swedberg K, Cleland JG, et al. Comparison of carvedilol and metoprolol on clinical outcomes in patients with chronic heart failure in the Carvedilol Or Metoprolol European Trial (COMET): randomised controlled trial. Lancet. 2003;362:7-13.

117. Packer M. Do beta-blockers prolong survival in heart failure only by inhibiting the beta1-receptor? A perspective on the results of the COMET trial. J Card Fail. 2003;9:429-43.

118. Klapholz M. Beta-blocker use for the stages of heart failure. Mayo Clinic proceedings. 2009;84:718-29.

119. Willenheimer R, van Veldhuisen DJ, Silke B, et al. Effect on survival and hospitalization of initiating treatment for chronic heart failure with bisoprolol followed by enalapril, as compared with the opposite sequence: results of

the randomized Cardiac Insufficiency Bisoprolol Study (CIBIS) III. Circulation. 2005;112:2426-35.

120. McAlister FA, Wiebe N, Ezekowitz JA, et al. Meta-analysis: beta-blocker dose, heart rate reduction, and death in patients with heart failure. Ann Intern Med. 2009;150:784-94.

121. Flannery G, Gehrig-Mills R, Billah B, et al. Analysis of randomized controlled trials on the effect of magnitude of heart rate reduction on clinical outcomes in patients with systolic chronic heart failure receiving beta-blockers. Am J Cardiol. 2008;101:865-9.

122. Maurer MS, Sackner-Bernstein JD, El-Khoury Rumbarger L, et al. Mechanisms underlying improvements in ejection fraction with carvedilol in heart failure. Circ Heart Fail. 2009;2:189-96.

123. Fonarow GC, Abraham WT, Albert NM, et al. Influence of beta-blocker continuation or withdrawal on outcomes in patients hospitalized with heart failure: findings from the OPTIMIZE-HF program. J Am Coll Cardiol. 2008;52:190-9.

124. Butler J, Young JB, Abraham WT, et al. Beta-blocker use and outcomes among hospitalized heart failure patients. Journal of the American College of Cardiology . 2006;47:2462-9.

125. Parameswaran AC, Tang WH, Francis GS, et al. Why do patients fail to receive beta-blockers for chronic heart failure over time? A "real-world" single-center, 2-year follow-up experience of beta-blocker therapy in patients with chronic heart failure. Am Heart J. 2005;149:921-6.

126. Lowes BD, Gilbert EM, Abraham WT, et al. Myocardial gene expression in dilated cardiomyopathy treated with beta-blocking agents. N Engl J Med. 2002;346: 1357-65.

127. Bristow MR, Murphy GA, Krause-Steinrauf H, et al. An alpha2C-adrenergic receptor polymorphism alters the norepinephrine-lowering effects and therapeutic response of the beta-blocker bucindolol in chronic heart failure. Circ Heart Fail. 2010;3:21-8.

Positive Inotropic Drugs: A Limited but Important Role

Carl V Leier, Garrie J Haas, Philip F Binkley

INTRODUCTION

Positive inotropic agents are drugs that increase the velocity and strength of contraction of the cardiomyocyte in which the myocardium and heart are the primary target organs. The classic measurement of cardiac function is ejection fraction, but it only indirectly represents a measurement of contractility. It is a way of determining the extent of contraction but does not account for the rate or strength of myocardial contraction. The more accurate measurements of myocardial contractility or inotropy include end-systolic elastance from the left ventricular (LV) pressure-velocity loop, ΔLV systolic upstroke pressure/Δtime, peak slope of LV developed pressure and velocity of circumferential fiber shortening.

The positive inotropes will also augment the magnitude of contraction (i.e., ejection fraction), but this effect can also be achieved to varying degrees by a wide variety of non-inotropic agents (e.g., angiotensin converting enzyme inhibitors (ACEIs), angiotensin II receptor blockers and vasodilators). Therefore, this is not a unique characteristic of positive inotropic agents.

This chapter will discuss the pharmacologic drugs employed clinically to directly enhance cardiac contractility or the inotropic state of the myocardium, the so-called positive inotropic drugs. These agents are directed at the patients whose overall cardiovascular function is impaired by loss of cardiac contractility to the extent that there are symptoms and signs of reduced stroke volume, cardiac output, hypotension and hypoperfusion of vital organs and systems.

Positive inotropic agents augment cardiac contractility through a number of different mechanisms, but most of them act by modulating calcium handling by the myocardial cell. The various mechanisms of action on the cardiomyocyte by the major positive inotropic drugs are presented in Figure 1.

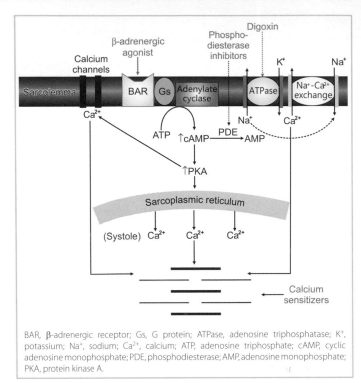

BAR, β-adrenergic receptor; Gs, G protein; ATPase, adenosine triphosphatase; K⁺, potassium; Na⁺, sodium; Ca²⁺, calcium; ATP, adenosine triphosphate; cAMP, cyclic adenosine monophosphate; PDE, phosphodiesterase; AMP, adenosine monophosphate; PKA, protein kinase A.

FIG. 1: Mechanisms of actions of positive inotropic drugs on cardiomyocytes. The major positive inotropic groups generally act through mechanisms that increase the concentration and availability of intracellular calcium for the actin-myosin contractile apparatus. β-adrenergic agonists attach to the β-adrenergic receptor, activating the Gs protein-adenylate cyclase complex to convert ATP to cAMP. cAMP activates protein kinase A, which phosphorylates several intracellular sites resulting in Ca^{2+} influx into the cell and Ca^{2+} release from sarcoplasmic reticulum to augment systole. Phosphodiesterase inhibitors impair the breakdown of cAMP. Calcium sensitizers act by making the troponin-actin-myosin complex more responsive to available intracellular Ca^{2+}. By blocking the Na^+/K^+ ATPase pump, digoxin increases intracellular Na^+ loading of the Na^+-Ca^{2+} exchanger, resulting in less extrusion of Ca^{2+} from the myocyte. Dashed arrow indicates inhibition. The comprehensive mechanisms of actions of these positive inotropic agents are considerably more numerous and complex.

Enhancement of cardiac contractility by these agents with resultant improvement of compromised hemodynamics is not achieved without a price to be paid. Unless the positive inotropic agent also has substantial cardiac unloading properties (preload- and afterload-reduction) and/or substantially causes other favorable effects (e.g., increase of diastolic perfusion time, improvement of autonomic imbalance), these agents invariably increase the metabolic and oxygen demands of the heart. This undesirable characteristic is accentuated by other pharmacologic properties not uncommonly associated with positive inotropes, such as positive chronotropy (increase in heart rate), an increase in systemic vascular resistance, and cardiac dysrhythmias. These unfavorable properties can be especially troublesome in the clinical setting of occlusive coronary artery disease (CAD), where the oxygen-metabolic supply to a threatened region can be limited by the coronary obstructing lesions. For these reasons, intravenous positive inotropic therapy should generally be directed at acute short-term intervention and must be administered properly.

At present, chronic oral inotropic therapy is primarily delivered by digoxin, an agent with a relatively mild positive inotropic effect. It is quite possible that any favorable response to digoxin is largely secondary to other accompanying beneficial properties (*See* the heading "Digoxin"). The development of newer orally administered positive inotropic agents to enhance cardiac function has received a lot of attention and research activity over the past four decades, but to date, most have been burdened with adverse effects and outcomes.

For the purpose of clinical application, this chapter is divided into those agents directed at the short-term support of cardiac contraction with the intravenous inotropes, followed by a discussion on chronic long-term inotropic therapy with digoxin.

INTRAVENOUS SHORT-TERM POSITIVE INOTROPIC THERAPY

The drugs placed under this category represent a wide spectrum of pharmacologic effects in addition to their positive inotropic properties. The predominant distinguishing feature among these agents is their effect on peripheral vasculature, which can range from vasodilatation (milrinone) to balanced vascular tone (dobutamine) to vasoconstriction (norepinephrine) (Fig. 2 and Table 1). The cellular mechanisms for the positive inotropic properties of these intravenous agents are centered on increasing intracellular cyclic adenosine monophosphate (cAMP) by either adrenergic receptor stimulation or inhibition of cAMP degradation with subsequent elevation of intracellular calcium available for contraction (Fig. 1).

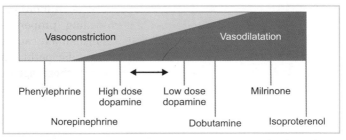

FIG. 2: Effects of short-term positive inotropic agents on peripheral vasculature. The wide range of vascular effects is presented for the agents currently available for short-term positive inotropy and cardiovascular support. The vascular properties are the major determinants for selection of these agents in individual patients.

TABLE 1: Hemodynamic profiles of the agents currently employed to deliver short-term inotropic and vasoactive support

	Phosphodiesterase inhibitor	Adrenergic agonists				
	Milrinone	Dobutamine	Dopamine Low dose	Dopamine Higher dose	Norepinephrine	Phenylephrine
Contractility (inotropy)	↑	↑↑↑	↑	↑↑	→↑	↗
Cardiac output	↑↑	↑↑↑	↑	↑	→↑	↗
Heart rate (chronotropy)	→↑	→↑	↗↑	↑↑	→↑	→↑
LV filling pressure	↓↓↓	↓↓	→	→↑	→↑	→↑
Systemic blood pressure	→↓	→↑	↑	↑↑	↑↑↑	↑↑↑
Systemic vascular resistance	↓↓↓	→↓	↑	↑↑	↑↑	↑↑↑
Pulmonary vascular resistance	↓↓↓	↓↓	↑	→↑	↑	↑

↓, decrease; →, minimal to no change; ↗, mild increase; ↑, increase.

ADRENERGIC AGENTS

Although the adrenergic receptor agonists can provoke tachycardia and dysrhythmias, they generally have a short elimination half-life. This is an ideal pharmacokinetic property for patients in the monitored critical care setting, where a quick onset and offset of cardiovascular effects allow immediate and tightly controlled hemodynamic support. An undesirable effect can be expected to be reversed shortly, within minutes, after the dose of the agent is lowered or discontinued.

The 3, 4-hydroxyphenyl ring is the essential structure of the catechols, the major component for the adrenergic agents employed for positive inotropic therapy. The molecular structures of the most commonly used adrenergic agents available and applied clinically are shown in Figure 3.

The adrenergic receptor agonists evoke most of their pharmacodynamic effects through activation of β-and α-adrenergic receptors. The myocardium is heavily populated with β-adrenergic receptors and, to a lesser extent, with α-adrenergic receptors; all capable of augmenting cardiac contraction in varying degrees. Stimulation-activation of both β1- and β2-adrenergic receptors augments the inotropic and, in some instances, the chronotropic states of the cardiac cell through mechanisms shown in Figure 1. β-adrenergic receptors are also present in other regions and organs of the body with the β2-adrenergic receptor being the most ubiquitous; accounting for concomitant vasodilatation and bronchodilation during β2-receptor agonism. α-adrenergic receptors are predominantly located in vasculature, such that their stimulation evokes vasoconstriction (also calcium-mediated) in excess of any positive inotropic effect.

The pharmacotherapeutic properties of the adrenergic receptor agonists used clinically for inotropic and hemo-dynamic support are individually presented under the heading of each. The pharmacologic properties are summarized in Table 1.

Dobutamine

Dobutamine is discussed first, because it is currently the agent most commonly employed for short-term intravenous positive inotropic support. Its overall cardiovascular effects in the setting of LV systolic dysfunction and failure result predominantly from positive inotropic enhancement of depressed cardiac contractility.

Dobutamine was formulated and developed in the laboratory by Tuttle and Mills[1] from a methodical manipulation and branch substitutions of the basic catechol-phenylethylamine molecule. Out of over 15 molecules developed and then studied

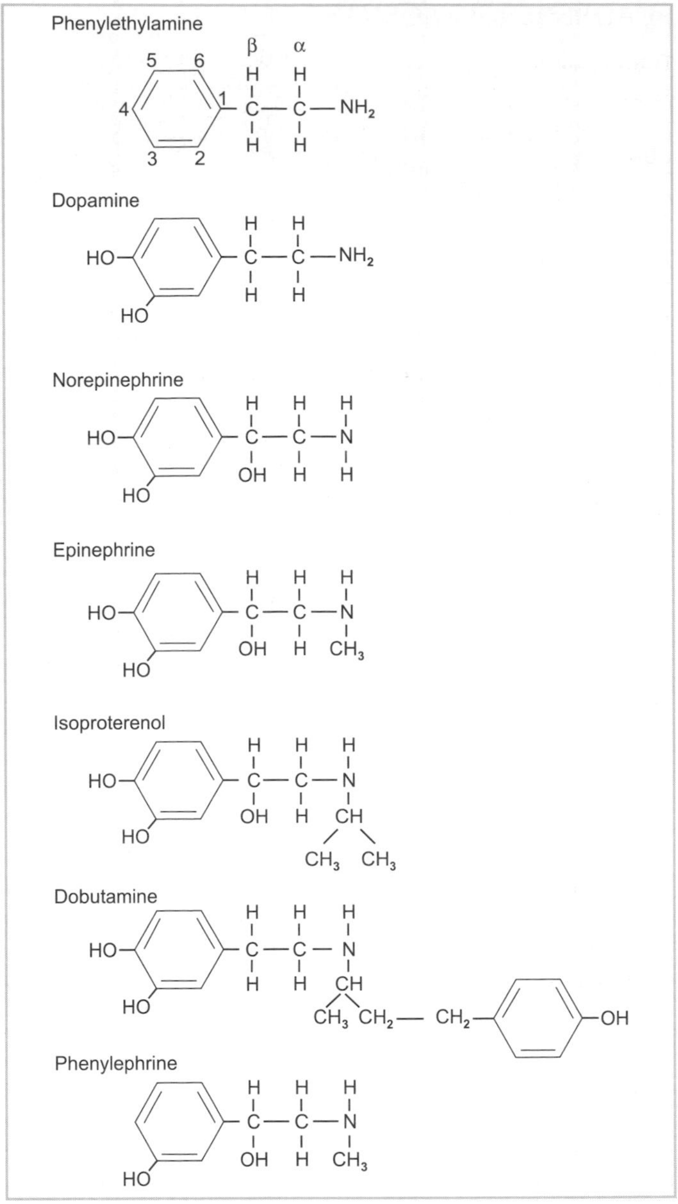

FIG. 3: The molecular structures of the most commonly used adrenergic agents. The phenylethylamine molecule is the basic molecular structure for the adrenergic compounds under discussion. Variations in the hydroxyl attachment at the β-site and the groups at the amino end determine many of the pharmacologic properties and consequent clinical applications of the catechols. Very little modification of the molecular structure is needed to change an intense vasodilator (isoproterenol) to a strong vasopressor (norepinephrine). Deletion of the 4-hydroxyl group from the epinephrine molecule results in phenylephrine, a powerful vasoconstrictor.

in large animal models, dobutamine achieved the greatest increase of cardiac contractility and performed with the least effect on vasculature and heart rate.

Pharmacologic Effects

Dobutamine is a racemic compound: dextro- and levo-isomers. It activates myocardial β1- and β2-adrenergic receptors to generate cAMP, which enhances calcium entry and release (the downstream mechanisms are depicted in Figure 1); thereby, increases the velocity and extent of myocardial contraction. In chronic heart failure (HF), the number and responsiveness of β1-adrenergic receptors are depleted such that dobutamine's cardiac effects in this clinical setting are largely rendered by activation of β2-receptors.[2] β-adrenergic receptor stimulation also accounts for the chronotropic properties and any dysrhythmias noted with higher dose dobutamine.

In the setting of LV systolic dysfunction and HF, dobutamine generally evokes a mild overall vasodilatory effect, reducing systemic and pulmonic vascular resistances through arteriolar β2-receptor stimulation (and secondary reduction of sympathetic vasoconstriction) exceeding the relatively modest vasoconstricting effects of its α-receptor agonism (Fig. 2 and Table 1). Studies by Binkley et al.[3-5] indicated that the pharmacology of dobutamine in human HF was considerably more complex. Their studies demonstrated that dobutamine favorably affected aortic impedance and vascular-ventricular coupling, allowing further enhancement of ventricular contractility and overall cardiac performance. In the total artificial heart model of the calf, dobutamine augmented cardiac output in the absence of myocardium and its associated positive inotropic mechanisms.[4] This response was the result of the vascular effects of dobutamine: its dextro-isomer (+ enantiomer) reduced systemic vascular resistance and afterload via β2-adrenergic receptor stimulation, and its levo-isomer (– enantiomer) reduced venous capacitance with enhanced venous return via α-receptor agonism.[4,6] The result is augmentation of cardiac output.

Clinical Effects

The major clinical indication for dobutamine administration is short-term positive inotropic support in patients afflicted with ventricular systolic dysfunction and failure, resulting in a problematic drop in blood pressure and systemic perfusion. Short-term support will vary somewhat, but generally, until the patient recovers adequately or is advanced into more definitive interventions (e.g., mechanical support, remedial cardiac surgery). The typical patient requiring inotropic support presents with acute systolic HF or decompensated chronic HF, a reduced stroke volume and cardiac output, elevated ventricular filling pressures, mild-to-moderate reduction in systemic pressure (systolic blood pressure 70–100 mmHg), and notably impaired systemic perfusion (e.g., prerenal azotemia, impaired mentation, elevated liver enzymes); the clinical setting is the "cold and wet" patient.[7]

Clinical Indications and Applications

Major indications

Short-term (hours to days) positive inotropic and hemo-dynamic support for patients with ventricular systolic dysfunction resulting in a depressed stroke volume and cardiac output, mild-to-moderate systemic hypotension (systolic blood pressures of 70–100 mmHg), systemic hypoperfusion and an elevated LV diastolic filling pressure (≥18 mmHg).

The support is maintained until the patient recovers or is directed into more advanced cardiovascular support (e.g., intra-aortic balloon counterpulsation and ventricular assist device) and/or remedial intervention (e.g., coronary artery intervention, valvular repair or replacement, and cardiac transplantation).

Additional considerations

- Pharmacologic support as needed for patients with severe HF undergoing major diagnostic or surgical procedures.
- Cardiovascular hemodynamic support for the HF patient as needed during the course of a major illness.
- Pharmacologic bridge in severe HF to standard therapies (e.g., ACEI, β-adrenergic blockade).
- As a continuous infusion via indwelling central venous catheter to provide the only means of stabilizing an unstable or decompensated HF patient to allow discharge from the hospital (to extended care, home or hospice).
- For hemodynamic support during weaning from cardiopulmonary bypass and during immediate recovery from cardiac surgery.
- To facilitate recovery of myocardial stunning in the setting of low-output cardiac failure.
- As a means of improving renal function and urine output in patients hospitalized for low-output, systemic hypoperfusion and volume-overloaded congestive HF when renal responsiveness to standard therapy and diuretics is impaired.
- For hemodynamic support during management of cardiac transplant-rejection complicated by hemodynamic low-output and volume-overloaded decompensation.
- To augment systolic function of problematic systolic failure of the right ventricle.
- To assess ventricular (right or left) contractile reserve.
- To evaluate the severity of aortic valvular stenosis in low-flow and low-gradient aortic stenosis.
- As pharmacologic stress for myocardial perfusion imaging or echocardiographic imaging.

The therapeutics in this general clinical setting can include diuretics for volume overload and elevated ventricular filling pressures (>18 mmHg), vasopressor infusion (e.g., norepinephrine, moderate-to-high dose dopamine, phenylephrine) for marked hypotension and shock, dobutamine for systemic systolic pressures of 70–100 mmHg, and combined with a positive inotrope—vasodilator or inodilator (e.g., milrinone) or a vasodilator (e.g., nitroprusside, nitroglycerin and nesiritide) for patients with systolic blood pressure more than 90–100 mmHg. It is relatively common to administer two or more of these agents simultaneously or in succession to attain and maintain the optimal and safest clinical and hemodynamic stability on the way to more definitive interventions. For example, a patient may be receiving a diuretic, dobutamine and nitroprusside, and yet another patient, dobutamine and norepinephrine.

With proper patient selection, specifically the patient with ventricular systolic dysfunction resulting in a fall in stroke volume and cardiac output, an abnormal rise in LV end-diastolic filling pressure, systemic hypoperfusion, and mild-to-moderate reduction in systemic blood pressure, dobutamine increases stroke volume, cardiac output, systemic systolic blood pressure and pulse pressure, and systemic perfusion, while decreasing the elevated LV filling pressure and pulmonary and systemic vascular resistances[8-10] (Fig. 4). In patients with concomitant mitral regurgitation, the reduction in systemic vascular resistance, ventricular volume and mitral orifice area likely account for the decrease in mitral regurgitation; the reduction in mitral regurgitation further augments stroke volume, and cardiac output during dobutamine administration.[10] While there appears to be a dose-related separation of positive inotropy or enhanced contractility with beneficial hemodynamic effects from the potential detrimental effects of positive chronotropy, higher dosing will elicit a faster heart rate and can provoke atrial and ventricular ectopic beats and various forms of tachydysrhythmias (Fig. 4).

Regional blood flow studies at rest in decompensated chronic HF revealed that dobutamine increases limb blood flow proportional to the increase in cardiac output. Dobutamine augments renal blood flow, but generally less than the proportional rise in cardiac output. However, dobutamine favorably affects renal function, glomerular filtration rate, and urine output, and can be expected to augment the renal effects (natriuretic and diuretic responses) of diuretics.[8] There is no statistical change in hepatic-splanchnic flow.[11]

In patients with LV systolic dysfunction and non-obstructed coronary arteries, dobutamine increases coronary blood flow proportional to or greater than the augmented cardiac output and myocardial oxygen consumption.[12,13] This favorable effect on myocardial oxygen balance is related to several mechanisms, including dobutamine-induced enhancement

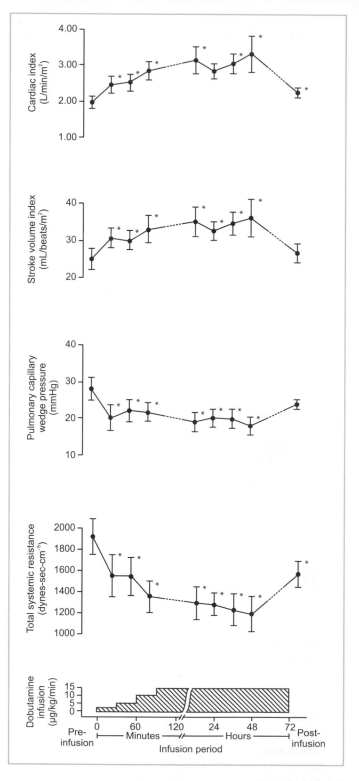

Figure 4 (*continued*)

(continued)

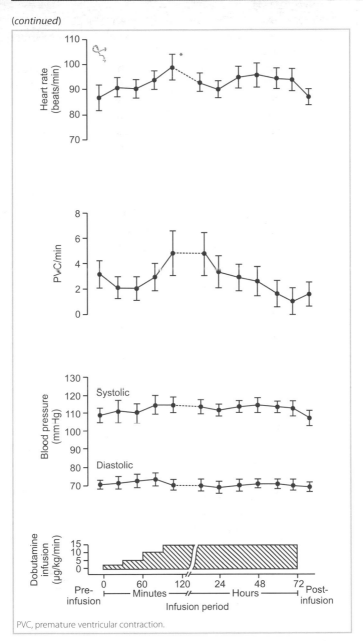

PVC, premature ventricular contraction.

FIG. 4: Pharmacodynamic curves for the dose-response and sustained infusions (72 hours) of dobutamine in chronic systolic heart failure. The infused dose is presented in the bottom panel.[8] $\overline{X} \pm SD$, n = 25, *p < 0.05 vs. preinfusion baseline.

of coronary perfusion pressure (reduction in LV diastolic pressure is more than the little to no drop in systemic diastolic pressure), an increase in coronary diastolic perfusion time, and a decrease in coronary vascular resistance.[8,12-14] Furthermore, the reduction in aortic impedance, systemic and pulmonary vascular resistances, ventricular afterload, and ventricular systolic volume with dobutamine lowers myocardial oxygen consumption. Positive inotropy as such increases myocardial oxygen consumption. At doses short of evoking a clinically significant elevation in heart rate (>10% above baseline), the coronary blood flow—myocardial oxygen delivery—is equal to or exceeds the increase in myocardial oxygen consumption caused by the enhanced contractility of dobutamine.[12,13]

However, these favorable coronary-myocardial energetic properties of dobutamine can be negated in the setting of high-grade occlusive CAD, where a fixed obstructive lesion can prevent an increase of coronary blood flow in its region to match the rise in myocardial contractility and associated oxygen consumption. Any substantial increase in heart rate (>10% above baseline) imposes a threat to coronary artery perfusion and the balance of oxygen demand—oxygen delivery by increasing myocardial oxygen—energy consumption of an ischemic region without an accompanying increase in coronary blood flow through the fixed coronary occlusion and by shortening of diastolic coronary perfusion time.[14] The positive chronotropic and inotropic properties of high-dose dobutamine are now regularly employed during dobutamine-stress echocardiographic, nuclear or magnetic resonance myocardial imaging to elicit evidence of inadequate coronary flow and myocardial ischemia in patients with occlusive CAD.

While the chronotropic properties of dobutamine are of major importance in all patients, they are particularly important in patients with occlusive CAD, where tachycardia will override the favorable coronary-myocardial energetic effects of dobutamine to evoke myocardial ischemia. For these reasons, proper patient and dose-selection is extremely important in patients with LV systolic dysfunction and occlusive coronary disease. Using the aforementioned pharmacologic considerations as a guide, dobutamine can be effectively and safely administered to decompensated HF patients with occlusive CAD to achieve and maintain a more stable, short-term, clinical and hemodynamic course until the patient is directed to more advanced intervention (e.g., intra-aortic balloon counterpulsation, catheter-based coronary intervention, coronary artery bypass surgery).[15-22] During this short-term "pharmacologic bridge", dobutamine has to be able to favorably alter the determinants of oxygen-metabolic consumption and supply (by reducing elevated ventricular diastolic pressures, pulmonic and systemic vascular resistances, ventricular volumes and wall stress, and increasing coronary artery perfusion pressure and diastolic perfusion time) comparable to and greater than the increase in myocardial oxygen-energy consumption of enhanced ventricular contraction. Nevertheless, even with proper patient-selection and dose-administration, a few patients with occlusive coronary disease can develop myocardial ischemia and potentially an infarction during dobutamine administration.[16,17,19]

Dobutamine appears to favorably affect and reverse myocardial stunning beyond the simple increase in coronary blood flow and myocardial perfusion of the affected region or whole heart.[23-25]

Clinical Indications

The most common clinical settings for appropriate dobutamine administration (to improve and then stabilize the patient's hemodynamic and clinical status) include patients treated for decompensated, hypoperfused, and typically hypotensive (generally systemic systolic blood pressure of 70–100 mmHg), chronic systolic HF, acute systolic HF (as can be seen with acute myocardial infarction or acute myocarditis), or immediately following cardiac surgery. The various considerations for the administration of dobutamine are presented.

Vasodilators or inodilators might be considered for augmentation and stabilization of hemodynamic- and clinical-status in symptomatic HF patients with systemic systolic pressures more than 90 mmHg.

2013 Guidelines for the Diagnosis and Management of Heart Failure in Adults[26]

Under the recommendations for management of patients with refractory end-stage HF (stage D):

Class I

1. Until definitive therapy (e.g., coronary revascularization, mechanical circulatory support, heart transplantation) or resolution of the acute precipitating problem, patients with cardiogenic shock should receive temporary intravenous inotropic support to maintain systemic perfusion and preserve end-organ performance. (*Level of Evidence: C*)

Class IIa

1. Continuous intravenous inotropic support is reasonable as "bridge therapy" in patients with stage D HF refractory to guideline-directed medical therapy and device therapy who are eligible for and awaiting mechanical circulatory support or cardiac transplantation. (*Level of Evidence: B*)

Class IIb

1. Short-term, continuous intravenous inotropic support may be reasonable in those hospitalized patients presenting with documented severe systolic dysfunction who present with low blood pressure and significantly depressed cardiac

output to maintain systemic perfusion and preserve end-organ performance. *(Level of Evidence: B)*

2. Long-term continuous intravenous inotropic support may be considered as palliative therapy for symptom control in selected patients with stage D HF despite optimal guideline-directed medical therapy and device therapy who are not eligible for either mechanical circulatory support or cardiac transplantation. (*Level of Evidence: B*)

Class III: Harm

1. Long-term use of either continuous or intermittent, intravenous parenteral positive inotropic agents, in the absence of specific indications or for reasons other than palliative care, is potentially harmful in the patient with HF. *(Level of Evidence: B)*

2. Use of parenteral inotropic agents in hospitalized patient without documented severe systolic dysfunction, low blood pressure, or impaired perfusion and evidence of significantly depressed cardiac output, with or without congestion, is potentially harmful. *(Level of Evidence: B)*

Administration and Dosing

Although the standard recommended dose range for dobutamine is 2.0–15.0 μg/kg/min, many patients can experience clinical and hemodynamic benefit at a lower initial dose of 0.5–1.0 μg/kg/min, and can achieve such with little to no increase in heart rate or the occurrence of dysrhythmias. Dosing can be increased incrementally by 1.0–2.0 μg/kg/min every 12–15 minutes (or more), until the desired clinical and hemodynamic responses are attained, but short of elevating heart rate more than 10% above baseline, provoking dysrhythmias, or inducing side effects. In the absence of β-adrenergic blockade, the inability to improve hemodynamic and clinical parameters in symptomatic, LV systolic dysfunction and HF during incremental dobutamine infusion dosing up to 15 μg/kg/min seems to be associated with a poor prognosis.[8]

To discontinue dobutamine, maintenance doses of less than 2.0 μg/kg/min can generally be withdrawn without difficulty. Higher infusion rates administered over an extended period usually require gradual weaning over 12–72 hours to avoid hemodynamic and clinical deterioration with rapid discontinuation.[8,27] Prolonged higher infusion rates in patients treated for decompensated, chronic systolic dysfunction, and HF often require a longer weaning period or incremented oral administration of hydralazine to effectively withdraw dobutamine with less difficulty.[27] Although tolerance can develop to a mild-moderate degree during a prolonged administration, it is generally not enough of a factor to facilitate withdrawal of dobutamine.[28]

The pharmacodynamic and pharmacokinetic properties of dobutamine support its role as a short-term, positive inotropic agent. Its half-life in HF patients (averages 2.37 ± 0.07 minutes)[29] indicates that steady-state blood level for any dose is achieved in about 12–13 minutes; an invaluable property if positive inotropic support of ventricular contraction is urgently needed. In human HF, there is a direct relationship between the infusion rate of dobutamine, the plasma levels of dobutamine, and its hemodynamic responses[30] (Fig. 5). Furthermore, the drug is eliminated from circulation within 12–13 minutes upon discontinuation of administration, thus allowing for a rapid reduction of undesirable side effects, if encountered during dobutamine administration.

The addition of a phosphodiesterase inhibitor (e.g., milrinone) augments the inotropic effect of dobutamine by impairing the metabolism of dobutamine-induced elevation of intracellular cAMP.[31] The inotropic-hemodynamic properties of dobutamine are blunted in patients taking β-adrenergic blocking agents, especially the nonselective adrenergic receptor blockers (e.g., carvedilol).[32-34] This effect can be reversed with incremental dosing of dobutamine, which competitively replaces the adrenergic receptor blocker at the receptor site. The β1-selective β-blockers (e.g., metoprolol) do not interfere with the β2-agonism and hemodynamic effects of dobutamine. It is generally not necessary to stop the β-blocker or to substitute a nonadrenergic agent (e.g., milrinone) for dobutamine in most of these patients.

Adverse Effects

The most common undesirable responses to dobutamine are an increase in heart rate and dysrhythmias. From comparative studies and various registries, it is clear that improper patient- or dose-selection will evoke tachycardia, atrial and ventricular dysrhythmias, poor clinical outcomes, and other adverse effects.[35-38] In a number of retrospective studies, the apparent dobutamine-induced undesirable effect on outcomes is largely attributable to improper dosing and/or to its administration in a sicker, more compromised patient population than that served by the comparator.[38-40] Nevertheless, these reports[35-40] emphasize the importance of appropriate selection of patient, drug and dose.

Other adverse effects, also usually dose-related, include anxiety, tremor, palpitations, headache and nausea. A hypertensive response (elevated systemic systolic blood pressure) can be observed when dobutamine is administered to patients with a history of hypertension or peripheral vascular disease, even though they can initially present with hypotension and systemic hypoperfusion. As noted above, patients with high-grade occlusive coronary disease

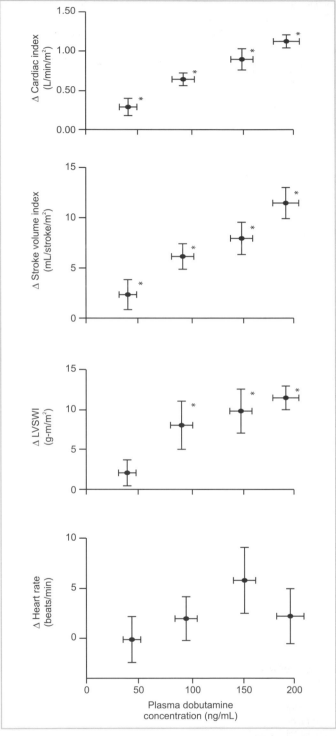

Figure 5 (*continued*)

(continued)

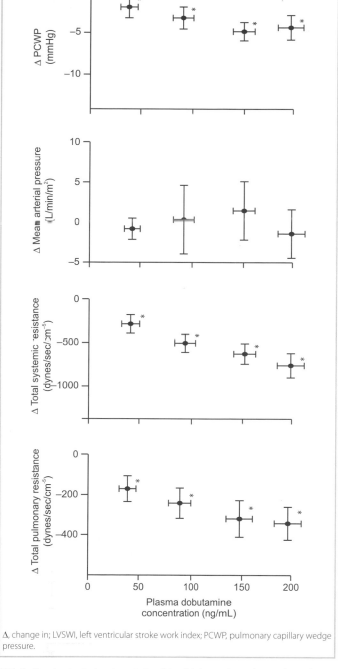

Δ, change in; LVSWI, left ventricular stroke work index; PCWP, pulmonary capillary wedge pressure.

FIG. 5: Graphs depicting the relationship of dobutamine infusion dose, plasma concentration and hemodynamic effects in patients with moderate to severe chronic systolic heart failure. The infusion rates for the four data points of each graph are 2.5, 5.0, 7.5 and 10.0 μg/kg/min, incremented every 20–30 minutes.[30] $\bar{X} \pm$ SED, *p < 0.05.

can develop angina, myocardial ischemia and infarction, particularly those who do not meet the primary indication for use, receive excessive initial dosing or excessively rapid advancement of dose. More prolonged dobutamine infusions can reduce plasma potassium concentrations.[41] Less common adverse effects include a generalized erythema-flushing, eosinophilia and hypersensitivity myocarditis.[42,43] These do not appear to be dose-related, and the reactions are probably related to the bisulfite adjuvant. Dobutamine has been reported to induce stress-cardiomyopathy (also known as Takotsubo cardiomyopathy) in rare patients undergoing pharmacologic stress-testing with this agent.[44]

Dopamine

Dopamine is the endogenous precursor of norepinephrine and epinephrine. Although it is the simplest molecule of the clinically available adrenergic drugs, it has the most complicated pharmacology (Figs 2 and 3, and Table 1).

Pharmacologic Effects

Dopamine evokes most of its effects through activation of the adrenergic receptors (β1, β2 and α), through the neuronal release and reduced neuronal uptake of endogenous norepinephrine, and via stimulation of dopaminergic receptors (D1 and D2).[45-47] In human HF, dopamine at lower infusion rates of less than 4.0 μg/kg/min can act as a mild vasodilator (dopaminergic), particularly of renal and visceral arterial-arteriolar vascular beds. At higher doses, this effect is modulated by dopamine's stimulation of adrenergic receptors directly and through its release of norepinephrine from nerve endings. Although individual responses vary widely, in general, vasodilatation gives way to a net-balanced vascular effect and some positive inotropy at moderate dosing of 4.0–8.0 μg/kg/min and to considerable vasoconstriction with some retained positive inotropy at doses of more than 8.0 μg/kg/min.

Clinical Effects

In states of reduced cardiac output, systemic hypoperfusion, and elevated ventricular filling pressures, dopamine administered at doses of less than 4.0 μg/kg/min can enhance ventricular contraction, stroke volume and cardiac output, and drop systemic and pulmonary vascular resistances—all to a modest degree without much change in systemic blood pressure.[11,48-50] As infusion dosing moves to more than 4.0 μg/kg/min, stroke volume and cardiac output tend to plateau, systemic and pulmonary vascular resistances even out or increase, and a substantial dose-related rise in systemic blood pressure occurs in a dose-related manner. A rise in heart rate and the development of dysrhythmias are also dose-related and often become undesirable effects at more than 6.0 µg/kg/min. LV filling pressure can decrease in some patients but usually does not change or can rise with higher dosing. Indices of positive inotropy or ventricular contractility are reduced at higher doses and during a continuous infusion.[11] This presumably is related to the increase in blood pressure, pulmonary and systemic vascular resistances, ventricular afterload, and via depletion of myocardial norepinephrine stores from dopamine-induced norepinephrine release and reduced reuptake at nerve endings during high dose or prolonged dopamine infusions.

Clinical Indications

The vasoconstricting effects of moderate to high doses of dopamine are employed clinically to increase and stabilize systemic blood pressure in the clinical settings of cardiogenic or vasodilatory (e.g., septic) hypotension and shock.[51-55] This clinical application should predominate over its use as a primary inotrope and, thus, is its principal indication (as a vasopressor).

Interestingly, the post-hoc analysis of a recently performed multicenter trial on shock suggests that dopamine may offer little advantage over norepinephrine and may be less effective in the cardiogenic shock group[55] (See the heading "Norepinephrine").

A multicenter study from Europe found that donor hearts from patients supported with dopamine (4.0 µg/kg/min) before harvest had an improved clinical course as allografts (less hemofiltration and graft failure) compared to the donor hearts not supported with dopamine infusions.[56]

Much of the clinical appeal for dopamine administration in problematic hypotension shock originates from what are thought to be favorable renal effects of dopaminergic stimulation. It has been demonstrated that dopamine, at lower doses of less than 5.0 µ/kg/min, can increase renal blood flow equal to or greater than the proportional increase in cardiac output.[11,57-59] Whether this increase in renal blood flow also evokes an increase in glomerular filtration rate, diuresis and natriuresis in HF, marked hypotension, or shock remains controversial and burdened by conflicting results of published reports.[11,48,57-63]

2013 Guidelines for the Diagnosis and Management of Heart Failure in Adults[26]

Refer to the 2013 guidelines presented under the above heading "Dobutamine".

In addition, under "The hospitalized Patient: Recommendations",

Diuretics in Hospitalized Patients

Class IIb

1. Low-dose dopamine infusion may be considered in addition to loop diuretic therapy to improve diuresis and better preserve renal function and renal blood flow. *(Level of Evidence B)*

Administration and Dosing

Due to considerable variation with respect to individual responses to dopamine, this drug is generally started at 2.0 µg/kg/min and advanced as needed to attain the necessary increase in systemic blood pressure. Doses more than 4.0 µg/kg/min are generally required to achieve and maintain a systemic pressure more than 80 mmHg. Dopamine, like dobutamine, is a rapid-onset and rapid-offset agent, which is ideal for the acute management of critically ill patients in the intensive care unit.

Adverse Effects

The most common adverse effects seen during dopamine administration are comparable to those of dobutamine, namely, a rise in heart rate and dysrhythmias, both dose-related.[11] Dopamine crosses the blood-brain barrier and can evoke nausea and vomiting in conscious, awake patients. Intense vasoconstriction by dopamine can result in ischemia of digits and organ systems. Subcutaneous infiltration at the intravenous site can elicit pain and local ischemic changes, partially reversible with local injections of phentolamine. Dopamine has been noted to depress minute ventilation in patients with HF.[64]

OTHER ADRENERGIC AGENTS

These agents are indicated in a variety of clinical settings. Although often categorized as "positive inotropes," these agents are rarely used as primary positive inotropic drugs because of their predominant vascular effects.

Isoproterenol

This drug is perhaps the most selective β-adrenergic receptor agonist (β1 and β2) available for clinical use. However, its positive inotropic properties are largely overwhelmed by its powerful vasodilatory and positive chronotropic effects (Fig. 2 and Table 1). Its clinical application is somewhat restricted, namely, to serve as a means to increase heart rate in the short-term, until recovery occurs or definitive intervention (e.g., pacemaker) is applied in patients with problematic bradycardia. This is particularly applicable in clinical situations where intravenous atropine is contraindicated, inadequate or ineffective. In view of other, generally safer vasodilating agents (e.g., milrinone and nitrates), isoproterenol is rarely employed as a primary vasodilator. Adverse effects during isoproterenol administration include flushing, anxiety, tremors, hypotension, tachycardia and dysrhythmias.

Epinephrine

This is another endogenous catecholamine, which acts by stimulating β1-, β2- and α1-adrenergic receptors. Epinephrine differs from dobutamine in that its β2 and α1 effects are more intense than those of dobutamine, and its administration is modulated by neuronal uptake. In cardiovascular medicine, epinephrine is most often used during cardiopulmonary resuscitation or employed as a general hemodynamic support drug during withdrawal from cardiopulmonary bypass and during immediate recovery from cardiac surgery. Undesirable effects include most of those described above for dobutamine, dopamine and isoproterenol.

Norepinephrine and Phenylephrine

Again, these agents are often placed under the "positive inotrope" category, but they are predominant α1-adrenergic stimulants with mild β-receptor agonism, and thus, they are also best categorized and viewed as vasopressors (Fig. 2 and Table 1). As such, these compounds are clinically applied for vasoconstriction to augment and stabilize systemic blood pressure in conditions of marked hypotension and shock (vasodilatory and cardiogenic forms).[55,65]

The results of a sizable multicenter trial (1,679 patients), conducted in Europe, on the management of shock-states demonstrated little difference in overall mortality at 28 days (primary endpoint) between norepinephrine and dopamine, when used to secure blood pressure and clinical status.[55] However, dopamine appeared to be more chronotropic and arrhythmogenic for comparable blood pressure responses. In a post-hoc analysis, the 28-day survival-outcome in the cardiogenic subgroup of 280 patients favored norepinephrine as the optimal stabilizing vasopressor[55] (Fig. 6).

Norepinephrine infusions in hypotension and shock generally range 0.02–0.08 µg/kg/min. In addition to the undesirable effects described for dopamine, norepinephrine can, if not carefully monitored, evoke dose-related systemic hypertension and consequent bradycardia.

More intense vasoconstriction with little-to-no positive inotropic effect is delivered by the intravenous administration of phenylephrine.

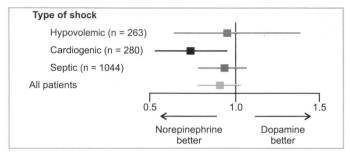

FIG. 6: A forest plot showing the hazard ratio (+95% confidence intervals) of dopamine versus norepinephrine support during shock management of the three major shock subgroups studied. There were no statistical differences between the two interventions for all shock patients combined or for the septic and hypovolemic subgroups. The hazard ratio for the cardiogenic shock subgroup favored norepinephrine over dopamine based on dysrhythmic events during treatment and on mortality at 28 days following the shock episode.[55]

PHOSPHODIESTERASE INHIBITORS

These drugs are often referred to as "inodilators," because vasodilation is a major part of their pharmacology. In fact, amrinone, studied initially in this general group, is predominantly a vasodilator with little enhancement of ventricular contraction beyond its vasodilating-unloading effects on the left ventricle.[66-68] Thrombocytopenia and arrhythmogenesis during prolonged oral administration of amrinone tempered both oral and intravenous application.[67,69] Amrinone has been replaced by milrinone as a therapeutic modality.

Milrinone

Although milrinone can enhance some positive inotropy through other cellular mechanisms (e.g., activation of calcium-release channel on the sarcoplasmic reticulum), its cardiovascular properties are principally caused by inhibition of phosphodiesterase III (PDE III) with subsequent delayed breakdown-metabolism of cAMP[69] (Fig. 1). As a PDE III inhibitor, milrinone may also improve ventricular diastolic function.[70] The vasodilatation of milrinone is mediated through PDE inhibition, causing an increase in cAMP to augment removal of intracellular calcium from vascular smooth muscle.

Pharmacologic and Clinical Effects and Clinical Indications

In contrast to dobutamine, a positive inotropic agent with mild vasodilating properties, milrinone is primarily a vasodilator with mild positive inotropic effects. Therefore, for any matched level of enhanced inotropy-contractility, milrinone elicits a greater decrease in pulmonary and systemic vascular resistances, pulmonary artery pressure, systemic blood pressure and biventricular filling pressures[71-82] (Figs 7 and 8). As a vasodilator, proper dosing of milrinone can augment hemodynamics with little-to-no increase in myocardial energetics-oxygen consumption.[76,77] Its ability to reduce pulmonary vascular

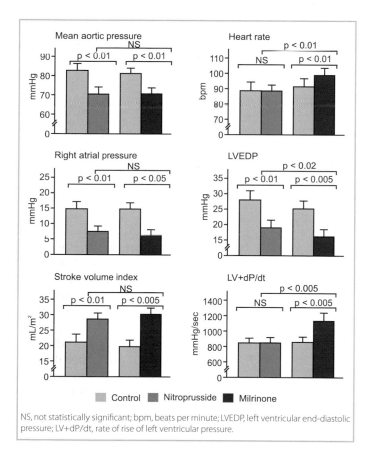

FIG. 7: Molecular structure of milrinone

NS, not statistically significant; bpm, beats per minute; LVEDP, left ventricular end-diastolic pressure; LV+dP/dt, rate of rise of left ventricular pressure.

FIG. 8: A comparison of the hemodynamic effects of milrinone at the maximal dose administered and nitroprusside at the dose selected to match the reduction in mean aortic pressure by milrinone. For comparable ventricular unloading, milrinone elicited positive inotropy (increased +dP/dt = change in LV developed systolic pressure over change in time) and positive chronotropy via a direct milrinone effect and perhaps an increase in reflex sympathetic tone from vasodilatory-hypotension.[72]

resistance, and pulmonary artery pressure makes it a favorable agent for augmentation of central hemodynamics in patients with high pulmonary artery pressures.[74,75]

Bolus milrinone is one of the vasodilating agents used to determine reversibility of elevated pulmonary artery pressures in patients with more severe HF under evaluation for cardiac transplantation.[78,79]

In patients with severe, low-output congestive HF, milrinone enhances the hemodynamic responses to dobutamine and vice versa. It is not unusual to employ the dobutamine-milrinone combination in patients with severely compromised hemodynamics, generally in the setting of end-stage HF, and often as a "pharmacologic bridge" to insertion of a ventricular assist device or cardiac transplantation.

Since milrinone acts distal to the activation of adrenergic receptors (Fig. 1), it can enhance hemodynamics in patients on β-adrenergic antagonists (β-blockers). This is particularly important for patients treated with nonselective β-blockers (e.g., carvedilol), which competitively interfere at the β-receptor site with low-dose dobutamine.[80]

Similar to dobutamine, milrinone may be required as palliative therapy to stabilize the end-stage HF (stage D) patient, who is not a candidate for cardiac transplant or a mechanical support device, and to allow discharge from the hospital, oftentimes to hospice care.[81]

2013 Guidelines for the Diagnosis and Management of Heart Failure in Adults[26]

Since milrinone is also placed under the heading of "positive inotropes," the guidelines for recommended use are generally considered similar to those of dobutamine, even though the drugs are pharmacologically and therapeutically quite different. *Refer to the 2013 guidelines presented under the above heading, "Dobutamine".*

Administration and Dosing

Milrinone is generally started at 0.10–0.30 μg/kg/min and advanced gradually as needed to arrive at the intended hemodynamic and clinical end-points but short of evoking hypotension, tachycardia and dysrhythmias. Milrinone has an elimination half-life of 1–3 hours,[83,84] and, thus, the onset of action, equilibration, and offset are not as prompt as that seen with the catechol-type of inotropes. Although rarely required, an initial intravenous bolus dose of 20–80 μg/kg delivered over 10–15 minutes accelerates the onset of action in conditions where a more rapid response is needed.[85] The relatively long elimination half-life (1–3 hours) results in a delayed recovery from undesirable effects after milrinone is discontinued; not an ideal pharmacokinetic profile for intensive or critical care medicine. Since milrinone is principally eliminated by the kidneys, its use in patients with renal dysfunction requires caution or avoidance. Some pharmacodynamic tolerance can occur during prolonged infusions.

Adverse Effects and Undesirable Responses

While vasodilatation is a favorable effect of milrinone, when administered properly to the appropriate patient, vasodilatation also offers its limitations. This drug is generally not used in patients with systemic systolic blood pressure below 90 mmHg and, therefore, milrinone is not a first-line agent used for low output hypotension or shock. Hypotension from extensive vasodilatation and inhibition of PDE III can elicit positive chronotropy and provoke dysrhythmias.[82] Some patients can experience flushing and generalized warmth at moderate-to-high infusion doses or during bolus administration. Fluid-volume retention is not uncommon during prolonged infusions.[82]

OTHER INTRAVENOUSLY ADMINISTERED POSITIVE INOTROPIC INTERVENTIONS

A number of additional agents are known to enhance positive inotropy and myocardial contractility.

Calcium Sensitizers

Calcium sensitizers (e.g., levosimendan) augment positive inotropy by "modulating" intracardiomyocyte mechanisms of contraction at the same levels of intracellular calcium (Fig. 1).

Levosimendan

Early studies reported that levosimendan's ability to increase myocardial contractility is via sensitization of the contractile apparatus to available intracellular calcium by augmenting and/or securing calcium binding to troponin C and by opening the ATP-sensitive potassium channels of myocardial mitochondria and vascular smooth muscle cells.[86-88] A recent report provided evidence that the positive inotropic effect of levosimendan is mostly rendered by PDE III inhibition.[89] (Fig. 1). The net hemodynamic effect is vasodilatation and some positive inotropy (i.e., inodilator).

Thus, levosimendan also behaves as an "inodilator" in human HF. As such, it lowers vascular resistances and ventricular filling pressures, and by vasodilatory unloading of the left ventricle and perhaps some positive inotropy, levosimendan increases stroke volume and cardiac output.[90-93] Levosimendan predictably causes a greater drop in systemic blood pressure during infusions compared to dobutamine.[92] Levosimendan, as an agent with vasodilating properties, theoretically, should have a favorable effect on myocardial energetics-oxygen balance, although this consideration has not been adequately investigated in human HF. For patients treated with nonselective adrenergic blockers (e.g., carvedilol), levosimendan can elicit its hemodynamic effects with mechanisms located beyond the adrenergic receptors with no need to compete for adrenergic receptor sites.[94] In decompensated HF, levosimendan may elicit a favorable effect on renal function.[95] Because of its vasodilating properties, levosimendan should not be employed as a first-line intervention for low output hypotension or shock.

The results of the Randomized Evaluation of Intravenous Levosimendan Efficacy (REVIVE) Trials I and II[96] in decompensated chronic HF showed that levosimendan (compared to placebo) improved HF symptoms and lowered serum BNP out to 5 days after a 24-hour infusion. However, the levosimendan group experienced more frequent hypotension and cardiac dysrhythmias. A numeric increase (but p = 0.29) in the risk of sudden death was also noted with levosimendan. The Survival of Patients with Acute Heart Failure in Need of Intravenous Inotropic Support (SURVIVE) Trial in decompensated chronic HF revealed that compared to dobutamine, levosimendan therapy did not alter mortality or secondary clinical endpoints at 180 days.[92]

The levosimendan molecule has an elimination half-life of 1–2 hours, but a primary active metabolite (OR-1896) has an elimination half-life of over 75 hours. A sustained hemodynamic effect is seen long after the infusion is discontinued and may be favorable in some instances, but when this is accompanied by hypotension, tachycardia, dysrhythmias, or other undesirable effects, this prolonged and somewhat unpredictable drug clearance is a major limitation, particularly in intensive-critical care medicine.

Levosimendan is approved for clinical use in some countries of Europe, South America and Asia.

Additional Intravenously Administered Positive Inotropes

The first-known, formulated cardiac myosin "activator" for administration in humans, omecamtiv mecarbil may have a role in systolic dysfunction HF. Early studies show that this agent renders a dose-related increase in LV ejection time, stroke volume, fractional shortening and ejection fraction.[97-99] No adverse effects were noted during standard intravenous infusions at effective doses, but myocardial ischemia became apparent during higher doses and higher plasma concentrations. Perhaps the lengthening of LV ejection time could shorten diastolic time and thus, jeopardize coronary perfusion time and coronary blood flow.

Initial studies of istaroxime, an inhibitor of sarcolemmal sodium/potassium adenosine triphosphatase (Na^+/K^+ ATPase) and activator of calcium ATPase of sarcoplasmic reticulum, demonstrated some promise as an agent to augment systolic and diastolic performance of the heart.[100]

Intravenously delivered thyroxine or triiodothyronine can improve hemodynamics as positive inotropes, even in patients with end-stage HF and cardiogenic shock.[101,102] However, the safety of parenteral thyroid therapy in euthyroid decompensated HF patients remains undetermined.

Historically, intravenously administered glucagon, another endogenous substance, has been used to augment myocardial contraction in patients with cardiogenic hypotension or shock refractory to or intolerant of adrenergic stimulation or in those treated with higher doses of β-blocking drugs.

ORALLY ADMINISTERED POSITIVE INOTROPIC AGENTS

While digitalis (now specifically digoxin) has been employed for over 200 years to treat the "dropsy" of HF, this coveted role has been curbed somewhat by the Digitalis Investigation Group (DIG) trial, published in 1997.[103] In general, newer oral inotropes have not fared well in clinical investigations over the past two to three decades as a means of improving myocardial contractility and cardiac performance. Several nondigitalis, orally administered agents have been formulated over the past four decades to replace digoxin in the pharmacotherapeutics of HF. A few examples include amrinone, oral milrinone, enoximone, vesnarinone and butopamine. In general, all were determined to be ineffective to evoke adverse effects or to adversely influence outcomes.

Digitalis-Digoxin

Pharmacologic and Clinical Effects

Much of the augmentation of myocardial contractility by digoxin appears to be generated by inhibiting the Na^+/K^+ ATPase pump of the cardiomyocyte sarcolemma (Fig. 1). This blocking effect results in a rise of intracellular sodium, which elevates (via impairment of the sodium-calcium exchanger) the intracellular calcium available for contraction.[104] Digitalis may also bring calcium into the cardiomyocyte to augment contractility by modulating the voltage-sensitive sodium channels.[104]

The therapeutic effects of digitalis are more complex and much of its clinical benefit probably occurs through noninotropic mechanisms. Digitalis in human HF reduces sympathetic nervous system tone. HF increases sympathetic tone and decreases parasympathetic tone, resulting in several undesirable effects, including increased systemic vascular resistance, tachycardia, increased renin release, and reduced baroreceptor sensitivity. Most of these undesirable responses in HF are suppressed by chronic digitalis administration.[105-112] It is likely that the clinical and hemodynamic benefits noted with chronic digoxin therapy are attributable to a combination of the improvement of autonomic tone and balance, and the direct effect on the cardiomyocyte.

Intravenously delivered digoxin in HF evokes a modest-mild increase in mean stroke volume, cardiac output and systemic blood pressure, with a modest-mild decrease in heart rate and ventricular filling pressures, and minimal change in vascular resistances. Although individual responses can vary widely, greater hemodynamic effects are noted in those who are more hemodynamically compromised.[111-114] The non-predictable variability of clinical and hemodynamic responses, potential undesirable effects (e.g., dysrhythmias) for an agent with a relatively low therapeutic index (the difference between therapeutic effect and toxicity), and a rather long elimination half-life have limited the regular use of intravenous digoxin and its congeners.

Intravenously administered digoxin is, therefore, reserved as an option to slow a fast ventricular rate to rapidly conducting atrial flutter or fibrillation in patients with decompensated HF.

Over the years, the results of mostly noncontrolled or relatively small (few number of patients) studies have suggested that chronic, orally administered digoxin in human HF can favorably alter clinical status, enhance LV ejection fraction, increase exercise performance, and augment hemodynamics at rest and during exercise.[115-121] Again, the clinical responses and hemodynamic effects are quite variable with improvement most noteworthy in HF patients with the most severe decompensation.[116-118,121,122]

Two studies looking at digoxin-withdrawal, both randomized, double-blind, and placebo-controlled, published around the same time (1993), provided reasonable evidence supporting the merits of chronic digoxin therapy in patients with mild-to-moderate HF (FC II–III) and sinus rhythm (it had always been assumed that HF patients in atrial fibrillation generally benefit from long-term digoxin).[123,124] The Prospective Randomized Study of Ventricular Failure and the Efficacy of Digoxin (PROVED) trial[123] was performed in HF patients treated primarily with diuretics and digoxin chronically and the Randomized Assessment of the effect of Digoxin in Inhibitors of the Angiotensin Converting Enzyme (RADIANCE) trial[124] in HF patients chronically treated with ACEIs, diuretics and digoxin. In both studies, compared to those randomized to continued digoxin therapy, the patients randomized to withdrawal of digoxin (to placebo therapy) experienced a fall in LV ejection fraction, impairment of clinical status, diminished functional capacity, and a documented decrease in exercise performance with an increase in heart rate and body weight over the 3-month study period. Again, this deterioration was greatest in patients with more severe HF, but also noteworthy in patients with a milder course.[125,126] It is important to remember that both trials were performed in an era before standard β-adrenergic blocker therapy (i.e., prior to background β-blockers).

Studies investigating either the intravenous or the chronic oral administration of digoxin in patients with LV dysfunction following acute myocardial infarction demonstrated minimal-to-no benefit with a high potential for adverse effects and undesirable outcomes.[127-133]

All prior studies regarding the use of long-term digitalis in patients with HF and sinus rhythm have now been somewhat overshadowed by the DIG trial.[103] This trial has now modified current digoxin use in this clinical setting (systolic HF in sinus rhythm) A total of 6,800 patients with the clinical features of HF LV ejection fraction less than 0.45 and in sinus rhythm were randomized 1:1 to digoxin or placebo. The median daily dose of digoxin for the patients randomized to this therapy was 0.25 mg. The average follow-up was 37 months. About 95% of the overall study population was chronically receiving an ACEI, 82% on a diuretic, 78% taking both agents, and an insignificant number received β-blockers. Patients with HF and relatively preserved ejection fraction (>0.45) were enrolled in a parallel ancillary study.[134]

Long-term digoxin therapy in the DIG trial did not affect total all-cause mortality. Digoxin tended to lower mortality (p = 0.06) attributable to HF, and also statistically lowered the combined end-points of HF mortality or HF hospitalization (largely driven by the reduced rate of hospitalization).[103] This benefit appeared to be greatest in patients with worse clinical status and lower ejection fractions.

The findings for patients with an LV ejection fraction more than 0.45 demonstrated no effect of digoxin on overall mortality and perhaps a minimal to no benefit in combined death or hospitalization reduction from HF.[103,134-136]

The DIG trial has since undergone extensive scrutiny, post-hoc analysis, and re-analysis. The trial has major limitations, including excessively high dosing of digoxin and consequent high serum levels (based on current standards and recommended practices) and performance in the pre-β-blocker era.

Two percent of patients on long-term digoxin were hospitalized for suspected digoxin toxicity compared to 0.9% in the placebo group (p < 0.001). Higher serum levels of digoxin (>1.2 ng/mL) were associated with increased mortality.[137] But importantly, improvement in HF mortality or hospitalization rates were present at lower digoxin concentrations (<1.0 ng/mL).[137-139]

The initial concern for worse outcomes (specifically higher mortality) for women[140] on chronic digoxin was also found to be linked to higher serum digoxin concentrations. Clinical outcomes improved at levels less than 1.0 ng/mL and a progressive increase in mortality and morbidity was noted at digoxin concentrations more than 1.2 ng/mL.[141]

In a select 3,405 elderly patients (age >65 years) of the DIG trial with chronic systolic HF, another post-hoc analysis showed that digoxin decreased 30 day cardiovascular and HF hospitalizations.[142] This favorable effect was not noted in the elderly with HF and preserved ejection fraction (HFpEF).[143]

Again, the DIG trial was performed before β-blocker therapy was used routinely in HF.[103] The results of two retrospective studies on relatively small populations (compared to that of the DIG trial) suggest that chronic digoxin administration in HF patients (in sinus rhythm) may be of little benefit when added on top of currently available, optimal management, including β-adrenergic blockade, ACE inhibition or angiotensin receptor blockade, a diuretic, spironolactone, and biventricular pacing for LV resynchronization.[144,145] But an adequately powered, prospective, controlled trial will have to be performed to address this question.

Clinical Indications and Guidelines

For the overall HF population, chronic digoxin therapy has a Class IIa indication (level of evidence: B) from the 2013 American College of Cardiology Foundation/American Heart Association Task Force, which states that "Digitalis can be beneficial in patients with HFrEF (heart failure with reduced LV ejection fraction) to decrease hospitalizations in HF".[26] Long-term oral digoxin therapy remains an option to control rapid ventricular rate in the HF patient with atrial fibrillation, although this consideration has also been challenged in the β-blocker era.[146]

Administration and Dosing

The initial and maintenance oral dose generally ranges 0.0625–0.25 mg/day. The 0.25 mg/day dose, considered for decades to be the standard daily dose, has largely been replaced by the 0.125 mg/day dose as the daily maintenance dose; because at the lower dose (0.125 mg), serum digoxin

TABLE 2: Agents known to alter serum digoxin concentrations

Reduced levels

- Cholestyramine
- Sucralfate
- Kaolin-pectin
- Antacids
- Salbutamol
- Rifampicin
- Thyroxine

Increased levels

Antiarrhythmics

- Amiodarone/dronedarone
- Propafenone
- Quinidine

Calcium channel blockers

- Verapamil
- Diltiazem
- Dihydropyridines

Potassium-sparing diuretics

- Spironolactone
- Triamterene
- Amiloride

Antimicrobials

- Macrolides
- Tetracycline
- Itraconazole

Others

- Captopril
- Carvedilol
- Cyclosporine
- Indomethacin
- Omeprazole
- St. John's wort

levels (drawn >8 hours after dosing) typically remain less than 1.0 ng/mL in HF patients with normal kidney function. Fifty to eighty percent of orally administered digoxin is absorbed by the gastrointestinal tract with an elimination half-life of 36–48 hours in large part by renal excretion. Drug discontinuation or dose reduction becomes important in patients with renal dysfunction and impaired digoxin clearance or during concomitant administration of medications known, via a number of different mechanisms, to elevate digoxin concentrations (Table 2).

With the exception of blocking atrioventricular (AV) nodal conduction in rapidly conducting atrial fibrillation or flutter, thereby, lowering a rapid ventricular rate in patients for whom other AV nodal blocking agents (e.g., β-adrenergic blockers and calcium-channel blockers) may be problematic (e.g., asthma, hypotension), there is rarely a need for high-dose digoxin administration (historically termed "digitalization").

Adverse Effects

The direct effect of digoxin on sinoatrial and AV nodal cells and its autonomic modulating properties (lowering sympathetic tone and augmenting parasympathetic tone) account for many of the manifestations of digoxin toxicity, including sinus bradycardia and AV nodal blockade, generally at serum levels more than 2.0 ng/mL. Other digoxin-induced or -toxic dysrhythmias include atrial tachycardia with AV nodal block ("paroxysmal atrial tachycardia with block"), other atrial tachydysrhythmias, ventricular ectopic beats, ventricular tachycardia and fibrillation, and accelerated conduction over accessory bypass tracts. Nausea, vomiting, mental disturbances, and visual aberrations are some of the systemic manifestations of digoxin toxicity. Digitalis is a sterol molecule with hormonal effects and, as such, is a common cause of gynecomastia and painful breasts in men receiving this agent chronically. To suppress some of the digoxin-induced dysrhythmias, the intravenous administration of atropine, potassium, and/ or magnesium can be employed, when appropriate, until serum digoxin levels fall to acceptable concentrations and the undesirable effects become less problematic. Severe life-threatening toxicity generally requires the administration of anti-digoxin fragment antigen-binding immunotherapy.[147,148]

OTHER ORALLY ADMINISTERED POSITIVE INOTROPIC AGENTS

In human HF, it has been demonstrated that hydralazine has positive inotropic properties, in addition to its known vasodilating, ventricular-unloading effects.[12,26,149] These positive inotropic and hemodynamic effects of hydralazine can be used to wean dobutamine from HF patients who appear to be clinically and hemodynamically dependent on this intravenous positive inotrope.[27]

Absolute and relative (subclinical) hypothyroidism can play a significant role in the clinical course of human HF and may impact outcomes.[150-157] Thyroid hormone replacement augments myocardial contractility through several mechanisms and is of clinical importance in these specific patient groups. However, its application as oral therapy in HF patients with subclinical hypothyroidism has not been adequately investigated.[157]

REFERENCES

1. Tuttle RR, Mills J. Dobutamine: development of a new catecholamine to selectively increase cardiac contractility. Circ Res. 1975;36(1):185-96.
2. Bristow MR, Ginsburg R, Umans V, et al. Beta 1- and beta 2-adrenergic-receptor subpopulations in nonfailing and failing human ventricular myocardium: coupling of both receptor subtypes to muscle contraction and selective beta 1-receptor downregulation in heart failure. Circ Res. 1986;59(3):297-309.
3. Binkley PF, VanFossen DB, Nunziata E, et al. Influence of positive inotropic therapy on pulsatile hydraulic load and ventricular-vascular coupling in congestive heart failure. J Am Coll Cardiol. 1990;15:1127-35.

4. Binkley PF, Murray KD, Watson KM, et al. Dobutamine increases cardiac output of the total artificial heart. Implications for vascular contribution of inotropic agents to augmented ventricular function. Circulation. 1991;84(3):1210-5.

5. Binkley PF, VanFossen DB, Haas GJ, et al. Increased ventricular contractility is not sufficient for effective positive inotropic intervention. Am J Physiol. 1996;271(4 Pt 2):H1635-42.

6. Ruffalo RR Jr, Spradlin TA, Pollock GD, et al. Alpha and beta adrenergic effects of the stereoisomers of dobutamine. J Pharmacol Exp Ther. 1981;219(2):447-52.

7. Nohria A, Tsang SW, Fang JC, et al. Clinical assessment identifies hemodynamic profiles that predict outcomes in patients admitted with heart failure. J Am Coll Cardiol. 2003;41(10):1797-804.

8. Leier CV, Webel J, Bush CA. The cardiovascular effects of the continuous infusion of dobutamine in patients with severe heart failure. Circulation. 1977;56(3):468-72.

9. Beregovich J, Bianchi C, D'Angelo R, et al. Hemodynamic effects of a new inotropic agent (dobutamine) in chronic heart failure. Br Heart J. 1975;37(6):629-34.

10. Keren G, Lanaido S, Sonnenblick EH, et al. Dynamics of functional mitral regurgitation during dobutamine therapy in patients with severe congestive heart failure: a Doppler echocardiographic study. Am Heart J. 1989;118(4):748-54.

11. Leier CV, Heban PF, Huss P, et al. Comparative systemic and regional hemodynamic effects of dopamine and dobutamine in patients with cardiomyopathic heart failure. Circulation. 1978;58(3 Pt 1):466-75.

12. Magorien RD, Unverferth DV, Brown GP, et al. Dobutamine and hydralazine: comparative influences of positive inotropy and vasodilation on coronary blood flow and myocardial energetics in nonischemic congestive heart failure. J Am Coll Cardiol. 1983;1(2 Pt 1):499-505.

13. Leier CV, Binkley PF. Parenteral inotropic support for advanced congestive heart failure. Prog Cardiovasc Dis. 1998;41(3):207-24.

14. Boudoulas H, Rittgers SE, Lewis RP, et al. Changes in diastolic time with various pharmacologic agents: implication for myocardial perfusion. Circulation. 1979;60(1):164-9.

15. Gillespie TA, Ambos HD, Sobel BE, et al. Effects of dobutamine in patients with acute myocardial infarction. Am J Cardiol. 1977;39(4):588-94.

16. Bendersky R, Chatterjee K, Parmley WW, et al. Dobutamine in chronic ischemic heart failure: alterations in left ventricular function and coronary hemodynamics. Am J Cardiol. 1981;48(3):554-8.

17. Pozen RG, DiBianco R, Katz RJ, et al. Myocardial and hemodynamic effects of dobutamine in heart failure complicating coronary artery disease. Circulation. 1981;63(6):1279-85.

18. Keung EC, Siskind SJ, Sonnenblick EH, et al. Dobutamine therapy in acute myocardial infarction. JAMA. 1981;245(2):144-6.

19. Pacold I, Kleinman B, Gunnar R, et al. Effects of low-dose dobutamine on coronary hemodynamics, myocardial metabolism, and anginal threshold in patients with coronary artery disease. Circulation. 1983;68(5):1044-50.

20. Fowler MB, Alderman EL, Osterle SN, et al. Dobutamine and dopamine after cardiac surgery: greater augmentation of myocardial blood flow with dobutamine. Circulation. 1984;70(3 Pt 2):I103-11.

21. Beanlands RS, Bach DS, Raylman R, et al. Acute effects of dobutamine on myocardial oxygen consumption and cardiac efficiency measured using carbon-11 acetate kinetics in patients with dilated cardiomyopathy. J Am Coll Cardiol. 1993;22(5):1389-98.

22. Krivokapich J, Czernin J, Schelbert HR. Dobutamine positive emission tomography: absolute quantitation at rest and dobutamine myocardial blood flow and correlation with cardiac work and percent diameter stenosis in patients with and without coronary artery disease. J Am Coll Cardiol. 1996;28(3):565-72.

23. Sun KT, Czernin J, Krivokapich J, et al. Effects of dobutamine on myocardial blood flow, glucose metabolism, and wall motion in normal and dysfunctional myocardium. Circulation. 1996;94(12):3146-54.

24. Rahimtoola SH. Hibernating myocardium has reduced blood flow at rest that increases with low-dose dobutamine. Circulation. 1996;94(12):3055-61.

25. Barilla F, DeVincentis G, Mangieri E, et al. Recovery of viable myocardium during inotropic stimulation is not dependent on an increase in myocardial blood flow in the absence of collateral filling. J Am Coll Cardiol. 1999;33(3):697-704.

26. Yancy CW, Jessup M, Bozkurt B, et al. 2013 ACCF/AHA Guideline for the Management of Heart Failure: Executive Summary. Circulation. 2013;128:1810-52.

27. Binkley PF, Starling RC, Hammer DF, et al. Usefulness of hydralazine to withdraw from dobutamine in severe congestive heart failure. Am J Cardiol. 1991;68(10):1103-6.

28. Unverferth DV, Blanford M, Kates RE, et al. Tolerance to dobutamine after a 72 hour continuous infusion. Am J Med. 1980;69(2):262-6.

29. Kates RE, Leier CV. Dobutamine pharmacokinetics in severe heart failure. Clin Pharmacol Therap. 1978;24(5):537-41.

30. Leier CV, Unverferth DV, Kates RE. The relationship between plasma dobutamine concentrations and cardiovascular responses in cardiac failure. Am J Med. 1979;66(2):238-42.

31. Colucci WS, Denniss AR, Leatherman GF, et al. Intracoronary infusion of dobutamine in patients with and without severe congestive heart failure. Dose-response relationships, correlation with circulating catecholamines, and effect of phosphodiesterase inhibition. J Clin Invest. 1988;81(4):1103-10.

32. Metra M, Nodari S, D'Aloia A, et al. Beta-blocker therapy influences the hemodynamic response to inotropic agents in patients with heart failure: a randomized comparison of dobutamine and enoximone before and after chronic treatment with metoprolol or carvedilol. J Am Coll Cardiol. 2002;40(7):1248-58.

33. Bollano E, Tang MS, Hjalmarson A, et al. Different responses to dobutamine in the presence of carvedilol or metoprolol in patients with chronic heart failure. Heart. 2003;89(6):621-4.

34. Waagstein F, Malek I, Hjalmarson AC. The use of dobutamine in myocardial infarction for reversal of the cardiodepressive effect of metoprolol. Br J Clin Pharmac. 1978;5(6):515-21.

35. Silver MA, Horton DP, Ghali JK, et al. Effect of nesiritide versus dobutamine on short-term outcomes in the treatment of acutely decompensated heart failure. J Am Coll Cardiol. 2002;39(5):798-803.

36. Gheorghiade M, Gattis Stough W, Adams K, et al. The pilot randomized study of nesiritide versus dobutamine in heart failure (PRESERVD-HF). Am J Cardiol. 2005;96(6A):18G-25G.

37. Burger AJ, Horton DP, LeJemtel TH, et al. Effect of nesiritide (B-type natriuretic peptide) and dobutamine on ventricular arrhythmias in the treatment of patients with acutely decompensated congestive heart failure: the PRECEDENT study. Am Heart J. 2002;144(6):1102-8.

38. Abraham WT, Adams KF, Fonarow GC, et al. In hospital mortality in patients with acute decompensated heart failure requiring intravenous vasoactive medications: an analysis from the acute decompensated heart failure national registry (ADHERE). J Am Coll Cardiol. 2005;46(1):57-64.

39. O'Connor CM, Gattis WA, Uretsky B, et al. Continuous dobutamine is associated with increased risk of death in patients with advance heart failure: insights from the Flolan International Randomized Trial (FIRST). Am Heart J. 1999;138(1 Pt 1):78-86.

40. Elkayam U, Tasissa G, Binanay C, et al. Use and impact of inotropes and vasodilator therapy in hospitalized patients with severe heart failure. Am Heart J. 2007;153(1):98-104.

41. Goldenberg IF, Olivari MT, Levine TB, et al. Effect of dobutamine on plasma potassium in congestive heart failure secondary to idiopathic or ischemic cardiomyopathy. Am J Cardiol. 1989;63(12):843-6.

42. El-Sayed OM, Abdelfattah RR, Barcelona R, et al. Dobutamine-induced eosinophilia. Am J Cardiol. 2004;93(8):1078-9.

43. Hawkins ET, Levine TB, Goss SJ, et al. Hypersensitivity myocardium in the explanted hearts of transplant recipients. Reappraisal of pathologic criteria and their clinical implications. Pathol Annu. 1995;30(Pt 1):287-304.

44. Abraham J, Mudd JO, Kapur NK, et al. Stress cardiomyopathy after intravenous administration of catecholamines and beta-agonists. J Am Coll Cardiol. 2009;53(15):1320-5.

45. Goldberg LI, Rajfer SI. Dopamine receptors: application in clinical cardiology. Circulation. 1985;72(2):245-8.

46. Brown L, Lorenz B, Erdmann E. The inotropic effects of dopamine and its precursor levodopa in isolated human ventricular myocardium. Klin Wochenschr. 1985;63(21):1117-23.

47. Anderson FL, Port JD, Reid BB, et al. Myocardial catecholamine and neuropeptide Y depletion in failing ventricles of patients with idiopathic dilated cardiomyopathy. Correlation with beta-adrenergic receptor downregulation. Circulation. 1992;85(1):46-53.

48. Beregovich J, Bianchi C, Rubler S, et al. Dose-related hemodynamic and renal effects of dopamine in congestive heart failure. Am Heart J. 1974;87(5):550-7.

49. Maskin CS, Kugler J, Sonnenblick EH, et al. Acute inotropic stimulation with dopamine in severe congestive heart failure: beneficial hemodynamic effect at rest and during maximal exercise. Am J Cardiol. 1983;52(8):1028-32.

50. Rajfer SI, Borow KM, Lang RM, et al. Effects of dopamine on left ventricular afterload and contractile state in heart failure. J Am Coll Cardiol. 1988;12(2):498-506.

51. MacCannell KL, McNay JL, Meyer MD, et al. Dopamine in the treatment of hypotension and shock. N Engl J Med. 1966;275(25):1389-98.

52. Loeb HS, Winslow EB, Rahimtoola SH, et al. Acute hemodynamic effects of dopamine in patients with shock. Circulation. 1971; 44(2):163-73.

53. Holzer J, Karliner JS, O'Rourke RA, et al. Effectiveness of dopamine in patients with cardiogenic shock. Am J Cardiol. 1973;32(1):79-84.

54. Winslow EJ, Loeb HS, Rahimtoola SH, et al. Hemodynamic studies and results of therapy in 50 patients with bacteremic shock. Am J Med. 1973;54(4):421-32.

55. De Backer D, Biston P, Devriendt J, et al. Comparison of dopamine and norepinephrine in the treatment of shock. N Engl J Med. 2010;362(9):779-89.

56. Benck U, Hoeger S, Brinkkoetter PT, et al. Effects of donor pre-treatment with dopamine on survival after heart transplant. J Am Coll Cardiol. 2011;58(17): 1768-77.

57. McDonald RH, Goldberg LI, McNay JL, et al. Dopamine in man: augmentation of sodium excretion, glomerular filtration rate and renal plasma flow. J Clin Invest. 1964;43:1116-24.

58. Elkayam U, Ng TM, Hatamizadeh P, et al. Renal vasodilatory action of dopamine in patients with heart failure. Circulation. 2008;117(2):200-5.

59. Ungar A, Fumagalli S, Marini M, et al. Renal, but not systemic hemodynamic effects of dopamine are influenced by the severity of congestive heart failure. Crit Care Med. 2004;32(5):1125-9.

60. Vargo DL, Brater DC, Rudy DW, et al. Dopamine does not enhance furosemide-induced natriuresis in patients with congestive heart failure. J Am Soc Nephrol. 1996;7(7):1032-7.

61. Varriale P, Mossavi A. The benefit of low-dose dopamine during vigorous diuresis for congestive heart failure associated with renal insufficiency: does it protect renal function? Clin Cardiol. 1997;20(7):627-30.

62. Giamouzis G, Butler J, Starling RC, et al. Impact of dopamine infusion on renal function in hospitalized heart failure patients: results of the Dopamine in Acute Decompensated Heart failure (DAD-HF) Trial. J Cardiac Fail. 2010;16:922-30.

63. Chen HH, Anstrom KJ, Givertz MM, et al. Low-dose dopamine or low-dose nesiritide in acute heart failure with renal dysfunction: the ROSE acute heart failure randomized trial. JAMA. 2013;310:2533-43.

64. van de Borne P, Oren R, Sowers VK. Dopamine depresses minute ventilation in patients with heart failure. Circulation. 1998;98(2):126-31.

65. Dellinger RP, Levy MM, Carlet JM, et al. Surviving sepsis campaign: international guidelines for management of severe sepsis and septic shock: 2008. Intensive Care Med. 2008;34(1):17-60.

66. Benotti JR, Grossman W, Braunwald E, et al. Hemodynamic assessment of amrinone. A new inotropic agent. N Engl J Med. 1978;299(25):1373-7.

67. Hermiller JB, Leithe ME, Magorien RD, et al. Amrinone in severe congestive heart failure: another look at an intriguing new cardioactive drug. J Pharmacol Exp Ther. 1984;228(2):319-26.

68. Wilmshurst PT, Thompson DS, Juul SM, et al. Effects of intracoronary and intravenous amrinone in patients with cardiac failure and patients with near normal cardiac function. Br Heart J. 1985;53(5):493-506.

69. Holmberg SR, Williams AJ. Phosphodiesterase inhibitors and cardiac sarcoplasma reticulum calcium release channel: differential effects of milrinone and enoximone. Cardiovasc Res. 1991;25(7):537-45.

70. Binkley PF, Shaffer PB, Ryan JM, et al. Augmentation of diastolic function with phosphodiesterase inhibition in congestive heart failure. J Lab Clin Med. 1989;114:266-71.

71. Baim DS, McDowell AV, Cherniles J, et al. Evaluation of a new bipyridine inotropic agent—milrinone—in patients with severe congestive heart failure. N Engl J Med. 1983;309(13):748-56.

72. Jaski BE, Fifer MA, Wright RF, et al. Positive inotropic and vasodilator actions of milrinone in patients with severe congestive heart failure. Dose-response relationships and comparison to nitroprusside. J Clin Invest. 1985;75(2):643-9.

73. Monrad ES, McKay RG, Baim DS, et al. Improvement in indices of diastolic performance in patients with severe congestive heart failure treated with milrinone. Circulation. 1984;70(6):1030-7.

74. Eichhorn EJ, Konstam MA, Weiland DS, et al. Differential effects of milrinone and dobutamine in right ventricular preload, afterload, and systolic performance in congestive heart failure secondary to ischemic or idiopathic dilated cardiomyopathy. Am J Cardiol. 1987;60(16):1329-33.

75. Monrad ES, Baim DS, Smith HS, et al. Milrinone, dobutamine, and nitroprusside: comparative effects on hemodynamics and myocardial energetics in patients with severe congestive heart failure. Circulation. 1986;73(3 Pt 2):III168-74.

76. Pfugfelder PW, O'Neill BJ, Ogilive RI, et al. Canadian multicenter study of a 48 hour infusion of milrinone in patients with severe heart failure. Can J Cardiol. 1991;7(1):5-10.

77. Monrad ES, Baim DS, Smith HS, et al. Effects of milrinone on coronary hemodynamics and myocardial energetics in patients with congestive heart failure. Circulation. 1985;71(5):972-9.

78. Givertz MM, Hare JM, Loh E, et al. Effect of bolus milrinone on hemodynamic variables and pulmonary vascular resistance in patients with severe left ventricular dysfunction: a rapid test for reversibility of pulmonary hypertension. J Am Coll Cardiol. 1996;28(7):1775-80.

79. Pamboukian SV, Carere RG, Webb JG, et al. The use of milrinone in pre-transplant assessment of patients with congestive heart failure and pulmonary hypertension. J Heart Lung Transplant. 1999;18(4):367-71.

80. Lowes BD, Tsvetkova T, Eichhorn EJ, et al. Milrinone versus dobutamine in heart failure subjects treated chronically with carvedilol. Int J Cardiol. 2001;81(2-3):141-9.

81. Gorodeski EZ, Chu EC, Reese JR, et al. Prognosis on dobutamine or milrinone for stage D heart failure. Circ Heart Fail. 2009;2:320-4.

82. Simonton CA, Chatterjee K, Cody RJ, et al. Milrinone in congestive heart failure: acute and chronic hemodynamic and clinical evaluation. J Am Coll Cardiol. 1985;6(2):453-9.

83. Benotti JR, Lesko LJ, McCue JE, et al. Pharmacokinetics and pharmaco-dynamics of milrinone in chronic congestive heart failure. Am J Cardiol. 1985;56(10):685-9.

84. Edelson J, Stroshane R, Benziger DP, et al. Pharmacokinetics of the bipyridines amrinone and milrinone. Circulation. 1986;73(3 Pt 2):III145-52.

85. Baruch L, Patacsil P, Hameed A, et al. Pharmacodynamic effects of milrinone with and without a bolus loading infusion. Am Heart J. 2001;141(2):266-73.

86. Endoh M. Cardiac Ca^{2+} signaling and Ca^{2+} sensitizers. Circ J. 2008;72(12): 1915-25.

87. Hasenfuss G, Pieske B, Castell M, et al. Influence of the novel inotropic agent levosimendan on isometric tension and calcium cycling in failing human myocardium. Circulation. 1998;98(20):2141-7.

88. Pathak A, Lebrin ML, Vaccaro A, et al. Pharmacology of levosimendan: inotropic, vasodilatory and cardioprotective effects. J Clin Pharmacy and Therapeutics. 2013;38:341-9.

89. Orstavik O, Ata SH, Riise J, et al. PDE3-inhibition by levosimendan is sufficient to account for its inotropic effect in failing human heart. Br J Pharmacol. 2014; doi: 10.1111 (bph 12647).

90. Slawsky MT, Colucci WS, Gottlieb SS, et al. Acute hemodynamic and clinical effects of levosimendan in patients with severe heart failure. Study Investigators. Circulation. 2000;102(18):2222-7.

91. Givertz MM, Andreon C, Conrad CH, et al. Direct myocardial effects of levosimendan in humans with left ventricular dysfunction: alteration of force-frequency and relaxation-frequency relationships. Circulation. 2007;115(10):1210-24.

92. Mebazaa A, Nieminen MS, Packer M, et al. Levosimendan vs dobutamine for patients with acute decompensated heart failure: the SURVIVE Randomized Trial. JAMA. 2007;297(17):1883-91.

93. Nieminen MS, Akkila J, Hasenfuss G, et al. Hemodynamic and neurohumoral effects of continuous Infusion of levosimendan in patients with congestive heart failure. J Am Coll Cardiol. 2000;36(6):1903-12.

94. Mebazza A, Nieminen MS, Filippatos GS, et al. Levosimendan vs. dobutamine: outcomes for acute heart failure patients on b-blockers in SURVIVE. J Heart Fail. 2009;11(3):304-11.

95. Fedele F, Bruno N, Brasolin B, et al. Levosimendan improves renal function in acute decompensated heart failure: possible underlying mechanisms. Eur J Heart Fail. 2014;16:281-8.

96. Packer M, Colucci W, Fisher L, et al. Effect of Levosimendan on the short-term clinical course of patients with acutely decompensated heart failure. J Am Coll Cardiol HF. 2013;1:103-11.

97. Malik FI, Hartman JJ, Elias KA, et al. Cardiac Myosin activation: a potential therapeutic approach for systolic heart failure. Science. 2011;331:1439-43.

98. Teerlink JR, Clarke CP, Saikaili KG, et al. Dose-dependent augmentation of cardiac systolic function with selective cardiac myosin activator, omecamtiv mecarbil: a first-in-man study. Lancet. 2011;378:667-75.

99. Cleland JGF, Teerlink JR, Senior R, et al. The effects of the cardiac myosin activator, omecamtiv mecarbil, on cardiac function in systolic heart failure: a double-blind, placebo-controlled, crossover, dose-ranging phase 2 trial. Lancet. 2011;378:676-83.

100. Gheorghiade M, Blair JE, Filippatos GS, et al. Hemodynamic, echocardiographic, and neurohormonal effects of istaroxime, a novel intravenous inotropic and lusitropic agent: a randomized controlled trial in patients hospitalized with heart failure. J Am Coll Cardiol. 2008;51(23):2276-85.

101. Malik FS, Mehra MR, Uber PA, et al. Intravenous thyroid hormone supplementation in heart failure with cardiogenic shock. J Card Fail. 1999;5(1):31-7.

102. Hamilton MA, Stevenson LW, Fonarow GC, et al. Safety and hemodynamic effects of intravenous triiodothyronine in advanced heart failure. Am J Cardiol. 1998;81(4):443-7.

103. The effect of digoxin on mortality and morbidity in patients with heart failure. The Digitalis Investigation Group. N Engl J Med. 1997;336(8):525-33.

104. Hauptman PJ, Kelly RA. Digitalis. Circulation. 1999;99(9):1265-70.

105. Ferrari A, Gregorini L, Ferrari MC, et al. Digitalis and baroreceptor reflexes in man. Circulation. 1981;63(2):279-85.

106. Ferguson DW, Berg WJ, Sanders JS, et al. Sympathoinhibitory responses to digitalis glycosides in heart failure patients: direct evidence from sympathetic neural recordings. Circulation. 1989;80(1):65-77.

107. Schobel HP, Oren RM, Roach PJ, et al. Contrasting effects of digitalis and dobutamine in baroreflex sympathetic control in normal humans. Circulation. 1991;84(3):1118-29.

108. Brouwer J, van Veldhuisen DJ, Man in 't Veld AJ, et al. Heart rate variability in patients with mild to moderate heart failure: effects of neurohormonal modulation by digoxin and ibopamine. The Dutch Ibopamine Multicenter Trial (DIMT) Study Group. J Am Coll Cardiol. 1995;26(4):983-90.

109. Newton GE, Tong JH, Schofield AM, et al. Digoxin reduces cardiac sympathetic activity in severe congestive heart failure. J Am Coll Cardiol. 1996;28(1):155-61.

110. Covit AB, Schaer GL, Sealey JE, et al. Suppression of the renin-angiotensin system by intravenous digoxin in chronic congestive heart failure. Am J Med. 1983;75(3):445-7.

111. Ribner HS, Plucinski DA, Hsieh AM, et al. Acute effects of digoxin on total systemic vascular resistance in congestive heart failure due to dilated cardiomyopathy: a hemodynamic-hormonal study. Am J Cardiol. 1985;56(13):896-904.

112. Krum H, Bigger JT Jr, Goldsmith RL, et al. Effect of long-term digoxin therapy on autonomic function in patients with chronic heart failure. J Am Coll Cardiol. 1995;25(2):289-94.

113. Gheorghiade M, St Clair J, St Clair C, et al. Hemodynamic effects of intravenous digoxin in patients with severe heart failure treated with diuretics and vasodilators. J Am Coll Cardiol. 1987;9(4):849-57.

114. Cohn K, Selzer A, Kersh ES, et al. Variability of hemodynamic responses to acute digitalization in chronic heart failure patients due to cardiomyopathy and coronary artery disease. Am J Cardiol. 1975;35:461-8.

115. Arnold SB, Byrd RC, Meister W, et al. Long-term digitalis therapy improves left ventricular function in heart failure. N Engl J Med. 1980;303(25):1443-8.

116. Lee DC, Johnson RA, Bingham JB, et al. Heart failure in outpatients: a randomized trial of digoxin versus placebo. N Engl J Med. 1982;306(12):699-705.

117. Comparative effects of therapy with captopril and digoxin in patients with mild to moderate heart failure. The Captopril-Digoxin Multicenter Research Group. JAMA. 1988;259(4):539-44.

118. Guyatt GH, Sullivan MJ, Fallen EL, et al. A controlled trial of digoxin in heart failure. Am J Med. 1988;61(4):371-5.

119. DiBianco R, Shabetai R, Kostuk W, et al. A comparison of oral milrinone, digoxin, and their combination in the treatment of patients with chronic heart failure. N Engl J Med. 1989;320(11):677-83.

120. Sullivan M, Atwood JE, Myers J, et al. Increased exercise capacity after digoxin administration in patients with heart failure. J Am Coll Cardiol. 1989;13(5):1138-43.

121. Davies RF, Beanlands DS, Nadeau C, et al. Enalapril versus digoxin in patients with congestive heart failure: a multicenter study. Canadian Enalapril Versus Digoxin Study Group. J Am Coll Cardiol. 1991;18(7):1602-9.

122. Ambrosy AP, Butler J, Ahmed A, et al. The Use of Digoxin in Patients with Worsening Heart Failure. J Am Coll Cardiol. 2014;63:1823-32.

123. Uretsky BF, Young JB, Shahidi FE, et al. Randomized study assessing the effect of digoxin withdrawal in patients with mild to moderate chronic congestive heart failure: results of the PROVED trial. PROVED Investigative Group. J Am Coll Cardiol. 1993;22(4):955-62.

124. Packer M, Gheorghiade M, Young JB, et al. Withdrawal of digoxin from patients with chronic heart failure treated with angiotensin-converting-enzyme inhibitors. RADIANCE study. N Engl J Med. 1993;329(1):1-7.

125. Adams KF Jr, Gheorghiade M, Uretsky BF, et al. Clinical predictors of worsening heart failure during withdrawal from digoxin therapy. Am Heart J. 1998;135(3):389-97.

126. Adams KF Jr, Gheorghiade M, Uretsky BF, et al. Patients with mild heart failure worsen during withdrawal from digoxin therapy. J Am Coll Cardiol. 1997;30(1):42-8.

127. Goldstein RA, Passamani ER, Roberts R. A comparison of digoxin and dobutamine in patients with acute infarction and cardiac failure. N Engl J Med. 1980;303(15): 846-50.

128. Hodges M, Friesinger GC, Riggins RC, et al. Effects of intravenously administered digoxin on mild left ventricular failure in acute myocardial infarction in man. Am J Cardiol. 1972;29(6):749-56.

129. Moss AJ, Davies HT, Conard DL, et al. Digitalis-associated cardiac mortality after myocardial infarction. Circulation. 1981;64(6):1150-6.

130. Madsen EB, Gilpin E, Henning H, et al. Prognostic importance of digitalis after acute myocardial infarction. J Am Coll Cardiol. 1984;3(3):681-9.

131. Bigger JT Jr, Fleiss JL, Rolnitzky LM, et al. Effect of digitalis treatment on survival after acute myocardial infarction. Am J Cardiol. 1985;55(6):623-30.

132. Muller JE, Turi ZG, Stone PH, et al. Digoxin therapy and mortality after myocardial infarction. Experience in the MILIS Study. N Engl J Med. 1986;314(5):265-71.

133. Ryan TJ, Bailey KR, McCabe CH, et al. The effects of digitalis on survival in high-risk patients with coronary artery disease: The Coronary Artery Surgery Study (CASS). Circulation. 1983;67(4):735-42.

134. Ahmed A, Rich MW, Fleg JL, et al. Effects of digoxin on morbidity and mortality in diastolic heart failure: the ancillary digitalis investigation group trial. Circulation. 2006;114(5):397-403.

135. Meyer P, White M, Mujib M, et al. Digoxin and reduction of heart failure hospitalization in chronic systolic and diastolic heart failure. Am J Cardiol. 2008;102(12):1681-6.

136. Gheorghiade M, Patel K, Filippatos G, et al. Fffect of oral digoxin in high-risk heart failure patients: a pre specified subgroup analysis of the DIG trial. Eur J Heart Fail. 2013;15(5): 551-9.

137. Rathore SS, Curtis JP, Wang Y, et al. Association of serum digoxin concentration and outcomes in patients with heart failure. JAMA. 2003;289(7):871-8.

138. Ahmed A, Pitt B, Rahimtoola SH, et al. Effects of low serum concentrations on mortality and hospitalization in heart failure: a propensity matched study of the DIG Trial. Int J Cardiol. 2008;123(2)138-46.

139. Digitalis Investigation Group, Ahmed A, Waagstein F, et al. Effectiveness of digoxin in reducing one-year mortality in chronic heart failure in the Digitalis Investigation Group Trial. Am J Cardiol. 2009;103(1):82-7.

140. Rathore SS, Wang Y, Krumholz HM. Sex-based differences in the effect of digoxin for treatment of heart failure. N Engl J Med. 2002;347(18):1403-11.

141. Adams KF Jr, Patterson JH, Gattis WA, et al. Relationship of serum digoxin concentration to mortality and morbidity in women in the digitalis investigation group trial: a retrospective analysis. J Am Coll Cardiol. 2005;46(3):497-504.

142. Bourge RC, Fleg JL, Fonarow GC, et al. Digoxin reduces 30-day all-cause hospital admission in older patients with chronic systolic failure. Am J Med. 2013;126:701-8.

143. Hashim T, Elbaz S, Patel K, et al. Digoxin and 30-day all-cause hospital admission in older patients with chronic diastolic heart failure. Am J Med. 2014;127:132-9.

144. Dhaliwal AS, Bredikis A, Habib G, et al. Digoxin and clinical outcomes in systolic heart failure patients on contemporary background heart failure therapy. Am J Cardiol. 2008;102(10):1356-60.

145. Georgiopoulou VV, Kalogeropoulus AP, Giamouzis G, et al. Digoxin therapy does not improve outcomes in patients with advanced heart failure on contemporary medical therapy. Circ Heart Fail. 2009;2(2):90-7.

146. Fauchier L, Grimard C, Pierre B, et al. Comparison of beta blocker and digoxin alone and in combination for management of patients with atrial fibrillation and heart failure. Am J Cardiol. 2009;103(2):248-54.

147. Smith TW, Haber E, Yeatman L, et al. Reversal of advanced digoxin intoxication with Fab fragments on digoxin-specific antibodies. N Engl J Med. 1976;294(15): 797-800.

148. Antman EM, Wenger TL, Butter VP, et al. Treatment of 150 cases of life-threatening digitalis intoxication with digoxin-specific Fab antibody fragments. Final report of a multicenter study. Circulation. 1990;81(6):1744-52.

149. Leier CV, Desch CE, Magorien RD, et al. Positive inotropic effects of hydralazine in human subjects: comparison with prazosin in the setting of congestive heart failure. Am J Cardiol. 1980;46(6):1039-44.

150. Ievasi G, Pingitore A, Landi P, et al. Low-T3 syndrome: a strong prognostic predictor of death in patients with heart disease. Circulation. 2003;107(5):708-13.

151. Ascheim DD, Hryniewicz K. Thyroid hormone metabolism in patients with congestive heart failure: the low triiodothyronine state. Thyroid. 2002;12(6):511-5.

152. Pingitore A, Galli E, Barison A, et al. Acute effects of triiodothyronine (T3) replacement therapy in patients with chronic heart failure and low-T3 syndrome: a randomized, placebo-controlled study. J Clin Endocrinol Metab. 2008;93(4):1351-8.

153. Iacoviello M, Guida P, Guastamacchia E, et al. Prognostic role of sub-clinical hypothyroidism in chronic heart failure outpatients. Curr Pharm Des. 2008;14(26): 2686-92.

154. Kahaly GJ, Dillmann WH. Thyroid hormone action in the heart. Endocr Rev. 2005;26(5):704-28.

155. Klein I, Danzi S. Thyroid hormone treatment to mend a broken heart. J Clin Endocrinol Metab. 2008;93(4):1172-4.

156. Grasiosi C, Peressotti B, Machado RA, et al. Improvement in functional capacity after levothyroxine treatment in patients with chronic heart failure and subclinical hypothyroidism. Endocrinol Nutr. 2013;60:427-32.

157. Mitchell JE, Hellkamp AS, Mark DB, et al. Thyroid function in heart failure and impact on mortality. J Am Coll Cardiol HF. 2013;1:48-55.

Antihypertensive Drugs

William J Lawton, Kanu Chatterjee

PHYSIOLOGY AND PATHOPHYSIOLOGY OF BLOOD PRESSURE REGULATION

Blood pressure, specifically systemic arterial pressure is the pressure of blood exerted against the walls of the arteries within the vessel. This pressure is generated by left ventricular systolic contraction, which produces forward blood flow against the resistance of the arterioles and arteries. The maximum blood pressure (systolic) occurs during systolic contraction of the left ventricle, and lowest blood pressure (diastolic) occurs during relaxation of the left ventricle. Normal blood pressure is determined by the cardiac output (CO) and the total peripheral resistance (TPR), (Blood pressure = CO × TPR). Normal blood pressure depends on the heart, blood vessels, extracellular fluid volume, the central and peripheral nervous system, kidneys, and circulating humoral factors.

Cardiac output is a complex function dependent on heart rate and stroke volume (L/min). Stroke volume depends on intravascular volume, which in turn is regulated by the kidneys as well as myocardial contraction. Stroke volume also depends on preload, afterload, and contractility. Decreased preload decreases stroke volume and lowers blood pressure. Decreased afterload and increased contractility increase stroke volume and blood pressure. Myocardial contraction is a complex process and depends on the intrinsic cardiac conduction system, membrane transport, and cellular events, including influx of calcium, effects of humoral substances, such as catecholamines and thyroxine, and sympathetic and parasympathetic regulation of heart rate.

The TPR is a complex integrated function, which depends on a number of factors, including neurohumoral substances, baroreflexes and the sympathetic nervous system, endothelial factors, electrolytes (sodium, potassium, calcium, magnesium, etc.), volume, and intracellular events mediated by receptors and signal transduction. Two major nervous system reflex arcs are recognized: (i) Low-pressure cardiopulmonary baroreceptors are present in cardiac ventricles and atria and (ii) high-pressure baroreceptors in the carotid sinus and aortic arch. These baroreceptors react to filling pressures (low pressure receptors) and to stretch (high pressure receptors). For example, if systemic blood pressure increases, high pressure baroreceptors increase tonic inhibition of sympathetic outflow (efferent pathways), resulting in a decrease in vascular resistance and heart rate. On the other hand, a decrease in blood pressure leads to less tonic inhibition of sympathetic outflow, which in turn, increases heart rate, peripheral vascular resistance, and systemic blood pressure increases.

Elevated blood pressure or hypertension can occur when CO or TPR are elevated. CO may be elevated in young people or in certain medical conditions, such as hyperthyroidism. In most cases, hypertension is due to increased TPR, which in turn is caused by dysregulation of one or a number of other factors discussed above. Hypertension is classified as either primary (essential), or secondary. In primary (essential) hypertension, a uniform mechanism cannot be found. Primary hypertension likely involves the interaction of genetic factors, environment, known regulatory systems (hormonal, neural, renal, vascular, and cardiac), and possibly factors yet undiscovered. In secondary hypertension, a cause can be identified and often the mechanism too can be traced. Some causes for secondary hypertension include chronic kidney disease (CKD) (volume expansion, increased activity of the renin-angiotensin-aldosterone system (RAAS), and overactive sympathetic nervous system), renal artery stenosis (increased activity of RAAS), endocrine disorders [hyperaldosteronism from adrenal adenomas or hyperplasia, pheochromoctyoma (increased catecholamines)], Cushing's syndrome (excess cortisol), hyperthyroidism, hypothyroidism, hyperparathyroidism (hypercalcemia), acromegaly (increased growth hormone), coarctation of aorta, drug-induced sleep apnea (sympathetic activation), obesity (sympathetic overactivity, possibly adipokines and others), and pregnancy (placental stimulus). About 90–95% of cases of hypertension are of primary (essential) hypertension and 5–10% are of secondary hypertension.

In this chapter, evidence-based drug therapy of essential hypertension is discussed.

DEFINITIONS AND CLASSIFICATIONS OF HYPERTENSION

For appropriate treatment of hypertension, adequate classification and definitions are necessary.

Report from the Panel Members Appointed to the Eighth Joint National Committee[1]

The 8th Joint National Committee (JNC) report was published in 2014. Definitions for hypertension are not addressed, but thresholds for pharmacologic treatment are defined. The definitions from JNC 7 continue to be accepted.

The 7th Report of the Joint National Committee on Prevention, Detection, Evaluation, and Treatment of High Blood Pressure[2]

The 7th report of the Joint National Committee on prevention, detection, evaluation, and treatment of high blood pressure (the JNC 7 report) was published in 2003 (Table 1). Major differences from JNC 6 (1997) included a new category of prehypertension and elimination of stage 3 hypertension as a separate category (Table 2).

The European Society of Hypertension and the European Society of Cardiology Guidelines for the Management of Arterial Hypertension (2013)[3]

The categories for defining office hypertension by the European Society of Hypertension (ESH) and by the European Society of Cardiology (ESC) 2013 are unchanged from 2003 and 2007, and are summarized in Tables 3 and 4.

There is ample evidence to suggest that adequate treatment of hypertension is associated with a substantial reduction in the risks of adverse cardiovascular events. The risks of stroke,

TABLE 1: Blood pressure classification (JNC 7)

Category	Blood pressure (mmHg)
Normal	<120 and <80
Prehypertension	120–139 or 80–89
Stage 1 hypertension	140–159 or 90–99
Stage 2 hypertension	≥160 or ≥100

TABLE 2: Blood pressure classification: comparison between JNC 6 and 7

SBP/DBP (mmHg)	JNC 7 category	JNC 6 category
<120/80	Normal	Optimal
120–129/80–84	Prehypertension	Normal
130–139/85–89	Prehypertension	Borderline
≥140/90	Hypertension	Hypertension
• 140–159/90–99	• Stage 1	• Stage 1
• 160–179/100–109	• Stage 2	• Stage 2
• ≥180/110	• Stage 2	• Stage 3

SBP, systolic blood pressure; DBP, diastolic blood pressure.

TABLE 3: Definitions and classification of blood pressure levels (mmHg): European Society of Hypertension (2013)

Category	Systolic blood pressure (mmHg)		Diastolic blood pressure (mmHg)
Optimal	<120	and	<80
Normal	120–129	and/or	80–84
High normal	130–139	and/or	85–89
Grade 1 hypertension	140–159	and/or	90–99
Grade 2 hypertension	160–179	and/or	100–109
Grade 3 hypertension	≥180	and/or	≥110
Isolated systolic hypertension	≥140	and	<90

TABLE 4: Blood pressure thresholds for defining hypertension with different types of measurements (ESH/ESC)

	Systolic blood pressure (mmHg)	Diastolic blood pressure (mmHg)
Office or clinic	140	90
24-hour (ambulatory)	125–130	80
Day	130–135	85
Night	120	70
Home	130–135	85

TABLE 5: Benefits of treating hypertension (JNC 7)

Cardiovascular events	Average reduction (%)
Stroke incidence	35–40
Myocardial infarction	20–25
Heart failure	50

myocardial infarction (MI), and heart failure decline with adequate treatment of hypertension as illustrated in Table 5. Also, treatment of hypertension in patients with chronic kidney disease (CKD) slows the progression of the CKD, especially when angiotensin I converting enzyme (ACE) inhibitors or angiotensin receptor blockers (ARBs) are used.[4-6]

RECOMMENDATIONS FOR TREATMENT OF HYPERTENSION

Several recommendations and guidelines for the diagnosis and management of hypertension are available. It should be noted, however, that no uniform approach for recognition and management of hypertension is available. In the following sections, the current approaches for selecting antihypertensive drugs are outlined.

Current Approach for Selecting Antihypertensive Medication

There is no "single approach". Hypertension experts in the United States, Europe, and other areas of the world offer recommendations based on clinical trials, pharmacology of the various drugs and personal experience. The clinical trials, however, do not show uniformly consistent results, and experts in hypertension do not have a uniform approach.

However, there is a general agreement that lifestyle modifications should be encouraged for every patient. There are also general principles that are recommended for management of hypertension (Table 6). Each patient needs to have a comprehensive evaluation for lifestyle modifications and the principles listed in Table 6. An algorithm representing treatment of hypertension is outlined in Figure 1.

TABLE 6: Principles for hypertension treatment

Evaluate for medical issues before considering the choice of anti-hypertensive drug therapy:

- Cardiovascular risks and disease
- Cerebrovascular risks and disease
- Glucose metabolism/diabetes mellitus
- Lipid profile
- Liver functions
- Renal functions
- Peripheral vascular disease
- Psychological factors and cognitive functions: Evaluation for compliance
- Weight
- Other diseases and medical concerns.

Other factors to evaluate:

- Lifestyle (diet, especially sodium and caloric intake, occupation, recreation and exercise, use of other medications, cigarette smoking, alcohol, use of illicit drugs and sexual practices)
- Socioeconomic factors (including ability to pay for medication, religious beliefs, family support, etc.)
- Race and ethnicity
- Age
- Gender

Start with a small dose of an antihypertensive drug: Once a day dosage preferred

Increase dose until goal blood pressure is achieved: To minimize side effects, an option is to not increase the single drug to maximum dose, but add another drug from a different class

May need to add multiple drugs with different modes of action to achieve goal blood pressure. When possible, use combination therapy to improve compliance

If two or more drugs are required to reach target blood pressure, reassess for secondary hypertension.

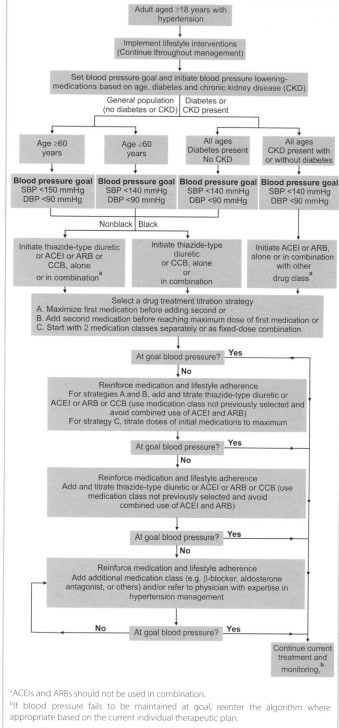

FIG. 1: 2014 hypertension guideline management algorithm (JNC-8).

At present, lifestyle management includes treatment of obesity/overweight, restriction of excessive salt intake, smoking cessation, and limitations on alcohol use. Regular exercise of moderate intensity is encouraged. Drugs which can increase blood pressure, such as steroidal and nonsteroidal anti-inflammatory agents should be avoided. Drugs containing catecholamines, such as some nasal decongestants should be discouraged. Recreational drugs like methamphetamine and cocaine can increase blood pressure, and should be avoided. Electrolyte imbalances, such as hypokalemia, need to be corrected.

Obesity is a risk factor not only for hypertension but also for diabetes, coronary artery disease (CAD) and heart failure. Reduction in body weight can be associated with a significant reduction in blood pressure.

Regular isotonic exercise, such as brisk walking is associated with decreased sympathetic tone and lower blood pressure. Isometric exercise, such as weight lifting, increases systemic resistance and blood pressure. Thus, isometric exercise should be avoided.

Excessive alcohol raises blood pressure through a number of mechanisms including activation of the sympathetic nervous system and release of corticotropin releasing hormone.[7] The benefits of lifestyle modifications are summarized in Table 7.

There are certain compelling indications for control of hypertension. There are different classes of antihypertensive drugs, and all are not suitable for all the special clinical circumstances.

TABLE 7: Lifestyle modifications (JNC 7)

- Optimize body weight, body mass index: 18.5–24.9 kg/m^2 (most effective, approximately 5–20 mmHg reduction in BP for every 10 kg weight loss)

- Reduce sodium intake: Not more than 100 mEq/day (2.4 g sodium or 6 g sodium chloride) (approximately 2–8 mmHg reduction in BP)

- Moderate alcohol intake: Limit to 2 drinks/day for men and 1 drink/day for women (approximately 2–4 mmHg reduction in BP)

- Manage stress: Counseling if needed

- Stop smoking: To reduce cardiovascular risk

- Graduated exercise program: Aerobic activity (e.g., brisk walking) at least 30 min/day, most days of the week (approximately 4–9 mmHg reduction in BP)

- Additional dietary management: Dietary Approaches to Stop Hypertension (DASH) diet: Advise diet rich in vegetables, fruits (ample potassium intake), low-fat dairy products, reduced total fat, saturated fat and no trans-fat (approximately 8–14 mmHg reduction in BP)

TABLE 8: Compelling indications for individual drug classes (JNC 7)

Indications	Drug classes
Heart failure	Thiazides, β-blockers, ACEIs, ARBs, ALDO antagonists
Post-MI	β-blockers, ACEIs, ALDO antagonists
High cardiovascular risk	Thiazides, β-blockers, ACEIs, CCBs
Diabetes mellitus	Thiazides, β-blockers, ACEIs, ARBs, CCBs
CKD	ACEIs, ARBs
Recurrent stroke prevention	Thiazides, ACEIs

ACEIs, angiotensin-converting enzyme inhibitors; ARBs, angiotensin II receptor blockers; CCBs, calcium channel blockers; ALDO, aldosterone; MI, myocardial infarction; CKD, chronic kidney disease.

In patients with systolic heart failure (SHF), β-blockers, angiotensin inhibitors and aldosterone antagonists are appropriate. In SHF, calcium channel blockers (CCBs) should be avoided. In patients with high-risk cardiovascular complications, β-blockers, angiotensin inhibitors, and CCBs should be considered. In patients with recent MI, β-blockers, angiotensin inhibitors, and aldosterone antagonists are preferable. In diabetics, all classes of antihypertensive drugs can be used. For renal protection in patients with CKD, drugs which inhibit the renin-angiotensin system are preferable. For prevention of recurrent strokes, thiazide diuretics and angiotensin-converting enzyme inhibitors (ACEIs) are recommended. The appropriate antihypertensive drugs for special clinical circumstances are summarized in Table 8.

The rationale for lowering of blood pressure is to reduce the risks of adverse cardiovascular and renal complications. Blood pressure should be reduced to at least 140/90 mmHg. New Guidelines from JNC-8 differ from JNC-7 and ESH/ESC Guidelines in 2013.[1] The major changes in JNC-8 compared to JNC-7 include recommendations for patients with diabetes mellitus and chronic kidney disease (CKD) to set the blood pressure goal at less than 140/90 mmHg. In addition, JNC-8 recommends for patients aged 60 years or above to set the blood pressure goal at less than 150/90 mmHg. For patients less than 60 years of age, the blood pressure goal is less than 140/90 mmHg.

Table 9 compares the Guidelines from JNC-8 (2014) with ESH/ESC (2013). Major differences:

1. For the elderly, defined as those older than 60 years old, JNC-8 recommends a goal BP of less than 150/90 mmHg. ESH/ESC recommends a goal BP of less than 150/90 mmHg in the elderly older aged 80 years or above and also in the "general elderly" less than 80 years old. However, the lower age limit for defining elderly is not specified (Table 10).

TABLE 9: Comparison of current recommendations from JNC 8 with JNC 7 guidelines

Topic	JNC 7	2014 Hypertension guideline
Methodology	<ul><li>Nonsystematic literature review by expert committee including a range of study designs</li><li>Recommendations based on consensus</li></ul>	<ul><li>Critical questions and review criteria defined by expert panel with input from methodology team</li><li>Initial systematic review by methodologists restricted to RCT evidence</li><li>Subsequent review of RCT evidence and recommendations by the panel according to a standardized protocol</li></ul>
Definitions	<ul><li>Defined hypertension and prehypertension</li></ul>	<ul><li>Definitions of hypertension and prehypertension not addressed, but thresholds for pharmacologic treatment were defined</li></ul>
Treatment goals	<ul><li>Separate treatment goals defined for "uncomplicated" hypertension and for subsets with various comorbid conditions (diabetes and CKD)</li></ul>	<ul><li>Similar treatment goals defined for all hypertensive populations except when evidence review supports different goals for a particular subpopulation</li></ul>
Lifestyle recommendations	<ul><li>Recommended lifestyle modifications based on literature review and expert opinion</li></ul>	<ul><li>Lifestyle modifications recommended by endorsing the evidence based recommendations of the Lifestyle Work Group</li></ul>
Drug therapy	<ul><li>Recommended 5 classes to be considered as initial therapy but recommended thiazide-type diuretics as initial therapy for most patients without compelling indication for another class</li><li>Specified particular antihypertensive medication classes for patients with compelling indications, i.e., diabetes, CKD, heart failure, myocardial infarction, stroke, and high CVD risk</li><li>Included a comprehensive table of oral antihypertensive drugs including names and usual dose ranges</li></ul>	<ul><li>Recommended selection among 4 specific medication classes (ACEI or ARB, CCB or diuretics) and doses based on RCT evidence</li><li>Recommended specific medication classes based on evidence review for racial, CKD, and diabetic subgroups</li><li>Panel created a table of drugs and doses used in the outcome trials</li></ul>

(continued)

Table 9 (continued)

Topic	JNC 7	2014 Hypertension guideline
Scope of topics	▪ Addressed multiple issues (blood pressure measurement methods, patient evaluation components, secondary hypertension, adherence to regimens, resistant hypertension, and hypertension in special populations) based on literature review and expert opinion	▪ Evidence review of RCTs addressed a limited number of questions, those judged by the panel to be of highest priority
Review process prior to publication	▪ Reviewed by the National High Blood Pressure Education Program Coordinating Committee, a coalition of 39 major professional, public, and voluntary organizations and 7 federal agencies	▪ Reviewed by experts including those affiliated with professional and public organizations and federal agencies; no official sponsorship by any organization should be inferred

ACEI, angiotensin-converting enzyme inhibitor; ARB, angiotensin receptor blocker; CCB, calcium channel blocker; CKD, chronic kidney disease; CVD, cardiovascular disease; JNC, Joint National Committee; RCT, randomized controlled trial

TABLE 10: Guideline comparisons of goal BP and initial drug therapy for adults with hypertension

Guideline	Population	Goal BP (mmHg)	Initial drug treatment options
2014 Hypertension guideline	General ≥60 years	<150/90	Nonblack: thiazide-type diuretic, ACEI, ARB, or CCB; black: thiazide-type diuretic or CCB
	General <60 years	<140/90	
	Diabetes	<140/90	
	CKD	<140/90	ACEI or ARB
ESH/ESC 2013	General nonelderly	<140/90	Diuretic, β-blocker, CCB, ACEI, or ARB
	General elderly <80 years	<150/90	
	General ≥80 years	<150/90	
	Diabetes	<140/85	ACEI or ARB
	CKD + no proteinuria	<140/90	ACEI or ARB
	CKD + proteinuria	<130/90	

ACEI, angiotensin-converting enzyme inhibitor; ARB, angiotensin receptor blocker; CCB, calcium channel blocker; CKD, chronic kidney disease; ESH, European Society of Hypertension; ESC, European Society of Cardiology.

2. For patients with CKD, JNC-8 recommends a goal BP of less than 140/90 mmHg for all CKD patients whereas the ESH/ESC advises a goal BP of less than 130/90 mmHg for CKD patients with proteinuria. The ESH/ESC recommendation in patients with CKD and proteinuria (24-hour urine protein generally 1,000 mg/day or higher) is supported by the MDRD Data,[8] and other studies.[9,10] A goal BP of less than 130/90 mmHg is now recommended for patients with CKD and proteinuria.

3. ESH/ESC, in contrast to JNC-8, includes β-blockers in the list of initial drug treatment options. This has been discussed further in section "Choice of Therapy in Essential Hypertension".

There are numerous other guidelines for hypertension management now published and in preparation. Some are listed in the Tables 10 and 11 from JNC-8. In general, the other guidelines are similar to either JNC-8 or ESH/ESC.

All hypertensive patients are not at the same risk to develop cardiovascular complications. Patients with blood pressure of 180/110 mmHg or higher or systolic blood pressure more than 160 mmHg with low diastolic pressure (<70 mmHg) are at higher risks of developing complications. Patients with metabolic syndrome, dyslipidemia and smokers are also high risks. Presence of overt or subclinical target organ damage, such as left ventricular hypertrophy (LVH), abnormal carotid artery wall thickening, and low estimated glomerular filtration

TABLE 11: Guideline comparisons of goal BP and initial drug therapy for adults with hypertension

Guideline	Population	Goal BP (mmHg)	Initial drug treatment options
CHEP 2013	General <80 years	<140/90	Thiazide, β-blocker (age <60 years), ACEI (nonblack), or ARB
	General ≥80 years	<150/90	
	Diabetes	<130/80	ACEI or ARB with additional CVD risk ACEI, ARB, thiazide, or DHPCCB without additional CVD risk
	CKD	<140/90	ACEI or ARB
ADA 2013	Diabetes	<140/80	ACEI or ARB
KDIGO 2012	CKD no proteinuria	≤140/90	ACEI or ARB
	CKD + proteinuria	≤130/80	
NICE 2011	General <80 years	<140/90	<55 years: ACEI or ARB
	General ≥80 years	<150/90	≥55 years or black: CCB
ISHIB 2010	Black, lower risk	<135/85	Diuretic or CCB
	Target organ damage or CVD risk	<130/80	

ADA, American Diabetes Association; ACEI, angiotensin-converting enzyme inhibitor; ARB, angiotensin receptor blocker; CCB, calcium channel blocker; CHEP, Canadian Hypertension Education Program; CKD, chronic kidney disease; CVD, cardiovascular disease; DHPCCB, dihydropyridine calcium channel blocker; ESC, European Society of Cardiology; ESH, European Society of Hypertension; ISHIB, International Society for Hypertension in Blacks; JNC, Joint National Committee; KDIGO, Kidney Disease: Improving Global Outcome; NICE, National Institute for Health and Clinical Excellence.

rate and creatinine clearance, and established cardiovascular or renal disease constitute high risks for developing cardiovascular complications. The definition of high- and very high-risk subjects are summarized in Table 12.

CHOICE OF MEDICATION FOR ESSENTIAL HYPERTENSION

There are multiple classes of antihypertensive drugs available for treatment of hypertension. For initiation of treatment, frequently one class of drugs is used. These drugs are known as first-line agents. Guidelines recommend thiazide diuretics as the initial agent. Other classes of drugs can also be used as first-line agents (Table 13). Frequently the use of the combination of several classes of antihypertensive drugs is required to obtain adequate control of hypertension. The recommendations for monotherapy versus multiple drugs combinations are outlined in Table 14.

TABLE 12: Definition of high- and very high-risk subjects

SBP ≥180 mmHg and/or DBP ≥110 mmHg
SBP >160 mmHg with DBP <70 mmHg
Diabetes mellitus

Metabolic syndrome: According to AHA and NHLBI, metabolic syndrome is present if three or more of the following signs are present:

- Blood pressure ≥130/85 mmHg
- Fasting blood glucose ≥100 mg/dL (5.6 mmol/L)
- Large waist circumference: Men ≥40 inches (102 cm), women ≥35 inches (88 cm)
- Low HDL: Men <40 mg/dL, Women <50 mg/dL
- Triglycerides ≥150 mg/dL

More than three cardiovascular risk factors: Cigarette smoking, high blood pressure, serum total cholesterol >190 mg/dL (5.0 mmol/L) and LDL >115 mg/dL (3.0 mmol/L), low HDL, advancing age (men >55 years and women >65 years), obesity, diabetes mellitus, and family history of premature heart disease

One or more of the following subclinical organ damages:

- Electrocardiographic LVH (Sokolow-Lyon >38 mm; Cornell >2,440 mm*ms) or
- Echocardiographic LVH* (LVMI: Men ≥125 g/m^2, women ≥110 g/m^2)
- Carotid wall thickening (IMT >0.9 mm) or plaque
- Carotid-femoral pulse wave velocity >12 m/s
- Ankle/brachial blood pressure index <0.9
- Slight increase in plasma creatinine: Men 115–133 μmol/L (1.3–1.5 mg/dL), Women: 107–124 μmol/L (1.2–1.4 mg/dL)
- Low estimated glomerular filtration rate** (<60 mL/min/1.73 m^2) or creatinine clearance*** (<60 mL/min)

Established cardiovascular or renal disease:

- Cerebrovascular disease: Ischemic stroke cerebral hemorrhage, transient ischemic attack
- Heart disease: MI, angina, coronary revascularization, heart failure
- Renal disease: Diabetic nephropathy, renal impairment [serum creatinine: men >133 μmol/L (1.5 mg/dL); women >124 μmol/L (1.4 mg/dL)]; proteinuria (>300 mg/day)
- Peripheral artery disease
- Advanced retinopathy: Hemorrhages or exudates, papilledema.

*Risk maximal for concentric left ventricular hypertrophy (LVH): Increased LVMI with a wall thickness/radius ratio >0.42.

**MDRD formula.

***Cockcroft-Gault formula.

SBP, systolic blood pressure; DBP, diastolic blood pressure; AHA, American Heart Association; NHLBI, National Heart, Lung, and Blood Institute; HDL, high-density lipoproteins; LDL, low-density lipoproteins; LVH, left ventricular hypotrophy; LVMI, left ventricular mass index; IMT, Intima media thickness; MI, myocardial infarction.

Choice of Therapy in Essential Hypertension (Monotherapy and Combination Therapy)[10]

The AHA and ESH/ESC guidelines on the management of hypertension and meta-analyses in 2008 and 2009 concluded that the major factor for reduction in cardiovascular risk was not the choice of antihypertensive drug but the magnitude

TABLE 13: Drugs which may be used as "first-line" agents

- ACEIs (long-acting)
- ARBs
- Beta-blockers (by ESH/ESC 2013 Guidelines; controversial—removed from UK Guidelines; not recommended as first-line in JNC-8 unless compelling indications)
- CCBs (long-acting dihydropyridines, diltiazem, verapamil)
- Diuretics (multiple)

ACEIs, angiotensin-converting enzyme inhibitors; ARBs, angiotensin II receptor blockers; CCBs, calcium channel blockers.

TABLE 14: Position statement: monotherapy versus combination antihypertensive therapy (ESH and ESC 2007)

- Regardless of the drug employed, monotherapy allows achievement of blood pressure target in only a limited number of hypertensive patients
- Use of more than one agent is necessary to achieve target blood pressure in the majority of patients. A vast array of effective and well-tolerated combinations are available
- During initial treatment, one can use monotherapy or combination of two drugs at low doses with a subsequent increase in drug doses or number, if needed
- Monotherapy could be the initial treatment for a mild blood pressure elevation with a low or moderate total cardiovascular risk. A combination of two drugs at low doses should be preferred as first step of treatment when initial blood pressure is in grade 2 or 3 range or total cardiovascular risk is high or very high (Fig. 2)
- Fixed combinations of two drugs can simplify treatment schedule and favor compliance. The possible and preferred combinations of antihypertensive drugs have been outlined in Figure 3
- If blood pressure control is not achieved by two drugs, a combination of three or more drugs is required
- In uncomplicated hypertensives and in the elderly, antihypertensive therapy should normally be initiated gradually. In higher-risk hypertensives, goal blood pressure should be achieved more promptly, which favors initial combination therapy and quicker adjustment of doses

of blood pressure reduction. The conclusion applied to those individuals who were at increased cardiovascular risk as seen in the Antihypertensive and Lipid Lowering Treatment to prevent Heart Attack Trial (ALLHAT),[11] Comparison of Amlodipine versus Enalapril to Limit Occurrences of Thrombosis (CAMELOT),[12] and Valsartan Antihypertensive Long-term Use Evaluation (VALUE)[13] clinical trials. Combination therapy, however, may be different. In avoiding cardiovascular events through combination therapy in Patients living with systolic hypertension (ACCOMPLISH)[14] trial, amlodipine plus benazepril was associated with a relative risk reduction of 19.6% in cardiovascular events compared to hydrochlorothiazide plus benazepril. The 24-hour blood pressure was slightly higher in the patients treated with amlodipine plus benazepril.

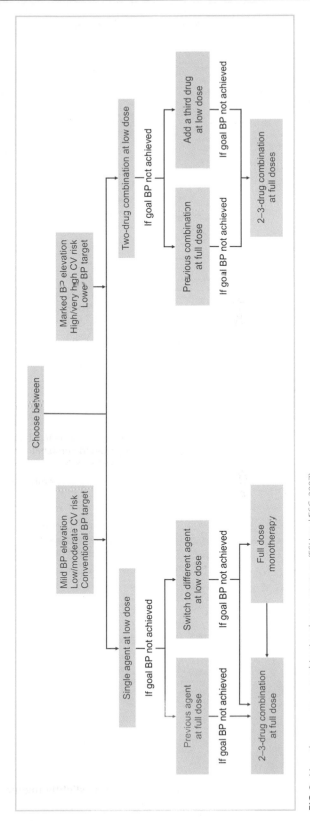

FIG. 2: Monotherapy versus combination therapy strategy (ESH and ESC, 2007).

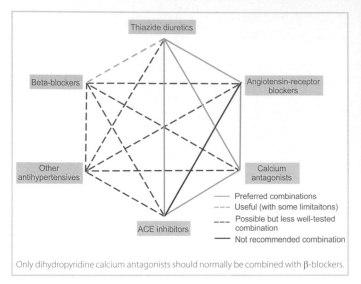

Only dihydropyridine calcium antagonists should normally be combined with β-blockers.

FIG. 3: Possible combinations of classes of antihypertensive drugs.

The following recommendations do not apply to patients with underlying conditions for which particular anti-hypertensive medications might be of benefit apart from blood pressure control (Compelling indications: Table 8).

Recommendations for Monotherapy

- In the absence of a compelling indication for the use of a specific antihypertensive medication, the major classes that have been used for monotherapy are: (a) low-dose thiazide diuretics, (b) long-acting ACEIs or (c) angiotensin II receptor blockers (ARBs), or (d) long-acting dihydropyridine CCBs.

  Monotherapy: From the ALLHAT Trial: 42,428 patients were followed with an average follow-up of 4.9 years. Chlorthalidone was shown to be superior to lisinopril or amlodipine in reducing cardiovascular disease events. The doxazosin arm was discontinued early due to excessive congestive heart failure.

- If a thiazide-type diuretic is used as an initial anti-hypertensive drug, chlorthalidone rather than hydro-chlorothiazide (HCTZ) is suggested. Chlorthalidone may be more likely to induce hypokalemia at the same dose as HCTZ. [Chlorthalidone produced hypokalemia in 7–8% of patients in ALLHAT and Systolic Hypertension in the Elderly Program (SHEP)[15] clinical trials]. Serum potassium needs to be monitored with both chlorthalidone and HCTZ.

- If the response to the initial antihypertensive drug is minimal, one option is treatment with a drug from a different class (sequential monotherapy).

- Beta-blockers are not recommended for first-line therapy unless underlying medical conditions warrant their use.

These conditions include: post-acute MI, stable heart failure, asymptomatic left ventricular dysfunction, rate control in atrial fibrillation, control of angina pectoris, migraine headaches and other disorders. Two meta-analyses concluded, in older patients, β-blockers showed an association with a higher risk of composite endpoints and strokes.[16,17]

- Alpha-blockers are not advised for initial monotherapy, based on the ALLHAT trial in which the doxazosin arm was stopped early due to a significantly increased risk for heart failure when compared to chlorthalidone.

- From the ACCOMPLISH trial, if combination therapy is required, amlodipine plus benazepril is preferred. Combination therapy is recommended for patients with a blood pressure greater than 20/10 above goal. Also, from this study, an ACEI/ARB or a dihydropyridine CCB is suggested for initial therapy. If this rationale is chosen, younger patients may find an ACEI/ARB more effective, and elderly and black patients may do better with a dihydropyridine CCB.

- If patients are at goal blood pressure during treatment with an ACEI/ARB and a thiazide-type diuretic, some experts would consider stopping the thiazide and replacing it with a long-acting dihydropyridine CCB, based on the ACCOMPLISH Trial.[14] If patients are well controlled on combination drugs other than an ACEI/ARB plus a thiazide diuretic, do not change the therapy. Many clinicians, however, would not change the combination of ACEI/ARB plus a thiazide-type diuretic in patients at goal pressure, and treatment must be individualized.

- If patients are not at goal blood pressure while taking a thiazide-type diuretic as monotherapy, it is recommended to switch to a long-acting ACEI/ARB plus a long-acting dihydropyridine CCB, with the goal of being able to stop the thiazide diuretic.

Bedtime and Evening versus Morning Dosing

Instead of taking all antihypertensive drugs in the morning, it is recommended to take at least one medication (but not the diuretic) at bedtime or evening. This may be especially important in patients who do not have the usual 15% decrease in blood pressure during sleep (these patients, in whom blood pressure does not decrease by at least 10% are termed "nondippers". Nondippers are at increased risk for cardiovascular events). However, use caution with PM drugs to avoid excessive hypotension during sleep, which will increase the risk for anterior ischemic optic neuropathy (AION). Ambulatory blood pressure monitoring is recommended if possible to determine which patients are "nondippers" and to avoid excessive nocturnal hypotension and AION. One option is to split the dose, giving, for example, two-thirds of antihypertensives in AM and one-third in PM.

SOME RECENT STUDIES, REVIEWS AND GUIDELINES FOR THE TREATMENT OF HYPERTENSION

- Trials with two drugs that interrupt the renin-angiotensin system: In the Ongoing Telmisartan Alone and in combination with Ramipril Global Endpoint Trial (ONTARGET) trial, worse renal outcomes were seen with the combination of an ACEI and ARB (ONTARGET study).[18] In addition, the ALTITUDE Trial showed that the addition of the renin-inhibitor aliskiren to ACEIs or ARBs may be harmful (Cardiorenal End Points in a Trial of Aliskiren for Type 2 Diabetes).[19]

- Meta-analysis in very elderly patients (>80 years) by Bejan-Angoulvant et al.[20] supported drug treatment for hypertension to decrease stroke, cardiovascular events and heart failure. Also, SBP target of 150 mmHg may be reasonable. In addition, a retrospective study by Lohr et al. of 15,221 veterans, aged 70 years or above, showed an optimal systolic pressure to prevent CKD was systolic blood pressure less than 140 mmHg but not lower than 130.[21]

- The ACCOMPLISH study[14] addresses treatment with a combination of benazepril plus hydrochlorothiazide versus benazepril plus amlodipine. The study enrolled 11,500 high-risk patients. Outcomes were significantly better in the benazepril plus amlodipine group with amlodipine plus benazepril associated with a relative risk reduction of 19.6% in cardiovascular events compared to hydrochlorothiazide plus benazepril. Also, the benazepril plus amlodipine group showed slowing of the progression of nephropathy compared to the benazepril plus hydrochlorothiazide group. The latter point, however, is controversial.

- *2011 guidelines update American College of Cardiology (ACC):*[22] When measuring blood pressure for elderly patients (>64 years), it should be measured after standing for 1–3 minutes to assess for orthostatic hypotension.

- *2011 guidelines update National Institute for Health and Clinical Excellence (NICE) (UK) clinical guideline 127:*[23] If clinic blood pressure is greater than 140/90 mmHg, offer monitoring of ambulatory blood pressure to confirm the diagnosis of hypertension. (Decision to recommend ambulatory blood pressure monitoring in all newly diagnosed patients with hypertension has not been recommended in the United States).

- 2012 Review of 13 RCTs which compared β-blockers to diuretics, or CCBs, or renin-angiotensin system inhibitors or placebo. Initiating hypertension treatment with β-blockers led to modest reductions in cardiovascular disease but no significant effect on mortality. β-blockers are inferior to other antihypertensive drugs.[17]

- 2015: A meta-analysis by Sundstrom et al. regarding effects of blood pressure reduction in more than 15,000 patients with uncomplicated mild hypertension (Grade 1) showed significant reduction for strokes, cardiovascular deaths and total deaths. Treatment reduced the odds ratios in adverse coronary events and heart failure, but did not reach statistical significance.[24]

- 2015: *First-line drugs inhibiting the renin angiotensin system (RAS) versus other first-line antihypertensive drug classes*: In analysis of 42 studies, involving 65,733 patients, all-cause mortality was similar between RAS inhibitors and other drugs. Thiazides caused less heart failure and stroke compared to RAS inhibitors. RAS inhibitors showed a lower risk of total cardiovascular events and stroke compared to β-blockers (quality of evidence was low). Compared to CCBs, RAS inhibitors reduced heart failure but increased stroke.[25]

PREFERRED ANTIHYPERTENSIVE DRUGS

The preferred antihypertensive drugs according to the class and compelling indications are discussed in Tables 15 to 18. The preferred antihypertensive drugs for other morbid conditions are discussed in Table 19. β-adrenergic receptor antagonists (β-blockers) have been used for many years for control of hypertension. Some β-blockers are selective. They only inhibit β1 receptors. Other β-blockers are nonselective and inhibit both β1 and β2 adrenoreceptors. Some β-blockers also possess α-adrenergic blocking property. Some β-blockers possess intrinsic sympathomimetic properties. Many β-blockers have local anesthetic effects. Table 20 summarizes the clinical uses of various β-blockers.

HYPERTENSION IN SPECIAL GROUPS

Resistant Hypertension

Despite multiple drugs therapy, some patients become resistant to drugs, and hypertension is poorly controlled. In patients who become resistant to drugs, proper investigation is necessary to identify the cause. In Table 21, the potential causes of resistant hypertension are outlined.

TABLE 15: Preferred antihypertensive drugs by class (ESH/ESC, 2007)

Drug class	Conditions favoring use	Compelling contraindications	Possible contraindications
Thiazide diuretics	Isolated systolic hypertension (elderly), HF, hypertension in Blacks	Gout	MS, glucose intolerance, pregnancy
Diuretics (antial-dosterone)	HF, post-MI	Renal failure, hyperkalemia	—
Loop diuretics	CKD (GFR <30 mL/min), end-stage renal disease, HF		—
β-blockers	Angina pectoris, post-MI, HF, tachyarrhythmias, glaucoma, pregnancy	Asthma, AV block (Grade 2 or 3)	Peripheral arterial disease, MS, glucose intolerance, athletes and physically active patients, COPD
Calcium antagonists (dihydro-pyridines)	Isolated systolic hypertension (elderly), angina pectoris, LVH, carotid/coronary atherosclerosis, pregnancy, hypertension in Blacks	—	Tachyarrhythmias, HF
Calcium antagonists (verapamil, diltiazem)	Angina pectoris, carotid atherosclerosis, supraventricular tachycardia	AV block (Grade 2 or 3), HF	—
ACEIs	HF, left ventricular dysfunction, post-MI, diabetic nephropathy, LVH, carotid atherosclerosis, proteinuria/microalbuminuria, atrial fibrillation, MS	Pregnancy, angioneurotic edema, hyperkalemia, bilateral renal artery stenosis	—
ARBs	HF, post-MI, diabetic nephropathy, proteinuria, LVH, atrial fibrillation, MS, ACEIs-induced cough	Pregnancy, hyperkalemia, bilateral renal artery stenosis	—

HF, heart failure; MS, multiple sclerosis; MI, myocardial infarction; CKD, chronic kidney disease; GFR, glomerular filtration rate; AV, atrioventricular; COPD, chronic obstructive pulmonary disease; LVH, left ventricular hypertrophy; ACEI, angiotensin-converting enzyme inhibitor; ARB, angiotensin receptor blocker.

TABLE 16: Drugs to be preferred in specific conditions (ESH/ESC 2013)

Condition	Drug
Asymptomatic organ damage	
LVH	ACE inhibitor, calcium antagonist, ARB
Asymptomatic atherosclerosis	Calcium antagonist, ACE inhibitor
Microalbuminuria	ACE inhibitor, ARB
Renal dysfunction	ACE inhibitor, ARB
Clinical CV event	
Previous stroke	Any agent effectively lowering BP
Previous myocardial infarction	BB, ACE inhibitor, ARB
Angina pectoris	BB, calcium antagonist
Heart failure	Diuretic, BB, ACE inhibitor, ARB, mineralocorticoid receptor antagonists
Aortic aneurysm	BB
Atrial fibrillation, prevention	Consider ARB, ACE inhibitor, BB or mineralocorticoid receptor antagonist
Atrial fibrillation, ventricular rate control	BB, non-dihydropyridine calcium antagonist
ESRD/proteinuria	ACE inhibitor, ARB
Peripheral artery disease	ACE inhibitor, calcium antagonist
Other	
ISH (elderly)	Diuretic, calcium antagonist
Metabolic syndrome	ACE inhibitor, ARB, calcium antagonist
Diabetes mellitus	ACE inhibitor, ARB
Pregnancy	Methyldopa, BB, calcium antagonist
Blacks	Diuretic, calcium antagonist

ACE, angiotensin-converting enzyme; ARB, angiotensin receptor blocker; BB, β-blocker; BP, blood pressure; CV, cardiovascular; ESRD, end-stage renal disease or renal failure; ISH, isolated systolic hypertension; LVH, left ventricular hypertrophy.

Hypertensive Emergencies

Although infrequent, hypertensive emergencies (ESH and ESC) are still encountered in clinical practice. As these complications are life-threatening, their early recognition is mandatory for adequate and appropriate management. The causes of hypertensive emergencies are summarized below:

- Hypertensive encephalopathy
- Hypertensive left ventricular failure
- Hypertension with MI and/or unstable angina
- Hypertension and dissection of the aorta
- Severe hypertension associated with subarachnoid hemorrhage or cerebrovascular accident
- Crisis associated with pheochromocytoma
- Use of recreational drugs, such as amphetamines, lysergic acid diethylamide (LSD), cocaine or ecstasy
- Perioperative hypertension
- Severe preeclampsia or eclampsia.

TABLE 17: Clinical trial and guideline basis for compelling indications for individual drug classes (JNC 7)

High-risk conditions with compelling indications*	Recommended drugs						Clinical trial basis**
	Diuretics	β-blockers	ACEIs	ARBs	CCBs	ALDO antagonists	
Heart failure	+	+	+	+		+	ACC/AHA Heart Failure Guideline, MERIT-HF,[26] COPERNICUS,[27] CIBIS,[28] SOLVD,[29] AIRE,[30] TRACE,[31] ValHEFT,[32] RALES,[33] CHARM[34]
Post-MI		+	+			+	ACC/AHA Post-MI Guideline, BHAT,[35] SAVE,[36] CAPRICORN,[37] EPHESUS[38]
High coronary disease risk	+	+	+		+		ALLHAT,[11] HOPE,[39] ANBP2,[40] LIFE,[41] CONVINCE,[42] EUROPA,[43] INVEST[44]
Diabetes mellitus	+	+	+	+	+		NKF-ADA Guideline, UKPDS,[45] ALLHAT[11]
CKD			+	+			NKF Guideline, Captopril trial, RENAAL,[46] IDNT,[47] REIN,[48] AASK[49]
Recurrent stroke prevention	+		+				PROGRESS[50]

*Compelling indications for antihypertensive drugs are based on benefits from outcome studies or existing clinical guidelines; the compelling indication is managed in parallel with the blood pressure.

**Conditions for which clinical trials demonstrate the benefit of specific classes of antihypertensive drugs used as part of an antihypertensive regimen to achieve blood pressure goal to test.

AASK, African American Study of Kidney Disease and Hypertension; ACC/AHA, American College of Cardiology/American Heart Association; ACEIs, angiotensin-converting enzyme inhibitors; AIRE, Acute Infarction Ramipril Efficacy; ALDO, aldosterone; ALLHAT, Antihypertensive and Lipid-lowering Treatment to prevent Heart Attack Trial; ANBP2, 2nd Australian National Blood Pressure study; ARBs, angiotensin II receptor blockers; BHAT, β-blocker Heart Attack Trial; CAPRICORN, CArvedilol Post-infarct survival control in left ventricular dysfunction; CCBs, calcium channel blockers; MI, myocardial infarction; CHARM, Candesartan in Heart failure Assessment of Reduction in Mortality and morbidity; CIBIS, Cardiac Insufficiency Bisoprolol Study; EPHESUS, Eplerenone Post-AMI Heart failure Efficacy and SUrvival Study; EUROPA, EUropean trial on Reduction Of cardiac events with Perindopril in stable coronary Artery disease; HOPE, Heart Outcomes Prevention Evaluation study; IDNT, Irbesartan Diabetic Nephropathy Trial; INVEST, the INternational VErapamil SR-trandolapril STudy; LIFE, Losartan Intervention For Endpoint reduction in hypertension study; MERIT-HF, Metoprolol CR/XL Randomized Intervention Trial in congestive Heart Failure; NKF-ADA, National Kidney Foundation-American Diabetes Association; PROGRESS, Perindopril pROtection aGainst REcurrent Stroke Study; RALES, Randomized Aldactone Evaluation Study; REIN, Ramipril Efficacy In Nephropathy study; RENAAL, Reduction of Endpoints in Non-insulin dependent diabetes mellitus with the Angiotensin II Antagonist Losartan study; SAVE, Survival And Ventricular Enlargement study; SOLVD, Studies of Left Ventricular Dysfunction; TRACE, TRAndolapril Cardiac Evaluation study; UKPDS, United Kingdom Prospective Diabetes Study; ValHEFT, Valsartan HEart Failure Trial.

TABLE 18: Antihypertensive drugs by compelling indications or contraindications[2,10]

Indication	Antihypertensive drugs
Compelling indication **(major improvement in outcome independent of blood pressure)**	
SHF	ACEIs or ARBs, β-blockers, diuretics, ALDO antagonist*
Post-MI	ACEIs, β-blockers, ALDO antagonists
Proteinuric chronic renal failure	ACEIs and/or ARBs
High coronary disease risk	Diuretics (ALLHAT), perhaps ACEIs (HOPE)
Diabetes mellitus (no proteinuria)	Diuretics (ALLHAT), perhaps ACEIs (HOPE)
Angina pectoris	β-blockers, CCBs
Atrial fibrillation, atrial flutter	β-blockers, nondihydropyridine CCBs
Likely to have a favorable effect on symptoms in comorbid conditions	
Benign prostatic hypertrophy	α-blockers
Essential tremor	β-blockers (noncardioselectives)
Hyperthyroidism	β-blockers
Migraine	β-blockers, CCBs
Osteoporosis	Thiazide diuretics
Perioperative hypertension	β-blockers
Raynaud's syndrome	Dihydropyridine CCBs
Contraindications	
Angioedema	ACEIs
Bronchospastic disease	β-blockers
Depression	Reserpine
Liver disease	Methyldopa
Pregnancy	ACEIs, ARBs (includes women likely to become pregnant)
Second or third degree heart block	β-blockers, nondihydropyridine CCBs
May have adverse effect on comorbid conditions	
Depression	β-blockers, central α-agonists
Gout	Diuretics
Hyperkalemia	ALDO antagonists, ACEIs, ARBs
Hyponatremia	Thiazide diuretics
Renovascular disease	ACEIs or ARBs

*A survival benefit from an ALDO antagonist has only been demonstrated in patients with advanced heart failure; in patients with less severe disease, an ALDO antagonist is primarily given for hypokalemia.

SHF, systolic heart failure; CCBs, calcium channel blockers; ALDO, aldosterone; ALLHAT, Antihypertensive and Lipid-Lowering treatment to prevent Heart Attack Trial; HOPE, Heart Outcomes Prevention Evaluation study; ACEIs, angiotensin-converting enzyme inhibitors; ARBs, angiotensin II receptor blockers; MI, myocardial infarction.

TABLE 19: Preferred antihypertensive drugs in other morbid conditions and cautions for the usage

Condition	Preferred drugs
Asthma, COPD	Diuretics, CCBs (dihydropyridines and diltiazem, possibly not verapamil), central sympatholytic agents (clonidine, guanabenz), direct vasodilators (hydralazine), ACEIs (may produce cough and infrequently bronchospasm), ARBs, α-adrenergic blockers (prazosin, terazosin, doxazosin, not as single agent or first-line drug) — Avoid or use with caution β-blockers, especially nonselectives (such as nadolol, propranolol, timolol, and others); in a patient without bronchospasm, may try β1 cardioselectives, β-blockers at low dose (such as metoprolol, atenolol, acebutolol, and others)
Atrial fibrillation/ atrial flutter	• Control of ventricular heart rate: β-adrenergic blockers [superior: atenolol (cardioselective) and nadolol and pindolol (nonselectives)], nondihydropyridine CCBs (verapamil, diltiazem) — Control of ventricular heart rate, labetalol no better than placebo • Prevention of relapse back into atrial fibrillation after cardioversion: β-adrenergic blockers [metoprolol, bisoprolol (cardioselectives) and carvedilol (nonselective β- and α-blockers)]
BPH	α-adrenergic blockers (doxazosin, prazosin, terazosin) (α-blockers used primarily for BPH—tamsulosin, silodosin, alfuzosin) — Diuretics, α-blockers may cause orthostatic hypotension, especially in elderly
Children and adolescents[51,52]	• Diagnostic evaluation for secondary hypertension is important in infants and school age children • New pediatric labeling since the Food and Drug Administration Modernization Act (FDAMA): Amlodipine, benazepril, enalapril, fenoldopam, fosinopril, irbesartan, losartan, lisinopril, metoprolol, valsartan • Prior pediatric labeling: Captopril, chlorothiazide, diazoxide, furosemide, hydralazine, hydrochlorothiazide, methyldopa, minoxidil, propranolol, spironolactone • Strongest evidence for use in pediatrics (Limited data compared to adults): ACEIs, ARBs, CCBs — ■ Nonpharmacologic treatment to be tried first and continued if drug therapy is needed ■ Cautions for various classes of antihypertensive drugs are the same as those for adults

(continued)

Table 19 (continued)

Condition	Preferred drugs	
CKD[53]	Varies with medical condition	• K+ sparing diuretics, β-blockers excreted by kidneys: Nadolol, atenolol, pindolol. ACEIs and ARBs may cause hyperkalemia, decrease GFR, and increase serum creatinine
	• CKD and proteinuria in nondiabetics or diabetics: ACEIs/ARBs, ALDO antagonists, β-adrenergic blockers (β-blockers not excreted primarily by kidneys—propranolol, metoprolol, timolol), may try dihydropyridines, although improvement in proteinuria is not predictable	• An increase in serum creatinine by of 30–35% is considered acceptable and associated with long-term stabilization, or slower decline, in renal function. ALDO antagonists may cause hyperkalemia
	• CKD in nondiabetics with normal urinary protein excretion: Diuretics (especially if edema, loop diuretics for GFR <30 mL/min), then ACEIs or ARBs, then nondihydropyridine or dihydropyridine	
	• CCBs, or β-adrenergic blockers (β-blockers not excreted primarily by kidneys—propranolol, metoprolol, timolol)	
	• CKD in kidney transplant patients: CCBs-first-line drug (dihydro-pyridines might be favored over verapamil and diltiazem), diuretics, or β-adrenergic blockers (β-blockers not excreted primarily by kidneys—propranolol, metoprolol, timolol)	
Chronic liver disease	Diuretics, CCBs, vasodilators, ACEIs, clonidine, guanabenz, α-adrenergic blockers (not as monotherapy or first-line drug)	β-blockers which depend on hepatic metabolism (major liver metabolism: metoprolol, nebivolol, oxprenolol, propranolol hepatic and renal metabolism: acebutolol, betaxolol, bisoprolol, penbutolol, pindolol, timolol), methyldopa, labetalol; CCBs (caution with severe hepatic impairment)
CAD[54]	• Varies with medical condition: angina pectoris: (RE: morning peak in ischemia within 3 hours after awakening) β-blockers (avoid ISA), ACEIs, ARBs, CCBs	• Angina pectoris: Hydralazine, minoxidil (unless adequately β-blocked), β-blockers with ISA activity (e.g., carteolol, pindolol, acebutolol, and others), guanethidine, guanadrel

(continued)

Table 19 (continued)

Condition	Preferred drugs	
	β-blockers (mortality reduced with: atenolol, carvedilol, metoprolol, propranolol, timolol, acebutolol, pindolol), ACEIs, ARBs, ALDO antagonists	Post-MI: Hydralazine, minoxidil (unless adequately β-blocked), postganglionic blockers (guanethidine, guanadrel)
	High coronary risk: Thiazide diuretics, β-blockers (atenolol, carvedilol, metoprolol, propranolol, timolol, acebutolol, and pindolol), ACEIs, CCBs (long-acting dihydropyridines, diltiazem, verapamil)	
Diabetes mellitus[55]	ACEIs and ARBs (with caution for increased K+ and BUN), CCBs, thiazide diuretics, central sympatholytic agents, β1-selective blockers and those with ISA (may still blunt tachycardia response to hypoglycemia)	If peripheral neuropathy: Avoid agents leading to orthostatic hypotension (guanethidine, guanadrel, α-adrenergic receptor antagonists), avoid nonselective β-blockers (hypoglycemia)
		If K+ increased: Avoid nonselective β-blockers, K+ sparing diuretics
Elderly and isolated systolic hypertension (ISH)	Diuretics (start low doses), CCBs, ACEIs and ARBs tend to be less effective	Drugs that cause orthostatic hypotension (guanabenz, guanfacine, guanadrel, guanethidine) or CNS side effects (clonidine, methyldopa, reserpine)
Emergencies (hypertensive)[56]	Parenteral drugs generally given by intravenous infusion: Nitroprusside (most effective), nitroglycerin, dihydropyridine CCBs (clevidipine, nicardipine), fenoldopam, β1 adrenergic blockers (labetalol as infusion or bolus), esmolol (useful during anesthesia), hydralazine (intravenous bolus—primarily used in pregnancy), phentolamine (limited to increased catecholamines (e.g., pheochromocytoma), tyramine ingestion in individual receiving MAOIs)	Enalaprilat response is variable and not predictable
		Nitroprusside—monitor for cyanide toxicity (risk increases at doses >2–4 μg/kg/min), avoid in pregnancy
		Nitroglycerin: Headache, tachycardia
		Labetalol: Avoid—asthma, chronic obstructive lung disease, heart failure, bradycardia, >first-degree heart block
		Additional side effects listed under individual drugs

(continued)

Table 19 (continued)

Condition	Preferred drugs	
Erectile dysfunction	ACEIs (<1%), ARBs (<1%), CCBs (<1–3%), α-adrenergic blockers (not as monotherapy or first-line drug) (<1–4%), thiazide diuretics (3–9%)	β-blockers (6–15%), methyldopa (7–19%), clonidine (11–24%), guanabenz, guanadrel (20–30%), guanethidine (54%)
Essential tremor	β-adrenergic blockers (noncardioselectives >cardioselective β1 blockers)	Direct vasodilators (hydralazine, minoxidil), β-adrenergic blockers with ISA
Exercise	CCBs, β-blockers with ISA, central α2 agonists, ACEIs or ARBs (if volume repleted)	<ul><li>Diuretics or ACEIs or ARBs in hot weather or during excessive sweating</li><li>β-blockers without ISA</li><li>Drugs that cause orthostatic hypotension (α1 antagonists: guanabenz, guanfacine, guanadrel, guanethidine)</li></ul>
Glaucoma	β-blockers (timolol, betaxolol and others—for specific glaucoma therapy, use topically), clonidine (use topically)	Avoid systemic hypotension with all antihypertensives
Gout	No recommendation	Thiazide diuretics may precipitate attack of gout
Heart block (second and third degrees)	Diuretics, ACEIs, ARBs, hydralazine/nitrates	β-blockers, CCBs (verapamil, diltiazem)
Heart failure[57]	Diuretics, ACEIs, ARBs, β-blockers (metoprolol, bisoprolol carvedilol, ALDO antagonists, hydralazine/nitrates	<ul><li>Other β-blockers: Bucindolol (did not reduce mortality), nebivolol (approved for heart failure in 71 countries but not approved by USFDA. Results not as robust for decreasing mortality as the other three β-blockers listed); all β-blockers in uncontrolled heart failure</li><li>CCBs especially verapamil or diltiazem, direct vasodilators (minoxidil), central acting sympatholytic agents, α-adrenergic antagonists (contraindicated in aortic stenosis)</li></ul>

(continued)

Table 19 (continued)

Condition	Preferred drugs	
Hyperthyroidism	β-adrenergic blockers (propranolol high dose, >160 mg/day), alprenolol (noncardioselevice), atenolol, and metoprolol (cardioselective) decrease T3 levels), CCBs if β-blockers are contraindicated (nondihydropyridines)	Nadolol does not decrease T3 levels
LVH	ACEIs, ARBs, ALDO antagonists (spironolactone, eplerenone), CCBs (diltiazem, verapamil, long-acting dihydropyridines), β-adrenergic blockers with α1 antagonist properties (carvedilol, labetalol), thiazide diuretics (used as additional drug), traditional β-adrenergic blockers	Direct vasodilators (hydralazine, minoxidil), β-adrenergic blockers with ISA
Menopausal symptoms	Clonidine, guanzabenz, methyldopa	Vasodilators
Metabolic syndrome	ACEI (lisinopril), ARBs, CCBs, β-blockers-vasodilating (carvedilol, nebivolol)	β-adrenergic blockers (without vadodilating properties), thiazide diuretics
Migraine headaches (prevention)	CCBs (verapamil, diltiazem, amlodipine, nicardipine), ACEI (lisinopril), ARB (candesartan) hydrochlorothiazide, β-blockers without ISA (atenolol, metoprolol, nadolol, propranolol, timolol) (not recommended as initial drug in patients >60 years due to increased rate of strokes)	Some CCBs are not effective (nifedipine, nimodipine), vasodilators
Peptic ulcer disease	ACEIs, ARBs, β-blockers, CCBs, diuretics, central sympatholytic agents	Spironolactone, reserpine, postganglionic blockers (guanethidine, guanadrel)
Peripheral vascular disease	CCBs, ACEIs, ARBs, α-adrenergic blockers (not as monotherapy or first-line drugs—prazosin, terazosin, doxazosin), hydralazine (usually used with diuretics and β-blockers)	Avoid nonselective β-blockers (such as nadolol, propranolol, timolol, and others). If compelling indications for a β-blocker, use β1-cardioselective β-blocker at low dose (such as metoprolol, atenolol, acebutolol, and others)

(continued)

Table 19 (continued)

Condition	Preferred drugs	
Pheochromocytoma; clonidine, guanabenz, or guanfacine rebound (with abrupt withdrawal); crisis in patient taking MAOIs	α-adrenergic blockers [phenoxybenzamine–irreversible α-blockers, preferred over prazosin, terazosin, or doxazosin], β-blockers after α-blocker is effective (e.g., propranolol, atenolol, metoprolol), preoperative treatment requires both α- and β-blockers, CCBs (e.g., nicardipine, amlodipine, diltiazem and others), α-methylparatyrosine (metyrosine), adequate/generous salt intake	Do not use β-blockers without adequate α-blockers first. Intravenous labetalol has been used successfully in patients with pheochromocytoma, but a small number of other patients have had a paradoxical hypertensive response, with MAOIs avoid methyldopa
Pregnancy[58]	▪ Varies with type of hypertension during pregnancy: Chronic hypertension: preferred methyldopa, second-line agents [labetalol, hydralazine β-adrenergic blockers, hydrochlorothiazide, clonidine, CCBs (nifedipine: avoid in 1st trimester, may be used in 2nd and 3rd trimesters)] ▪ Mild preeclampsia: Methyldopa, labetalol, other β-adrenergic blockers, CCBs ▪ Severe hypertension in preeclampsia: Usually requires intravenous hydralazine or labetalol, or peroral nifedipine, rarely sodium nitroprusside	▪ ACEIs and ARBs (increase fetal mortality, renal agenesis, cardiac defects, oligohydramnios) ▪ Avoid Aliskiren ▪ No antihypertensive drugs are proven to be safe during the first trimester [β-blockers may lead to intrauterine growth retardation (labetalol, atenolol), diuretics—not first-line, CCBs—limited data beyond nifedipine] may inhibit labor. Sympatholytic agents with hydralazine may lead to neonatal thrombocytopenia ▪ Severe hypertension in preeclampsia: Nifedipine can cause a marked drop in blood pressure if used with magnesium sulfate; sodium nitroprusside may lead to fetal cyanide poisoning ▪ Eclampsia: Avoid diuretics

(continued)

Table 19 (continued)

Condition	Preferred drugs	
Psychiatric comorbidity[59]	▪ Eclampsia: After control of seizures and hypertension with magnesium sulfate, control hypertension with intravenous hydralazine or labetalol ▪ Varies with psychiatric condition: depression: CCBs, ACEIs, ARBs, diuretics ▪ Panic disorder, anxiety: β-adrenergic blockers ▪ Schizophrenia, other major psychiatric disorders (little data), suggested drugs that have little entry into CNS: ACEIs, ARBs, CCBs (verapamil-mania), possibly diuretics	▪ Depression: β-blockers [lipid soluble, fewer side effects with hydrophilic β-blockers], central α2 agonists (clonidine, guanabenz, methyldopa and others), reserpine ▪ Caution: Interaction between vasodilating β-blockers (nebivolol, labetalol, and others) and SSRIs (increased blood pressure lowering effect) ▪ Panic disorder (anxiety): α-adrenergic blockers, possibly direct vasodilators ▪ Schizophrenia, other major psychiatric disorders: Caution with diuretics if patients are compulsive water drinkers
Race: African-Americans, ancestry-black Africans	Diuretics, CCBs (often three drugs are required): Add an ACEI or ARB or β-blocker for compelling indications or vasodilating β-blocker (carvedilol—cardioprotective in African-Americans)	▪ β-blockers may be less effective and require higher doses ▪ Note: In the ALLHAT study, African-Americans randomized to the ACEI group had a 40% increased risk of stroke and a 32% increased risk of heart failure compared to patients randomized to the diuretic group. These differences disappeared when the ACEI was combined with a diuretic
Raynaud's phenomenon	CCB (long-acting dihydropyridines, diltiazem), ARB (losartan), α-adrenergic blockers, methyldopa, nitroglycerin cream	β-blockers
Renovascular disease (renal artery stenosis)	If choice is for medical therapy: ACEIs, ARBs, CCBs (often with ACEIs or ARBs), diuretic added to ACEIs or ARBs (chlorthalidone, loop diuretic for GFR <30 mL/min), β-adrenergic blockers	ACEIs and ARBs may lead to rise in BUN and creatinine, especially with bilateral renal artery stenosis, or renal artery stenosis in solitary kidney, renal dysfunction may be worsened by diuretics, need to monitor renal function

(continued)

Table 19 (continued)

Condition	Preferred drugs	
Resistant hypertension (AHA 2008 definitions: ■ Blood pressure above goal despite 3 antihypertensive drugs of different classes, including one diuretic ■ Blood pressure requiring 4 different drugs for control)[60]	■ Three or more drugs are required, including a diuretic. Chlorthalidone recommended, plus ACEIs or ARBs and CCBs (long-acting dihydropyridine), then add ALDO antagonist (eplerenone or spironolactone). If still hypertensive: may add, one at a time—vasodilating β-blocker (carvedilol, labetalol, nebivolol), centrally acting sympatholytic agents (clonidine, guanfacine), or direct vasodilator (minoxidil or hydralazine) ■ Experimental invasive treatments: – Radiofrequency ablation of renal sympathetic nerves: Efficacy not confirmed in the symplicity HTN-3 trial (2014)[61] – Electrical activation of carotid sinus baroreceptors	■ Evaluate and treat secondary hypertension (if present) ■ Include nonpharmacologic treatment as part of regimen ■ Standard β-blockers may be less effective than vasodilating β-blockers ■ Monitor patients for orthostatic hypotension
Stroke[62-63]	Varies with medical condition ■ Risk of stroke: Primary prevention—diuretics (hydrochlorothiazide, indapamide, chlorthalidone, bendrofluazide), amlodipine (exact place in therapy controversial) ■ Recurrent stroke prevention: Thiazide diuretics, thiazide diuretics plus ACEI combined (ACEI alone not as effective), possibly ARB (nimodipine for subarachnoid hemorrhage)	■ Avoid drugs which produce an abrupt drop or orthostatic decrease in blood pressure—direct vasodilators ■ Risk of stroke – Primary prevention—β-adrenergic blockers are not as effective for primary prevention of stroke as other drugs (risk of stroke is higher in patients >60 years) ■ Caution: Large artery stenosis (e.g., carotid artery stenosis)

(continued)

Table 19 (continued)

Condition	Preferred drugs	
Hypertension control in acute stroke:	• Candidates for fibrinolysis: Blood pressure >185/110 mmHg labetalol intravenously or nitropaste or nicardipine infusion • Noncandidates for fibrinolysis: Blood pressure >220/120 mmHg labetalol intravenously or nicardipine infusion	• Recurrent stroke prevention: β-adrenergic blockers not recommended unless compelling indication • Caution: Large artery stenosis (e.g., carotid artery stenosis) • Avoid volume depletion with diuretics • Hypertension control in acute stroke*

*Additional information: Jauch EC, et al. Based on ACLS Guidelines, 2005 and American Stroke Association Scientific Statement, 2007. ESH/ESC 2013; Fuentes P, et.al. Ther Adv Chronic Dis 2012; 3:163-171.

COPD, chronic obstructive pulmonary disease; CCBs, calcium channel blockers; ACEIs, angiotensin-converting enzyme inhibitors; ARBs, angiotensin II receptor blockers; BPH, benign prostatic hypertrophy; CKD, chronic kidney disease; GFR, glomerular filtration rate; ISA, intrinsic sympathomimetic activity; BUN, blood urea nitrogen; MAOIs, monoamine oxidase inhibitors; SSRIs, selective serotonin reuptake inhibitors; MI, myocardial infarction; CAD, coronary artery disease; LVH, left ventricular hypertrophy.

TABLE 20: Clinical uses of β-adrenoreceptor blockers[64]

Class/Drug	Clinical uses					Comments
	HTN	Angina	Arrhy	MI	CHF	
Nonselective β1/β2						
Carteolol	X					ISA; long acting; also used for glaucoma
Carvedilol	X				X	α-blocking activity
Labetalol	X	X				ISA; α-blocking activity
Nadolol	X	X	X	X		Long-acting
Penbutolol	X	X				ISA
Pindolol	X	X				ISA; MSA
Propranolol	X	X	X	X		MSA; proto-typical beta-blocker
Sotalol			X			Several other significant mechanisms
Timolol	X	X	X	X		Primarily used for glaucoma
β1 selective						
Acebutolol	X	X	X			ISA
Atenolol	X	X	X	X		
Betaxolol	X	X	X			MSA
Bisoprolol	X	X	X			
Esmolol	X		X			Ultra short acting; intra- or postoperative HTN
Metoprolol	X	X	X	X	X	MSA
Nebivolol	X					Relatively selective in most patients; vaso-dilating (NO release)

HTN, hypertension; Arrhy, arrhythmias; MI, myocardial infarction; CHF, congestive heart failure; ISA, intrinsic sympathomimetic activity; NO, nitric oxide; MSA, membrane stabilizing activity.

End-organ damage may occur in some hypertensive patients. Cerebrovascular and cardiovascular complications have been discussed. Renal dysfunction is another complication that may occur in hypertensive patients.

Proteinuria and albuminuria are manifestations of renal dysfunction. In Table 22, definitions of proteinuria and albuminuria are summarized.

TABLE 21: Causes of resistant hypertension (JNC 7 and ESH/ESC)

Volume overload

- Excess sodium intake
- Volume retention from kidney disease
- Inadequate diuretic therapy

Drug-related, drug-induced or other causes

- Nonadherence
- Inadequate doses
- Inappropriate combinations
- Nonsteroidal anti-inflammatory drugs, cyclooxygenase 2 inhibitors
- Cocaine, amphetamines, other illicit drugs
- Sympathomimetics (decongestants, anorectics)
- Oral contraceptive hormones
- Adrenal steroid hormones
- Cyclosporine and tacrolimus
- Erythropoietin
- Licorice (including some chewing tobacco)
- Selected over-the-counter dietary supplements and medicines (e.g., ephedra, ma huang, bitter orange)
- Unsuspected secondary hypertension, including obstructive sleep apnea

Associated conditions

- Obesity
- Excess alcohol intake (including binge drinking)

Causes of spurious resistant hypertension

- Isolated office (white-coat) hypertension
- Failure to use large cuff on large arm (improper measurement)
- Pseudohypertension (arterial stiffening, more common in the elderly)

Hypertension in Children and Adolescents

Hypertension is recognized in children and adolescents too. It is more frequently observed in children and adolescents with hypertensive parents. There are other risk factors, such as obesity, culture, environment, and family history for development of hypertension in children and adolescents. It is highly desirable to recognize those at risk of developing hypertension.

In Table 23, the blood pressure values in children and adolescents that require further evaluation are summarized.

Dyslipidemia

Dyslipidemia has been recognized as a potential side effect of antihypertensive therapy for several years. However, not all

TABLE 22: Definitions of proteinuria and albuminuria[65] (Measurement is more accurate with a 24-hour urine collection, or by factoring urine protein or albumin per gram creatinine)

	Urine collection	Normal	Microalbuminuria	Albuminuria or proteinuria
Total protein	24-hour excretion	<300 mg/day (usually <150 mg/day)	—	>300 mg/day
	"Spot" urine dipstick	<30 mg/dL	—	>30 mg/dL
	"Spot" or random urine protein-to-creatinine ratio	<200 mg/g	—	>200 mg/g
Albumin	24-hour excretion	<30 mg/day	30–299 mg/day	>300 mg/day
	"Spot" urine dipstick (albumin-specific dipstick)	<30 mg/dL	>30 mg/dL	—
	"Spot" or random urine albumin-to-creatinine ratio	<17 mg/g (men) <25 mg/g (women)	17–250 mg/g (men) 25–355 mg/g (women) or 30–299 mg/g	>250 mg/g (men) >355 mg/g (women)

TABLE 23: Blood pressure values* requiring further evaluation according to age and gender in children and adolescents[52]

Age (years)	Blood pressure values (mmHg)			
	Male		Female	
	Systolic	Diastolic	Systolic	Diastolic
3	100	59	100	61
4	102	62	101	64
5	104	65	103	66
6	105	68	104	68
7	106	70	106	69
8	107	71	108	71
9	109	72	110	72
10	111	73	112	73
11	113	74	114	74
12	115	74	116	75
13	117	75	117	76
14	120	75	119	77
15	120	76	120	78
16	120	78	120	78
17	120	80	120	78
≥18	120	80	120	80

*These values represent the lower limits for abnormal blood pressure ranges, according to age and gender. Any blood pressure readings equal to or greater than these values represent blood pressures in the prehypertensive, stage 1 hypertensive, or stage 2 hypertensive range and should be further evaluated by a physician.

antihypertensive agents exert similar effects on lipid profile. Some agents can produce deleterious effects and others have beneficial effects. The effects of antihypertensive drugs on serum lipids are summarized in Table 24.

ANTIHYPERTENSIVE DRUGS AND DOSING RECOMMENDATIONS

Dosing recommendations for various classes of antihypertensive drugs are summarized in Tables 25 to 27 and 29 to 37. The actions of β-adrenergic receptors on various organs are summarized in Table 28.

Dosing recommendations for various combinations of antihypertensive drugs are summarized in Tables 25 to 49. The tables show dose ranges according to the drug manufacturers, from Micromedex, and other pharmacologic sources. Table 50, from JNC-8 shows evidence-based dosing from Randomized

TABLE 24: Antihypertensive drugs and their effects on serum lipids[66]

Favorable effects

β1-adrenergic receptor blockers: Lower total cholesterol (3–5%) and triglycerides (3–4%) and raise HDL (mild effect)

CCBs: May increase HDL and decrease triglycerides (mild effect), or have no effect on lipids (diltiazem may have the most favorable effects compared to verapamil and dihydropyridines)

Unfavorable effects (may be mild)

Thiazide diuretics: May raise LDL (5–10%) and increase triglycerides. This may occur with short-term use and may not be present after a year

β-adrenergic receptor blockers (nonselective and β1-selective):

- *Without ISA:* May lower HDL (10%) and raise triglycerides (20–40%)
- *With ISA:* Less effect to lower HDL or raise triglycerides, or changes in lipids nonsignificant

No effect (or mild beneficial effect)

Central sympatholytic action (α2 adrenergic agonists)—methyldopa, clonidine, guanabenz, guanfacine: Lipid (neutral), guanabenz, small decreases in total cholesterol and triglycerides and reduction in HDL

β-blockers with vasodilating properties: Generally lipid neutral, nebivolol may increase triglycerides and decrease HDL

ACEIs and ARBs: Lipid neutral, or mild effect to increase HDL, decrease LDL and triglycerides

Vasodilators (hydralazine, minoxidil): Lipid neutral or mild effect to increase HDL and decrease LDL, no effect on triglycerides

Potassium channel openers: Lipid neutral or mild effect to decrease LDL and triglycerides and increase HDL

HDL, high-density lipoproteins; LDL, low-density lipoproteins; ACEIs, angiotensin-converting enzyme inhibitors; ARBs, angiotensin II receptor blockers; ISA, intrinsic sympathomimetic activity; CCBs, calcium channel blockers.

Control Trials (RCTs). The Food and Drug Administration (FDA), United States of America, last approved a single drug, "azilsartan" in 2011. No other antihypertensives have been approved since then until January 2015, with the approval of the combination drug perindopril arginine and amlodipine besylate (Prestalia).

ANTIHYPERTENSIVE DRUGS: SIDE EFFECTS AND CAUTIONS[67-72]

Antihypertensive drugs are prone to produce minor or serious adverse effects. The serious side effects are important causes of noncompliance. Some side effects are common. The major and minor side effects are summarized in the Tables 51 to 54, 56 to 59, and 61 to 65. The lipid solubility of some β-blockers is summarized in Table 55. Effects of various CCBs on selected cardiac and vascular functions are summarized in Table 60.

TABLE 25: Dosing recommendations for diuretics[67-72]

Drugs	Starting adult daily dose [oral unless specified]	Daily dose range	Frequency/day
Thiazides (benzothiadiazine derivatives) [Ineffective in patients with GFR <30 mL/min, serum creatinine >2.5 mg/dL (221 µmol/L)]			
Bendroflumethiazide (only in combination tablet)	1.25–2.5 mg	1.25–20 mg	1
Benzthiazide	50 mg	50–200 mg	1–2
Butizide or buthiazide	2.5 or 5 mg	2.5–15 mg	1–2
Chlorothiazide	500 mg	500–1000 mg	1–2
Clopamide	10–40 mg	Initial: 10–40 mg, maintenance: 5–20 mg daily or every other day	1 or for maintenance: once every other day
Cyclopenthiazide	0.25 mg	0.25–1.5 mg	1
Cyclothiazide	2 mg	2–6 mg	1–3
Hydrochlorothiazide (HCTZ)	12.5 or 25 mg	12.5–50 mg (up to 100 mg)	1–2
Hydroflumethiazide	12.5–25 mg	12.5–50 mg	1–2
Mefruside	10 mg	10–50 mg	1–2 (maintenance: daily or every other day)
Methyclothiazide	2.5 mg	2.5–5 mg	1
Meticrane	150 mg	150–300 mg	1
Polythiazide	1.0 mg	1–4 mg	1
Trichlormethiazide	1–2 mg	1–4 mg	1
Xipamide	20 or 40 mg	10–80 mg (for maintenance, may decrease to 10–20 mg)	1

(continued)

Table 25 (continued)

Drugs	Starting adult daily dose [oral unless specified]	Daily dose range	Frequency/day
Diazoxide (nondiuretic/nonsaluretic thiazide)	Intravenous use only for malignant hypertension	1–2 mg/kg (maximum dose: bolus = 150 mg)	May repeat every 5–15 minutes until diastolic pressure <100 mmHg
Phthalimidine derivatives			
Chlorthalidone	12.5 or 25 mg	12.5–50 mg	1
	15 mg	15–45 mg	
Quinazoline derivatives			
Metolazone	2.5 mg	2.5–10 mg (20 mg CKD)	1
Metolazone (bioavail)	0.5 mg	0.5–1.0 mg	1
Quinethazone	25 mg	25–100 mg	1–2
Indoline derivatives			
Indapamide	1.25–2.5 mg	1.25–5 mg	1
Metipamide	1.25–2.5 mg	1.25–5 mg	1 (For maintenance: once/day or every other day)
Tripamide	15 mg	15–30 mg	1–2
Loop diuretics [Diuretics of choice in patients with GFR <30 mL/min or serum creatinine >2.5 mg/dL (221 mmol/l)]			
Azosemide (similar - furosemide; may also act in proximal tubule)	30–60 mg (azosemide 30 mg = furosemide 20 mg)	30 mg or 60 mg (maximum dose not established)	1
Bumetanide	0.5 mg	0.5–10 mg	1–2

Table 25 (continued)

Drugs	Starting adult daily dose [oral unless specified]	Daily dose range	Frequency/day
Ethacrynic acid	25 mg	25–100 mg (max: 200 mg or 400 mg)	1–2
Etozolin	200 mg	200–400 mg	1
Furosemide	20–40 mg	Oral: 40–480 mg (max: 600 mg), intravenous 0.05 mg/kg/hour and titrate or 20–40 mg intravenous over 1–2 minutes, may repeat in 2 hours (usually for edema)	1, 2, or more
Piretanide	6 mg (piretanide 6 mg = furosemide 40 mg)	6–12 mg	1
Torsemide	5 mg	5–200 mg	1, 2, or more
Potassium sparing diuretics			
Amiloride	5 mg	5–20 mg	1–2
Triamterene	50–100 mg	50–300 mg	1 or 2 or every other day
ALDO antagonists			
Canrenone (major metabolite of spironolactone)	50 mg	50–300 mg	1
Eplerenone	25–50 mg	25–100 mg	1–2
Potassium canrenoate (prodrug for canrenone)	100 mg	100–400 mg (in one or two divided doses)	1–2
Spironolactone	25 mg	25–100 mg (maximum 400 mg)	1–2

CKD, chronic kidney disease; GFR, glomerular filtration rate; ALDO, aldosterone; HCTZ, hydrochlorothiazide.

TABLE 26: Dosing recommendations for central sympatholytic agents, imidazoline receptor antagonist[67-72]

Drugs	Starting adult daily dose [oral unless specified]	Daily dose range	Frequency/day
Central sympatholytic agents (α2 adrenergic agonists)			
Clonidine			
▪ Oral tablets	0.1 mg	0.1–0.6 mg (max 1.2 mg)	1–2 (up to 4)
▪ Transdermal patch (TTS)	TTS-1 (1 patch/week = 0.1 mg/day)	One TTS-1 to two TTS-3	1 patch/week
Guanabenz	4 mg	4–32 mg	2
Guanfacine	1 mg	1–3 mg	1 (HS)
Methyldopa	250 mg	250–3,000 mg	2–3 (or 4)
	(*Intravenous use*: 250–500 mg QID, infuse slowly over 1/2–1 hour, maximum 1 g QID)		
Central depleting agents of catecholamines and 5-hydroxytryptophan (Rauwolfia alkaloids)			
Reserpine 0.1 mg; 0.25 mg	0.05–0.1 mg	0.05–0.25 mg	1
Central imidazoline receptor agonists (α2-adrenergic agonists)			
Moxonidine	0.1–0.2 mg	0.1–0.6 mg	1 (or 2)
Rilmenidine	1 mg	1–2 mg	1 (or 2)

TABLE 27: Dosing recommendations for ganglionic and post-ganglionic blockers[67-72]

Drugs	Starting adult daily dose [oral unless specified]	Daily dose range	Frequency of dose/day
Ganglionic blockers			
Trimethaphan	Continuous intravenous only, 1 g/L (1 mg/mL), titrated, start 0.5–1 mg/min, range: 0.5–6 mg/min (used for malignant hypertension, acute aortic dissection)		
Mecamylamine	2.5 mg	2.5–25 mg	2 (or 3 or 4)
Postganglionic blockers			
Bethanidine	5 or 10 mg	15 mg or 30–200 mg	3
Debrisoquine	10 mg	10 mg or 20–120 mg	1–2
Guanadrel	5 mg	10–75 mg	2 (or 3 or 4)
Guanethidine	10 mg	10–100 mg	1–2
Pargyline (monoamine oxidase inhibitor)	10 mg	10–25 mg	1

TABLE 28: Actions of β-adrenergic receptors

β1-receptors

- Heart
  - Increase heart rate via SA node
  - Increase conduction velocity via AV node
  - Increase contractility via atria and ventricles
  - Increase conduction velocity and automaticity of cardioventricular pacemakers via ventricles
- Kidneys
  - Increase renin
- Posterior pituitary
  - Increase vasopressin (ADH)
- Parathyroid gland
  - Increase parathormone secretion
- Stomach
  - Increase ghrelin

β2-receptors

- Heart
  - β2-receptors are also present on heart with similar functions to β1-receptors
- Lungs
  - Relax bronchiolar smooth muscle
- Blood vessels
  - Relax smooth muscles (arterioles, veins)
- Intestines
  - Decrease motility
- Stomach
  - Decrease motility
- Skeletal muscle
  - Increase contractility, K^+ uptake
- Liver
  - Increase glycogenolysis and gluconeogenesis
- Fat cells
  - Lipolysis (also, β3-receptors)
- Pancreas
  - Stimulate insulin secretion
- Urinary bladder
  - Detrusor relaxation
- Uterus
  - Relaxation
- Thyroid
  - Promote conversion of T4 to T3

SA, sinoatrial; AV, atrioventricular; ADH, antidiuretic hormone; K^+, potassium; T3, tri-iodothyronine; T4, thyroxine.

TABLE 29A: Dosing recommendations for adrenergic receptor blocking drugs

Drugs	Half-life (hours)	Starting adult daily dose	Daily dose range	Frequency of dose/day
β-blockers				
Nonselective (β1- and β2-receptor antagonists)				
Alprenolol	2–3	25 mg BD	50–800 mg	2
Bopindolol* (prodrug for pindolol)	4–6	0.5–1.0 mg	0.5–2 mg (has been used up to 8 mg)	1
Bupranolol (similar to propranolol)	2–4	50 mg BD	50 mg BD to100 mg QID	2–4
Carteolol*	5–6	2.5 mg	2.5–60 mg	1
Indenolol*	7	60 mg	60–120 mg	1
Mepindolol* (analog of pindolol)	3–4.5	5 mg	5–15 mg	1
Nadolol	20–24	20–40 mg	20–320 mg	1
Oxprenolol*	2	160 mg	160–480 mg	4
Penbutolol*	5–6	10 mg	10–20 mg	1
Pindolol*	3–4	5 mg BD	10–60 mg	2
Propranolol				
Regular preparation	4	20–40 mg BD	40–480 mg (maximum 640 mg)	2–4
Long-acting preparation	8–11	80 mg	80–480 mg (maximum 640 mg)	1
Extended-release preparation		80 mg at bedtime	80–120 mg	1
Propranolol (intravenous use)		(Intravenous: 1 mg/min; total 1–3; electrocardiographic monitoring)		

(continued)

Table 29A (continued)

Drugs	Half-life (hours)	Starting adult daily dose	Daily dose range	Frequency of dose/day
Tertatolol	3–9	5 mg	5–10 mg	1
Timolol	4–5	10 mg BD	20–60 mg	2
Cardioselective (β1-selective antagonists)				
Acebutolol*	3–4	200 mg BD	200–1200 mg	Usually 2 (or 1)
Atenolol	6–7	25 mg	25–100 mg	1
Betaxolol	14–22	5 mg	5–20 mg (or 40 mg)	1
Bisoprolol	9–12	2.5 mg	2.5–20 mg	1
Celiprolol*	5.1–5.8	200 mg	200–400 mg (or 600 mg)	1
Esatenolol (isomer of atenolol)	6–7	25 mg	25–100 mg	1
Metoprolol (tartrate)	3–7	50–100 mg	50–450 mg	1–2
Metoprolol (succinate) extended release	3–7	25–100 mg	50–400 mg	1
Talinolol	12	50–100 mg in morning and 50 mg in evening	100–300 mg	2
Esmolol (intravenous use)	Approximately 9 minutes	Intravenous load: 500 mg/kg over 1 min followed by 25 mg/kg/min; increase by 25–50 mg/kg/min every 5 minutes Usual maintenance: 100 mg/kg/min; maximum: 200 mg/kg/minute		

Table 29A (continued)

Drugs	Half-life (hours)	Starting adult daily dose	Daily dose range	Frequency of dose/day
β-blockers with vasodilating properties				
Amosulalol (β-nonselective, α-antagonist)	5	10 mg BD	20–60 mg (effective dose range in clinical studies)	2
Arotinolol* (β-nonselective, α-antagonist)	10–11.2	10 mg BD	20–40 mg in 2 divided doses, or 30 mg OD	1–2
Bevantolol (β1-selective, α1-selective antagonist)	1–2	75 mg BD	150–400 mg in 2 divided doses	2
Bucindolol (β-nonselective, very weak α1-selective antagonist)	4–12	10–50 mg TID	50–200 mg TID (optimal dose not established)	3
Carvedilol (β-nonselective, α1-selective antagonist)	7–10	6.25 mg BD	12.5–50 mg	2
Labetalol* (β-nonselective, α1-selective antagonist)	6–8	100 mg BD per oral Intravenous use: Start bolus 20 mg; then 20–80 mg every 10 minutes to maximum of 300 mg or infusion: start 0.5–2 mg/min to total 30 mg	200–1,200 mg (maximum 2,400 mg)	2
Nebivolol (β1-selective plus vasodilator through nitric oxide pathway)	12–19	5 mg	5–40 mg	1
Tilisolol (β-nonselctive, vasodilator properties, possibly K⁺ channel opener)	12	10 mg	10–30 mg	1

*Intrinsic sympathomimetic activity.

OD, once a day; BD, twice a day; TID, thrice a day; QID, four times a day.

TABLE 29B: Dosing recommendations for adrenergic receptor antagonists

Drugs	Starting adult daily dose [oral unless specified]	Daily dose range	Frequency/day
α-adrenergic receptor antagonists			
Bunazosin (competitive α1 antagonists)	Start 6 mg at bedtime; then 6 mg every morning	6–12 mg	1
Doxazosin (competitive α1 antagonists) ▪ Regular preparation ▪ Extended-release preparation (GITS)	Start 1 mg Start 4 mg	1–16 mg 4–8 mg	1
Indoramin (competitive α1 antagonists)	25 mg BD	50–200 mg/day	2
Prazosin (competitive α1 antagonists)	Start 1 mg at bedtime, then 1 mg every morning	2–30 mg	2–3
Terazosin (competitive α1 antagonists)	Start 1 mg at bedtime, then 1 mg every morning	1–20 mg (maximum 40 mg)	1–2
Tolazoline (competitive α1 antagonists) (for pulmonary hypertension)	Intravenous: 10–50 mg QID	40–200 mg	4
Phenoxybenzamine (noncompetitive α1 and 2 antagonists)	10 mg BD	20–40 mg	2–3
Phentolamine (competitive α1 and 2 antagonists)	Intramuscular: 5–10 mg; intravenous: 5–10 mg, bolus: may repeat every 5 minutes to 20–30 mg, infusion: 0.1–100 mg/kg/min		

GITS, gastrointestinal therapeutic system; OD, once a day; BD, twice a day; TID, thrice a day; QID, four times a day.

TABLE 30A: Dosing recommendations for direct vasodilators (Oral acting)

Drugs	Starting adult daily dose [oral unless specified]	Daily dose range	Frequency of dose/day
Cadralazine	10 mg	10–30 mg	1
Dihydralazine	12.5 mg BD	25–100 mg (maximum 150 mg)	2–3
Endralazine	10 mg	10–40 mg	1–2
Hydralazine	10 mg BD to QID	50–300 mg	2–4
	(Intravenous or intramuscular use: start 10 mg, may use to 40 mg every 4–6 hours)		
Minoxidil (also listed under K⁺ channel openers)	2.5–5 mg	2.5–100 mg	1–2
Todralazine	20 mg BD	40–120 mg	2–4

BD, twice a day; QID, four times a day; K⁺, potassium.

TABLE 30B: Dosing recommendations for direct vasodilators (Intravenous use for hypertensive emergencies)

Drugs	Dose
Sodium nitroprusside	Continuous intravenous infusion (in dextrose 5% in water only): 0.3–10.0 mg/kg/min, average dose: 3 mg/kg/min. Risk of cyanide toxicity increased at >2–4 mg/kg/min
Diazoxide (also listed under K⁺ channel openers)	Intravenous bolus injection: 1–3 mg/kg (max: 150 mg); bolus repeated every 5–15 minutes as needed

K⁺, potassium.

TABLE 31: Dosing recommendations for inhibitors of the renin-angiotensin system

Drugs	Half-life (hours)	Starting adult daily dose	Daily dose range	Frequency of dose/day
ACEIs				
Alacepril (converted to captopril)	1.9	12.5 mg	12.5–100 mg	1
Benazepril	10	5 or 10 mg	5–80 mg	1 (or 2)
Captopril (sulfhydryl-containing)	<3	12.5–25 mg BD or TID	12.5–450 mg	2–3
Cilazapril	30–50	2.5 mg	2.5–10 mg	1
Delapril	1/2	15 mg BD	30–120 mg in 2 divided doses	2
Enalapril	11	2.5 or 5 mg	2.5–40 mg	1 (or 2)
Enalaprilat	11	Intravenous use: 0.625 mg or 1.25 mg every 6 hours, given over a 5 minute period. Maximum dose: 5 mg QID		
Fosinopril (phosphonate-containing)	11.5–12	10 mg	10–80 mg	1 (or 2)
Imidapril	1.1–2.5	5 mg	10 mg	1
Lisinopril	12	5 or 10 mg	5–80 mg	1
Moexipril	9.8	7.5 mg	7.5–60 mg	1 (or 2)
Perindopril	20–120	4 mg	4–16 mg	1 (or 2)
Quinapril	25	10–20 mg	10–80 mg	1 (or 2)
Ramipril	13–17	2.5 mg	2.5–20 mg	1 (or 2)
Spirapril	30–35	6 mg	6 mg	1
Temocapril	1.6	1 mg	1–4 mg	1

(continued)

Table 31 (*continued*)

Drugs	Half-life (hours)	Starting adult daily dose	Daily dose range	Frequency of dose/day
Trandolapril	10	1 mg (non-Blacks) 2 mg (Blacks)	1–8 mg	1 (or 2)
Zofenopril	5	15 mg	15–60 mg	1
ARBs				
Azilsartan	11	40–80 mg	40–80 mg	1
Candesartan	9	8 mg	8–32 mg	1 (or 2)
Eprosartan	20	400–600 mg	400–800 mg	1 (or 2)
Irbesartan	11–15	75–150 mg	75–300 mg	1
Losartan	6–9	25 or 50 mg	25–100 mg	1 (or 2)
Olmesartan	12–18	20 mg	20–40 mg	1
Telmisartan	24	20–40 mg	20–80 mg	1
Valsartan	6–9	80 mg	80–320 mg	1
DRIs				
Aliskiren*	40	150 mg	150–300 mg	1

*As of December 20, 2011, the randomized ALTITUDE study with aliskiren has been terminated due to increased adverse events among high-risk patients taking aliskiren in addition to conventional antihypertensive drugs (ACEIs or ARBs). Patients had type 2 diabetes mellitus and CKD.

Historical note: Teprotide is a nonapeptide isolated from venom of the snake *Bothrops jararaca*. It was the first ACEI observed by Sergio Ferreira in 1965 and required intravenous use. Saralasin is a competitive angiotensin II inhibitor used intravenously as a test for renin-dependent hypertension. It was discontinued in 1984.

ACEIs, angiotensin-converting enzymes inhibitors; ARBs, angiotensin II receptor blockers; DRIs, direct renin inhibitors; BD, twice a day; TID, thrice a day; QID, four times a day.

TABLE 32: Dosing recommendations for calcium channel blockers

Drugs	Starting adult daily dose	Daily dose range	Frequency of dose/day
Benzothiazepines (block L-type channels)			
Diltiazem	30 mg QID	120–360 mg	3–4
Diltiazem injectable	Intravenous use: 0.25 mg/kg over 2 minutes. After 15 minutes, repeat 0.35 mg/kg over 2 minutes, or intravenous infusion 5–10 mg (up to 15 mg/hr)		
Diltiazem sustained-release	60–120 mg BD	120–360 mg	2
Diltiazem extended-release capsule	120–240 mg	120–480 mg*	1
Diltiazem extended-release tablet	120–240 mg	120–540 mg	1
Dihydropyridines (block L-type channels)			
1st Generation: may suppress myocardial contractility or suppress SA node			
Nifedipine immediate-release	10 mg TID	30–180 mg	3–4
	For angina pectoris, not recommended for hypertension treatment		
Nifedipine slow-release	30–60 mg	30–120 mg	1
	30 mg	30–90 mg	1
2nd Generation dihydropyridines			
Benidipine	2 mg	2–4 mg (8 mg)	1
Felodipine	2.5 or 5 mg	2.5–10 mg	1
Isradipine			
▪ Capsule	2.5 mg BD	5–20 mg	2
▪ Tablet	5 mg	5–20 mg	1

(continued)

Table 32 (continued)

Drugs	Starting adult daily dose	Daily dose range	Frequency of dose/day
Nicardipine immediate-release	20 mg TID	60–120 mg	3
Nicardipine slow-release	30 mg BD	60–120 mg	2
Nisoldipine			
▪ Hydrogel tablet	17 mg	17–34 mg	1
▪ Coatcore tablet	20 mg	20–60 mg	1
Nitrendipine	5–10 mg	10–40 mg	1–2
Nimodipine	60 mg six times a day	360 mg/day	6
(USFDA approved for subarachnoid hemorrhage (SAH) from ruptured intracranial aneurysm. Begin within 96 hours after SAH and continue for 21 days)			
3rd generation dihydropyridines			
Amlodipine	2.5 mg or 5 mg	2.5–10 mg	1
Aranidipine	5 mg	5–20 mg	1
Azelnidipine	8 mg	8–16 mg	1
Barnidipine	5–10 mg	5–20 mg	1
Cilnidipine	5 mg	5–20 mg	1
Efonidipine	10 mg BD	20–40 mg	(1)–2
Lacidipine	2–4 mg	2–6 mg (8 mg)	1
Lercanidipine	10 mg	10–30 mg	1
Manidipine	10 mg	10–20 mg	1
Nilvadipine	8 mg	8–16 mg	1

(continued)

Table 32 (continued)

Drugs	Starting adult daily dose	Daily dose range	Frequency of dose/day
Pranidipine	1 mg	1–4 mg	1
Clevidipine	Intravenous use: 1–2 mg/hour. May double dose every 90 seconds, increase of 1–2 mg/hour decreases systolic blood pressure by 2–4 mmHg. Maximum dose: 21 mg/hour		
Phenylalkylamines (block L-type channels)			
Gallopamil	50 mg BD	50–200 mg	2–4
Verapamil (immediate-release)	80 mg TID	240–480 mg	3
Verapamil (sustained-release)	(120 mg or) 180 mg	(120 mg or) 180–480 mg	1 (or 2)
Verapamil (extended-release at bedtime)	200 mg	200–400 mg	1
Verapamil (intravenous)	Intravenous use: 5–10 mg over 2–3 minutes; repeat in 30 minutes if necessary. Used for PSVT		
Diarylaminopropylamine ester			
Bepridil (US FDA approved for angina pectoris)	200 mg	200–400 mg	1

*The daily dose can go up to 540 mg depending on the preparation of the drug.

BD, twice a day; TID, thrice a day; QID, four times a day; PSVT, paroxysmal supraventricular tachycardia.

TABLE 33: Dosing recommendations for nitrates

Drugs	Starting adult daily dose	Daily dose range	Frequency of dose/day
Nitroglycerin (intravenous)		5–100 mg/min	
Nicorandil (used for angina pectoris; also is a K$^+$ channel opener activator—see **Table 35**)	10 mg BD	20–80 mg	2

BD, twice a day; K$^+$, potassium.

TABLE 34: Dosing recommendations for catecholamine synthesis inhibitor (Tyrosine hydroxylase blocker) (for pheochromocytoma only)

Drugs	Starting adult daily dose	Daily dose range	Frequency of dose/day
Metyrosine	250 mg QID	1,000–4,000 mg (decrease catecholamines by 35–80%)	4

QID, four times a day.

TABLE 35: Dosing recommendations for potassium channel openers or activators

Drugs	Starting adult daily dose	Daily dose range	Frequency of dose/day
Cromakalim, levcro-makalim and others	Under investigation		
Minoxodil	2.5–5 mg	2.5–100 mg	1–2
Nicorandil (used for angina pectoris, also has nitrate-like actions—see **Table 33**)	10 mg BD	20–80 mg	2
Pinacidil (sustained-release)	12.5 mg BD	25–150 mg (200 mg) (preliminary)	2
Diazoxide	Intravenous bolus injection: 1–3 mg/kg (max: 150 mg) Bolus repeated every 5–15 minutes as needed		

BD, twice a day.

TABLE 36: Dosing recommendations for serotonin receptor agents

Drugs	Starting adult daily dose	Daily dose range	Frequency of dose/day
Ketanserin (antagonizes serotonin S2 receptor in peripheral vasculature and α1 adrenergic receptors)	20 mg BD	40–80 mg	2
	Intravenous dose for hypertensive emergencies: (a) 5–30 mg infused at 3 mg/min, or (b) repeated injections of 5 mg every few minutes, or (c) 5 mg bolus doses every 10 minutes followed by infusion of 5–10 mg/hour		
Urapidil (stimulates central serotonin 1A receptors and antagonizes peripheral α1 adrenergic receptors)	30 mg OD or BD	30–180 mg (above 30 mg, use BD)	1–2
	Intravenous dose for hypertensive emergencies: 25 mg over 20 seconds. May repeat 25 mg after 5 minutes and 50 mg after another 5 minutes, then continuous infusion 9–30 mg/hour		

OD, once a day; BD, twice a day.

TABLE 37: Dosing recommendations for dopamine agonists (peripheral D1 receptor)

Drugs	Starting adult daily dose	Daily dose range	Frequency of dose/day
Fenoldopam mesylate (severe hypertension)	Intravenous use: 0.03–0.1 mg/kg/min	Usual effective dose: 0.1–1.6 mg/kg/min	Increase or decrease by 0.05–0.1 mg/kg/min no sooner than every 15 minutes, use up to 48 hours

TABLE 38: Major drug combinations used in trials of antihypertensive treatment in a step-up approach or as a randomized control

Trial	Comparator	Type of patients	SBP diff (mmHg)	Outcomes
ACE-I and diuretic combination				
PROGRESS	Placebo	Previous stroke or TIA	−9	−28% strokes (P <0.001)
ADVANCE	Placebo	Diabetes	−5.6	−9% micro/macro vascular events (P = 0.04)
HYVET	Placebo	Hypertensives aged ≥80 years	−15	−34% CV events (P <0.001)
CAPPP	BB + D	Hypertensives	+3	+5% CV events (P = NS)
Angiotensin receptor blocker and diuretic combination				
SCOPE	D + placebo	Hypertensives aged ≥70 years	−3.2	−28% non fatal strokes (P = 0.04)
LIFE	BB + D	Hypertensives with LVH	−1	−26% stroke (P <0.001)
Calcium antagonist and diuretic combination				
FEVER	D + placebo	Hypertensives	−4	−27% CV events (P <0.001)
ELSA	BB + D	Hypertensives	0	NS difference in CV events
CONVINCE	BB + D	Hypertensives with risk factors	0	NS difference in CV events
VALUE	ARB + D	High-risk hypertensives	−2.2	−3% CV events (P = NS)

(continued)

Table 38 (continued)

Trial	Comparator	Type of patients	SBF diff (mmHg)	Outcomes
ACE-I and calcium antagonist combination				
SystEur	Placebo	Elderly with ISH	−10	−31% CV events (P <0.001)
SystChina	Placebo	Elderly with ISH	−9	−37% CV events (P <0.004)
NORDIL	BB + D	Hypertensives	+3	NS difference in CV events
INVEST	BB + D	Hypertensives with CHD	0	NS difference in CV events
ASCOT	BB + D	Hypertensives with risk factors	−3	−16% CV events (P <0.001)
ACCOMPLISH	ACE-I + D	Hypertensives with risk factors	−1	−21% CV events (P <0.001)
BB and diuretic combination				
Coope & Warrender	Placebo	Elderly hypertensives	−8	−42% strokes (P <0.03)
SHEP	Placebo	Elderly with ISH	−3	−36% strokes (P <0.001)
STOP	Placebo	Elderly hypertensives	−23	−40% CV events (P = 0.003)
STOP	ACE-I or CA	Hypertensives	0	NS difference in CV events
CAPPP	ACE-I + D	Hypertensives	−3	−5% CV events (P = NS)
LIFE	ARB + D	Hypertensives with LVH	+1	+26% stroke (P <0.001)
ALLHAT	ACE-I + BB	Hypertensives with risk factors	−2	NS difference in CV events
ALLHAT	CA + BB	Hypertensives with risk factors	−1	NS difference in CV events

(continued)

Table 38 (*continued*)

Trial	Comparator	Type of patients	SBP diff (mmHg)	Outcomes
CONVINCE	CA + D	Hypertensives with risk factors	0	NS difference in CV events
NORDIL	ACE-I + CA	Hypertensives	−3	NS difference in CV events
INVEST	ACE-I + CA	Hypertensives with CHD	0	NS difference in CV events
ASCOT	ACE-I + CA	Hypertensives with risk factors	+3	+16% CV events (P <0.001)
Combination of two renin-angiotensin-system blockers / ACE-I + ARB or RAS blocker + renin inhibitor				
ONTARGET	ACE-I or ARB	High-risk patients	−3	More renal events
ALTITUDE	ACE-I or ARB	High-risk diabetics	−1.3	More renal events

ACE-I, angiotensin-converting-enzyme inhibitor; ARB, angiotensin receptor blocker; BB, β-blocker; CA, calcium antagonist; CHD, coronary heart disease; CV, cardiovascular; D, diuretic; ISH, isolated systolic hypertension; LVH, left ventricular hypertrophy; NS, not significant; RAS, renin angiotensin system; TIA, transient ischemic attack.

TABLE 39: Dosing recommendations for combinations with two diuretics

Drugs (Dose in mg)	Starting adult daily dose	Daily dose range	Frequency of dose/day
Altizide/spironolactone (15/25)	1/2–1 tab	1/2–2 mg	1
Bemetizide/triamterene (10/20, 25/50)	10/20 mg	10/20–25/50 mg	1
Butizide/spironolactone (2.5/25)	2 tab	2–4 tab (max: 8 tab/day)	1
Cyclopenthiazide/amiloride (0.25/2.5)	1 tab	1–2 mg	1
Epitizide/triamterene (4/50)	1 mg tab	1–4 mg	1
HCTZ/amiloride (50/5)	1/2 tab	1/2–2 tab	1
HCTZ/triamterene (25/37.5)	1 cap	1–2 cap	1–2
HCTZ/triamterene			
(50/75)	1/2 tab	1/2–1 tab	1
(25/37.5)	1 tab	1–2 tab	1
HCTZ/spironolactone			
(25/25)	1 tab	1–4 tab	1–2
(50/50)	1 tab	1–2 tab	1–2

HCTZ, hydrochlorothiazide; tab, tablet(s); cap, capsule(s).

TABLE 40: Dosing recommendations for combinations of β-blockers with diuretics

Drugs (Dose in mg)	Starting adult daily dose	Daily dose range	Frequency of dose/day
Atenolol/chlorthalidone (50/25, 100/25)	50/25 mg	Start 1 tab Increase to 100/25 mg	1 1
Bisoprolol/HCTZ (2.5/6.25, 5/6.25, 10/6.25)	2.5/6.25 mg	2.5/6.25–20/12.5 mg	1
Mepindolol/HCTZ (5/12.5)	1 tab	1–3 tab	1
Metoprolol/HCTZ (50/25, 100/25, 100/50)	50/25 mg 100/25 mg 100/50 mg	1 or 2 tab 1 or 2 tab 1 tab	1–2 1–2 1
Nadolol/bendroflumethazide (40/5, 80/5)	40/5 mg	Start 1 tab Increase to 80/5 mg	1 1
Pindolol/clopamide (10/5)	1/2–1 tab	Start 1/2 or 1 tab Increase to BD (maximum TID)	1
Propranolol/HCTZ (40/25, 80/25)	40/25 mg	Start BD Increase to 80/25 mg BD	2
Propranolol (extended-release)/HCTZ (80/50, 120/50, 160/50)	80/50 mg 120/50 mg 160/50 mg	Start OD Increase OD Increase OD	1 1 1
Timolol/HCTZ (10/25)	1 tab	1 tab BD or 2 tab OD	1–2

HCTZ, hydrochlorothiazide; tab, tablet(s); OD, once aday; BD, twice a day; TID, thrice a day.

TABLE 41: Dosing recommendations for combinations of angiotensin-converting enzyme inhibitors with diuretics

Drugs (Dose in mg)	Starting adult daily dose (mg)	Daily dose range (mg)	Frequency of dose/day
Benazepril/HCTZ (5/6.25, 10/12.5, 20/12.5, 20/25)	5/6.25 10/12.5	Start with 5/6.25 Titrate to maximum of each: benazepril 80 HCTZ 50	1 1
Captopril/HCTZ (25/15, 25/25, 50/15, 50/25)	25/15	Start OD Titrate to maximum 150/50	1 1 or 2
Enalapril/HCTZ (5/12.5, 10/25)	5/12.5 10/25	Start OD Titrate to maximum 20/50	1 1 (or 2)
Fosinopril/HCTZ (10/12.5, 20/12.5)	10/12.5	Start with 10/12.5 Maximum dose: fosinopril 80, HCTZ 50	1
Lisinopril/HCTZ (10/12.5, 20/12.5, 20/25)	10/12.5 20/12.5	Start OD Titrate to maximum 80/50	1 1
Moexipril/HCTZ (7.5/12.5, 15/12.5, 15/25)	7.5/12.5	3.75/6.25 (1/2 tab) or 7.5/12.5 to start, titrate to maximum 30/50	1 (or 2)
Quinapril/HCTZ (10/12.5, 20/12.5, 20/25)	10/12.5	Start with 20/12.5, titrate to maximum dose: quinapril 80, HCTZ 50	1 (or 2)

HCTZ, hydrochlorothiazide; OD, once a day.

TABLE 42: Dosing recommendations for combinations of angiotensin II receptor blockers with diuretics

Drugs (Dose in mg)	Starting adult daily dose (mg)	Daily dose range (mg)	Frequency of dose/day
Candesartan/HCTZ (16/12.5, 32/12.5, 32/25)	16/12.5	16/12.5–32/25	1
Azilsartan/chlorthalidine (40/12.5, 40/25)	40/12.5	40/12.5–40/25	1
Eprosartan/HCTZ (600/12.5, 600/25)	600/12.5	600/12.5–600/25	1
Irbesartan/HCTZ (150/12.5, 300/12.5, 300/25)	150/12.5	150/12.5–300/25	1
Losartan/HCTZ (50/12.5, 100/12.5, 100/25)	50/12.5	50/12.5–100/25	1
Olmesartan/HCTZ (20/12.5, 40/12.5, 40/25)	20/12.5	20/12.5–40/25	1
Telmisartan/HCTZ (40/12.5, 80/12.5, 80/25)	40/12.5	40/12.5–80/25	1
Valsartan/HCTZ (80/12.5, 160/12.5)	80/12.5 or 160/12.5	80/12.5–320/25	1

HCTZ, hydrochlorothiazide..

TABLE 43: Dosing recommendations for combinations of direct renin inhibitors with other antihypertensives

Drugs (Dose in mg)	Starting adult daily dose (mg)	Daily dose range (mg)	Frequency of dose/day
Aliskiren/amlodipine (150/5, 150/10, 300/5, 300/10)	150/5	150/5–300/10	1
Aliskiren/HCTZ (150/12.5, 150/25, 300/12.5, 300/25)	150/12.5	150/12.5–300/25	1
Aliskiren/valsartan (150/160, 300/320)	150/160	150/160–300/320	1

HCTZ, hydrochlorothiazide.

TABLE 44: Dosing recommendations for combinations of calcium channel blockers and angiotensin-converting enzymes inhibitors

Drugs (Dose in mg)	Starting adult daily dose	Daily dose range	Frequency of dose/day
Perindopril/amlodipine 3.25/2.5, 7/5, 14/10	3.25/2.5 mg	Maximum: Perindopril 14 mg/amlodipine 10 mg	1
Amlodipine/benazepril (2.5/10, 5/10, 5/20, 5/40, 10/20, 10/40)	2.5/10 mg	2.5/10–10/40 mg	1
Diltiazem/enalapril (180/5)	1 tab	1–2 tab	1
Felodipine extended-release/enalapril (2.5/5, 5/5)	2.5/5 mg or 5/5 mg	Increase to 10/10 mg	1
Verapamil extended-release/trandolapril (180/2, 240/1, 240/2, 240/4)	180/2 mg or 240/1 mg	Increase to maximum for each: Verapamil 480 mg, trandolapril 4 mg	1–2

tab, tablet(s)

TABLE 45: Dosing recommendations for combinations of calcium channel blockers and angiotensin II receptor blockers

Drugs (Dose in mg)	Starting adult daily dose (mg)	Daily dose range (mg)	Frequency of dose/day
Amlodipine/olmesartan (5/20, 5/40, 10/20, 10/40)	5/20	5/20–10/40	1
Amlodipine/telmisartan (5/40, 5/80, 10/40, 10/80)	5/40	5/40–10/80	1
Amlodipine/valsartan	5/160	5/160–10/320	1

TABLE 46: Dosing recommendations for combinations of Rauwolfia alkaloids and other antihypertensive agents

Drugs (Dose in mg)	Starting adult daily dose	Daily dose range	Frequency of dose/day
Chlorthalidone/reserpine (50/0.25) (25/0.125)	50/0.25 mg 25/0.125 mg	1 tab 1–2 tab	1 1
Chlorothiazide/reserpine (250/0.125) (500/0.125)	1 tab OD 1 tab OD	1 or 2 tab OD or BD 1 tab OD or BD (avoid chronic reserpine dose above 0.25 mg/day)	1–2 1–2
Hydrochlorothiazide/reserpine (25/0.125) (50/0.125)	1 tab 1 tab	1–2 tab 1 tab	1 1
Methyclothiazide/deserpidine (5/0.25) (5/0.5)	1/2 or 1 tab 1/2 or 1 tab	1/2 to 2 tab 1/2 to 2 tab	1 1
Polythiazide and reserpine	1/2 or 1 tab	1/2–2 tab (avoid chronic reserpine dose above 0.25 mg/day)	1

OD, once a day; BD, twice a day; tab, tablet(s).

TABLE 47: Dosing recommendations for other combinations of two antihypertensive drugs

Drugs (Dose in mg)	Starting adult daily dose	Daily dose range	Frequency of dose/day
Clonidine/chlorthalidone (0.1/15, 0.2/15, 0.3/15)	0.1/15 mg OD	0.1/15 mg OD to maximum 0.3/15 mg ED	1–2
Guanethidine/HCTZ (10/25)	1 tab	1–2 tab (average dose for guanethidine is 25–50 mg/day and HCTZ dose usual maximum 50 mg/day) Increase to maximum for each: Hydralazine 300 mg, HCTZ 50 mg	1–2
Hydralazine/HCTZ (25/25, 50/50, 100/50)	25/25 mg BD	(100 mg)	2
Methyldopa/HCTZ (250/15, 500/30, 500/50)	250/15 mg BD (or TID)	Increase to maximum HCTZ dose of 50 mg	2–3
Prazosin/polythiazide (1/0.5, 2/0.5, 5/0.5)	1/0.5 mg BD (or TID)	Increase daily dose to maximum: Prazosin 20 mg and/or polythiazide 4 mg	2–3

HCTZ, hydrochlorothiazide; OD, once a day; BD, twice a day; TID, thrice a day; tab, tablet(s).

TABLE 48: Dosing recommendations for combinations of three antihypertensive drugs

Drugs (Dose in mg)	Starting adult daily dose	Daily dose range	Frequency of dose/day
Amlodipine and olmesartan and HCTZ 5/20/12.5, 5/40/12.5, 5/40/25, 10/40/12.5, 10/40/25	5/20/12.5 mg	5/20/12.5 mg, titrate to maximum 10/40/25 mg	1
Amlodipine and valsartan and HCTZ 5/160/12.5, 10/160/12.5, 5/160/25, 10/160/25, 10/320/25	5/160/12.5 mg	5/160/12.5 mg, titrate to maximum 10/320/25 mg	1
Aliskiren and amlodipine and HCTZ 150/5/12.5, 300/5/12.5, 300/5/25, 300/10/12.5, 300/10/25	150/5/12.5 mg	150/5/12.5 mg, titrate to maximum 300/10/25 mg	1
Hydralazine and HCTZ and reserpine 25/15/0.1	1 tab	1 or 2 tab (avoid chronic reserpine dose above 0.25 mg/day)	1

HCTZ, hydrochlorothiazide; tab, tablet(s).

TABLE 49: Dosing recommendations for combinations which include antihypertensive drugs

Drugs (Dose in mg)	Starting adult daily dose	Daily dose range	Frequency of dose/day
Amlodipine and atorvastatin 2.5/10, 2.5/20, 2.5/40, 5/10, 5/20, 5/40, 5/80, 10/10, 10/20, 10/40, 10/80	2.5/10 or 5/10 mg	2.5/10 mg, increase to maximum 10/80 mg	1
Hydralazine and isosorbide dinitrate 37.5/20	37.5/20 mg TID	1/2 tab up to 2 tab TID	3

TID, thrice a day; tab, tablet(s).

TABLE 50: Evidence-based dosing for antihypertensive drugs (JNC-8)

Antihypertensive medication	Initial daily dose, mg	Target dose in RCTs reviewed, mg	No. of doses per day
ACE inhibitors			
Captopril	50	150–200	2
Enalapril	5	20	1–2
Lisinopril	10	40	1
Angiotensin receptor blockers			
Eprosartan	400	600–800	1–2
Candesartan	4	12–32	1
Losartan	50	100	1–2
Valsartan	40–80	160–320	1
Irbesartan	75	300	1

(continued)

Table 50 (*continued*)

Antihypertensive medication	Initial daily dose, mg	Target dose in RCTs reviewed, mg	No. of doses per day
β-Blockers			
Atenolol	25–50	100	1
Metoprolol	50	100–200	1–2
Calcium channel blockers			
Amlodipine	2.5	10	1
Diltiazem extended release	120–180	360	1
Nitrendipine	10	20	1–2
Thiazide-type diuretics			
Bendroflumethiazide	5	10	1
Chlorthalidone	12.5	12.5–25	1
Hydrochlorothiazide	12.5–25	25–100[a]	1–2
Indapamide	1.25	1.25–2.5	1

ACE, angiotensin-converting enzyme; RCT, randomized controlled trial. [a]Current recommended evidence-based dose that balances efficacy and safety is 25–50 mg daily.

TABLE 51: Diuretics—Side effects and cautions

Drugs	Frequent or severe side effects	Caution
Thiazides (multiple) chlorthalidone	Decreases serum K$^+$, Mg^{2+}, Na$^+$, HDL. Increases glucose, serum effective at GFR <30 mL/min), pancreatitis, hyponatremia, lithium (decreased uric acid, Ca^{2+}, triglycerides, LDL. Pancreatitis, erectile dysfunction	Digitalis and hypokalemia (arrhythmias), gout, renal insufficiency (may not be excretion), sulfa allergy*
Loop-furosemide, ethacrynic acid, bumetanide, torsemide	Decreases serum K$^+$, Mg^{2+}, Ca^{2+}, HDL. Increases glucose, serum uric acid, triglycerides, LDL. Volume depletion, metabolic alkalosis	Digitalis and hypokalemia (arrhythmias), gout, excessive diuresis, ototoxicity (ethacrynic acid worse than furosemide, torsemide and bumetanide), hyponatremia, lithium (decreased excretion), effect blunted by NSAIDs, sulfa allergy*
Potassium sparing diuretics spironolactone, eplerenone	Increases serum K$^+$, gynecomastia (men), hair growth (women) (less with eplerenone). Decreases HDL, triglycerides (modest effect). Libido, gastrointestinal symptoms (gastric hemorrhage-spironolactone), impotence, menstrual irregularities, agranulocytosis, tumorigenic in rats	Hyperkalemia, CKD (GFR <50 mL/min), use with cyp3a4 inhibitors (multiple drugs), ACEIs, ARBs, renin inhibitors, other K$^+$ sparing diuretics, lithium, NSAIDs, type 2 diabetes mellitus. Safety in pregnancy (teratogenic in animal studies), peptic ulcer disease (upper gastrointestinal bleeding)
Trimaterene	Increases serum K$^+$, nausea	Nephrolithiasis, hyperkalemia, CKD (GFR <50 mL/min), ACEIs, ARBs, renin inhibitors, other K$^+$ sparing diuretics, lithium, NSAIDs, cyclosporine, black licorice
Amiloride	Increases serum K$^+$	Hyperkalemia, CKD (GFR <50 mL/min), ACEIs, ARBs, renin inhibitors, other K$^+$ sparing diuretics, lithium, NSAIDs, cyclosporine, tacrolimus, black licorice

*If sulfa allergy is present, may use: amiloride, eplerenone, ethacrynic acid, spironolactone, triamterene.
NSAIDs, nonsteroidal anti-inflammatory drugs; GFR, glomerular filtration rate; ACEIs, angiotensin-converting enzyme inhibitors; HDL, high-density lipoproteins; LDL, low-density lipoproteins; ARBs, angiotensin II receptor blockers; CKD, chronic kidney disease; K$^+$, potassium; Mg^{2+}, magnesium; Na$^+$, sodium; Ca^{2+}, calcium.

TABLE 52: Central sympatholytic agents and central depleting agents of catecholamines and 5-hydroxytryptophan—side effects and cautions

Drugs	Frequent or severe side effects	Caution
Central sympatholytic action (α2 adrenergic agonists)		
Clonidine*	Dry mouth, somnolence, sedation, drowsiness, fatigue, dizziness, constipation, AV block, lipid (neutral) with patches—contact dermatitis (5–47%), erythema (26%)	Rebound hypertension and arrythmias with abrupt withdrawal, use with other depressants
Guanabenz Guanfacine	Dry mouth, somnolence, sedation, weakness, dizziness, arrhythmias, orthostatic hypotension, impotence, small decrease in total cholesterol and triglycerides, similar to clonidine, reduction in HDL with guanabenz	Rebound hypertension with abrupt withdrawal
Methyldopa	Drowsiness, fatigue, dizziness, dry mouth, fever, edema, hepatotoxicity, bone marrow depression, red cell aplasia, abnormal cardiac conduction, parkinsonism, impotence, reduces HDL	Hepatic disease, hemolytic anemia (Coombs' positive), fever
Central depleting agents of catecholamines and 5-hydroxytryptophan (Rauwolfia alkaloids)		
Reserpine	Depression (6–30%), nasal congestion, lethargy, hematemesis, nausea, vomiting, dry mouth atrial fibrillation, arrhythmias, orthostatic hypotension, wheezing	Mental depression, peptic ulcer disease, asthma

*Except clonidine, centrally acting sympatholytic drugs are not used for treatment of hypertension.

AV, atrioventricular; HDL, high-density lipoproteins.

TABLE 53: Central imidazoline receptor agonists—side effects and cautions

Drugs	Frequent or severe side effects	Caution
Moxonidine Rilmenidine	Dry mouth, somnolence, headache, dizziness, vertigo, edema, nervousness, diuresis	Severe coronary insufficiency, SA and AV conduction defects, CKD (especially serum creatinine >1.8 mg/dL (159.1 μmol/L) and GFR <30 mL/min), angioedema, claudication, Raynaud's disease, Parkinson's disease, depression

SA, sinoatrio; AV, atrioventricular; CKD, chronic kidney disease; GFR, glomerular filtration rate.

TABLE 54: Ganglionic and postganglionic blockers—side effects and cautions

Drugs	Frequent or severe side effects	Caution
Ganglionic blockers*		
Trimethaphan (intravenous) Mecamylamine (oral tablet)	Intravenous use in emergencies (e.g., acute aortic dissection), postural hypotension, syncope, paralytic ileus, constipation, nausea, vomiting, dry mouth, angina pectoris, urinary retention, blurred vision (mydriasis, diplopia), respiratory depression (fatal respiratory arrest with dose >5 mg/min), asthma, impaired cognition, weakness	CAD, heart failure, CKD, cerebral vascular disease, chronic lung disease, bladder outlet obstruction, gastrointestinal obstruction, abrupt withdrawal (rebound hypertension)
Postganglionic blockers*		
Guanethidine	Postural hypotension, dizziness, weakness, drowsiness, fluid retention, diarrhea, leg cramps, inhibition of ejaculation, impotence, blurred vision, nasal congestion	Heart failure, CKD, CAD, bradycardia, cerebral vascular disease, peptic ulcer disease, anesthesia (stop guanethidine 48–72 hours before), asthma, patients with pheochromocytoma
Bethanidine	As with guanethidine	As with guanethidine
Debrisoquine	As with guanethidine	As with guanethidine
Guanadrel	Shorter-acting than guanethidine	As with guanethidine
MAOIs	Rarely used. CNS disturbances—dizziness, headache, blurred vision, vertigo, insomnia. Postural hypotension, vomiting, muscle twitching, fever	Foods with tryamine produce increased blood pressure (extensive list includes most cheese, alcohol, chocolate, and foods that are pickled, aged, fermented, or smoked), never use with methyldopa

*Presently ganglionic and postganglionic blockers are seldom used for long-term treatment of hypertension because of their side effects.

MAOIs, monoamine oxidase inhibitors; CNS, central nervous system; CKD, chronic kidney disease; CAD, coronary artery disease.

TABLE 55: Lipid solubility of β-adrenergic receptors

Low lipid solubility/hydrophilic

Atenolol	Labetalol*	Carteolol*	Nadolol
Esmolol	Sotalol		

Lipophilic

Acebutolol*	Betaxolol	Bisoprolol	Bucindolol*
Carvedilol	Celiprolol, metoprolol	Penbutolol*	Pindolol*
Propranolol	Timolol		

*Intrinsic sympathomimetic activity.

TABLE 56: Adrenergic receptor blockers—side effects and cautions

Drugs	Frequent or severe side effects	Caution
β-blockers		
Nonselective (β1 and β2 receptor antagonists: tend to be lipophilic and metabolized by the liver)		
Nadolol	Similar to propranolol but hydrophilic and low CNS concentration with less CNS side effects, longer half-life	Similar to propranolol, acute kidney injury, CKD
Carteolol, penbutolol, pindolol and other nonselective β-blockers with ISA	Similar to propranolol but has ISA, less bradycardia, less effect on lipids, may not be cardioprotective after MI	Similar to propranolol, carteolol—renal insufficiency, penbutolol—hepatic dysfunction

(continued)

Table 56 (continued)

Drugs	Frequent or severe side effects	Caution
Propranolol, timolol, and other nonselective β-blockers without ISA	Bradycardia, anorexia, fatigue, sleep disturbance, dizziness, depression, first-degree AV block, bronchospasm, hypoglycemia, hypotension, reduces exercise tolerance, raises or does not affect total cholesterol and LDL, lowers HDL, increases triglycerides, cardioprotective after MI, timolol—less CNS effect (propranolol and timolol are lipophilic and CNS concentrations are higher compared to hydrophilic β-blockers)	Heart failure, second- or third-degree heart block, ventricular dysrhythmias, COPD, asthma, peripheral vascular disease, insulin dependent diabetics (may mask hypoglycemia), hyperkalemia (K^+ translocation into cells is mediated in part by β2 receptors), avoid abrupt withdrawal especially in CAD
Cardioselective (β1 selective: tend to be hydrophilic and removed by the kidneys)		
Acebutolol and other cardio-selective β-blockers with ISA	Relatively selective β1 blocker once a day, similar to atenolol but has ISA, less bradycardia, overall fewer side effects than atenolol, less effect on lipids, may not be cardioprotective after MI	Similar to atenolol, avoid abrupt withdrawal especially in CAD
Atenolol, metoprol, betaxolol, bisoprolol, and other cardioselective β-blockers without ISA	Relatively selective β1 blocker at lower doses. Bradycardia, somnolence, dizziness, depression (less than propranolol), cold extremities, bronchospasm, hypoglycemia, hypotension, reduced exercise tolerance. Raises or does not affect total cholesterol and LDL, lowers HDL, increases triglycerides. Cardioprotective after MI. Atenolol preferred in hepatic insufficiency. Metoprolol preferred in CKD	COPD, asthma, peripheral vascular disease (at low doses, less effect on bronchial and vascular smooth muscle than nonselective β-blockers), heart failure, second- or third-degree heart block ventricular dysrhythmias, insulin dependent diabetics (may mask hypoglycemia), hyperkalemia, atenolol with GFR <35 mL/min. Avoid abrupt withdrawal, especially in CAD
β-blockers with vasodilating properties		
Labetalol (with ISA), carvedilol, and other β-blockers with vasodilating properties	From nonselective β-blockade: Dizziness, somnolence, GI (nausea 14%), hypotension, postural hypotension (5%), wheezing, bronchospasm. From α-blockade: nasal stuffiness, sexual dysfunction, urinary retention, lipid neutral, may not be cardioprotective after MI	Similar to propranolol. Concomitant diuretics and high doses produce dizziness. Heart failure, second- or third-degree heart block, COPD, asthma, insulin dependent diabetics (may mask hypoglycemia), hepatic impairment, hyperkalemia. Peripheral vascular disease. Avoid abrupt withdrawal, especially in CAD

(continued)

Table 56 (continued)

Drugs	Frequent or severe side effects	Caution
Nebivolol	Similar to labetalol, increases triglycerides, decreases HDL	Similar to abetalol, peripheral vascular disease. Avoid concomitant use with other β-blockers, verapamil, diltiazem, clonidine. Avoid use with CYP2D6 inhibitors which raise nebivolol levels)
		Strong inhibitors: Fluoxetine, paroxetine (SSRIS), bupropion (non-SSRI antidepressant), quinidine (class i antiarrhythmic agent), cinacalcet (calcimimetic), ritonavir (antiretroviral)
		Moderate inhibitors: Sertraline (SSRI), duloxetine, terbinafine, and others)
α-adrenergic receptor antagonists		
Prazosin, terazosin, doxazosin, and other α-blockers	"1st dose phenomenon" (syncope within 30–90 minutes of first dose due to excessive postural hypotension), postural hypotension, dizziness, asthenia, somnolence, palpitations, tachycardia, fluid retention. Nasal congestion, vasculitis, intraoperative floppy iris syndrome. Reduces total cholesterol, triglycerides, LDL and elevates HDL	Avoid use as first-line treatment and single agent treatment (excessive risk of heart failure shown with doxazosin (ALLHAT clinical trial). 1st dose syncope, increased potential for hypotension when used with other antihypertensives (β-blockers and diuretics). Cataract surgery [intraoperative floppy iris syndrome, especially with α-blockers used for BPH (tamsulosin, silodosin)]
Phentolamine, phenoxybenzamine	Similar to prazosin; postural hypotension, tachycardia (used in pheochromocytoma or clonidine rebound)	Cerebral or coronary atherosclerosis, angina pectoris, MI, exercise, volume depletion

ISA, intrinsic sympathomimetic activity; CNS, central nervous system; AV, atrioventricular; HDL, high-density lipoproteins; LDL, low-density lipoproteins; COPD, chronic obstructive pulmonary disease; GFR, glomerular filtration rate; ALLHAT, antihypertensive and lipid-lowering treatment to prevent heart attack trial; SSRIs, selective serotonin reuptake inhibitors; CKD, chronic kidney disease; BPH, benign prostatic hypertrophy; MI, myocardial infarction; CAD, coronary artery disease; GI, gastrointestinal.

TABLE 57: Direct vasodilators—side effects and cautions

Drugs	Frequent or severe side effects	Caution
Oral acting		
Hydralazine and other direct vasodilators	Headaches, tachycardia, palpitations, angina pectoris, anorexia, nausea, hypotension (intravenous), SLE, fluid retention, peripheral neuritis, hepatitis. No effect on triglycerides. May increase HDL and decrease LDL	Contraindicated in aortic dissection Caution: History of CAD, cerebrovascular disease, SLE, systemic hypertension reported in pulmonary hypertension
Minoxidil	Tachycardia, palpitations, edema, hypertrichosis, hirsutism, hypotension, may be associated with pericardial effusion, pericardial tamponade (especially in CKD), thrombocytopenia, leukopenia. Effect on lipids same as hydralazine	Avoid: Pheochromocytoma, use with guanethidine Caution: CAD, cerebrovascular disease, CHF, pericarditis, CKD hemodialysis
Intravenous use for hypertensive emergencies (vasodilators)		
Diazoxide	Hypotension, palpitations, tachycardia, MI, dizziness, weakness, salt and water retention, hyperglycemia, ketoacidosis, nonketotic hyperosmolar coma, extrapyramidal signs, increased uric acid, hypertrichosis	Marked hypotension with other antihypertensives, concomitant use with coumarin anticoagulants (warfarin and others—increased risk of bleeding), CAD, gout, CKD
Sodium nitroprusside	Hypotension, nausea, vomiting, dizziness, somnolence, headache, palpitations, tachycardia	Cyanide toxicity (can be lethal)—monitor acidosis, thiocyanate toxicity, CHF with decreased peripheral vascular resistance rebound hypertension after cessation of drug, hypothyroidism

LDL, low-density lipoprotein; HDL, high-density lipoprotein; SLE, systemic lupus erythematosus; CKD, chronic kidney disease; CAD, coronary artery disease; CHF, congestive heart failure; MI, myocardial infarction.

TABLE 58: Inhibitors of renin-angiotensin system*—side effects and cautions

Drugs	Frequent or severe side effects	Caution
ACEIs		
Captopril	Cough, bronchospasm, acute renal failure with bilateral renal artery stenosis, or unilateral renal artery stenosis in solitary kidney, worsening renal insufficiency, hypotension if volume depleted, dysgeusia, rash, SLE-like syndrome, bone marrow depression, hyperkalemia, angioedema, cholestatic jaundice. Effect on lipids: Some studies, no effect; others, increase HDL and lowered LDL and triglycerides	Avoid: Pregnancy, discontinue as soon as possible (causes fetal injury and increased fetal mortality), angioedema history Caution: Bilateral renal artery stenosis, volume depletion or severe CHF, CKD-reduce dose for GFR <50 mL/min, CKD and/or, collagen vascular disease (may lead to blood dyscrasia), hemodialysis with high-flux membranes [pan (polyacrylonitrile)] may produce anaphylactoid reaction, aortic stenosis
Benazepril, enalapril, fosinopril, lisinopril, moexipril, perindopril, quinapril, ramipril, trandolapril, and other ACEIs	Side effects are similar to captopril but may be less as enalapril and others lack S-H group. Enalapril: pancreatitis (half cases due to enalapril; others due to captopril, lisinopril: lysine analogue of enalapril), otherwise similar to captopril	Same as captopril, creatinine clearance <30–40 mL/min, may need to decrease dose
ARBs		
Azilsartan, candesartan, eprosartan, irbesartan, losartan, olmesartan, telmisartan, valsartan	Headache, dizziness, asthenia, fatigue, dysgeusia, acute kidney injury (acute renal failure) with bilateral renal artery stenosis, or unilateral renal artery stenosis in solitary kidney, worsening renal insufficiency, hypotension if volume depleted, cough and angioedema are significantly less than ACEIs. Losartan uniquely lowers serum uric acid. Effect on lipids: some studies, no effect; others, studies show, increases in HDL cholesterol and decreases in LDL and triglycerides	Avoid: Pregnancy, discontinue as soon as possible (causes oligohydramnios, fetal injury and increased fetal mortality) May increase serum K+, BUN, creatinine (especially in CKD, bilateral renal artery stenosis), orthostatic hypotension if volume depleted, severe CHF, angioedema history. Losartan use with rifampin or fluconazole

(continued)

Table 58 (continued)

Drugs	Frequent or severe side effects	Caution
DRI		
Aliskiren	Dizziness, headache, hyperkalemia (especially in CKD), hypotension (especially with volume depletion or other anti-hypertensive drugs), increased BUN and creatinine (minor), acute kidney injury (similar to ACEIs and ARBs), rash, diarrhea, angioedema (rare), less cough than ACEIs	Avoid: Pregnancy, discontinue as soon as possible (causes fetal injury and increased fetal mortality); avoid with ACEIs, cyclosporine, itraconazole Caution: Volume depletion

*Renin-angiotensin inhibitors are valuable armamentarium for management of hypertension. Combination of ACEIs and ARBs and direct renin inhibitors are not recommended (may produce worse renal outcomes).

SLE, systemic lupus erythematosus; CKD, chronic kidney disease; LDL, low-density lipoproteins; HDL, high-density lipoproteins; BUN, blood urea nitrogen; ACEIs, angiotensin-converting enzyme inhibitors; ARBs, angiotensin II receptor blockers; GFR, glomerular filtration rate; CHF, congestive heart failure; DRI, direct renin inhibitor.

TABLE 59: Calcium channel blockers*—side effects and cautions

Drugs	Frequent or severe side effects	Caution
Benzothiazepines (block L-type channels)		
Diltiazem	Bradyarrhythmia, cardiac conduction defect, hypotension, gingival hyperplasia (21%), edema (4.6–8%), dizziness, headache, asthenia, agranulocytosis, SLE, cognitive decline, acute renal failure (rare). Lipids (neutral) or may increase HDL and decrease triglycerides	General comments: (i) cimetidine (and drugs that decrease hepatic blood flow) may increase drug levels, (ii) CCBs may increase digoxin levels. Contraindicated: acute MI with pulmonary congestion, atrial fibrillation or flutter with accessory bypass tract (Wolff-Parkinson-White), cardiogenic shock, second or third degree heart block, ventricular tachycardia, aortic stenosis.

(continued)

Table 59 (continued)

Drugs	Frequent or severe side effects	Caution
		Caution: CKD, use with β-blockers, impaired hepatic function, cyclosporine (levels increased), (many drug-drug interactions) (grape-fruit juice does not increase plasma levels of diltiazem)
Dihydropyridines (block L-type channels)		
Dihydropyridines: Amlodipine, felodipine, isradipine, nicardipine, nifedipine, nisoldipine and others Note: Side effects are mainly due to powerful vasodilation. Short-acting nifedipine has the highest frequency of side effects, which are less with sustained-release nifedipine and newer longer-acting dihydropyridines. In general, the minimal influence on cardiac conduction and decreased heart contractility are less in 2nd and 3rd generation dihydropyridines compared to 1st generation	Peripheral edema (7–29%), reflex tachycardia (most likely with 1st generation nifedipine), palpitations, hypotension (5%, especially with β-blockers), dizziness (4–10%), flushing (4%), headache (19–23%), increased angina pectoris, acute MI, CHF (tight aortic stenosis, with β-blockers), asthenia (4–12%), nausea (10%), gastrointestinal obstruction (bezoar), gingval hyperplasia [especially nifedipine, nicardipine, felodipine (40%)], increased BUN and creatinine (in CKD), Parkinson-like syndrome, tremor (8%), agranulocytosis (rare, fatal cases). Nicardipine may cross the blood-brain barrier and produce cerebral vasodilation. Lipids (neutral) or increase HDL	Contraindications: Cardiogenic shock, flecainide (increased flecainide side effects), concomitant use of strong cyp3a4 inducers (carbamazepine, phenytoin, oxcarbazepine, barbiturates, St John's wort, rifampicin, rifabutin, efavirenz, nevirapine, pioglitazone, troglitazone, glucocorticoids, modafinil, and others) Caution: Aortic stenosis, heart failure, surgery with high dose fentanyl anesthesia, abrupt withdrawal (may lead to rebound hypertension), hepatic impairment Some drug-drug interactions: cyclosporine levels increased with amlodipine, felodipine, and nicardipine, but not with isradipine or nifedipine, grape-fruit juice increases plasma levels
Nimodipine US FDA indication: Subarachnoid hemorrhage, from ruptured intracranial berry aneurysms (Hunt and Hess grades 1–5)	Greater effect to dilate cerebral vessels compared to coronary or peripheral vessels (crosses blood-brain barrier), excess bleeding during elective heart valve surgery, rarely thrombocytopenia, hypotension, similar to nifedipine, both tachycardia and bradycardia	Warning: Do not give intravenously or parenterally (deaths reported). Do not use perioperatively Caution: Hepatic impairment, similar to nifedipine

(continued)

Table 59 (*continued*)

Drugs	Frequent or severe side effects	Caution
Phenylalkylamines (block L-type channels)		
Verapamil	Negative inotropic effect, CHF, decreased SA node discharge and AV conduction, bradyarrhythmias, ventricular tachycardia, hypotension, cardiogenic shock, atrial fibrillation (especially with paroxysmal atrial fibrillation), dizziness (3–5.9%), headache (2.2–12.1%), constipation (8.8–42%), nausea, gingival hyperplasia (20%), dyspnea, cough Lipids (neutral) or increase HDL	Contraindications: Atrial fibrillation or flutter with accessory bypass tract (Wolff-Parkinson-White), left ventricular dysfunction (left ventricular ejection fraction <30%), CHF; 2nd or 3rd degrees heart block, sick sinus syndrome Caution: Hepatic impairment, abrupt withdrawal—increased angina pectoris in some, hypertrophic cardiomyopathy Drug-drug interactions: Quinidine produces hypotension and ventricular arrhythmias, decreased clearance of digoxin, β-blockers—left ventricular dysfunction and possible heart failure, cyclosporine levels increased (and many others) Grape-fruit juice increases plasma levels
Diarylaminopropylamine ester		
Bepridil (blocks slow calcium channel and fast sodium channel)	Proarrhythmic, including ventricular tachycardia (torsade de pointe) or fibrillation, prolongation QTC interval, death, lengthening of QRS, decreased left ventricular function, flushing, gingival hyperplasia, nausea, nervousness, dizziness (15%), asthenia (10%), headache (7%), tremor	Contraindications: Heart block, sick sinus, serious ventricular arrhythmias, QT prolongation, uncompensated cardiac insufficiency Caution: CHF, MI, hepatic and renal impairment, hypokalemia, sinus bradycardia, left bundle branch block

*CCBs are important antihypertensive drugs and are frequently used in clinical practice. These agents are also used for treatment of angina. Nondihydropyridine CCBs are also used for treatment of supraventricular tachycardias. In general, CCBs are contraindicated in patients with systolic heart failure (SHF).

**Dihydropyridines which cross the blood-brain barrier: Amlodipine, azelnidipine, clevidipine, clinidipine, felodipine, isradipine, nicardipine, nifedipine, nimodipine.

CCBs, calcium channel blockers; SLE, systemic lupus erythematosus; HDL, high-density lipoproteins; BUN, blood urea nitrogen; CKD, chronic kidney disease; SA, sinoatrial; AV, atrioventricular; CHF congestive heart failure; SHF, systolic heart failure; MI, myocardial infarction.

TABLE 60: Effects of various calcium channel blockers on selected cardiac and vascular functions

Drugs	Coronary vasodilation	Suppression		Negative inotropic effect	Vascular vasodilation	Side effects	Frequency of dose/day
		SA node	AV node				
Dihydropyridines							
Nifedipine*	5	0–1	0	1	3	3	1
Nimodipine*	5	0–1	0	0	3 (cerebral)	3	6
Nicardipine**	5	0–1	0	0	3	3	3
Nisoldipine**	5	0–1	0	0	3	3	1
Isradipine**	5	0	0	0	3	3	2
Felodipine**	5	0	0	0	3	3	1
Amlodipine***	5	0	0	0–1	3	3	1
Diltiazem*	3	5	4	2	2	1	1
Verapamil*	4	5	5	4	2	2	1

*, first generation; **, second generation; ***, third generation; numbers 0–5 indicate relative values of the effect; e.g., 0–1= least effect; 4–5 = greatest effect.

TABLE 61: Nitrates—side effects and caution

Drugs	Frequent or severe side effects	Caution
Nitroglycerin (intravenous)*	Headache (>60%), hypotension and severe orthostatic hypotension, increased angina pectoris, paradoxical bradyarrhythmia, fatal ventricular tachycardia (torsades de pointes)	Contraindications: Concomitant use of phosphodiesterase-5 inhibitors (sildenafil, tadalafil, vardenafil), other nitrates, constrictive pericarditis, pericardial tamponade, restrictive cardiomyopathy, early MI, increased intracranial pressure Caution: Volume depletion, CAD

*Intravenous nitroglycerin is occasionally used to control hypertension. It is more frequently used as an adjunctive treatment for acute coronary syndromes.

PDE-5i, phosphodiesterase-5 inhibitors; CAD, coronary artery disease; MI, myocardial infarction.

TABLE 62: Catecholamine synthesis inhibitor (tyrosine hydroxylase blocker) (for pheochromocytoma only)—side effects and cautions

Drugs	Frequent or severe side effects	Caution
Metyrosine	Diarrhea (10%), nausea, extrapyramidal symptoms (10%) (drooling, tremor, speech difficulty), lethargy, metyrosine crystalluria (needles or rods), slight gynecomastia, galactorrhea (infrequent)	Increased sedation with ethanol, CNS depressants, need for liberal fluid intake (>2 L/day) (to minimize crystalluria), rebound insomnia when discontinued

CNS, central nervous system.

TABLE 63: Potassium channel openers or activators—side effects and cautions

Drugs	Frequent or severe side effects	Caution
Minoxidil*	See vasodilators (oral acting) (Table 57)	
Nicorandil (also has nitrate-like actions—see Table 61)	Headache (22–48%), postural hypotension, palpitations, aphthous ulcers of the mouth (and infrequent ulcers in other parts of gastrointestinal tract), dizziness, fatigue, angioneurotic edema (rare), lipid (neutral)	Recent MI, hypotension, AV or intraventricular conduction disturbance, severe liver impairment, cerebral hemorrhage, recent head trauma, concomitant treatment with nitrates
Pinacidil	Peripheral edema (23.5–45.2%), reflex tachycardia, palpitations, headache, dizziness, somnolence, chest pain, depression. Effect on lipids: decreased LDL, and triglycerides, increased HDL	CAD, acutely after MI, cerebrovascular accidents, severe renal impairment
Diazoxide	See intravenous use for hypertensive emergencies (vasodilators) (Table 57)	

*Direct acting vasodilator minoxidil is used in patients with severe hypertension. Hair growth limits its use. It can also produce pericardial effusion. Potassium channel opener, such as nicorandil has been used in patients with angina. It is seldom used for treatment of hypertension.

AV, atrioventricular; LDL, low-density lipoproteins; HDL, high-density lipoproteins; MI, myocardial infarction; CAD, coronary artery disease.

TABLE 64: Serotonin receptor agents—side effects and cautions

Drugs	Frequent or severe side effects	Caution
Ketanserin	Sedation, fatigue, light-headedness, dizziness, headache, dry mouth, gastrointestinal disturbance, edema (better tolerated in the elderly compared to younger patients)	Contraindication: Second- and third-degrees atrioventricular heart block Caution: If QT is prolonged, ventricular arrhythmias (including torsades de pointes), liver cirrhosis Concomitant drugs: Diuretic use—avoid hypokalemia, β-blockers (may produce profound hypotension), other antiarrhythmic drugs
Urapidil	Dizziness, headache, fatigue, nausea, enuresis, palpitations (no tachycardia), edema, orthostatic hypotension, sleep disturbance, increased liver function tests, lipid (neutral)	Contraindication: Aortic stenosis Caution: Liver disease, moderate-to-severe renal impairment, head trauma (increased intracranial pressure), elderly Concomitant drugs: Cimetidine (need to reduce dose of urapidil)

*Serotonin receptor agents are seldom used for treatment of hypertension. They are prone to produce undesirable side effects.

TABLE 65: Dopamine agonists* (peripheral d1 receptors)—side effects and cautions

Drug	Frequent or severe side effects	Caution
Fenoldopam mesylate	Headache (10–54.5%), hypotension (5–18.2%), tachycardia (18.2%), atrial fibrillation, angina pectoris, MI, ECG changes (~12.9%) (ST-t changes, t-wave inversion), CHF, peripheral edema, hypokalemia, nausea (10%), vomiting (~18.2%), dizziness (~7.1%), flushing (~27.3%), increased IOP, backache (~18.2%), oliguria (~5%), increased serum creatinine (6.5%), reaction at injection site (3.8–18.2%), increased blood sugar (~5%)	Contraindication: Sensitivity to sulfites Caution: Glaucoma, hypotension, hypokalemia, tachycardia, liver disease Concomitant drugs: β-blockers (may cause severe hypotension)

*Dopamine agonists are used only acutely to control severe hypertension. Activation of dopamine 1 receptors induces peripheral vasodilatation and reduction in blood pressure.

ECG, electrocardiography; MI, myocardial infarction; IOP, intraocular pressure.

CONCLUSION

Hypertension is a common disorder and is frequently asymptomatic. It is a risk factor for CAD, stroke, peripheral vascular disease and chronic kidney disease (CKD). Adequate control of hypertension is associated with a reduction in the incidence of MI, stroke, congestive heart failure and progression of CKD. The desirable level of blood pressure varies according to comorbidity. For example, in diabetics with proteinuria, blood pressure should be reduced to a lower level than in nondiabetics or diabetics without proteinuria.

Several classes of antihypertensive drugs are available for treatment of hypertension. Frequently a combination of several classes of antihypertensive agents needs to be used for adequate control of hypertension. All classes of antihypertensive drugs can produce side effects. Some side effects are unique to a particular class of antihypertensive drugs. The dosing regimens of different drugs in the same class are variable. Constant vigilance is necessary to avoid side effects.

INVESTIGATIONAL, NONPHARMACOLOGIC MODALITIES FOR TREATING HYPERTENSION

Renal artery denervation: The Symplicity HTN-3 study was a blinded trial in 535 patients and did not show a significant reduction of systolic blood pressure in patients with resistant hypertension 6 months after renal-artery denervation as compared with a sham control. The future of this technique is uncertain.[61]

Baroreflex activation by carotid artery baroreceptor stimulation: This technique continues to be investigational with the Rheos Pivotal Trial and others supporting continued clinical research.[73-74]

Central iliac arteriovenous anastomosis: Investigational: A study was completed in which 195 patients with uncontrolled hypertension were randomized to implantation of an arteriovenous coupler device plus drug treatment or drug treatment alone. The A-V anastomosis significantly reduced blood pressure (ROX control HTN study).[75]

REFERENCES

1. James PA, Oparil S, Carter BL, et al. 2014 evidence-based guideline for the management of high blood pressure in adults: report from the panel members appointed to the Eighth Joint National Committee (JNC 8). JAMA. 2014;311(5):507-20.
2. Chobanian AV, Bakris GL, Black HR, et al. The Seventh Report of the Joint National Committee on Prevention, Detection, Evaluation, and Treatment of High Blood Pressure: the JNC 7 report. JAMA. 2003;289(19):2560-72.

3. Mancia G, De Backer G, Dominiczak A, et al. 2007 Guidelines for the Management of Arterial Hypertension: The Task Force for the Management of Arterial Hypertension of the European Society of Hypertension (ESH) and of the European Society of Cardiology (ESC). J Hypertens. 2007;25(6):1105-87.

4. Casas JP, Chua W, Loukogeorgakis S, et al. Effect of inhibitors of the renin-angiotensin system and other antihypertensive drugs on renal outcomes: systematic review and meta-analysis. Lancet. 2005;366(9502):2026-33.

5. Kent DM, Jafar TH, Hayward RA, et al. Progression risk, urinary protein excretion, and treatment effects of angiotensin-converting enzyme inhibitors in nondiabetic kidney disease. J Am Soc Nephrol. 2007;18(6):1959-65.

6. Lohr JW, Golzy M, Carter RL, et al. Elevated systolic blood pressure is associated with increased incidence of chronic kidney disease but not mortality in elderly veterans. J Am Soc Hypertens. 2015;9(1):29-37.

7. Randin D, Vollenweider P, Tappy L, et al. Suppression of alcohol-induced hypertension by dexamethasone. N Engl J Med. 1995;332(26):1733-7.

8. Klahr S, Levey AS, Beck GJ, et al. The effects of dietary protein restriction and blood-pressure control on the progression of chronic renal disease. Modification of Diet in Renal Disease Study Group. N Engl J Med. 1994;330:877-84.

9. Appel LJ, Wright JT, Greene T, et al. Intensive blood-pressure control in hypertensive chronic kidney disease. N Engl J Med. 2010;363(10):918-29.

10. Mann JFE. (2015). Choice of drug therapy in primary (essential) hypertension: Recommendations. [online] Available from: http://www.uptodate.com/contents/choice-of-drug-therapy-in-primary-essential-hypertension-recommendations. [Accessed in February, 2015].

11. ALLHAT Officers and Coordinators for the ALLHAT Collaborative Research Group. The Antihypertensive and Lipid-Lowering Treatment to Prevent Heart Attack Trial. Major outcomes in high-risk hypertensive patients randomized to angiotensin-converting enzyme inhibitor or calcium channel blocker vs diuretic: The Antihypertensive and Lipid-Lowering Treatment to Prevent Heart Attack Trial (ALLHAT). JAMA. 2002;288(23):2981-97.

12. Nissen SE, Tuzcu EM, Libby P, et al. Effect of antihypertensive agents on cardiovascular events in patients with coronary disease and normal blood pressure: the CAMELOT study: A randomized controlled trial. JAMA. 2004;292(18):2217-25.

13. Julius S, Kjeldsen SE, Weber M, et al. Outcomes in hypertensive patients at high cardiovascular risk treated with regimens based on valsartan or amlodipine: the VALUE randomized trial. Lancet. 2004;363(9426):2022-31.

14. Jamerson K, Weber MA, Bakris GL, et al. Benazepril plus amlodipine or hydrochlorothiazide for hypertension in high-risk patients. N Engl J Med. 2008;359(23):2417-28.

15. Prevention of stroke by antihypertensive drug treatment in older persons with isolated systolic hypertension. Final results of the Systolic Hypertension in the Elderly Program (SHEP). SHEP Cooperative Research Group. JAMA. 1991;265(24):3255-64.

16. Khan N, McAlister FA. Re-examining the efficacy of beta-blockers for the treatment of hypertension: a meta-analysis. CMAJ. 2006;174(12):1737-42.

17. Wiysonge CS, Bradley H, Mayosi BM, et al. Beta-blockers for hypertension. Cochrane Database Syst Rev. 2007;(1):CD002003.

18. ONTARGET Investigators, Yusuf S, Teo KK, et al. Telmisartan, ramipril, or both in patients at high risk for vascular events. N Engl J Med. 2008;358(15):1547-59.

19. Parving HH, Brenner BM, McMurray JJ, et al. Cardiorenal end points in a trial of aliskiren for type 2 diabetes. N Engl J Med. 2012;367(23):2204-13.

20. Bejan-Angoulvant T, Saadatian-Elahi M, Wright JM, et al. Treatment of hypertension in patients 80 years and older: the lower the better? A meta-analysis of randomized controlled trials. J Hypertens. 2010;28(7):1366-72.

21. Lohr JW, Golzy M, Carter RL, et al. Elevated systolic blood pressure is associated with increased incidence of chronic kidney disease but not mortality in elderly veterans. J Am Soc Hypertens. 2015;9(1):29-37.

22. Aronow WS, Fleg JL, Pepine CJ, et al. ACCF/AHA 2011 expert consensus document on hypertension in the elderly: a report of the American College of Cardiology Foundation Task Force on Clinical Expert Consensus Documents. Circulation. 2011;123(21):2434-506.

23. Hypertension: Clinical management of primary hypertension in adults. NICE clinical guideline 127. Available from: www.nice.org.uk/guidance/ CG127. Aug 2011.

24. Sundström J, Arima H, Jackson R, et al. Effects of Blood Pressure Reduction in Mild Hypertension: A Systematic Review and Meta-analysis. Ann Intern Med. 2015;162(3):184-91.

25. Xue H, Lu Z, Tang WL, et al. First-line drugs inhibiting the renin-angiotensin system versus other first-line antihypertensive drug classes for hypertension. Cochrane Database Syst Rev. 2015;1:CD008170.

26. Tepper D. Frontiers in congestive heart failure: Effect of Metoprolol CR/ XL in chronic heart failure: Metoprolol CR/XL Randomised Intervention Trial in Congestive Heart Failure (MERIT-HF). Congest Heart Fail. 1999;5(4):184-5.

27. Packer M, Coats AJ, Fowler MB, et al. Effect of carvedilol on survival in severe chronic heart failure. N Engl J Med. 2001;344(22):1651-8.

28. A randomized trial of beta-blockade in heart failure. The Cardiac Insufficiency Bisoprolol Study (CIBIS). CIBIS Investigators and Committees. Circulation. 1994;90(4):1765-73.

29. Effect of enalapril on survival in patients with reduced left ventricular ejection fractions and congestive heart failure. The SOLVD Investigators. N Engl J Med. 1991;325(5):293-302.

30. Effect of ramipril on mortality and morbidity of survivors of acute myocardial infarction with clinical evidence of heart failure. The Acute Infarction Ramipril Efficacy (AIRE) Study Investigators. Lancet. 1993;342(8875):821-8.

31. Køber L, Torp-Pedersen C, Carlsen JE, et al. A clinical trial of the angiotensin-converting-enzyme inhibitor trandolapril in patients with left ventricular dysfunction after myocardial infarction. Trandolapril Cardiac Evaluation (TRACE) Study Group. N Engl J Med. 1995;333(25):1670-6.

32. Cohn JN, Tognoni G, Valsartan Heart Failure Trial Investigators. A randomized trial of the angiotensin-receptor blocker valsartan in chronic heart failure. N Engl J Med. 2001;345(23):1667-75.

33. Pitt B, Zannad F, Remme WJ, et al. The effect of spironolactone on morbidity and mortality in patients with severe heart failure. Randomized Aldactone Evaluation Study Investigators. N Engl J Med. 1999;341(10):709-17.

34. Granger CB, McMurray JJ, Yusuf S, et al. Effects of candesartan in patients with chronic heart failure and reduced left-ventricular systolic function intolerant to angiotensin-converting-enzyme inhibitors: the CHARM-Alternative trial. Lancet. 2003;362(9386):772-6.

35. A randomized trial of propranolol in patients with acute myocardial infarction. I. mortality results. JAMA. 1982;247(12):1707-14.

36. Hager WD, Davis BR, Riba A, et al. Absence of a deleterious effect of calcium channel blockers in patients with left ventricular dysfunction after myocardial infarction: the SAVE Study Experience. SAVE Investigators. Survival and Ventricular Enlargement. Am Heart J. 1998;135(3):406-13.

37. Dargie HJ. Effect of carvedilol on outcome after myocardial infarction in patients with left-ventricular dysfunction: the CAPRICORN randomised trial. Lancet. 2001;357:1385-90.

38. Pitt B, Remme W, Zannad F, et al. Eplerenone a selective aldosterone blocker, in patients with left ventricular dysfunction after myocardial infarction. N Engl J Med. 2003;348:1309-21.

39. Yusuf S, Sleight P, Pogue J, et al. Effects of an angiotensin-converting enzyme inhibitor, ramipril, on cardiovascular events in high risk patients. The Heart Outcomes Prevention Evaluation Study Investigators. N Engl J Med. 2000;342(3):145-53.

40. Wing LM, Reid CM, Ryan P, et al. A comparison of outcomes with angiotensin-converting enzyme inhibitors and diuretics for hypertension in elderly. N Engl J Med. 2003;348(7):583-92.

41. Dahlöf B, Devereux RB, Kjeldsen SE, et al. Cardiovascular morbidity and mortality in the Losartan intervention for endpoint reduction in hypertension study (LIFE): a randomized trial against atenolol. Lancet. 2002;359(9311):995-1003.

42. Black HR, Elliott WJ, Grandits G, et al. Principal results of the Controlled Onset Verapamil Investigation of Cardiovascular End Points (CONVINCE) trial. JAMA. 2003;289:2073-82.

43. Fox KM, European trial on reduction of cardiac events with Perindopril in stable coronary Artery disease Investigators. Efficacy of perindopril in reduction of cardiovascular events among patients with stable coronary artery disease: randomised, double-blind, placebo-controlled, multicentre trial (the EUROPA study). Lancet. 2003;362 (9386):782-8.

44. Pepine CJ, Handberg EM, Cooper-DeHoff RM, et al. INVEST investigators. A calcium antagonist vs a non-calcium antagonist hypertension treatment strategy for patients with coronary artery disease. The International Verapamil-Trandolapril Study (INVEST): a randomized controlled trial. JAMA. 2003;290(21):2805-1646.

45. Tight blood pressure control and risk of macrovascular and microvascular complications in type 2 diabetes: UKPDS 38. UK Prospective Diabetes Study Group. BMJ. 1998;317(7160):703-13.

46. Brenner BM, Cooper ME, de Zeeuw D, et al. RENAAL study investigators. Effects of losartan on renal and cardiovascular outcomes in patients with type 2 diabetes and nephropathy. N Engl J Med. 2001;345(12):861-9.

47. Lewis EJ, Hunsicker LG, Clarke WR, et al. Collaborative Study Goup. Renoprotective effect of the angiotensin-receptor antagonist irbesartan in patients with nephropathy due to type 2 diabetes. N Engl J Med. 2001;345(12):851-60.

48. Randomised placebo-controlled trial of effect of ramipril on decline in glomerular filtration rate and risk of terminal renal failure in proteinuric, non-diabetic nephropathy. The GISEN (Gruppo Italiano di Studi Epidemiologici in Nefrologia) Group. Lancet. 1997;349(9069):1857-63.

49. Wright JT, Bakris G, Greene T, et al. Effect of blood pressure lowering and antihypertensive drug class on progression of hypertensive kidney disease: results from the AASK trial. JAMA. 2002;288(19):2421-31.

50. PROGRESS Collaborative Group. Randomised trial of a perindopril-based BP-lowering regimen among 6105 individuals with previous stroke or transient ischaemic attack. Lancet. 2001;358:1033-41.

51. National High Blood Pressure Education Program Working Group on High Blood Pressure in Children and Adolescents. The fourth report on the diagnosis, evaluation, and treatment of high blood pressure in children and adolescents. Pediatrics. 2004;114:555-76.

52. Kaelber DC, Pickett F. Simple table to identify children and adolescents needing further evaluation of blood pressure. Pediatrics. 2009;123(6):e972-4.

53. Kidney Disease Outcomes Quality Initiative (K/DOQI). K/DOQI Clinical Practice Guidelines on Hypertension and Antihypertensive Agents in Chronic Kidney Disease. Am J Kidney Dis. 2004;43(5 Suppl 1):S1-290.

54. Rosendroff C, Black HR, Cannon CP, et al. American Heart Association Council for High Blood Pressure Research; American Heart Association Council on Clinical Cardiology; American Heart Association Council on Epidemiology and Prevention. Treatment of hypertension in the prevention and management of ischemic heart disease: a scientific statement from the American Heart Association Council for High Blood Pressure Research and the Councils on Clinical Cardiology and Epidemiology and Prevention. Circulation. 2007;115(21):2761-88.

55. Bakris GL, Kaplan NM, Nathan DM, et al. (2011). Treatment of hypertension in patients with diabetes mellitus. [online] Available from http://www.uptodate com/contents/treatment-of-hypertension-in-patients-with-diabetes-mellitus. [Accessed in February, 2015].

56. Kaplan NM, Rose BD, Bakris GL, et al. (2010). Drug treatment of hypertensive emergencies. [online] Available from: http://www.uptodate.com/contents/drug-treatment-of-hypertensive-emergencies?source=search. [Accessed February, 2015].

57. Hunt SA, Abraham WT, Chin MH, et al. 2009 focused updates incorporated into the acc/aha 2005 guidelines for the diagnosis and management of heart failure in adults: a report of the American College of Cardiology Foundation/ American Heart Association Task Force on Practice Guidelines: developed in collaboration with the International Society for Heart and Lung Transplantation. Circulation. 2009;119(14):e391-479.

58. Podymow T, August P. Update on the use of antihypertensive drugs in pregnancy. Hypertension. 2008;51(4):960-9.

59. Esler M, Schwarz R. Management of hypertension complicated by psychiatric comorbidity. J Clin Hypertens (Greenwich). 2007;9(9):708-13.

60. Kaplan NM, Calhoun DA, Bakris GL, et al. (2012). Treatment of resistant hypertension. [online] Available from: http://www.uptodate.com/contents/treatment of reisistant hypertension?source=search_result&search. [Accessed in February 2015].

61. Bhatt DL, Kandzari DE, O'Neill WW, et al. A controlled trial of renal denervation for resistant hypertension. N Engl J Med. 2014;370(15):1393-401.

62. Sacco RL, Adams R, Albers G, et al. Guidelines for prevention of stroke in patients with ischemic stroke or transient ischemic attack: a statement for healthcare professionals from the American Heart Association/American Stroke Association Council on Stroke: co-sponsored by the Council on Cardiovascular Radiology and Intervention: the American Academy of Neurology affirms the value of this guideline. Stroke. 2006;37(2):577-617.

63. Jauch EC, Kissela B, Stettler B. (2011). Acute Management of Stroke. [online] Available from: http://emedicine.medscape.com/article/1159752-overview. [Accessed in February, 2015].

64. Klabunde RE. (2010). Cardiovascular Pharmacology Concepts: Beta-Adrenoceptor Antagonists (Beta-Blockers). [online] Available from: http://www. cvpharmacology. com/cardioinhibitory/beta-blockers.htm. [Accessed in February, 2015].

65. Toto RD. Microalbuminuria: definition, detection, and clinical significance. J Clin Hypertens (Greenwich). 2004;6(11 Suppl 3):2-7.

66. Tziomalos K, Athyros VG, Karagiannis A, et al. Dyslipidemia induced by drugs used for prevention and treatment of vascular diseases. Open Cardiovasc Med J. 2011;5:85-9.

*67. Facts and Comparison. Drug Facts and Comparison, 60th Edition. Philadelphia: Wolters Kluwer Health: Lippincott Williams & Wilkins; 2006.

*68. Hamilton RJ (Ed). Tarascon Pocket Pharmacopoeia. Burlington, MA: Jones and Bartlett Learning; 2012.

*69. Kaplan NM, Victor RG. Clinical Hypertension, 10th Edition. Philadelphia:Wolters Kluwer Health: Lippincott Williams & Wilkins; 2010.

*70. Montvale NJ. Physicians' Desk Reference, 65th Edition. Montvale, NJ: Thomson; 2011.

*71. Micromedex 2.0. (2015). Domestic and international trademarks and/or service marks of OCLC Online Computer Library Center, Inc. and its affiliates. [online] Available from http://www.thomsonhc.com/micromedex2/librarian. [Accessed in March, 2015].

*72. US Food and Drug Administration; [online] Available from http://www.accessdata. fda.gov/scripts/cder/drugsatfda/ [Accessed in March, 2015].

73. Bakris GL, Nadim MK, Haller H, et al. Baroreflex activation therapy provides durable benefit in patients with resistant hypertension: results of long-term follow-up in the Rheos Pivotal Trial. J Am Soc Hypertens. 2012;6(2):152-8.

74. Gassler JP, Bisognano JD1. Baroreflex activation therapy in hypertension. J Hum Hypertens. 2014;28(8):469-74.

75. Lobo MD, Sobotka PA, Stanton A, et al. Central arteriovenous anastomosis for the treatment of patients with uncontrolled hypertension (the ROX CONTROL HTN study): a randomised controlled trial. Lancet. 2015. pii: S0140-6736(14)62053-5.

---

*For drugs not available in the United States and not available in references 67-72, internet websites were carefully searched. Every effort has been taken to assure the accuracy of information. However, practitioners should check current information from medication inserts, local pharmacies and appropriate texts and websites before prescribing.

Diuretics

Michael E Ernst

INTRODUCTION

Diuretic compounds promote the fractional excretion of sodium, leading to an increased rate and extent of urine formation and altering of long-term sodium balance. They are fundamental therapies in the management of several cardiac and edematous disorders, including congestive heart failure, hypertension, and renal disease. The selection of an individual diuretic agent is based on several key features, including its site of action in the nephron, pharmacokinetic and pharmacodynamic properties, and adverse effect profile.

DIURETIC CLASSIFICATION AND OVERVIEW OF USE

Modern diuretic compounds are grouped into one of four categories on the basis of their primary site of action in the nephron (Fig. 1):

1. *Carbonic anhydrase inhibitors* (e.g., acetazolamide) interfere with carbonic anhydrase activity in the proximal tubule brush border and inside the epithelial cells, leading to impaired sodium, bicarbonate, and water reabsorption. The resulting alkaline diuresis is of limited therapeutic value because sodium rejected proximally continues downstream where it is reabsorbed in the thick ascending limb of the loop of Henle. Acetazolamide is the prototype in the class, but is rarely used because of its minimal diuretic capability as well as the development of metabolic acidosis occurring with long-term use. Acetazolamide use is now primarily for noncardiac conditions, such as in decreasing intraocular pressure in patients with glaucoma, and in the prophylaxis of acute mountain sickness.

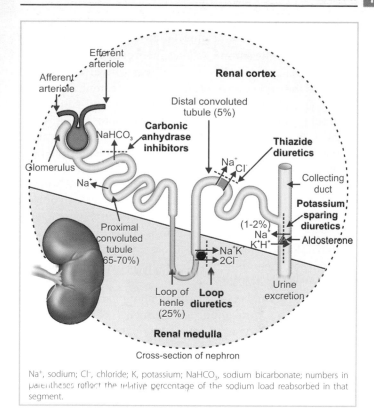

Na+, sodium; Cl-, chloride; K, potassium; NaHCO₃, sodium bicarbonate; numbers in parentheses reflect the relative percentage of the sodium load reabsorbed in that segment.

FIG. 1: Diuretic sites of action in the nephron.

2. *Loop, or high-ceiling diuretics* (e.g., furosemide, torsemide) bind to the Na^+-K^+-2Cl^- co-transporter, found within the apical membrane of epithelial cells of the thick ascending limb of the loop of Henle. This transporter passively carries sodium, potassium, and chloride ions into the cell based on the electrochemical Na^+ gradient generated by the Na^+-K^+-ATPase pump of the basolateral membrane. Inhibition of this transporter by loop-acting agents causes a diuresis of Na^+Cl^- and K^+Cl^-. Loop diuretics are also referred to as 'high-ceiling' diuretics due to the substantial diuresis they induce resulting from their ability to block nearly all sodium reabsorption (~25%) occurring in the loop of Henle. These are the preferred diuretics for relieving edematous states such as in congestive heart failure and nephrotic syndrome.

3. *Thiazide, and thiazide-like diuretics* (e.g., hydrochloro-thiazide, chlorthalidone) inhibit sodium reabsorption from the luminal side in the early segments of the distal tubule, by interfering with the electroneutral Na^+Cl^- symporter located in the apical membrane. The increased delivery of sodium to the collecting duct results in a modest diuresis, but one which is prolonged at a low-level and alters cardiovascular hemodynamics over the long-term.[1] The reduction in total

peripheral resistance shifts blood pressure downward, making thiazides and thiazide-like agents the optimal diuretics for the chronic management of hypertension.

4. *Potassium-sparing diuretics* act primarily at the cortical part of the collecting duct and, to a lesser extent, in the final segment of the distal convoluted tubule and connecting tubule. They are further subdivided into those acting as direct antagonists of cytoplasmic mineralocorticoid receptors (e.g., spironolactone), and those acting independent of mineralocorticoids (e.g., triamterene). The latter exert their action via blocking of the epithelial sodium channels in the luminal membrane. Because only a small amount of sodium is reabsorbed here, these agents provide only limited natriuresis (excluding states of mineralocorticoid excess). Their primary clinical utility resides in their ability to prevent potassium wasting from thiazides and loops.

5. *Osmotic agents (e.g., mannitol),* interfere with sodium reabsorption throughout all segments of the nephron by creating an osmotic force throughout the length of the renal tubule. The prevailing diuresis resembles the glucose-mediated osmotic polyuria observed in patients with uncontrolled diabetes.[2] The use of mannitol is limited to neurosurgical procedures, head trauma, and in other conditions of increased intracranial pressure. It has also been used as a preventive measure against kidney injury in patients receiving iodinated contrast agents. Because its main use is not in cardiac disorders, it will not be discussed further.

LOOP DIURETICS

Loop diuretics (Table 1) were developed in the 1960s while developing more tolerable and effective replacements to organic mercurials. Furosemide, the most commonly used loop diuretic in the United States, was the first to be developed, followed later by bumetanide and torsemide.

Mechanism of Action

All loop diuretics bind to the Na^+-K^+-$2Cl^-$ co-transporter in the thick ascending limb of the loop of Henle. This segment is responsible for concentrating urine; solute removal from this area generates the hypertonic medullary interstitium that serves as the osmotic force driving water reabsorption across the collecting duct. Inhibition of this reabsorptive process by loop diuretics impairs the ability of the kidney to generate concentrated urine, causing sodium, chloride, and potassium ions to remain intraluminally and be lost in the urine.

TABLE 1: High-ceiling or loop diuretics[1,2]

Agent	Oral bioavailability (%)	V_d (L/kg)	Protein binding (%)	Fate	Normal $T_{1/2}$ (hr)	Normal duration of natriuresis (hr)
Furosemide	10–100	0.15	91–99	R (50%), 50% conjugated in kidneys	1.5*	6
Bumetanide	80–100	0.15	90–99	R (60%), M (40%)	1.5*	3–6
Torsemide	80–100	0.2	99	R (20%), M (80%)	3–4*	8–12
Ethacrynic acid**	100	—	90	R (67%), M (33%)	1	4–8

*Prolonged in renal insufficiency.

**Higher risk of ototoxicity; reserve for patients with documented allergy to other loops.

R, renal excretion as intact drug; M, hepatically metabolized; V_d, volume of distribution; $T_{1/2}$, elimination half-life; —, insufficient data.

Pharmacology

Pharmacokinetics

All loop diuretics are extensively bound to serum albumin (>95%).[3] Consequently, to obtain access to their site of action, they must be actively secreted into the tubular lumen through probenecid-sensitive organic anion transporters located in the proximal tubule. This process may be slowed by elevated levels of endogenous organic acids, such as in chronic kidney disease, as well as some commonly prescribed drugs that share the same transporter, including salicylates and nonsteroidal anti-inflammatories.

Bioavailability, half-life, and routes of metabolism differ among the available loop diuretics. Furosemide is the most widely used, but it does not possess the most favorable pharmacokinetic profile within the class; absorption is erratic and ranges from 10 to 100%.[4] Coadministration with food can further decrease the bioavailability. The absorption of bumetanide and torsemide is more predictable, ranging from 80 to 100%.[5]

The duration of action and frequency of dosing for loop diuretics are determined by their half-lives. Furosemide and bumetanide are rapidly acting, with very short half-lives (~1.5 hours). Therapeutic response occurs within minutes after intravenous administration, while peak response from oral administration occurs in about 30–90 minutes. With both routes of administration, diuretic effects continue for approximately 2–3 hours, lasting up to 6 hours.[2] Because their action is brief, loop diuretics are subject to a significant anti-natriuretic period after the dose falls below the threshold necessary to trigger diuresis; this post dose rebound sodium retention can offset their therapeutic benefit such that furosemide and bumetanide must be given multiple times per day, to ensure adequate amounts of drug are maintained at the site of action. Torsemide has a longer plasma half-life and duration of action, and can be dosed less frequently.

Furosemide is excreted both unchanged in the urine (approximately 50% of the dose), with the remainder conjugated to glucuronic acid in the kidney.[6] Bumetanide and torsemide are primarily hepatically metabolized.[7] In hepatic disease, the plasma half-life of bumetanide and torsemide are prolonged, and their therapeutic effects may be paradoxically enhanced.[8] Similarly, renal insufficiency alters the pharmacokinetics of furosemide by prolonging both the plasma half-life and duration of action, due to decreased urinary excretion and renal conjugation.

Pharmacodynamics

Specific hemodynamic changes in both systemic and renal microcirculations occur subsequent to administration of a loop diuretic. Initially, intravenous administration stimulates the renin-angiotensin-aldosterone system at the macula densa, causing vasoconstriction, increased afterload and decreased renal blood flow.[9] This may account for lack of response to a bolus dose. This action is temporary, however, as a second-phase response occurs within 5–15 minutes. The second-phase is characterized by an increase in renal release of vasodilating prostaglandins, leading to venodilation, decreased preload and ventricular filling pressures.[10] The latter effects may explain the nearly immediate symptomatic improvement often noted in patients with acute pulmonary edema, which may precede the onset of actual diuresis.[2] With prolonged use, a compensatory activation of the sympathetic nervous system occurs and can lead to chronic adaptations known as the *braking* effect. These changes are natural compensations intended to protect intravascular volume. Their net result is to stabilize volume losses, leading to *tolerance* of the diuretic effect. Diuretic tolerance should be distinguished clinically from diuretic *resistance* states; the latter more appropriately refer to what is observed in conjunction with pathophysiologic conditions such as renal failure, nephrotic syndrome, congestive heart failure, and cirrhosis.[3]

Dosing

Diuresis is dependent upon achieving a diuretic threshold specific within the individual patient. Once the threshold is met, there is an optimal rate of drug delivery leading to maximal response (Fig. 2). Because diuretic response is not linearly related to dose, once the dose and rate of delivery leading to maximal response is determined, additional diuretic administration will not increase diuresis. To identify the point of maximal response, it is best to start first with small doses then titrate upward according to response. This can be achieved by sequentially doubling the dose until response is observed or a ceiling dose is reached (Table 2).

Intravenous furosemide is usually started with a 40 mg loading dose, followed by a repeated dose an hour later or a continuous infusion. The wide degree of variability in absorption of furosemide makes it difficult to reliably predict response; thus, one must try different doses before the drug is determined to be ineffective.[2] With its short duration of action (4–6 hours), oral dosing must be given twice daily, usually early morning and mid-afternoon, to avoid nocturia. Given the wide bioavailability range for furosemide, if one assumes an average absorption of 50%, the oral dose should be approximately twice the intravenous dose when switching routes of administration. Because absorption of bumetanide and torsemide is more reliable, the dose is approximately the same when switching from intravenous to oral dosing.

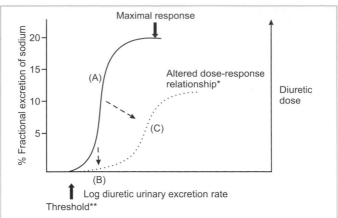

* Nephrotic syndrome, congestive heart failure, cirrhosis
** Determinants of diuretic threshold and efficacy include: dose, bioavailability, tubular secretory capacity, rate of absorption, and time course of delivery. After identifying the threshold dose to achieve effect, a higher diuretic concentration (A) leads to significant natriuresis. When severe sodium retention occurs or sodium intake is reduced, the curve shifts to the right and the previous diuretic serum concentration achieved by the dose in (A) is no longer effective; (B) The dose of the diuretic must be increased to achieve clinically effective natriuresis; and (C) Increasing the frequency of doses has no effect on sodium excretion as long as each dose is below the threshold.

FIG. 2: Relationship between loop diuretic dose and response.

Larger doses of all loops may be necessary in the presence of renal disease to effectively reach the site of action since they compete with accumulated endogenous organic acids for delivery into the tubular lumen.

Clinical Evidence/Indications

Loops are the most effective agents when strictly evaluated according to the level of diuresis they produce; they are agents of choice for symptomatic relief in patients with edematous disorders such as congestive heart failure, cirrhosis, and nephrotic syndrome.

General Therapeutic Considerations

The removal of excess extracellular fluid volume with loop diuretics should generally be gradual to minimize electrolyte imbalances as well as avoid reductions in blood volume that may impair adequate perfusion to the kidneys and other vital tissues and organs. Initial losses in response to diuretic administration occur from the plasma volume. The rate at which vascular space is refilled by fluid mobilized from the interstitium is variable, and this will direct the maximal rate of diuresis that can be tolerated.[11] For generalized edema, interstitial fluid is rapidly mobilized and a diuresis of 1–2 L/day can be safely achieved.[11] Mobilization is much slower, and diuresis must, therefore, be approached more gradually, for edema that is sequestered as ascites or in the pleural space.

TABLE 2: Intravenous and oral dosing of loop diuretics[3,13]

	Furosemide IV	Furosemide PO	Bumetanide IV and PO	Torsemide IV and PO
Continuous infusion (mg/hr)				
Loading dose	40 mg load	–	1 mg load	20 mg load
CrCl <25	20, then 40	–	1, then 2	10, then 20
CrCl 25–75	10, then 20	–	0.5, then 1	5, then 10
CrCl >75	10	–	0.5	5
Single-dose ceilings (mg)				
Renal insufficiency				
Moderate (CrCl 20–50)	80–160	160	2–3	20–50
Severe (CrCl <20)	160–200	400	8–10	50–100
Congestive heart failure	40–80	80–150	1–2	20–40
Cirrhosis	40	80	1	10–20
Nephrotic Syndrome	80–120	240	2–3	40–60

IV, intravenous; PO, per oral; CrCl: creatinine clearance (mL/min).

The short half-lives of loop diuretics limit their effectiveness as a treatment for hypertension, unless there is impaired renal function [glomerular filtration rate (GFR) <40 mL/min/1.73m^2], where thiazides may lose efficacy (*See Thiazide Diuretics* section).

Renal Disease

Renal disease impairs the ability of the diuretic to reach its site of action, so there is a need to administer larger doses to attain adequate amounts to reach the threshold for diuresis (Fig. 2).[12] This is accomplished by giving gradually increasing doses of the loop diuretic until an effective dose is identified, or a specific ceiling dose achieved (Table 2). Once the effective dose is identified, it should be given as frequently as necessary to maintain response, which will be influenced by the duration of action of the drug in the particular patient as well as the degree of sodium restriction employed.[3] Continuous infusions can be tried if intermittent doses are not sufficient. However, before using a continuous infusion, a loading dose should be given first to reduce the time necessary to achieve a steady state therapeutic drug concentration. The rate of the continuous infusion is then determined based on renal function.[3]

Patients with inadequate natriuresis despite the use of maximal doses of loop diuretics may benefit from using a combination of diuretic agents—a strategy commonly referred to as *sequential nephron blockade* (Table 3).[13] Addition of a

TABLE 3: Clinical considerations with diuretic use in renal disease[12]

Consideration (Cause)	Solution
Diuretic resistance	
Renal Disease (impaired delivery of diuretic to site of action)	• Use larger doses; increase frequency or use continuous infusion • Try sequential nephron blockade (i.e., addition of distally-acting agent such as thiazide)
Nephrotic syndrome (diminished nephron response and increased binding of diuretic to urinary albumin → reduced delivery of drug to site of action)	Need to obtain sufficiently high dose to reach diuretic threshold → increase frequency of effective dose; co-administration with albumin
Proteinuria despite maximized renin-angiotensin-aldosterone blockade	Add spironolactone
Hypertension in chronic kidney disease	Loop diuretic (usually twice daily unless torsemide) preferred when GFR ≤40 mL/min/1.73 m^2

GFR, glomerular filtration rate.

distally-acting diuretic, such as a thiazide, to the loop agent is the most common strategy. Several mechanisms contribute to the enhanced response with combination use in refractory states. First, the longer half-life of distally-acting agents may decrease the effect of the post-dose sodium retention observed with the shorter-acting loops. Secondly, chronic administration of loop diuretics can induce hypertrophy of distal tubule cells, enhancing reabsorption of sodium at this site and blunting the response to loops.[13]

Congestive Heart Failure

Several factors influence responsiveness to oral loop diuretics in patients with heart failure, and include the extent of gastrointestinal absorption and rate of tubular secretion. The absolute bioavailability of the diuretic is usually unchanged, but the rate of absorption is slowed such that the peak response may not be observed for several hours after the dose is administered.[3] Torsemide has a higher bioavailability than furosemide, and evidence exists for less fatigue and readmittance for decompensated heart failure in patients receiving torsemide compared to furosemide.[14]

As long as normal renal function is intact, delivery of diuretic into the tubular fluid remains normal in heart failure. However, renal responsiveness to loops as measured by the natriuretic response to maximally effective doses can be one-third to one-fourth that of healthy individuals.[15] Larger doses will therefore not overcome this diminished response, unless renal insufficiency is present. Rather, the natriuretic response may be increased by giving moderate doses more frequently.[3] In this manner, intravenous therapy is often appropriate in patients with severe heart failure or acute pulmonary edema. In addition to avoiding troughs in drug concentration that can lead to intermittent periods of positive sodium balance, it also has the added advantage of bypassing the delayed gut absorption of the diuretic. A loading dose followed by a continuous infusion (Table 2) is preferred, as they seem to provide greater natriuresis with a lower incidence of toxicity than intermittent bolus injections.[16]

THIAZIDE DIURETICS

While developing more potent inhibitors of carbonic anhydrase, researchers serendipitously discovered chloro-thiazide.[1] Rather than the usual alkaline diuresis expected from a carbonic anhydrase inhibitor, an unanticipated finding with chlorothiazide was that it increased chloride excretion. Chlorothiazide was quickly made available for clinical use in 1957, marking the beginning of the modern era of effective oral diuretic therapy.

Mechanism of Action

Thiazide, and the thiazide-like, diuretics (Table 4) are also referred to as benzothiadiazines, as most compounds are analogs of 1,2,4-benzothiadiazine-1,1-dioxide.

The primary mechanism of action of thiazides is by interfering with the electroneutral Na^+Cl^- symporter located in the apical membrane in the early segments of the distal tubule. The increased delivery of sodium to the collecting duct also increases the exchange with potassium, leading to potassium depletion. Magnesium excretion is also increased as a result of thiazide administration. As the normal Na^+Cl^- reabsorption in the distal tubule contributes to tubular fluid dilution, thiazides impair the diluting capacity of the kidney, but preserve urinary concentrating mechanisms.

There is significant heterogeneity within the class in their structure-activity relationships, and thiazides can be further designated as *thiazide-type* or *thiazide-like*; however, the general designation of *thiazide diuretic* is considered inclusive of all diuretics with a primary action in the distal tubule.[1] Although all thiazides retain an unsubstituted sulfonamide group in common with the carbonic anhydrase inhibitors and retain varying degrees of potency against carbonic anhydrase, this activity is not believed to contribute to their diuretic effect.[1]

Pharmacology

Pharmacokinetics

All thiazides are orally absorbed, have volumes of distribution equal to or greater than equivalent body weight, and are extensively bound to plasma proteins.[1] As with loop agents, thiazides must be actively secreted into the proximal tubule to access their site of action, because they are highly protein bound and subject to limited glomerular filtration.

The average onset of action for thiazides is approximately 2–3 hours, peaking at 3–6 hours, with progressively diminishing natriuretic effect occurring beyond 6 hours for most agents, except chlorthalidone.[1] There is significant variation in the metabolism, bioavailability, and plasma half-lives of the thiazides (Table 4). Hydrochlorothiazide, the most commonly used thiazide, is well absorbed (approximately 60–70%).[17] Co-administration with food slightly enhances absorption, most likely through interference with gastric emptying.

Several thiazides undergo hepatic metabolism (e.g., bendro-flumethiazide, polythiazide, methyclothiazide, indapamide), while others are excreted nearly completely intact in urine (e.g., chlorothiazide, hydrochlorothiazide). Metabolism of chlorthalidone and metolazone are mixed, primarily renal (50–80%), with minor biliary excretion (10%).[17] Other than

TABLE 4: Thiazide, and thiazide-like diuretics[1,2]

Agent	Daily dosage (dosing schedule)	Oral bioavailability (%)	V_d (L/kg)	Protein binding (%)	Fate	Normal $T_{1/2}$ (hr)	Normal duration of natriuresis (hr)
Chlorothiazide	125–500 mg (OD or BID)	15–30	1	70	R (100%)	1.5–2.5	6–12
Hydrochlorothiazide	12.5–50 mg (OD)	60–70	2.5	40	R (100%)	3–10	6–12
Bendroflumethiazide	2.5–5 mg (OD)	90	1–1.5	94	R (30%), M (70%)	2–5	18–24
Chlorthalidone*	12.5–25 mg (OD)	65	3–13	99	R (65%)	50–60	24–72
Metolazone*	2.5–10 mg (OD)	65	113 (total)	95	R (80%)	8–14	12–24
Indapamide*	1.25–5 mg (OD)	71–79	25 (total)	75	M (70%), R (5%)	14	24–36

*considered 'thiazide-like'.

BID, twice a day; OD, once a day; R, renal excretion as intact drug; M, hepatically metabolized; V_d, volume of distribution; $T_{1/2}$, elimination half-life.

a 50% reduction in hydrochlorothiazide absorption noted in patients with heart failure, the influence of disease on the pharmacokinetics of thiazides is not well-described.[17]

Because the distal tubule is responsible for reabsorbing only about 5% of the filtered sodium load, the potential for appreciable volume removal with thiazides in edematous disorders is limited. However, relative to loops and other diuretics, an advantage of the thiazides is their long duration of action (minimum of 8–12 hours). This property is the major determinant in their usefulness as antihypertensive agents. Chlorthalidone distinguishes itself from other thiazides as a naturally long-acting agent, as it possesses a significantly longer elimination half-life averaging 50–60 hours with chronic dosing.[18] It has a larger volume of distribution than other thiazides, with ≥99% of drug sequestered within erythrocyte carbonic anhydrase. In effect, this functions as a storage reservoir and enables a constant backflow of drug into the plasma, which may sustain a more constant, low-level diuresis and minimize the post dose antinatriuretic period.[1]

Pharmacodynamics

The dose-response curve of thiazides is much shallower than that of loops, such that there is little difference in efficacy between the lowest and maximally effective doses. Although the various analogs differ by potency in the dose required to produce their therapeutic effects, there are minimal differences between individual agents with respect to their optimal therapeutic or maximal responses when equipotent doses are employed.

The antihypertensive efficacy of thiazides does not directly stem from strict diuresis, but rather, the long-term hemodynamic changes which accompany their administration. These hemodynamic changes are induced by a protracted low-level of diuresis and allow the duration of antihypertensive effect to exceed that of their diuretic effect. Hemodynamic effects of thiazides can be separated into acute (1–2 weeks) and chronic (several months) periods (Fig. 3).[19] In the acute period, blood pressure-lowering is initially attributed to extracellular fluid contraction and reduction in plasma volume.[20] The accompanying decrease in venous return depresses cardiac preload and output, thereby reducing blood pressure. With chronic use, effects on plasma volume and cardiac output dissipate and these parameters return to near-normal levels, suggesting other reasons for sustained antihypertensive efficacy.[21] The most likely explanation for the long-term effects of thiazides in lowering blood pressure is an overall reduction in total peripheral resistance induced by a modest, but protracted state of volume contraction.[1]

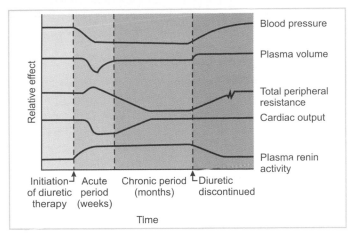

FIG. 3: Time course of hemodynamic responses to thiazides.

Dosing

Originally, it was believed that thiazide efficacy depended explicitly on the amount of renal sodium excretion and reduction in plasma volume that could be obtained; thus, larger doses were assumed to provide greater reductions in blood pressure.[22] A more thorough understanding of the dose-response relationship of thiazides has since led to use of significantly lower doses; generally, 12.5–25 mg/day of hydrochlorothiazide or its equivalent.[1]

Approximately, 50% of patients will respond initially, even to these small doses. Increasing the dose of hydrochlorothiazide to 25 mg/day may add approximately 20% to the responders, while at 50 mg/day 80–90% of possible responders should experience measurable blood pressure decreases.[23] A dose of 50 mg/day will result in significant hypokalemia (50% or higher) for most patients, and may require potassium supplementation or co-administration with a potassium-sparing diuretic. Thus, many clinicians do not routinely exceed 25 mg/day, although increasing the dose to 50 mg/day should be considered for certain patients with resistant hypertension or in those who exhibit signs of volume expansion despite being on a low-dose diuretic (often seen in obesity and in blacks). The risk of excessive potassium-wasting can be lessened when diuretics are co-administered with renin-angiotensin-aldosterone system blockers such as angiotensin-converting enzyme (ACE) inhibitors or angiotensin receptor blockers (ARBs), and when patients restrict their dietary sodium intake.[24]

Clinical Evidence/Indications

Diuretic-based therapy has been an essential part of the treatment of hypertension for many years. Thiazides are the preferred agents for chronic therapy in most hypertensive patients where a diuretic is indicated.[1]

General Therapeutic Considerations

Randomized placebo-controlled trials over the last 40 years involving nearly 50,000 hypertensive patients show that lowering of blood pressure with diuretic-based regimens leads to a reduction in cardiovascular events. Combined meta-analyses and systematic review suggest that thiazide-based regimens reduce relative rates of heart failure by 41–49%, stroke by approximately 29–38%, coronary heart disease by 14–21%, and overall mortality by 10–11% compared to placebo.[1] Effect sizes are consistent when examined by gender, age, and presence of diabetes.[25-27] The results of these studies have collectively formed the basis for national treatment recommendations advocating thiazides as a foundation of therapy for most patients.

The efficacy of thiazides in reducing hypertensive-related cardiovascular events has typically been considered a *class effect,* although there are no direct comparison studies within the class.[1] On the basis that it has reduced cardiovascular events in every study where used, chlorthalidone is often recommended, since other thiazide regimens (particularly hydrochlorothiazide-based) have resulted in less consistent benefit in clinical trials.[1] The few trials of hydrochlorothiazide in which it has successfully lowered cardiovascular disease events have typically used higher doses ($\geq$ 25–50 mg/day) than commonly used today, while lower-dose regimens in clinical use today have been found inferior to comparator regimens.[28,29] The reason for these differences is unexplained, but could relate to differences in potency between the two drugs at the low doses commonly employed today. It is now becoming more widely appreciated that chlorthalidone is 1.5–2 times more potent than hydrochlorothiazide, when evaluated with respect to doses required to achieve similar levels of blood pressure reduction.[30-33] In addition, there are also a number of indirect comparisons suggesting superiority of chlorthalidone-based regimens to hydrochlorothiazide-based regimens.[34-36]

Like chlorthalidone, indapamide is another thiazide-like diuretic that is not widely used but has favorable clinical trial outcome data. In the Hypertension in the Very Elderly Trial, indapamide-based regimen resulted in significant reductions in a 39% reduction in the rate of death from stroke, 21% reduction in death from any cause, and 64% reduction in heart failure rates.[37]

Hypertension

Thiazide administration typically results in a 10–15/5–10 mmHg placebo-adjusted reduction in blood pressure.[1] Thiazide responders are often referred to as having *low-renin* or *salt-sensitive* hypertension, reflecting the large dependence of blood pressure on volume and sodium in these individuals. These patients typically include the elderly, blacks, and high cardiac output states such as obesity. Although they are more likely to respond to thiazides, thiazides can be effectively combined with nearly any antihypertensive to achieve an antihypertensive effect that is usually additive of the two individual components.[1] Racial differences observed in the monotherapy response to ACE inhibitors or ARBs (blacks often do not respond as well to monotherapy with these agents) are minimized with the addition of a thiazide.

Thiazides are generally considered ineffective when GFR falls below 40 mL/min/1.73 m^2 since less drug is delivered to the site of action in the distal tubule, and the distal tubule is only responsible for a small portion of sodium reabsorption even under normal circumstances.[17] However, the exact level of GFR at which point the efficacy of each thiazide compound is obliterated has not been thoroughly investigated. Larger doses of thiazides have been shown to induce diuresis in patients with chronic kidney disease,[38,39] but increasing the doses of thiazides is often impractical given the risk of metabolic and electrolyte side effects. There is recent evidence that chlorthalidone, at usual doses prescribed for hypertension, retains efficacy in patients with poorly controlled hypertension and chronic kidney disease.[40,41]

Nevertheless, in patients with chronic kidney disease and hypertension, a loop diuretic is preferred, usually dosed two or three times daily to maintain efficacy. One thiazide-like agent, metolazone, is an exception among thiazides as it retains efficacy in patients with renal insufficiency and other diuretic-resistance states. It has slow and erratic absorption, so the more predictable bioavailability of other thiazides makes them better suited for chronic therapy of hypertension. Metolazone is reserved in combination with loop diuretics in volume-overloaded patients undergoing close monitoring of fluid and electrolyte balance. It is usually administered daily for a short period (3–5 days) to achieve euvolemia, then reduced to approximately three times weekly.[13]

POTASSIUM-SPARING DIURETICS

Potassium-sparing diuretics (Table 5) can be classified into one of two groups: (1) epithelial sodium channel blockers and (2) mineralocorticoid receptor antagonists. Generally, both types are only modestly effective in lowering blood pressure and with minimal exception, are primarily used in the general hypertensive population to offset potassium and magnesium loss in patients receiving a loop or thiazide diuretic.

Mechanism of Action

Sodium reabsorption in the distal tubule and collection ducts is mediated through an aldosterone-sensitive sodium channel and by activation of an ATP-dependent sodium-potassium pump. To preserve electroneutrality, potassium and hydrogen are concurrently secreted into the lumen.[1] Spironolactone and eplerenone (Table 5) are competitive antagonists of aldosterone, and interfere with the aldosterone-mediated exchange of sodium for potassium and hydrogen. Amiloride and triamterene are pteridine derivatives. They block epithelial sodium channels in the luminal membrane, which causes the electrical potential across the tubular epithelium to fall and reduces the driving force for secretion of potassium into the lumen.[2]

Pharmacology

Pharmacokinetics/Pharmacodynamics

Spironolactone is the prototypical mineralocorticoid receptor antagonist. It is orally absorbed (~65%) and highly protein bound (90%). It has a short half-life of only 1.5 hours, but undergoes extensive metabolism in the liver into several active metabolites.[2] The two most well-characterized are 7-α-thiomethylspirolactone and canrenone; both have half-lives of about 15–20 hours and are responsible for the majority of spironolactone's therapeutic effect. Eplerenone is very similar to spironolactone, with the exception that its activity is not due to active metabolites, and it has >100-fold less affinity for androgen and progesterone receptors. Spironolactone retains efficacy in renal impairment since it is not dependent on glomerular filtration to reach its site of action.

Triamterene and amiloride are also orally absorbed (~50%). Triamterene has a short half-life (3–6 hours) and duration of action.[3] Both renal and liver disease significantly affect the disposition of triamterene since it is conjugated in the liver and the metabolite then secreted into the proximal tubular fluid.[3] Triamterene must be used carefully with other potential nephrotoxins, as it is associated with formation of crystals, nephrolithiasis, interstitial nephritis, and acute renal failure.

Amiloride has a much longer half-life (17–26 hours) than triamterene, achieving steady state in approximately 2 days.[2] It is preferred in patients with liver disease since it is not metabolically activated. However, it is extensively renally cleared, and accumulates rapidly when administered in patients with chronic kidney disease. In these situations, the dose and/or dosing frequency of amiloride should be reduced to avoid the potential for hyperkalemia.

TABLE 5: Potassium-sparing diuretics[1,2]

Agent	Daily dosage (dosing schedule)	Oral bioavailability (%)	V_d (L/kg)	Protein binding (%)	Fate	Normal $T_{1/2}$ (hr)	Normal duration of natriuresis (hr)
Amiloride	5–10 mg (QD)	15–25	350 (total)	0	R (50%), 50% fecal	17–26*	24
Triamterene	50–150 mg (QD)	50	—	55–67	M (80%) R (10)	3	7–9
Spironolactone	12.5–50 mg (up to 200 mg for ascites) (QD)	65	—	90	M (extent unknown)	1.5 (15 hours for active metabolite, canrenone)	16–24
Eplerenone	25–100 mg (QD)	69	43–90 (total)	50	M (extent unknown)	5	24

* $T_{1/2}$ = 100 hours in end stage renal disease.

R, renal excretion as intact drug; M, hepatically metabolized; V_d, volume of distribution; $T_{1/2}$, elimination half-life; —, insufficient data.

Dosing

The active metabolites of spironolactone have half-lives, which are sufficiently long-enough to allow spironolactone to be dosed once daily. Because time must be allowed to accumulate these active metabolites, spironolactone has a characteristically slow onset, taking up to 48 hours before becoming maximally effective.[2] Usual dosing is to begin with 12.5 mg/day, titrating up to 50 mg/day (Table 5). Adverse effects such as gynecomastia and hyperkalemia are dose-related, and doses above 50 mg/day are generally reserved for cirrhotic patients with ascites. Eplerenone is naturally long-acting and can be dosed once daily, usually 25–100 mg.

Triamterene should ideally be dosed multiple times per day, but because it is rarely prescribed alone (most commonly used in a fixed-dose combination with hydrochlorothiazide), once-daily dosing is usually employed. The use of lower doses of thiazides, with less electrolyte disturbances, has led to lower overall use of triamterene. Amiloride can be dosed once- or twice-daily due to its long half-life. Amiloride is also usually given as part of a fixed-dose combination with hydrochlorothiazide.

Clinical Evidence/Indications

In the absence of states of mineralocorticoid excess or certain rare genetic conditions, the primary role of potassium-sparing diuretics in the treatment of hypertension is that of an ancillary to help offset the potassium and magnesium wasting induced by thiazides.

Hypertension

Spironolactone and eplerenone are indicated for treating low-renin forms of hypertension. They are particularly effective in combination with a thiazide-type diuretic. Spironolactone has shown significant additive hypotensive effects in patients resistant to treatment regardless of ethnicity or baseline aldosterone level.[42] In doses ≤50 mg/day, spironolactone is effective and well-tolerated. Direct antihypertensive efficacy comparisons between spironolactone and eplerenone in patients with resistant hypertension are lacking. Amiloride, an epithelial sodium channel blocker, has demonstrated greater efficacy than spironolactone in blacks resistant to treatment.[43]

It is generally assumed that angiotensin blockade will secondarily suppress aldosterone. However, "aldosterone escape" (unsuppressed aldosterone levels while on an ACE inhibitor or ARB), may be an important contributor of disease progression in patients with chronic kidney disease as evidenced by the finding that many hypertensive patients with chronic kidney disease and proteinuria do not have resolution of proteinuria despite treatment with ACE inhibitors or ARBs. Several studies have indicated that the addition of spironolactone to an ACE inhibitor or ARB can reduce proteinuria and progression of chronic kidney disease, independent of additional blood pressure-lowering effects induced.[44,45] Aldosterone is profibrotic, including to kidney, and animal models have shown that unopposed aldosterone increases glomerulosclerosis.[44]

Other Conditions

The addition of spironolactone 25 mg/day to the standard regimen of an ACE-inhibitor and loop diuretic in patients with severe heart failure (ejection fraction <35%) reduced death by 30% and hospitalizations by 35% in a pivotal trial.[46] Similarly, eplerenone has also shown reductions in mortality in both mild and severe heart failure patients.[47,48] However, these benefits do not seem to occur in patients with heart failure with preserved ejection fraction.[49,50]

Liddle's syndrome, a rare autosomal dominant disorder characterized by severe hypertension, hypokalemia, hypoaldosteronism, is treated with amiloride or triamterene. Mineralocorticoid antagonist therapy in this condition is ineffective.

DIURETIC ADVERSE EFFECTS

Several predictable adverse effects occur with diuretics (Table 6). The majority of these involve electrolyte and metabolic disturbances. Their clinical impact can be lessened by using the lowest effective dose and insuring a regular monitoring schedule.

TABLE 6: Electrolyte and metabolic effects of diuretics

Category	Thiazides	Loops	Potassium-sparing
Electrolytes			
Potassium	↓	↓	↑
Magnesium	↓	↓	↑
Sodium	↓	↓	—
Metabolic			
Glucose	↑	↑	—
Lipids	↑	↑	—
Other			
Uric acid	↑	↑	—

—, minimal/no effect; ↑, increased; ↓, decreased.

Electrolytes

Thiazide and loop diuretics increase potassium and magnesium excretion in a dose-related manner. An average potassium fall of 0.2–0.4 mEq/L with typical dosing in monotherapy can be expected.[1] In the Antihypertensive and Lipid-Lowering to Prevent Heart Attack Trial (ALLHAT), the average potassium level for chlorthalidone-treated patients (12.5–25 mg/day) over four years went from 4.3 mEq/L to 4.1 mEq/L.[51] Concurrent administration of an ACE inhibitor or ARB can reduce incident hypokalemia with thiazides. If hypokalemia should occur, it can be managed by co-administering a potassium-sparing diuretic, or oral potassium supplements. Potassium-sparing diuretics are preferred since they correct the underlying etiology, and have the additional effect of correcting hypomagnesemia, which itself must be normalized before hypokalemia can be effectively remedied. Dietary sodium restriction should also be recommended for those on a diuretic, as it can help reduce the loss of potassium occurring with diuretics.[24] It should be noted that in the Systolic Hypertension in the Elderly Program (SHEP), the benefit of the diuretic in reducing coronary events was nullified in those patients experiencing potassium levels of less than 3.5 mEq/L.[52] Thus, maintenance of normokalemia should be a priority in patients treated with diuretics.

Amiloride, triamterene, spironolactone, and eplerenone can all cause hyperkalemia. Caution is advised when they are co-administered with ACE inhibitors, ARBs, or other potentially nephrotoxic agents (e.g., NSAIDs), or in the presence of preexisting renal disease.

Hyponatremia is often asymptomatic, but careful monitoring of serum sodium should occur and patients should be advised to avoid excessive free-water intake while on a diuretic. Thiazides are more frequently implicated than loops, but both are equally capable of causing hyponatremia.[53] Thiazide-induced hyponatremia usually manifests within the first 2 weeks of therapy, while loops can occur after a longer interval. Risk factors for diuretic-induced hyponatremia include older age, female gender, psychogenic polydipsia, and concurrent antidepressant use (in particular, selective serotonin reuptake inhibitors).[53]

Metabolic

Diuretics can increase plasma glucose levels, and data suggest that receipt of thiazides in the treatment of hypertension over several years may lead to an excess of 3–4% in new diabetes cases compared to other antihypertensives.[54] These data must be interpreted cautiously, since the diagnosis of diabetes is a dichotomous endpoint: a change from 124 mg/dL to

127 mg/dL would establish a new diagnosis of diabetes, despite being an absolute glucose change of only 3 mg/dL. The etiology for incident diabetes with diuretics may lie in reduced insulin release secondary to hypokalemia, but definitive studies have not been performed.[54]

The clinical significance of glucose changes with diuretics has been the subject of intense debate. New cases of diabetes are recognized over time in many hypertensive patients, regardless of which class of antihypertensive is used. For example, in ALLHAT, new-onset diabetes occurred in 11.6% of chlorthalidone-treated patients, but occurred in 9.8% and 8.1% of amlodipine and lisinopril-treated patients, respectively.[55] To date, analyses from several different studies indicate that diabetics treated with diuretics, and individuals who develop diabetes while on a diuretic, experience as great or greater decrease in cardiovascular events than nondiabetics.[55,56]

Diuretics can cause atherogenic changes in blood lipids, namely by increasing total cholesterol and low-density lipoproteins. Estimates are approximately 5–7% in the first 3–12 months of therapy.[57] However, these changes are short-lived, as evidenced from long-term follow-up in clinical trials. A low-fat diet and regular monitoring are advised.

Hyperuricemia

Thiazides compete with uric acid for secretion into the proximal tubule by the organic acid secretory system; this leads to reduced uric acid excretion and can precipitate gout in predisposed individuals. If a patient experiences gout while taking a diuretic, the diuretic should be discontinued if possible. Uric acid can be rechecked after resolution of the attack and the need for prophylaxis or alternate antihypertensive therapy assessed. If the diuretic remains necessary to control blood pressure and the serum urate rises more than 10 mg/dL, allopurinol may be used.

Drug Interactions

Diuretics are relatively free of significant drug-drug interactions. Most drug interactions are pharmacodynamic in nature, relating to antagonism of effect or synergistic adverse effects, rather than in specific pharmacokinetic interferences. Nonsteroidal anti-inflammatory drugs and steroids can antagonize the therapeutic effects of diuretics by causing sodium retention. They also lessen the renal response to loop diuretics, probably by decreasing the formation of vasodilatory prostaglandins. Co-administration of NSAIDs increases the risk of hyperkalemia when used with potassium-sparing diuretics because they decrease secretion of renin and aldosterone. Lithium clearance can be decreased by thiazides (but not loops). Co-therapy with certain antibiotics such as aminoglycosides can potentiate nephrotoxicity.

Others

A number of other adverse effects of diuretics are described, including hypovolemia, ototoxicity (particularly with high-dose loop therapy), urinary frequency, and erectile dysfunction. Thiazide diuretics retain calcium through an increase in proximal tubular reabsorption. This is not generally harmful, but in fact, may be protective in fractures.[58] However, hyperparathyroid patients may be at risk for hypercalcemia. Lastly, there appears to be no specific cross-sensitivity between sulfa-antibiotic allergy and other non-antibiotics that have a sulfa-moiety, such as thiazides.[59]

REFERENCES

1. Ernst ME, Moser M. Use of diuretics in patients with hypertension. N Engl J Med. 2009;361:2153-64.
2. Brater DC. Pharmacology of diuretics. Am J Med Sci . 2000;319:38-50.
3. Brater DC. Diuretic therapy. N Engl J Med . 1998;339:387-95.
4. Murray MD, Haag KM, Black PK, et al. Variable furosemide absorption and poor predictability of response in elderly patients. Pharmacotherapy . 1997;17:98-106.
5. Vargo DL, Kramer WG, Black PK, et al. Bioavailability, pharmacokinetics, and pharmacodynamics of torsemide and furosemide in patients with congestive heart failure. Clin Pharmacol Ther. 1995;57:601-9.
6. Pichette V, du SP. Role of the kidneys in the metabolism of furosemide: its inhibition by probenecid. J Am Soc Nephrol. 1996;7:345-9.
7. Brater DC, Leinfelder J, Anderson A. Clinical pharmacology of torasemide: a new loop diuretic. Clin Pharmcol Ther. 1987;42:187-92.
8. Schwartz S, Brater DC, Pound D, et al. Bioavailability, pharmacokinetics, and pharmacodynamics of torsemide in patients with cirrhosis. Clin Pharmacol Ther. 1993;54:90-7.
9. Francis GS, Siegel RM, Goldsmith SR, et al. Acute vasoconstrictor response to intravenous furosemide in patients with chronic congestive heart failure. Activation of the neurohumoral axis. Ann Intern Med. 1985;103:1-6.
10. Dikshit K, Vyden JK, Forrester JS, et al. Renal and extrarenal hemodynamic effects of furosemide in congestive heart failure after acute myocardial infarction. N Engl J Med. 1973;288:1087-90.
11. Rasool A, Palevsky PM. Treatment of edematous disorders with diuretics. Am J Med Sci. 2000;319:25-37.
12. Ernst ME, Gordon JA. Diuretic therapy: key aspects in hypertension and renal disease. J Nephrol . 2010;23:487-93.
13. Ellison DH. Diuretic resistance: physiology and therapeutics. Sem Nephrol. 1999;19:581-97.
14. Murray MD, Deer MM, Ferguson JA, et al. Open-label randomized trial of torsemide compared with furosemide therapy for patients with heart failure. Am J Med. 2001;111:513-20.
15. Brater DC, Chennavasin P, Seiwell R. Furosemide in patients with heart failure: shift in dose-response curves. Clin Pharmacol Ther. 1980;28:182-6.
16. Dormans TP, van Meyel JJ, Gerlag PG, et al. Diuretic efficacy of high dose furosemide in severe heart failure: bolus injection versus continuous infusion. J Am Coll Cardiol. 1996;28:376-82.
17. Welling PG. Pharmacokinetics of the thiazide diuretics. Biopharm Drug Dispos. 1986;7:501-35.
18. Riess W, Dubach UC, Burckhardt D, et al. Pharmacokinetic studies with chlorthalidone (Hygroton) in man. Eur J Clin Pharmacol. 1977;12:375-82.

19. Tarzi RC, Dustan HP, Frohlich ED. Long-term thiazide therapy in essential hypertension. Evidence for persistent alterations in plasma volume and renin activity. Circulation. 1970;41:709-17.

20. Wilson IM, Freis ED. Relationship between plasma and extracellular fluid volume depletion and the antihypertensive effect of chlorothiazide. Circulation . 1959;20:1028-36.

21. Roos JC, Boer P, Koomans HA, et al. Haemodynamic and hormonal changes during acute and chronic diuretic treatment in essential hypertension. Eur J Clin Pharmacol. 1981;19:107-12.

22. Ernst ME, Grimm RH Jr. Thiazide diuretics: 50 years and beyond. Curr Hypertens Rev. 2008;4:256-65.

23. Materson BJ, Reda DJ, Cushman WC, et al. Single-drug therapy for hypertension in men. A comparison of six antihypertensive agents with placebo. N Engl J Med. 1993;328:914-21.

24. Ram CV, Garrett BN, Kaplan NM. Moderate sodium restriction and various diuretics in the treatment of hypertension. Arch Intern Med. 1981;141:1015-9.

25. Turnbull F, for the Blood Pressure Lowering Treatment Trialists' Collaboration. Effects of different blood-pressure-lowering regimens on major cardiovascular events: results of prospectively-designed overviews of randomised trials. Lancet. 2003;362:1527-35.

26. Blood Pressure Lowering Treatment Trialists' Collaboration. Do men and women respond differently to blood pressure-lowering treatment? Results of prospectively designed overviews of randomized trials. Eur Heart J. 2008;2:2669-80.

27. Blood Pressure Lowering Treatment Trialists' Collaboration. Effects of different regimens to lower blood pressure on major cardiovascular events in older and younger adults: meta-analysis of randomised trials. BMJ. 2008;336:1121-3.

28. Wing LM, Reid CM, Ryan P, et al. A comparison of outcomes with angiotensin-converting enzyme inhibitors and diuretics for hypertension in the elderly. N Engl J Med. 2003;348:583 02.

29. Jamerson K, Weber MA, Bakris GL, et al. for the ACCOMPLISH trial investigators. Benazepril plus amlodipine or hydrochlorothiazide for hypertension in high-risk patients. N Engl J Med. 2008;359:2417-28.

30. Carter BL, Ernst ME, Cohen JD. Hydrochlorothiazide versus chlorthalidone: evidence supporting their interchangeability. Hypertension. 2004;43:4-9.

31. Ernst ME, Carter BL, Goerdt CJ, et al. Comparative antihypertensive effects of hydrochlorothiazide and chlorthalidone on ambulatory and office blood pressure. Hypertension. 2006;47:352-8.

32. Ernst ME, Carter BL, Zheng S, et al. Meta-analysis of dose-response characteristics of hydrochlorothiazide and chlorthalidone: effects on systolic blood pressure and potassium. Am J Hypertens. 2010;23:440-6.

33. Peterzan MA, Hardy R, Chaturvedi N, et al. Meta-analysis of dose-response relationships for hydrochlorothiazide, chlorthalidone, and bendroflumethiazide on blood pressure, serum potassium, and urate. Hypertension. 2012;59:1104-9.

34. Ernst ME, Neaton JD, Grimm RH Jr, et al. Long-term effects of chlorthalidone versus hydrochlorothiazide on electrocardiographic left ventricular hypertrophy in the multiple risk factor intervention trial. Hypertension . 2011;58:1001-7.

35. Dorsch MP, Gillespie BW, Erickson SR, et al. Chlorthalidone reduces cardiovascular events compared with hydrochlorothiazide: a retrospective analysis. Hypertension. 2011;57:689-94.

36. Roush GC, Holford TR, Guddati AK. Chlorthalidone compared with hydro-chlorothiazide in reducing cardiovascular events: systematic review and network meta-analyses. Hypertension. 2012;59:1110-7.

37. Beckett NS, Peters R, Fletcher AE, for the HYVET Study Group. Treatment of hypertension in patients 80 years of age or older. N Engl J Med. 2008;358:1887-98.

38. Knauf H, Mutschler E. Diuretic effectiveness of hydrochlorothiazide and furosemide alone and in combination in chronic renal failure. J Cardiovasc Pharmacol. 1995;26: 394-400.

39. Dussol B, Moussi-Frances J, Morange S, et al. A randomized trial of furosemide vs hydrochlorothiazide in patients with chronic renal failure and hypertension. Nephrol Dial Transplant. 2005;20:349-53.

40. Agarwal R, Sinha AD, Pappas MK, et al. Chlorthalidone for poorly controlled hypertension in chronic kidney disease: an interventional pilot study. Am J Nephrol. 2014;39:171-82.

41. Cirillo M, Marcarelli F, Mele AA, et al. Parallel-group 8-week study on chlorthalidone effects in hypertensives with low kidney function. Hypertension. 2014;63:692-7.

42. Nishizaka MK, Zaman MA, Calhoun DA. Efficacy of low-dose spironolactone in subjects with resistant hypertension. Am J Hypertens. 2003;16:925-30.

43. Saha C, Eckert GJ, Ambrosius WT, et al. Improvement in blood pressure with inhibition of the epithelial sodium channel in blacks with hypertension. Hypertension. 2005;46:481-7.

44. Bomback AS, Kshirsagar AV, Amamoo MA, et al. Change in proteinuria after adding aldosterone blockers to ACE inhibitors or angiotensin receptor blockers in CKD: a systematic review. Am J Kidney Dis. 2008;51:199-211.

45. Navaneethan SD, Nigwekar SU, Sehgal AR, et al. Aldosterone antagonists for preventing the progression of chronic kidney disease. Cochrane Database Syst Rev. 2009; Jul 8;(3):CD007004.

46. Pitt B, Zannad F, Reme WJ, et al. The effect of spironolactone on morbidity and mortality in patients with severe congestive heart failure. N Engl J Med. 1999;341:709-17.

47. Pitt B, Remme W, Zannad F, et al. Eplerenone, a selective aldosterone blocker, in patients with left ventricular dysfunction after myocardial infarction. N Engl J Med. 2003;348:1309-21.

48. Zannad F, McMurray JJ, Krum H, et al. Eplerenone in patients with systolic heart failure and mild symptoms. N Engl J Med. 2011;364:11-21.

49. Edelmann F, Wachter R, Schmidt AG, et al. Effects of spironolactone on diastolic function and exercise capacity in patients with heart failure with preserved ejection fraction: the Aldo-DHF randomized controlled trial. JAMA. 2013;309:781-91.

50. Pitt B, Pfeffer MA, Assmann SF, et al. Spironolactone for heart failure with preserved ejection fraction. N Engl J Med. 2014;370:1383-92.

51. ALLHAT Officers and Coordinators for the ALLHAT Collaborative Research Group. Major outcomes in high-risk hypertensive patients randomized to angiotensin-converting enzyme inhibitor or calcium channel blocker vs diuretic: the Antihypertensive and Lipid-Lowering Treatment to Prevent Heart Attack Trial (ALLHAT). JAMA. 2002;288:2981-97.

52. Franse LV, Pahor M, Di Bari M, et al. Hypokalemia associated with diuretic use and cardiovascular events in the Systolic Hypertension in the Elderly Program. Hypertension. 2000;35:1025-30.

53. Sarafidis PA, Georgianos PI, Lasaridis AN. Diuretics in clinical practice. Part II: electrolyte and acid-base disorders complicating diuretic therapy. Expert Opin Drug Saf. 2010;9:259-73.

54. Carter BL, Einhorn PT, Brands M, et al. Thiazide-induced dysglycemia: review of the literature and call for research: a report from a working group from the National Heart, Lung, and Blood Institute. Hypertension. 2008;52:30-6.

55. Barzilay JI, Davis BR, Cutler JA, et al. for the ALLHAT Collaborative Research Group. Fasting glucose levels and incident diabetes mellitus in older nondiabetic adults randomized to receive 3 different classes of antihypertensive treatment. A report from the Antihypertensive and Lipid-Lowering Treatment to Prevent Heart Attack Trial (ALLHAT). Arch Intern Med. 2006;166:2191-201.

56. Kostis JB, Wilson AC, Freudenberger RS, et al. ,for the SHEP Collaborative Research Group. Long-term effect of diuretic-based therapy on fatal outcomes in subjects with isolated systolic hypertension with and without diabetes. Am J Cardiol. 2005;95:29-35.

57. Savage PJ, Pressel SL, Curb JD, et al. Influence of long-term, low-dose, diuretic-based, antihypertensive therapy on glucose, lipid, uric acid, and potassium levels in older men and women with isolated systolic hypertension: the systolic hypertension in the elderly program. Arch Intern Med. 1998;158:741-51.

58. LaCroix AZ1, Wienpahl J, White LR, et al. Thiazide diuretic agents and the incidence of hip fracture. N Engl J Med. 1990;322:86-90.

59. Strom BL, Schinnar R, Apter AJ, et al. Absence of cross-reactivity between sulfonamide antibiotics and sulfonamide nonantibiotics. N Engl J Med. 2003;349:1628-35.

Drugs for Dyslipidemias

Byron Vandenberg

INTRODUCTION

The treatment of lipid disorders is directed at preventing progression and promoting regression of atherosclerosis. Atherosclerosis is primarily a lipid storage disease involving the retention of apolipoprotein-B (apo-B) containing lipoproteins which subsequently induce chronic inflammation, cell death, and thrombosis resulting in heart disease and stroke. Clinical studies have demonstrated that elevated levels of the apo-B lipoprotein, low-density lipoprotein (LDL), promote human atherosclerosis. Cardiovascular (CV) morbidity and mortality vary directly with the level of total cholesterol and LDL, although the association is not linear, as risk rises more steeply with increasing LDL concentrations.[1-4] LDL is one of the lipoprotein complexes involved in cholesterol and triglyceride transport (Fig. 1).[5] The lipoprotein complexes include LDL, high-density lipoprotein (HDL), very low-density lipoprotein (VLDL), and intermediate density lipoprotein (IDL).

The atherogenic triad of elevated triglycerides, low HDL, and small LDL particle size is frequently part of the metabolic syndrome which is associated with a two-fold increase in CV outcomes.[6] While isolated plasma triglyceride levels have not consistently been shown to be an independent risk factor for coronary heart disease (CHD), CV morbidity and mortality vary inversely with the level of HDL.[7]

STATINS

Introduction

Statin therapy is recommended for individuals at increased atherosclerotic cardiovascular disease (ASCVD) risk who are most likely to experience a net benefit in terms of the potential for ASCVD risk reduction and the potential for adverse

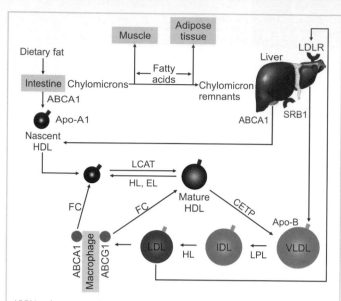

ABCA1, adenosine triphosphate-binding cassette A1; SRB1, scavenger receptor B1; LCAT, lecithin cholesterol acyltransferase; HL, hepatic lipase; EL, endothelial lipase; HDL, high-density lipoprotein; LDL, low-density lipoprotein; LDLR, low-density lipoprotein receptor; IDL, intermediate density lipoprotein; LPL, lipoprotein lipase; VLDL, very low-density lipoprotein; CETP, cholesteryl ester transfer protein; ABCG1, adenosine triphosphate-binding cassette G1; Apo-A1, apolipoprotein-A1; Apo-B, apolipoprotein-B.

FIG. 1: Schematic diagram of lipoprotein metabolism. The intestine absorbs dietary fat and packages it into chylomicrons (large triglyceride-rich lipoproteins), which are transported to peripheral tissues through the blood. In muscle and adipose tissues, the enzyme LPL breaks down chylomicrons, and fatty acids enter these tissues. The chylomicron remnants are subsequently taken up by the liver. The liver loads lipids onto apo-B and secretes VLDL, which undergoes lipolysis by LPL and HL to form LDL. LDL is then taken up by the liver through binding to the LDLR, as well as through other pathways. By contrast, HDL is generated by the intestine and the liver through the secretion of lipid-free apolipoprotein-A1 (apo-A1). Apo-A1 then recruits cholesterol from these organs through the ABCA1 transporter, forming nascent HDL, and this protects apo-A1 from being rapidly degraded in the kidneys. In the peripheral tissues, nascent HDL promotes the efflux of cholesterol from tissues, including from macrophages, through the actions of ABCA1. Mature HDL also promotes this efflux but through the actions of ABCG1. The free (unesterified) cholesterol in nascent HDL is esterified to cholesteryl ester by the enzyme LCAT, creating mature HDL. The cholesterol in HDL is returned to the liver both directly through uptake by the SRB1, and indirectly, by transfer to LDL and VLDL through the CETP. The lipid content of HDL is also altered by the enzymes HL and EL.

effects. Other approaches to treatment of blood cholesterol have been advocated, including "treat to target" [such as low density lipoprotein cholesterol (LDL-C) <70 mg/dL or LDL-C <100 mg/dL].[3,4] While this strategy has been widely used over the past 15 years, current clinical trial data and guidelines do not indicate specific targets.[1]

High-intensity statin therapy (Table 1) should be initiated or continued as first-line therapy in women and men ≤75 years of age with clinical ASCVD, unless contraindicated.[1] The

TABLE 1: High-, moderate- and low-intensity statins

High-intensity statins (>50% reduction in LDL-C)	Moderate-intensity statins (30% to < 50% reduction in LDL-C)	Low-intensity statins (<30% reduction in LDL-C)
• Atorvastatin, 40–80 mg • Rosuvastatin, 20–40 mg	• Atorvastatin, 10–20 mg • Rosuvastatin, 5–10 mg • Simvastatin, 20–40 mg • Pravastatin, 40–80 mg • Lovastatin, 40 mg • Fluvastatin, XL 80 mg • Fluvastatin, 40 mg BID • Pitavastatin, 2–4 mg	• Simvastatin, 10 mg • Pravastatin, 10–20 mg • Lovastatin, 20 mg • Fluvastatin, 20–40 mg • Pitavastatin, 1 mg

LDL-C, low density lipoprotein cholesterol; BID, twice a day.

efficacy and safety of more intensive lowering of LDL has been reviewed by "Cholesterol Treatment Trialists" Collaboration.[8] Clinical ASCVD includes acute coronary syndromes, history of myocardial infarction (MI), stable or unstable angina, coronary or other arterial revascularization, stroke, transient ischemic attack, or peripheral arterial disease presumed to be of atherosclerotic origin. When high-intensity statin therapy is contraindicated or when characteristics predisposing to statin-associated adverse effects are present, a moderate-intensity statin should be used as the second option if tolerated. Moderate-intensity statin therapy should be considered for individuals greater than 75 years of age with clinical ASCVD, since it is not clear that there is additional reduction in ASCVD events from high-intensity statin therapy.[1]

In patients not currently on a statin, initial evaluation includes a fasting lipid panel, hepatic transaminase [alanine transaminase (ALT)], creatinine kinase (CK) (if indicated, such as those with a personal or family history of statin intolerance or muscle disease, clinical presentation, or concomitant drug therapy that might increase the likelihood of myopathy) and evaluation for other secondary causes of LDL-C elevation.

During statin therapy, it is reasonable to measure CK in individuals with muscle symptoms and liver function tests if symptoms suggesting hepatotoxicity arise (e.g., unusual fatigue or weakness, loss of appetite, abdominal pain, dark-colored urine or jaundice).

After initiation of statin therapy, a follow-up lipid panel is recommended 4–12 weeks later to determine the patient's adherence. Then, surveillance testing should be performed every 3–12 months as clinically indicated.

Decreasing the statin dose may be considered when two consecutive values of LDL-C are less than 40 mg/dL, although there is no evidence that an excess of adverse events occurs when LDL-C is below this level.[1]

Statins are listed as pregnancy category X, and should not be used in women of childbearing potential unless these women are using effective contraception and are not nursing.

For primary prevention, a global ASCVD risk assessment is recommended to guide initiation of statin therapy. The Pooled Cohort Risk Assessment Equation is recommended to predict stroke as well as coronary heart disease events in women and men aged 40–79 years with or without diabetes who have LDL-C levels 70–189 mg/dL. In patients with high estimated 10-year ASCVD risk, primary prevention with statins reduces total mortality as well as nonfatal ASCVD events. Recent guidelines selected 7.5% as a threshold for statin treatment.[1] A downloadable spreadsheet enabling estimation of 10-year and lifetime risk for ASCVD and a web-based calculator are available at http://my.americanheart.org/cvriskcalculator.

Prior to initiating statin therapy, patients should be screened for characteristics that may be associated with an increased risk of adverse side effects with statin therapy, as discussed in the secondary prevention section. Significant statin adverse effects are rare but should be considered especially in the evaluation of their use for primary prevention in low-risk groups.

The rate of excess diabetes varies by statin intensity. For moderate-intensity statins, approximately 0.1 excess case of diabetes per 100 statin-treated individuals per year has been observed, and approximately 0.3 excess cases of diabetes per 100 statin-treated individuals per year have been observed for high-intensity statins. The long-term adverse effects of statin-associated cases of diabetes over a 10-year period are unclear and are unlikely to be equivalent to an MI, stroke, or ASCVD death. Myopathy (~0.01 excess case per 100) and hemorrhagic stroke (~0.01 excess case per 100) make minimal contributions to excess risk from statin therapy.[1]

Although ASCVD events are reduced by moderate- and high-intensity statin therapy for those with a 5% to less than 7.5% estimated 10-year ASCVD risk, the potential for adverse effects may outweigh the potential for ASCVD risk reduction benefit when high-intensity statin therapy is used in this risk group. However, for moderate-intensity statin therapy the ASCVD risk reduction exceeds the potential for adverse effects.[1]

Drugs Under the Category

The currently available statins are atorvastatin,[9] fluvastatin,[10] lovastatin,[11] pitavastatin,[12] pravastatin,[13] rosuvastatin,[14] and simvastatin.[15]

Mechanism of Action

Statins are competitive inhibitors of 3-hydroxy-3-methylglutaryl coenzyme A (HMG-CoA) reductase that is responsible for the conversion of HMG-CoA to mevalonate, a precursor of sterols, including cholesterol (Fig. 2). The inhibition in the cholesterol biosynthesis pathway reduces the cholesterol in hepatic cells, which further stimulates the synthesis of LDL receptors thereby increasing LDL uptake. The pleiotropic effects are probably related to a decrease in protein prenylation in peripheral cells with a subsequent decrease in activation and release of growth factors and a decrease in platelet aggregation or activation[16] (Fig. 3).

Pharmacology

Statins mimic the HMG moiety substrate of HMG-CoA reductase and competitively bind to the enzyme, although the binding site residues are different between statins and this affects their relative potency. The lipophilicity also varies and may influence side effects, such as an increase in the risk for muscle-related adverse effects (Table 2).[9-15,17]

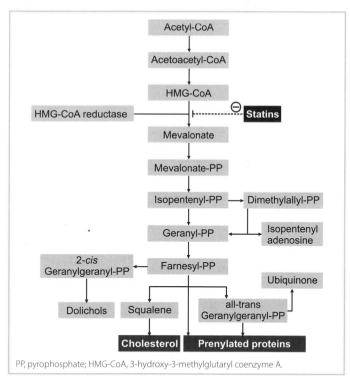

PP, pyrophosphate; HMG-CoA, 3-hydroxy-3-methylglutaryl coenzyme A.

FIG. 2: The mevalonate pathway and the beneficial effects of statins. The inhibition of HMG-CoA reductase results in a decrease in cholesterol and upregulation of LDL receptors. Mevalonic acid is the product of the effect of HMG-CoA reductase on HMG-CoA and is the precursor of numerous metabolites. The inhibition of HMG-CoA reductase has the potential to inhibit signaling pathways that require prenylated proteins resulting in decreased cell growth, an example of the pleiotropic effects of statins. In addition, isoprenoids such as isopentenyl adenosine, dolichols and ubiquinone are vital for diverse cellular functions.

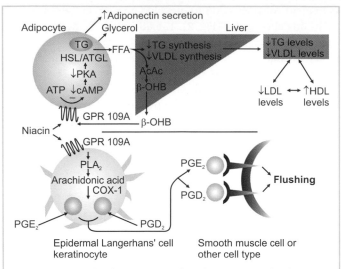

ATP, adenosine triphosphate; cAMP, cyclic adenosine monophosphate; PKA, protein kinase A; HSL, hormone sensitive lipase; ATGL, adipose triglyceride lipase; GPR, G protein-coupled receptor; TG, triglyceride; FFA, free fatty acid; VLDL, very low-density lipoprotein; AcAc, acetoacetate; β-OHB, β-hydroxybutyrate; LDL, low-density lipoprotein; HDL, high-density lipoprotein; PLA$_2$, phospholipase A$_2$; COX-1, cyclooxygenase-1; PGE$_2$, prostaglandin E$_2$; PGD$_2$, prostaglandin D$_2$.

FIG. 3: Mechanism of action of niacin for causing changes in lipids and flushing. GPR109A is a receptor for endogenous (β-OHB) and exogenous (e.g., niacin) ligands. Activation of the GPR109A (top panel) in the adipocyte results in inhibition of adenylate cyclase activity and subsequent reduction in cAMP levels and PKA, and HSL/ATGL activity. This results in reduced hydrolysis of TG and subsequent suppression of FFA and glycerol release from the adipocyte. At the same time, adipocyte secretion of adiponectin is increased. The reduction of substrate availability to the liver limits TG and VLDL synthesis and subsequently reduces serum concentrations of TG and LDL and increases HDL. In epidermal Langerhans' cells and keratinocytes (bottom panel), GPR109A activation results in arachidonic acid-mediated prostaglandin synthesis which will initiate a flushing response.[65]

All statins are absorbed rapidly with time to peak absorption within 4 hours.[18,19] However, their elimination half-lives vary considerably. Since atorvastatin and rosuvastatin have longer elimination half-lives, their cholesterol lowering efficacy is similar throughout the day.[19]

All statins, with the exception of pravastatin, are highly plasma protein bound and these statins are more likely to displace albumin-bound drugs, such as warfarin. For example, rosuvastatin or simvastatin coadministration can result in an increased prothrombin time.[14,15]

The cytochrome P450 (CYP) enzymes in the gastrointestinal (GI) tract and liver are responsible for statin metabolism, although some statins are more dependent on these enzymes for their metabolism than other statins. Interactions between statins and other drugs occur because of the interference with the CYP isoenzymes by either induction or inhibition of

TABLE 2: Pharmacology of statins[9-15,17]

	Atorvastatin	Fluvastatin	Lovastatin	Pitavastatin	Pravastatin	Rosuvastatin	Simvastatin
Lipophilicity Log P	Lipophilic 1.11	Lipophilic 1.27	Lipophilic 1.70	Lipophilic 1.43	Hydrophilic −0.84	Hydrophilic −0.33	Lipophilic 1.60
Metabolizing CYP enzymes	3A4	2C9 (75%) 2C8 (~5%) 3A4 (~20%)	3A4	Minimal (2C9 >2C8)	—	2C9	3A4
$t_{1/2}$ (hours)	14	0.5–2.3	2.9	12	1.3–2.8	19	1.9–3
Renal excretion (%)	<2	5	10	15	20	10	13
Protein binding (%)	>98	98	>95	>99	50	88	95

CYP, cytochrome P450; $t_{1/2}$, half-life.

the CYP enzymes. Induction of these enzymes may lead to a reduced bioavailability and therapeutic effect of the statin. In contrast, CYP enzyme inhibitors may raise the plasma concentration of statins and increase the risk of adverse effects, such as myopathy.[19]

Indications

Statins are indicated to:

- Lower LDL in patients with mixed (combined) dyslipidemias or familial hypercholesterolemia.
- Lower triglyceride levels in patients with mixed (combined) dyslipidemias or primary dysbetalipoproteinemia.

In addition, some of the statins are indicated for the reduction in the risk of total mortality by reducing CHD deaths and to reduce the risk of nonfatal MI, stroke, and the need for revascularization procedures in patients at high risk of coronary events.[9,13,15]

Dosage

Pravastatin

The recommended starting dose for pravastatin is 40 mg once a day. If this dose does not achieve desired cholesterol levels, 80 mg once a day can be used. However, a starting dose of 10 mg daily is recommended in patients with significant renal impairment.

Pravastatin can be administered as a single dose at any time of the day, irrespective of meal timings. Since the maximal effect of a given dose is seen within 4 weeks, periodic lipid determination should be performed at this time and dosage adjusted according to the patient's response to therapy and established guidelines.[13]

The dose of pravastatin should be initiated at 10 mg and not exceed 20 mg/day when administered along with cyclosporine. The dose should not exceed 40 mg/day when administered along with clarithromycin. Pravastatin should be avoided in patients taking gemfibrozil and used with caution on patients taking other fibrates or colchicine. A dose reduction should be considered in patients on niacin.[13]

Lovastatin

The usual recommended starting dose is 20 mg once a day given with the evening meal. The dose range is 10–80 mg/day in a single or two divided doses. A starting dose of 10 mg may be considered for patients requiring less than 20% reduction in LDL. Dose adjustments should be made at intervals of 4 weeks or more. In patients with severe renal insufficiency [i.e., glomerular filtration rate (GFR) <30 mL/min/1.73 m²], dosage above 20 mg/day should be implemented with caution.[11]

The use of lovastatin with strong inhibitors of CYP3A4 is contraindicated (*See* the heading "Contraindications" for the specific contraindicated drugs). The concomitant use of gemfibrozil or cyclosporine should be avoided. The lovastatin dose should not exceed 20 mg/day when administered along with danazol, diltiazem, dronedarone or verapamil and should not exceed 40 mg/day when administered with amiodarone. Caution should be exercised when coadministered with colchicine or ranolazine because of the risk of myopathy, including rhabdomyolysis.[11]

Simvastatin

The usual dosage range is 5–40 mg/day. The recommended starting dose is 10 or 20 mg once a day in the evening. However, for patients at high risk of a CHD event (e.g., patient with existing CHD, diabetes mellitus, peripheral vessel disease, history of stroke, or other cerebrovascular disease), the recommended starting dose is 40 mg/day. Due to the increased risk of myopathy, including rhabdomyolysis, particularly during the first year of treatment, use of 80 mg dose should be restricted to patients who have been taking the dose for 12 months or more without evidence of muscle toxicity. Patients receiving 80 mg dosing who need to be initiated on a drug with potential interaction that is contraindicated or associated with a dose maximum for simvastatin should be switched to an alternative statin with a lower potential for drug-drug interaction. Patients unable to achieve their LDL goal utilizing 40 mg dose should not be titrated to 80 mg dose, but should be placed on alternative LDL lowering therapy.[15]

The combined use of simvastatin with strong CYP3A4 inhibitors, gemfibrozil, cyclosporine, or danazol is contra-indicated (*See* the heading "Contraindications"). The daily dose should not exceed 10 mg/day when taken with verapamil, diltiazem or dronedarone and should not exceed 20 mg/day when taken with amiodarone, amlodipine, or ranolazine.[15]

Caution should be used when treating Chinese patients with simvastatin in doses exceeding 20 mg/day, while coadministering with lipid modifying doses of niacin (i.e., ≥1 g/day) because of the increased risk of myopathy. It is not known if the increased risk applies to other Asian patients.[15]

Atorvastatin

The recommended starting dose is 10 or 20 mg once a day. Patients who require greater than 45% reduction in LDL levels may be directly started on 40 mg once a day. The dosage range is 10–80 mg once a day. Atorvastatin can be administered as a single dose at any time of the day, irrespective of meal timings. Lipid levels should be analyzed within 2–4 weeks and dose should be adjusted as required. Renal disease does not affect the plasma concentration of atorvastatin, so dose adjustment in patients with renal dysfunction is not necessary.[9]

Atorvastatin should be avoided in patients taking cyclosporine, the human immunodeficiency virus (HIV) protease inhibitor combination, tipranavir plus ritonavir, or the hepatitis C protease inhibitor, telaprevir. Caution (and the lowest dose necessary) should be taken when prescribing atorvastatin in combination with the HIV protease inhibitor combination, lopinavir plus ritonavir. The atorvastatin dose should be limited to 20 mg/day when used with clarithromycin, itraconazole, or in patients with HIV taking a combination of saquinavir plus ritonavir, darunavir plus ritonavir, fosamprenavir, or fosamprenavir plus ritonavir. In HIV patients taking nelfinavir or the hepatitis C protease inhibitor, boceprevir, atorvastatin dosage should not exceed 40 mg/day.[9]

Atorvastatin is a substrate of the organic anion transport polypeptide transporter, organic anion transport protein 1B1 (OATP1B1). Therefore, inhibitors of OATP1B1 (e.g., cyclosporine) can increase the bioavailability of atorvastatin.[9]

Fluvastatin

For patients requiring LDL reduction to a goal of greater than 25%, the recommended starting dose is 40 mg in the evening, 80 mg as one extended-release (XR) tablet administered as a single dose at any time of the day, or 80 mg in divided doses of the 40 mg capsule given twice a day. The XR tablets should not be crushed or broken. For patients requiring LDL reduction to a goal of less than 25%, a starting dose of 20 mg may be used. The recommended dosing range is 20–80 mg/day.[10]

The fluvastatin dose should be limited to 20 mg twice a day for those patients who are also receiving cyclosporine or fluconazole. Fluvastatin should be cautiously used when patients are also taking fibrates, niacin, glibenclamide, phenytoin, or coumarin anticoagulants.[10]

Fluvastatin has not been studied at doses greater than 40 mg in patients with severe renal impairment, so caution should be exercised when treating such patients at higher doses. Fluvastatin may be taken without regard to meals. The maximal reduction in LDL is seen within 4 weeks.[10]

Rosuvastatin

The dose range is 5–40 mg once a day. The recommended starting dose of rosuvastatin is 10–20 mg once a day administered at any time of the day, with or without food. For patients with marked hyperlipidemia (e.g., LDL >190 mg/dL) and aggressive lipid targets, a 20 mg starting dose may be considered. After initiation or upon titration of rosuvastatin, lipid levels should be analyzed within 2–4 weeks and the dosage adjusted accordingly. The 40 mg dose should be used only for those patients who have not achieved their LDL goal utilizing the 20 mg dose. Initiation of rosuvastatin therapy with 5 mg once a day should be considered for Asian patients.[14]

The use of rosuvastatin with gemfibrozil should be avoided and the dose limited to 10 mg/day if used. The dose of rosuvastatin should not exceed 5 mg/day when used with cyclosporine. Caution should be exercised when coadministering rosuvastatin with protease inhibitors in combination with ritonavir. The rosuvastatin dose should be limited to 10 mg/day when given with combination therapy of ritonavir plus lopinavir or ritonavir plus atazanavir. Caution should also be exercised with dosing when patients are also taking niacin, fenofibrate, colchicine or coumarin anticoagulants.[14]

In patients with severe renal impairment (i.e., GFR <30 mL/min/1.73 m²) and not on hemodialysis, rosuvastatin should be started at 5 mg once a day and not exceed 10 mg once a day. In patients on hemodialysis, plasma concentrations were approximately 50% greater compared with healthy volunteers. Dose reduction should be considered in patients on rosuvastatin with unexplained proteinuria or hematuria found on routine urinalysis testing.[14]

Pitavastatin

The dose range for pitavastatin is 1–4 mg once a day irrespective of meals. The recommended starting dose is 2 mg once a day. After initiation or titration, lipid levels should be analyzed at 4 weeks and the dose adjusted accordingly. Patients with moderate and severe renal impairment (i.e., GFR 30–59 mL/min/1.73 m² and 15–29 mL/min/1.73 m², respectively) as well as end-stage renal disease receiving hemodialysis, should receive a starting dose of 1 mg once a day, and a maximum dose of 2 mg once a day.[12]

Pitavastatin is contraindicated in patients simultaneously receiving cyclosporine (See the heading "Contraindications"). The dose should not exceed 1 mg/day in patients receiving erythromycin and not exceed 2 mg/day in patients on rifampicin. Pitavastatin should be avoided with gemfibrozil and used with caution in patients on fibrates. A dose reduction should be considered in patients on niacin, and colchicine should be coadministered with caution because of reports of myopathy when used with statin therapy.[12]

Contraindications

Statins are contraindicated in:[9-15]

- Women who are or may become pregnant because of the potential hazard to the fetus. They are also contraindicated in nursing mothers because of the potential for serious adverse effects in nursing infants. Statins are pregnancy category X drugs.
- Patients with active liver disease or unexplained persistent elevation in hepatic transaminase elevations.
- Patients with hypersensitivity to any component of the medication.

Simvastatin and lovastatin are contraindicated for coadministration with strong CYP3A4 inhibitors (e.g., itraconazole, ketoconazole, posaconazole, voriconazole, HIV protease inhibitors, boceprevir, telaprevir, the macrolide antibiotics erythromycin and clarithromycin, the ketolide antibiotic telithromycin, the antidepressant nefazodone or cobicistat-containing products). Simvastatin is contraindicated in patients also taking gemfibrozil, cyclosporine, or danazol. Pitavastatin is contraindicated during concomitant administration of cyclosporine.[11,12,15]

Adverse Effects

Statins may cause myopathy (i.e., muscle ache or weakness) in conjunction with increases in creatine phosphokinase (CPK) greater than 10 times the upper limit of normal (ULN), although rare (i.e., <4 events/10,000 patient years[19]). Myopathy may take the form of rhabdomyolysis with or without acute renal failure secondary to myoglobinuria. The use of statins with CYP inhibitors increases the risk of myopathy and rhabdomyolysis and they should be discontinued if markedly elevated CPK levels occur or myopathy is diagnosed or suspected.[19] Statin dose adjustment is recommended when taking gemfibrozil, cyclosporine, or drugs that inhibit the CYP3A4 or 2C9 pathways (Table 3). Large quantities of grapefruit juice should be avoided while taking statins that are metabolized by CYP3A4 pathway.[9,11,15]

Statins should be temporarily withheld or discontinued during an acute, serious condition, suggesting myopathy or having a risk factor predisposing to the development of renal failure secondary to rhabdomyolysis (e.g., severe acute infection, hypotension, major surgery, trauma, severe metabolic, endocrine and electrolyte disorders, and uncontrolled seizures). Statins should be prescribed with caution in patients with predisposing factors for myopathy: Age greater than 65 years, female gender, undertreated hypothyroidism, or renal impairment. The risk of myopathy

TABLE 3: Statin interactions: Maximum recommended statin doses (mg) and cautions[9-15]

	Simvastatin	Lovastatin	Pravastatin	Atorvastatin	Rosuvastatin	Fluvastatin	Pitavastatin
Itraconazole	0[h]	0[h]	—	20 mg[a]	—	—	—
Ketoconazole	0[h]	0[h]	—	b	—	—	—
Posaconazole	0[h]	0[h]	—	b	—	—	—
Fluconazole	—	—	—	b	—	20 mg BD	—
Erythromycin	0[h]	0[h]	—	b	—	—	1 mg
Clarithromycin	0[h]	0[h]	40 mg	20 mg[a]	—	—	—
Telithromycin	0[h]	0[h]	—	—	—	—	—
HIV protease inhibitors	0[h]	0[h]	—	0–40 mg[c]	10 mg[c,d]	—	—
Telaprevir	0[h]	0[h]	—	Avoid	—	—	—
Boceprevir	0[h]	0[h]	—	—	—	—	—
Nefazodone	0[h]	0[h]	—	—	—	—	—
Gemfibrozil	0[h]	Avoid	Avoid	b,d	Avoid or 10 mg	d	d
Other fibrates	d	20 mg	d	b,d	d	d	d
>1 g niacin/day	b,d	20 mg	b	b	d	b	b
Cyclosporine	0[h]	Avoid	20 mg	Avoid	5 mg	20 mg BD	0[h]
Danazol	0[h]	20 mg	—	d	—	—	—
Amiodarone	10 mg	40 mg	—	—	—	—	—

(continued)

Table 3 (*continued*)

	Simvastatin	Lovastatin	Pravastatin	Atorvastatin	Rosuvastatin	Fluvastatin	Pitavastatin
Dronedarone	10 mg						
Verapamil	10 mg	20 mg	✓	✓	✓	✓	✓
Diltiazem	10 mg	20 mg	✓	✓	✓	✓	✓
Amlodipine	20 mg	✓	✓	✓	✓	✓	✓
Ranolazine	20 mg	✓	✓	✓	✓	✓	✓
Digoxin	✓	✓	✓	e	✓		
Warfarin	f	f	✓	✓	d	f	f
Rifampicin	✓	✓	✓	g	✓	✓	2
Phenytoin	✓	✓	✓	✓	✓	d	✓
Colchicine	d	✓	d	✓	✓	✓	✓

a Caution should be used at doses above this dose (lowest dose necessary should be used).

b Consider statin dose reduction when coadministering this drug.

c Refer to the section "Statin Dosage".

d Coadminister with caution.

e Coadministration of atorvastatin and digoxin can increase digoxin level by 20%, these patients should be monitored appropriately.

f Monitor INR when statin started.

g Administration of atorvastatin with inducers of CYP 450 3A4 (e.g., rifampicin and efavirenz) can lead to variable reduction in plasma concentration of atorvastatin. Thus, atorvastatin should be administered simultaneously with drugs that are 3A4 inducers since delaying the statin administration can result in reduced statin plasma concentration.

h Not to be used in this particular combination.

i No specific USFDA recommendation.

HIV, human immunodeficiency virus; CYP, cytochrome P450; INR, International Normalized Ratio; BD, twice a day.

is dose-related. About 5–10% of patients may report myalgias without CPK elevation during statin therapy. These symptoms typically resolve within 2 months of statin discontinuation.[20]

Myalgias are a common adverse effect of statins. If the symptoms are mild-to-moderate, the statin can be discontinued until the symptoms can be evaluated. Initial evaluation should include assessment for other conditions that might increase the risk for muscle symptoms (e.g., hypothyroidism, reduced renal or liver function, rheumatologic disorders such as polymyalgia rheumatica, steroid myopathy, vitamin D deficiency or a primary muscle disease).

If muscle symptoms resolve, and if no contraindication exists, the patient may be given the original or a lower dose of the same statin to establish a causal relationship between the muscle symptoms and statin therapy. If a causal relationship exists, the statin should be discontinued, and when muscle symptoms resolve, start a low dose of a different statin or an intermittent dose of a long-acting statin (such as atorvastatin or rosuvastatin). Then, if a low or intermittent dose is tolerated, the dose can be gradually increased as tolerated. However, if muscle symptoms or elevated CK level do not resolve completely after 2 months, consider another etiology of the muscle symptoms.

If the muscle symptoms are severe, the statin should be discontinued and the patient evaluated for the possibility of rhabdomyolysis by checking CK, creatinine, and urinalysis for myoglobinuria.

Nonstatin cholesterol-lowering drugs [such as ezetimibe, bile acid sequestrants (BASs) and niacin] are alternative pharmacologic agents to lower LDL-C in statin intolerant patients.

Statins have been associated with biochemical abnormalities of liver function with alanine aminotransferase (ALT) elevations in less than 1.2%, although increasing to 2.3% with higher doses. Liver enzyme changes generally occur in the first 3 months of therapy (possibly related to changes in the lipid components of the hepatocyte membrane, leading to an increase in permeability).[21] ALT and aspartate aminotransferase (AST) should be checked prior to the initiation of therapy and when clinically indicated. Serious liver injury with statins is rare and unpredictable in patients. Routine periodic monitoring of liver enzymes does not appear to be effective in detecting or preventing serious liver injury. However, if liver injury occurs and an alternative etiology is not found, statin therapy should not be restarted.[22]

Patients who develop increased transaminase levels should be monitored until the abnormalities resolve. Nearly 70% of cases resolve spontaneously.[21] Statins should be used with caution in patients who consume substantial quantities of alcohol and/or have a history of liver disease.

Strategies to improve statin tolerance include decreasing the statin dose, intermittent dosing of long-acting statins (e.g., atorvastatin and rosuvastatin), or alternative LDL-lowering agents (e.g., niacin, BASs, or ezetimibe).[20]

Memory loss and confusion have been reported with statin use; however, these symptoms are not common, generally not serious, do not lead to cognitive decline, and resolve when the statin is discontinued. The time to onset is highly variable, ranging from one day to years after exposure. The reported cases do not appear to be associated with dementia, such as Alzheimer's disease.[22]

Statin therapy has been associated with a 9–13% increased risk of diabetes mellitus. However, the United States Food and Drug Administration (USFDA) believes that the CV benefits of statins outweigh the small increased risk associated with an elevation in glucose levels.[22]

Clinical Evidence

In general, the reduction in LDL increases with statin dose. For example, fluvastatin XR 80 mg, lovastatin 40 mg, pravastatin 20–40 mg, simvastatin 20 mg, atorvastatin 10 mg, and pitavastatin 1–2 mg are equivalent in decreasing LDL by 30–40%. Greater than 40% reduction is expected with atorvastatin greater than 20 mg, rosuvastatin greater than 5 mg, and pitavastatin 4 mg. The HDL elevating and triglyceride lowering effects are similar among different statins of equivalent dose (Table 4).[23]

Secondary prevention trials have demonstrated that statin therapy reduces coronary morbidity and mortality as well as overall mortality (Table 5).[9,10,13,15,24] Primary prevention trials have expanded the populations shown to benefit from statins to include patients without CHD.[9,11,13,14,24] Generic pricing has ameliorated concerns over cost effectiveness. In a meta-analysis of 10 primary prevention trials, statin therapy was associated with a significant 12% relative risk reduction (RRR) in all-cause mortality, a 30% RRR in major coronary events and a 19% RRR in major cerebrovascular events. Moreover, statin use was not associated with an increased risk of cancer.[25]

Choice of Therapy/Guidelines

Statins are recommended as first-line therapy for secondary prevention in patients with clinical ASCVD, familial hyper-cholesterolemia (i.e., LDL >190 mg/dL), diabetes mellitus and for primary prevention with a greater than 7.5%, 10-year risk of heart disease or stroke (Table 6).

TABLE 4: Changes in lipoprotein levels with statin therapy[9-15]

Statin	Dose (mg)	Low-density lipoprotein cholesterol (% change)	High-density lipoprotein cholesterol (% change)	Triglycerides (% change)
Lovastatin				
—	10	–21	5	–10
	20	–27	6	9
	40	–31	5	–8
Fluvastatin				
Baseline triglycerides ≤200	20	–22	3	–12
	40	–25	4	–14
	40 BD	–36	6	–18
	80 XR	–35	7	–19
Baseline triglycerides >200	20	–22	6	–17
	40	–24	7	–20
	40 BD	–35	9	–23
	80 XR	–33	11	–25
Rosuvastatin				
Baseline triglycerides ≤250	5	–45	13	–35
	10	–52	14	–10
	20	–55	8	–23
	40	–63	10	–28

(continued)

Table 4 (continued)

Statin	Dose (mg)	Low-density lipoprotein cholesterol (% change)	High-density lipoprotein cholesterol (% change)	Triglycerides (% change)
Baseline triglycerides >250	5	−28	3	−21
	10	−45	8	−37
	20	−31	22	−37
	40	−43	17	−43
Pravastatin				
Baseline triglycerides ≤200	10	−22	7	−15
	20	−32	2	−11
	40	−34	12	−24
	80	−37	3	−19
Baseline triglycerides >200	40	−32	7	−21
Dysbetalipoproteinemia	40	−30 to −41	5 to 6	−12 to −24
Pitavastatin				
—	1	−32	8	−15
	2	−36	7	−19
	4	−43	5	−18
Atorvastatin				
Baseline triglycerides ≤250	10	−39	6	−19
	20	−43	9	−26
	40	−50	6	−29
	80	−60	5	−37

(continued)

Table 4 (*continued*)

Statin	Dose (mg)	Low-density lipoprotein cholesterol (% change)	High-density lipoprotein cholesterol (% change)	Triglycerides (% change)
Baseline triglycerides >250	10	−26	14	−41
	20	−30	11	−39
	80	−40	8	−52
Dysbetalipoproteinemia	10	—	—	−39
	80	—	—	−53
Simvastatin				
—	5	−26	10	−12
	10	−30	12	−15
	20	−38	8	−19
	40	−41	9	−18
	80	−47	8	−24
Baseline triglycerides elevated (median, 404)	40	−28	11	−29
	80	−37	15	−34
Dysbetalipoproteinemia	40		7	−41
	80		7	−38

BD, twice a day; XR extended release.

TABLE 5: Statin prevention trials

Statin	Trial (Year)	Dose (mg)	Population (Number of patients)	Baseline LDL	Duration (Years)	End-points	Relative risk reduction (p value)
Primary prevention							
Pravastatin	West of Scotland (1995)[13]	40	LDL >155 (6,595 men)	272	4.8	CHD death, non-fatal MI	31% (p = 0.0001)
Atorvastatin	ASCOT (2003)[9]	10	Hypertensive and >3 other risk factors [10,305 (81% men)]	132	3.3	Fatal and non-fatal CHD	36% (p = 0.0005)
Atorvastatin	CARDS (2004)[9]	10	Diabetes mellitus + >1 additional risk factor [2,838 (68% men)]	117	3.9	MI, CHD death, unstable angina, coronary revascularization, and stroke	37% (p = 0.001)
Rosuvastatin	JUPITER (2008)[14]	20	LDL <130, hs-CRP >2 mg/dL (17,802)	108	2	CV death, nonfatal MI, nonfatal stroke, hospitalization for unstable angina or arterial revascularization	44% (p < 0.001)
Lovastatin	AFCAPS/TexCAPS (1998)[11]	20–40	LDL 130–190; 63% with >1 risk factor (6,605)	150	5.1	MI, unstable angina, and sudden cardiac death	37% (p < 0.001)
Secondary prevention							
Fluvastatin	LIPS (2002)[10]	40 BD vs. placebo	CAD after PCI (1,677)	131	3.9	Recurrent cardiac events	22% (p = 0.013)

(continued)

Table 5 (continued)

Statin	Trial (Year)	Dose (mg)	Population (Number of patients)	Baseline LDL	Duration (Years)	End-points	Relative risk reduction (p value)
Pravastatin	LIPID (1998)[13]	40 OD vs. placebo	CAD (MI or unstable angina) (7,498 men, 1,516 women)	150	5.6	CHD death	24% (p = 0.0004)
Pravastatin	CARE (1996)[13]	40 OD vs. placebo	Previous MI (3,583 men, 576 women)	139	4.9	CHD death and non-fatal MI	24% (p = 0.003)
Atorvastatin	TNT (2005)[9]	80 vs. 10 OD	CAD and LDL <130 mg/dL (on atorvastatin 10)[10,001 (81% men)]	<130	4.9	CHD death, non-fatal MI, resuscitated cardiac arrest, and fatal/non-fatal stroke	22% (p = 0.0002)
Simvastatin	4S (1994)[15]	20 [could titrate to 10 (n = 2) or 40 (37%)]	CAD [4,444 (81% men)]	188	5.4	Overall mortality	30% (p = 0.0003)
Simvastatin	HPS (2002)[15]	40	CAD, occlusive non-CAD arterial diease, or DM [20,536 (75% men)]	132	5	Overall mortality and CHD mortality	13% (p = 0.0003) 18% (p = 0.0005)

ASCOT, Anglo-Scandinavian Cardiac Outcomes Trial; CARDS, Collaborative Atorvastatin Diabetes Study; JUPITER, Justification for the Use of Statins in Prevention: an Intervention Trial Evaluating Rosuvastatin; AFCAPS/TexCAPS, Air Force/Texas Coronary Atherosclerosis Prevention Study; LIPS, Lescol Intervention Prevention Study; LIPID, Long-term Intervention with Pravastatin in Ischemic Disease; CARE, Cholesterol and Recurrent Events; TNT, Treating to New Target; 4S, Scandinavian Simvastatin Survival Study; HPS, Heart Protection Study; LDL, low-density lipoprotein cholesterol; MI, myocardial infarction; CV, cardiovascular; CHD, coronary heart disease; CAD, coronary artery disease; hs-CRP, high-sensitivity C-reactive protein; PCI, percutaneous coronary intervention; DM, diabetes mellitus; BD, twice a day; OD, once a day.

TABLE 6: Recommendations for statin use

	Moderate-intensity statin	High-intensity statin
Clinical ASCVD	Age >75 years, or Not candidate for high-intensity statin	Age ≤75 years
LDL-C >190 mg/dL	Not candidate for high-intensity statin	Yes
Diabetes mellitus, type 1 or 2 (age 40–75 years), and no ASCVD	10 years risk score <7.5%	10 years risk score ≥7.5%
10 years risk >7.5%, no ASCVD and LDL-C 70–189 mg/dL	Moderate to high-intensity statin	

ASCVD, arteriosclerotic cardiovascular disease; LDL-C, low-density lipoprotein-cholesterol.

FIBRATES

Introduction

Fibrates are considered first-line therapy for severe hypertriglyceridemia.[26] Fibrates decrease triglyceride levels by 20–50%, with a more significant effect when baseline levels are higher.[27] HDL increases in the range of 10–20%, and is also related to the severity of the baseline abnormality. LDL may decrease by 5–20%, but LDL may increase if high triglycerides are present.[1-4] Fibrates also reduce small, dense LDL by promoting a shift to larger, more buoyant particles, which are less susceptible to oxidation and possess higher binding affinity for the LDL receptor.[28,29] Fibrates reduce triglycerides and increase HDL, but their impact on improving outcome in patients with metabolic syndrome already on a statin is controversial.

For patients presenting with baseline triglycerides greater than 500 mg/dL, the goal of therapy is a reduction in the risk of pancreatitis and not CV risk.[1-4] When fasting triglycerides are greater than 1,000 mg/dL, there is usually a secondary cause of hypertriglyceridemia (e.g., diabetes mellitus, hypothyroidism, or medications known to increase triglycerides, such as β-blockers or thiazide diuretics) occurring in individuals with one or more common genetic hypertriglyceridemia disorders, such as familial hypertriglyceridemia or familial combined hyperlipidemia. Excess body weight and alcohol intake may be important factors in hypertriglyceridemia and should be addressed prior to therapy.[1]

Fibrates are agonists for the peroxisome proliferator activated receptor-α (PPAR-α) group of nuclear receptors, which control expression of genes that play important roles in lipid cholesterol transport and metabolism. The PPAR-α receptors are located in liver, kidney, heart, and skeletal muscle cells where higher amounts of fatty acids are metabolized.[29]

Fibrates also have pleiotropic effects on endothelial function, vascular inflammation, and coagulation or fibrinolytic pathways.[26]

Drugs Under the Category

Fenofibrate, fenofibric acid, gemfibrozil, and bezafibrate are the currently available fibrates. There are many available dosing formulations of fenofibrate for patients with and without renal dysfunction. The differences among strengths are in part related to bioavailability, which varies with particle size (i.e., micronized formulations have lower dose strengths because of improved bioavailability of the smaller particles).

Mechanism of Action

Multiple mechanisms are involved through which fibrates lower plasma triglycerides levels.[29,30]

- Suppression of fatty acid synthesis.
- Increase in fatty acid catabolism by stimulation of mitochondrial uptake and β-oxidation of fatty acids.
- Decrease in production of triglycerides by inhibition of diacylglycerol acyltransferase 2 (DGAT2), an enzyme that catalyzes formation of triglyceride from diglyceride.
- Increase in triglyceride hydrolysis of VLDL (and chylomicrons) by stimulation of lipoprotein lipase (LPL) expression. LPL action is also potentiated by the decreased expression of hepatic apolipoprotein-C3, a lipoprotein that attenuates LPL activity.

As VLDL level is reduced, plasma cholesteryl ester transfer protein (CETP) activity is attenuated. This results in a shift of smaller to larger, more buoyant, LDL particles and diminished triglyceride content in HDL particles with increased cholesterol ester content (Fig. 4). The formation of LDL particles with a higher affinity for the LDL receptor increases their removal and large HDL is less vulnerable to renal excretion.[31]

Fibrates promote reverse cholesterol transport (RCT) and increase HDL-C in part through an increase in tissue production of apo-A1 and apo-A2. Apo-A1 is a structural protein for HDL and an activator of lecithin cholesterol acyltransferase. Apo-A2 is also a structural protein for HDL and an activator of hepatic lipase. The HDL particle profile then shifts from a predominance of small, protein-rich, lipid-poor HDL3 to large, cholesterol ester rich HDL2 particles. Fibrates may upregulate adenosine triphosphate (ATP) binding cassette A1 (ABC A1) on the surface of macrophages (which promotes conversion of unstable nascent HDL to stable spherical particles) and scavenger receptor B1 (SRB1) on the surface of hepatocytes.[29-31]

Nonlipid changes with fibrates may help account for the decreased risk of CV disease with their use. For example,

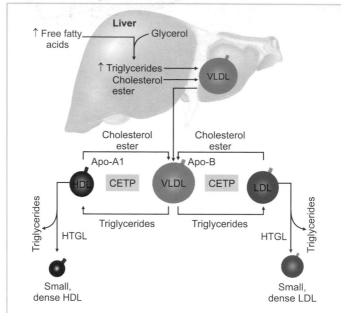

Apo-A1, apolipoprotein-A1; Apo-B, apolipoprotein-B100; HDL, high-density lipoprotein; HTGL, hepatic triglyceride lipase; LDL, low-density lipoprotein; VLDL, very low-density lipoprotein; CETP, cholesteryl ester transfer protein.

FIG. 4: Metabolic consequences of hypertriglyceridemia and the metabolic syndrome. In the setting of insulin resistance and mixed dyslipidemia, there is increased free fatty acid flux to the liver and increased VLDL secretion. Higher VLDL output activates CETP that results in enrichment of LDL and HDL. The triglyceride content within these particles is hydrolyzed by hepatic triglyceride lipase which results in small, dense LDL and HDL particles.

fibrates reduce the inflammatory and prothrombotic markers, including C-reactive protein (CRP) and lipoprotein-associated phospholipase A2.[29]

Fibrate therapy appears to have a synergistic effect with niacin on HDL, since their mechanisms of action are complementary. Fibrates stimulate hepatic production of apo-A1 while niacin inhibits its catabolism.[31]

The decreased uric acid levels seen in the fenofibrate trials are related to an increase in the urinary excretion of uric acid.

Pharmacology

Gemfibrozil is completely absorbed after oral administration, reaching peak plasma concentration 1–2 hours after dosing. Both the rate and extent of absorption of the drug are increased when administered 0.5 hour before meals, so dosing is recommended before meals. Approximately 70% of an administered dose is excreted in the urine, mostly as the glucuronide conjugate, while less than 2% is excreted as unchanged gemfibrozil. Gemfibrozil is highly bound to plasma proteins and there is a potential for displacement interactions with other drugs. The elimination half-life is approximately 1.1 hours.[29,32]

Fenofibrate is a prodrug of the active moiety, fenofibric acid. Fenofibrate is converted by ester hydrolysis to fenofibric acid. Protein binding is approximately 99%. Fenofibric acid is metabolized by conjugation with glucuronic acid and primarily excreted in the urine (60%) in the form of fenofibric acid and fenofibric acid glucuronide. Approximately 25% is excreted in the feces. Neither fenofibrate nor fenofibric acid undergo oxidative metabolism by CYP P450 to a significant extent. The elimination half-life is approximately 20 hours.[29,33-35]

Bezafibrate has an elimination half-life of 1–2 hours and protein binding of 94–96%. Excretion is almost exclusively renal, with 95% recovered in the urine.[36]

Indications

Fibrates are indicated as adjunctive therapy to diet for treatment of adult patients with severe hypertriglyceridemia.[32-36]

As noted above, fibrates have a variable effect on LDL and may increase LDL in patients with atherogenic dyslipidemia (i.e., elevated triglycerides and low HDL). Therefore, the potential benefit of a fibrate in treating patients with elevation of LDL only is not likely to outweigh the risk of potential side effects.

Fibrates are not indicated for the treatment of patients with isolated low HDL as their only lipid abnormality.[32]

Dosage

Fenofibrate

The recommended dose of fenofibrate will vary on the product used. In the USA, the initial dose is 120–160 mg once a day, depending on the trade name. The recommended initial dose of fenofibric acid is 135 mg once a day.[35]

For severe hypertriglyceridemia, the initial recommended dosing is between the low and high dose, "individualized according to patient response".[33-36]

For patients with impaired renal function, the initial dose of fenofibrate or fenofibric acid should be lowered. A low dose is recommended when GFR is less than 60 mL/min/1.73 m^2 and may be given without regard to meals.[33,34] Fenofibrate and fenofibric acid should not be used if moderate or severe renal impairment is present (i.e., if GFR <30 mL/min/1.73 m^2). Renal status should be evaluated before the fibrate initiation. If, during follow-up, the GFR decreases persistently to levels ≤30 mL/min/1.73 m^2, the fibrate should be discontinued.

Caution should be exercised when coadministering with colchicine because of cases of myopathy, including rhabdomyolysis that have been reported with the combination.[35]

Gemfibrozil

The recommended dose of gemfibrozil is 600 mg twice a day, given 30 minutes before the morning and evening meals.[32] Dose adjustment is recommended according to GFR with a dose decrease to 600 mg once a day when GFR is less than 60 mL/min/1.73 m^2. However, since half-life is independent of renal function, dose adjustment may not be necessary in patients with renal transplant or chronic renal disease.[37,38] Fibrate use is not recommended in patients who undergo long-term dialysis, because of the narrow margin between effective and toxic doses.[37]

When combining gemfibrozil with anticoagulants, caution should be exercised and the dose of anticoagulant reduced to maintain the prothrombin time at the desired level to prevent bleeding complications.

There have been reports of worsening renal function in patients with baseline creatinine greater than 2.0 mg/dL and there should be consideration of a lower dose versus alternative therapy.

Bezafibrate

The recommended dosage of bezafibrate is 200 mg twice or thrice a day (or 400 mg sustained release formula daily), with a dose adjustment according to renal function. The sustained release form is contraindicated if GFR is less than 60 mL/min/1.73 m^2.[36]

Since BAS may bind other drugs given concurrently, patients should take fibrates at least 1 hour before or 4–6 hours after a BAS to avoid impeding its absorption. An interval of 2 hours should be maintained between intake of a BAS and the sustained release formulation.

Fibrate therapy should be withdrawn in patients who do not have an adequate response after 2 months of treatment with the maximum dose.

Contraindications

Contraindications include hypersensitivity reactions to the medication or history of active liver disease (including those with primary biliary cirrhosis) and unexplained persistent liver function abnormalities, severe renal dysfunction (including patients receiving dialysis), or preexisting gallbladder disease.

The combination of gemfibrozil with the oral hypoglycemic agent repaglinide is contraindicated because of the risk of severe hypoglycemia.

Fibrates are pregnancy category C drugs and should be used during pregnancy only if the benefit justifies the potential risk to the fetus. Fibrates are contraindicated in nursing mothers because of the tumorigenicity seen in animal studies.[32-36]

Adverse Effects

Myopathy and rhabdomyolysis have been reported with fibrate use and the risk is increased when fibrates are coadministered with a statin, particularly in elderly patients and in patients with diabetes mellitus, renal failure, or hypothyroidism.[27,32-36] Approximately 1% of patients in fibrate trials withdrew because of muscle discomfort.[31] The risk of rhabdomyolysis is increased when fibrates, in particular gemfibrozil, are coadministered with a statin. The rate of myopathy for gemfibrozil with a statin is estimated to be 33 times more than that of a statin with fenofibrate.[37] The combination should be avoided unless the benefit of further alterations in lipid levels is likely to outweigh the increased risk of this drug combination. The increased risk associated with the gemfibrozil-statin combination is likely related to the inhibition of statin glucuronidation by gemfibrozil. If gemfibrozil is necessary, fluvastatin may be an appropriate option, since there is no significant effect of gemfibrozil on its concentration.[27,31,37]

In the Fenofibrate Intervention and Event Lowering in Diabetes (FIELD) trial, there were no cases of rhabdomyolysis reported in approximately 1,000 patients taking combination fenofibrate-statin therapy.[38] In the Action to Control Cardiovascular Risk in Diabetes (ACCORD) trial, 40% of participants reported muscle symptoms during the trial, but the number reporting such symptoms was essentially identical in both the fenofibrate or statin and placebo or statin groups.[39] In addition, such complaints were rarely associated with an elevation in CPK greater than 10 times ULN (0.4% in fenofibrate and 0.3% in placebo).[39,40]

Fenofibrate at doses of 96–145 mg/day has been associated with increases in serum hepatic transaminases. In a pooled analysis of 10 placebo-controlled trials, increases to greater than 3 times the ULN occurred in 5.3% of patients taking fenofibrate (compared to 1.1% on placebo).[33,34] The incidence of increases in transaminases related to fenofibrate therapy appears to be dose-related. When transaminase determinations have been followed either after discontinuation of treatment or during continued treatment, a return to normal has usually been observed. Liver function tests, including ALT, should be periodically monitored during therapy and therapy discontinued if enzyme levels persist greater than 3 times the ULN.

Fenofibrate can reversibly increase serum creatinine levels by 10–20%,[41] so renal function should be monitored periodically in patients with renal impairment. The etiology of the reversible increase in creatinine is uncertain, although fibrates may increase creatinine production with no attenuation of GFR.[37] Fenofibrate and bezafibrate are more likely than gemfibrozil to increase creatinine.[29] In the ACCORD trial, the study drug was discontinued by 2.4% in fenofibrate and 1.1% in the placebo group because of a decrease in the estimated GFR. This effect of fenofibrate was also seen in the FIELD trial. A serum creatinine should be checked before initiating fibrate therapy, and routine creatinine monitoring is recommended in patients with preexisting chronic kidney disease.[37]

Fibrates alter biliary composition, reducing bile acid content and increasing cholesterol content. Increased biliary secretion of cholesterol may be a major mechanism for cholesterol removal from the body, but it increases lithogenicity of bile.[27,37] While an early clinical trial with clofibrate demonstrated that cholecystectomies occurred 2–3 times more often than in placebo-treated patient, the association with gemfibrozil and fenofibrate is less clear. A recent meta-analysis demonstrated no increased risk of gallbladder disease.[42] However, fibrate therapy should be discontinued if gallstones are found and are not recommended in the presence of preexisting gallbladder disease.[31]

Pancreatitis has been reported in patients on fenofibrate or gemfibrozil. This may represent a failure of efficacy in patients with severe hypertriglyceridemia, a direct drug effect, or a secondary phenomenon, mediated by biliary tract stone or sludge formation with common bile duct obstruction.[32-36]

Pulmonary embolism occurred in 1% of the fenofibrate group, compared to 0.7% in the placebo group (p = 0.022) in the FIELD trial.[39] Treatment with fibrates and fenofibrate, in particular, is known to increase homocysteine levels, an effect which may be mediated by a direct PPAR-α action.[37] However, gemfibrozil does not appear to raise homocysteine and no change in thromboembolic events was reported in the Helsinki Heart Study (HHS) or Veterans Affairs HDL Intervention Trial (VA-HIT).[27,43,44] The dosage of coumarin anticoagulants may need to be adjusted during fibrate therapy to prevent bleeding complications.[37]

Severe reductions in HDL-C (to as low as 2 mg/dL) have been reported in patients initiated on fenofibrate and fenofibric acid therapy. The decrease in HDL-C is accompanied by a decrease in apo-A1 and occurs within 2 weeks of fibrate initiation. The low HDL-C increases rapidly once the fibrate is withdrawn. The clinical significance of the HDL-C decrease is not known.[33,35]

Clinical Evidence

Lipid effects of fibrates are generally additive to those of statin monotherapy,[45,46] especially with respect to improvements in triglycerides and HDL, making the combination a useful option to manage patients with combined dyslipidemia and metabolic syndrome (Table 7).[27,30] However, the addition of gemfibrozil rather than fenofibrate (or fenofibric acid) to a statin is associated with an increased risk of rhabdomyolysis (*See* the heading "Adverse Effects").

Angiographic trials have shown that fibrates retard progression of atherosclerotic coronary artery disease (CAD).[31] Results from clinical trials have not been consistent in their finding of impact on CV events and mortality. While fibrate therapy is associated with a clinically important decrease in nonfatal MI, they have little effect, if any, on all-cause mortality.[42,47] However, subgroup analyses have demonstrated that in patients with atherogenic dyslipidemia (i.e., high triglyceride levels and low HDL), fibrates may exert a greater cardioprotective effect than in the general populations studied (Table 8).[26,39-41,43,44,48-50] A meta-analysis of the five major fibrate trials found that fibrate-treated patients with atherogenic dyslipidemia had a 30% RRR of major CV events.[51]

Fibrate therapy is associated with a reduction in micro vascular complications of diabetes mellitus, including progression of albuminuria and diabetic retinopathy.[42] The reduced risk of progression of diabetic retinopathy appears to be mainly restricted to patients with baseline retinopathy.[26]

Choice of Therapy/Guidelines

Treatment of elevated triglyceride levels depends on the cause and severity of elevation. In patients with triglycerides greater than 500 mg/dL, fibrate therapy should be started to prevent

TABLE 7: Changes in lipoprotein levels with fenofibrate (or fenofibric acid) as monotherapy and in combination with statin therapy

Trials	LDL (% change)	HDL (% change)	Triglycerides (% change)
SAFARI (2005)[45]			
Simvastatin 20 mg	−26	10	−20
Simvastatin 20 mg + Fenofibrate 160 mg/day	−31*	19*	−43*
Goldberg et al. (2009)[46]			
Atorvastatin 20 mg	−37	6	−16
Atorvastatin 20 mg + Fenofibric acid 135 mg/day	−34	14**	−46*

*p < 0.001 vs. statin. **p = 0.005 vs. statin.
LDL, low-density lipoprotein; HDL, high-density lipoprotein; SAFARI, simvastatin plus fenofibrate for combined hyperlipidemia.

TABLE 8: Fibrate clinical trials

Trial (Year)/ duration (Years)	Fibrate (Dose)	Patients (Number)	Population	Primary outcome	LDL (% change)	HDL (% change)	TG (% change)	RRR in primary end-point: entire cohort (p value)	Lipid subgroup criterion	RRR in primary end-point: subgroup (p value)
									Outcomes	
HHS (1987, 1992)[43,48]/5	Gemfibrozil (600 mg BD)	4,081 M (1° prevention)	Non-HDL ≥200 + No CAD	Fatal or nonfatal MI, cardiac death	−11	11	−35	−34% (0.02)	TG ≥204, HDL <42, BMI >26 kg/m²	−78% (0.005)
VA-HIT (1999)[44]/5.1	Gemfibrozil (600 mg BD)	2,531 M (2° prevention)	HDL ≤40 + LDL ≤140 + CAD	Nonfatal MI, death from CHD	0	6	−31	−22% (0.006)	HDL <31.5 TG ≥151	−30% (0.003)* −27 (0.01)*
BIP (2000)[49]/6.2	Bezafibrate (400 mg/day)	3,090 (91% M) (2° prevention)	HDL ≤45 + LDL ≤180 + TG ≤300 + CAD	Fatal or non-fatal MI or sudden death	−6	18	−21	−7.3% (0.24)	TG ≥200 + HDL <35	−42% (0.02)
FIELD (2005, 2009)[39,50]/5	Fenofibrate (200 mg/day)	9,795 M) (1° + 2° prevention)	Diabetic + TC 116–251 + HDL >4 or TG 87–443	Nonfatal MI or CHD death	−12	5	−29	−11% (0.16)	TG ≥204 + HDL ≤42	−27% (0.005)
ACCORD (2010)[40]/4.7	Fenofibrate (160 mg/day)	5,518 (69% M) (1° + 2° prevention)	Diabetic on statin + LDL 60–180 + HDL<50–55 + TG <400	Nonfatal MI, nonfatal stroke, or cardiac death	−11	6	−21	−8% (0.32)	TG ≥204 + HDL ≤34	−31% (0.057)

*Includes confirmed stroke.

HHS, Helsinki Heart Study; VA-HIT, Veterans Affairs High-density Lipoprotein Cholesterol Intervention Trial; BIP, Bezafibrate Infarction Prevention; FIELD; Fenofibrate Intervention and Event Lowering in Diabetes; ACCORD; Action to Control Cardiovascular Risk in Diabetes, BD, twice a day; HDL, high-density lipoprotein; LDL, low-density lipoprotein; CAD, coronary artery disease; TG, triglyceride; MI, myocardial infarction; BMI, body mass index; RRR, relative risk reduction; TC, total cholesterol; M, men.

pancreatitis. Only after triglycerides are less than 500 mg/dL, should attention be turned to LDL lowering in order to reduce the risk of CHD.[1-4]

In patients with mixed dyslipidemia, after achieving goal LDL, the addition of a fibrate to patients with triglycerides in the range of 200–499 mg/dL already on a statin is debatable since there is, at best, a trend in improved outcomes when a fibrate is added. Aside from weight reduction and increased physical activity, if additional triglyceride is desired, a consensus guideline preferred the combination of statin and niacin over statin and fibrate because of better evidence for the former in reducing CV risk and the potential for myopathy with combination statin and fibrate therapy (especially if the fibrate is gemfibrozil).[52]

Subgroup and post hoc analyses imply mortality benefits for treating patients with elevated triglycerides and low HDL. However, there are no studies that prospectively examine a patient population with the metabolic syndrome and, therefore, the true mortality benefit of fibrates remains to be determined.[31] The combination of statin and fibrate should be reserved for high-risk patients, only after optimal control of LDL has been achieved with statin therapy.[53]

BILE ACID SEQUESTRANTS

Introduction

Bile acid sequestrants are large polymers that bind the negatively charged bile acids and bile salts in the small intestine. As bile acids decrease, hepatic cholesterol is converted to bile acid and there is a compensatory increase in LDL receptors. Monotherapy with BAS lowers LDL by 5–30% in a dose-dependent manner.[54]

Cholestyramine and colestipol were initially available as water-insoluble powder, but colestipol was subsequently developed as a tablet form to improve palatability and compliance.[55] Colesevelam was developed with a unique polymer structure accounting for its gelatinous structure (in contrast to the sandy consistency of cholestyramine and colestipol) and is a high-capacity bile acid-binding molecule.

Mechanism of Action

During normal digestion, bile acids are secreted in the bile from the liver and gallbladder into the intestine. Bile acids emulsify the fat and lipid material present in food, facilitating dietary fat and lipid-soluble vitamin absorption. A major portion of the secreted bile acid is reabsorbed from the intestines and returned to the liver via portal circulation, thus, forming the

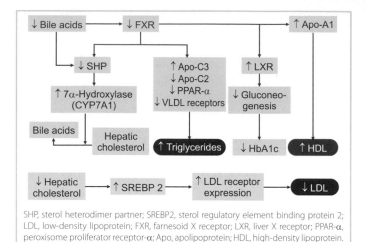

SHP, sterol heterodimer partner; SREBP2, sterol regulatory element binding protein 2; LDL, low-density lipoprotein; FXR, farnesoid X receptor; LXR, liver X receptor; PPAR-α, peroxisome proliferator receptor-α; Apo, apolipoprotein; HDL, high-density lipoprotein.

FIG. 5: Mechanism of action of bile acid sequestrants (BASs). The reduction in bile acids by BASs reduces activity of the FXR. LDL levels are reduced due to increased clearance by receptors which compensates for the reduced hepatic cholesterol (due to conversion to bile acids). HDL increases with increased expression of apo-A1. Triglycerides increase due to reduced expression of PPAR-α and changes in the cofactors apo-C2 and C3 activity. Improvement in glucose levels is related to increased expression of the LXR.

enterohepatic cycle.[56] However, about 5% escape absorption and additional bile acids are synthesized from cholesterol by the liver.

Bile acids are ligands for the nuclear receptor farnesoid X receptor (FXR), and as bile acid levels and FXR activity decrease during BAS therapy, there is increased conversion of cholesterol into bile acids by increased 7α-hydroxylase activity (which is regulated by the nuclear receptor sterol heterodimer partner)[55,56] (Fig. 5). The resulting decrease in hepatocyte cholesterol content promotes an increase in LDL receptors and increased clearance of LDL from the circulation.[56]

Bile acid sequestrant increases HDL by increasing synthesis of apo-A1 (the major lipoprotein of HDL),[55,56] ABCA1, and hepatic lipase (an enzyme involved in the catabolism of HDL). While the expression of SRB1 and CETP activity may be increased with the potential to decrease HDL, the net effect of BAS is a modest increase in HDL.[55,57]

The likely mechanism for improvement in glucose levels during BAS therapy is deactivation of FXR and increased liver X receptor activity, which may increase insulin secretion from the pancreas and improve adipose tissue functionality.[55]

Pharmacology

Bile acid sequestrants are not absorbed (<0.2% is excreted in the urine) or metabolized, and there is no interference with systemic drug metabolizing enzymes.[54,58,59]

Indication

Bile acid sequestrants are indicated to reduce elevated LDL as monotherapy or in combination with a statin. BASs improve glycemic control in adults with type 2 diabetes mellitus, and colesevelam is approved for use as an adjunct to diet and exercise; however, it has not been studied as monotherapy or in combination with a dipeptidyl peptidase-4 inhibitor and has not been extensively studied in combination with thiazolidinediones.[58]

In addition to combining statins with BAS, the combination of niacin and BAS may achieve greater LDL reduction than BAS alone.[54]

Dosage

Cholestyramine

The recommended starting dose is 4 g (i.e., one 4 g packet or scoop of the bulk form) once or twice a day. The recommended maintenance daily dose is 8–16 g, divided into 2 doses. *See* "Adverse Effects" section for recommendations regarding timing of dosing when other medications are also taken. Dose increments should be gradual with periodic assessment of lipid levels at intervals of 4 weeks. The maximum recommended daily dose is 24 g. The suggested time of administration is mealtime but may be modified to avoid absorption of other medications. Although the recommended dosing schedule is twice a day, cholestyramine may be administered in 1–6 divided doses during the day.[60]

Colestipol

The starting doses should be 5 g (i.e., approximately 1 teaspoon) of granules once or twice a day, or two 1 g tablets once or twice a day. Dosage increases of one 5 g dose/day of granules, or 2 g/day of tablets should occur every 1–2 months. The dose is 5–30 g/day of granules or 2–16 g/day of tablets given once or in divided doses.[59]

Colesevelam

The dosage is six 625 mg tablets once a day or divided in two doses. The medication should be taken with a meal and liquid. It can be dosed at the same time as a statin or the two drugs can be dosed apart. Colesevelam has greater bile acid-binding capacity and affinity than that of cholestyramine or colestipol, so it can be used at lower doses. After initiation, lipids should be checked in 4–6 weeks. No specific recommendation or dosage adjustments are recommended when colesevelam is administered to patients with hepatic impairment.[58] The oral suspension of colesevelam contains 13.5 mg phenylalanine per 1.875 g of drug, so warning is provided to phenylketonurics.

The decline in LDL-C is usually evident within 2 weeks with colesevelam and by 1 month with colestipol and cholestyramine.[58-60]

Contraindications

Bile acid sequestrants are contraindicated in patients with a history of bowel obstruction, complete biliary obstruction, elevated triglycerides greater than 500 mg/dL, and a history of triglyceride-induced pancreatitis or hypersensitivity.

Cholestyramine and colestipol are pregnancy category C drugs. Their use during pregnancy or lactation, or by women of childbearing age requires that potential benefit be weighed against hazard to mother or child.[59,60]

Colesevelam is a pregnancy category B drug and should be used during pregnancy only if clearly needed. It is not expected to be excreted in human milk because it is not absorbed systemically from the GI tract.[58]

The effect of BAS on the absorption of fat-soluble vitamins has not been studied in pregnant women.[58-60]

Adverse Effects

Bile acid sequestrants may produce or worsen preexisting constipation. To minimize GI side effects with BAS, low initial doses are suggested. For constipation, increased fluid and dietary fiber intake are recommended and stool softeners may be added as needed. Less frequent adverse effects include abdominal discomfort and/or pain, flatulence, nausea, and vomiting. BASs are not recommended in patients with gastroparesis, other GI motility disorders, in those who have had major GI motility tract surgery or who may be at risk of bowel obstruction and those with complete biliary tract obstruction. Because of tablet size, colesevelam and colestipol should be used with caution in patient with dysphagia or swallowing disorders, since they may cause dysphagia or esophageal obstruction.[58-60]

Bile acid sequestrants can increase triglycerides. For example, colesevelam may increase triglycerides by 5% in patients with primary hyperlipidemia; however, median increases in triglycerides of 18–22% have been reported in clinical studies treating patients with type 2 diabetes mellitus.[58] Decreased FXR activity decreases apo-C2 activity (which is an activator of LPL) and increases apo-C3 activity (which is an inhibitor of LPL). The net effect of BAS on these cofactors is to decrease LPL and, therefore, the lipolysis of triglyceride rich particles, such as VLDL and chylomicrons. A decrease in PPAR-α activity also results in decreased fatty oxidation.[56] It is reasonable to use BAS with caution if baseline triglyceride levels are less than 300 mg/dL, but a fasting lipid panel should be evaluated 4–6 weeks after initiation of therapy. BAS should not be used in individuals with baseline fasting triglyceride levels ≥300 mg/dL or type III hyperlipoproteinemia, because severe triglyceride elevations might occur. A fasting lipid panel should be obtained before BAS is initiated, 3 months after initiation, and every 6–12 months thereafter. BAS should be discontinued if triglycerides exceed 400 mg/dL.[1]

Chronic use of BAS may be associated with increased bleeding tendency due to hypoprothrombinemia and vitamin K deficiency. In addition, a reduction of serum or red cell folate has been reported with chronic use of cholestyramine and colestipol.[59,60]

Prolonged use of cholestyramine or colestipol may produce hyperchloremic acidosis, since they are chloride forms of an anion exchange resin. The chloride anion of the resin can be replaced by other anions, usually those with greater affinity for the resin than chloride. Caution should be exercised in patients with renal insufficiency, volume depletion, and on spironolactone therapy.[59,60]

Bile acid sequestrants may decrease absorption of fat-soluble vitamins [58-60] Patients on vitamin therapy should take vitamins at least 4 hours before the BAS.

If a patient is taking other medications in addition to cholestyramine or colestipol, the other medications should be taken 1 hour before or 4 hours after the BAS. Colesevelam is a more specific BAS, but may reduce GI absorption of some drugs. Drugs with a known interaction that should be taken at least 4 hours prior to a colesevelam dose are: cyclosporine, glyburide, l-thyroxine, oral contraceptive containing ethinyl estradiol and norethindrone, and phenytoin.[58]

Clinical Evidence

Randomized controlled trials using coronary arteriography have demonstrated that BAS as monotherapy or in combination with niacin or lovastatin slows progression and promotes regression of atherosclerotic lesions in the coronary arteries of patients with CHD[55,59,60] (Table 9).

The most significant outcome trial was the Lipid Research Clinics Coronary Primary Prevention Trial (LRC-CPPT), which demonstrated a 19% decrease in risk of combined CHD death and nonfatal MI in men with elevated cholesterol treated with 24 g/day of cholestyramine.[61] The effect of colesevelam on CV morbidity and mortality has not been determined.[58]

In combination trials, the addition of colesevelam to a statin resulted in an additional 10–16% reduction in LDL above that seen by the statin alone (Table 10). Advantages of the

TABLE 9: Clinical studies of bile acid sequestrants

Study (Year)	Type of study	Number of patients	Heart disease	Duration (Years)	Study drug	LDL (% change)	HDL (% change)	Results
LRC-CPPT (1984)	Outcome	3,806 men	Without CHD	7.4	Cholest 24 g/day	−20.3	1.6	19% reduction in fatal and nonfatal MI in treated group
NHLBI (1984)	Angiography	116 men + women	CHD	5	Cholest 24 g/day	−26	8	Significant decreased progression in coronary artery lesions >50% stenosis at baseline
CLAS 1 (1987)	Angiography	162 men	CABG	2	Colest 30 g/day + niacin 4.3 g/day	−43	37	Significant increased regression and decreased progression in treated group than placebo group
CLAS 2 (1990)	Angiography	103 men	CABG	4	Colest 30 g/day + niacin 4.2 g/day	−40	37	Significant increased regression and decreased progression in treated group than placebo group
FATS (1990)	Angiography	38 men	CAD + FH of CVD	2.5	Colest 30 g/day + lovastatin 40 mg/day	−46	15	Significant increased regression, decreased progression, and decreased CHD events compared with conventional therapy
FATS (1990)	Angiography	36 men	CAD + FH of CVD	2.5	Colest 30 g/day + niacin 4 g/day	−32	43	Significant increased regression, decreased progression, and decreased CHD events compared with conventional therapy
UCSF-SCOR (1990)	Angiography	72 men + women	Type IIa	2	Colest, niacin ± lovastatin	−39	26	Mean within-patient change in percent area of stenosis was significantly greater in diet than drug intervention group with the treatment group demonstrating mean regression and the diet group demonstrating mean progression
STARS (1992)	Angiography	90 men	CHD	3	Cholest16 g/day	−35.7	4	Greater increase in coronary diameter with cholest + diet than diet alone

Colest, colestipol; cholest, cholestyramine; FH, family history; CHD, coronary heart disease; type IIa, familial hypercholesterolemia; LRC-CPPT, Lipid Research Clinics Coronary Primary Prevention Trial; NHLBI, National Heart, Lung and Blood Institute; CLAS, Cholesterol Lowering Atherosclerosis Study; CABG, coronary artery bypass graft; FATS, Familial Atherosclerosis Treatment Study; UCSF-SCOR, University of California, San Francisco Specialized Center of Research; STARS, St Thomas Atherosclerosis Regression Study.

TABLE 10: Changes in lipoprotein levels with bile acid sequestrant therapy[58]

Therapy	LDL (% change)	HDL (% change)	Triglycerides (% change)
Monotherapy			
Colesevelam 3.8 g/day	−15	3	10
Combination therapy			
Simvastatin 10 mg/day	−26	3	−17
Simvastatin 10 mg/day + colesevelam 3.8 g/day	−42	10	−12
Atorvastatin 10 mg/day	−38	8	−24
Atorvastatin 10 mg/day + colesevelam 3.8 g/day	−48	11	−1

LDL, low-density lipoprotein; HDL, high-density lipoprotein.

statin-BAS combination are that both drug classes have been shown to improve LDL and outcomes (although not studied with colesevelam) and there may be reduced blood glucose in diabetics with the addition of a BAS. Disadvantages are the need to avoid absorption interference of statins if taken simultaneously with colestipol and cholestyramine.[58]

Colesevelam in combination with ezetimibe reduces LDL by 32% with nonsignificant increases in HDL and triglyceride levels.[55]

Choice of Therapy/Guidelines

If treatment with a statin does not achieve the LDL goal selected for a patient, intensification of LDL lowering drug therapy with a BAS is reasonable.[1] In addition, BAS provides an alternative to statins as initial drug therapy for LDL-lowering. Recommendations for limiting use in patients with elevated triglycerides are discussed in the "Adverse Effects" section above.

The combination of BAS and ezetimibe can have additive effects on LDL lowering, and is useful for patients who do not tolerate a statin or for whom statins are contraindicated.[54]

NIACIN

Introduction

Niacin reduces apoB-containing particles, including LDL, VLDL, triglycerides, and lipoprotein(a).[62-64] Niacin may also exert beneficial pleiotropic effects independent of changes in lipid levels, such as improving endothelial function and attenuating vascular inflammation.[62,65]

Drugs Under the Category

Several niacin products are available, including immediate release (IR) and extended release (ER) formulations. Niacin products are also available as over-the-counter dietary supplements, and include intermediate-release, sustained release, and "no-flush" formulations. However, "no-flush" niacin preparations may contain several niacin compounds (e.g., inositol hexanicotinate) that neither contain nor metabolize to nicotinic acid.

Mechanism of Action

Niacin acts via the G protein-coupled receptor (GPR109A) in the adipocyte which inhibits the formation of intracellular cyclic adenosine monophosphate and downregulates lipolysis (by reduced activation of lipases, such as hormone sensitive lipase) and production of free fatty acids[62,65,66] (Fig. 3). This leads to a reduction in the amount of free fatty acids released from the adipocyte that are available to the liver for triglycerides and VLDL production. Decreased levels of VLDL lead to diminished hepatic and peripheral production of IDL and LDL. Niacin also inhibits hepatocyte DGAT-2 and the reduction in intrahepatic triglyceride synthesis decreases the availability of triglycerides to be incorporated within VLDL.[29,62,65-67]

Although the precise mechanism by which niacin increases HDL is unclear, it is likely multifaceted. Niacin increases apo-A1 by decreasing its cellular uptake.[62] HDL may also interact with SRB1 which primarily acts as a docking station to allow downloading of cholesterol ester.[65] Niacin interferes with HDL holoparticle endocytosis by interfering with the β-chain of adenosine triphosphate synthase.[29,65-67] Niacin inhibits plasma hepatic lipase activity and promotes the formation of mature HDL.[2,63] The reduction in VLDL production that occurs with niacin therapy limits the activity of plasma CETP to exchange triglycerides in VLDL (and LDL) particles for cholesterol esters in HDL particles. Thus, niacin therapy favors carriage of cholesterol esters in HDL particles.[67] Finally, niacin may improve RCT efficiency through GPR109A activation and increased expression of ABCA1 and ABCG1 cholesterol transporters in macrophages (and ABCA1 transporters in adipocytes) resulting in cholesterol efflux to HDL.[62,64,66]

Pharmacology

The absorption (i.e., peak plasma concentration after ingestion) of IR formulation of niacin is about 30–60 minutes and 5 hours for the ER formulation. Approximately 60–76% of ER formulation of niacin (or its metabolites) and 88% of IR formulation is excreted in the urine. The plasma elimination half-life of IR formulation is 20–45 minutes.[68,69]

Niacin is metabolized in the liver by two independent, saturable pathways. One is a low-affinity, high-capacity conjugation (with glycine) pathway resulting in the production of nicotinuric acid. The other pathway is a high-affinity, low-capacity amidation pathway resulting in the production of nicotinamide, which does not have lipid lowering properties and may be associated with hepatotoxicity,[62] although there is controversy.[70] IR formulations provide a short-lived bolus of niacin; overwhelming the high-affinity, low-capacity pathway, resulting in more nicotinuric acid production via the conjugation pathway. Sustained release niacin formulations lengthen the dissolution of niacin and, therefore, provide substrate for the high-affinity amidation pathway and may have higher rates of hepatotoxicity.[29,62,69]

Indications

Niacin is indicated to reduce elevated LDL and triglycerides, and to increase HDL in patients with primary hypercholesterolemia or mixed dyslipidemia. Niacin is an alternative to statin as therapy for LDL-C lowering.[1-4] Niacin is also indicated as adjunctive therapy to lower triglycerides in patients with severe hypertriglyceridemia.[68,69]

Dosage

Immediate Release Niacin

The usual dose range of IR niacin is 1–2 g twice or thrice a day. The starting dose of 250 mg as a single daily dose is given following the evening meal. The frequency of dosing and total daily dose can be increased every 4–7 days until the desired LDL-C and/or triglyceride level is achieved or the dose of 1.5–2 g is achieved. If goals are not achieved after 2 months, the dose can be increased at 2–4 weeks interval to 1 g thrice a day.[68]

Extended Release Niacin

The usual dose range of ER niacin is 0.5–2 g once a day, taken at bedtime with a low-fat snack. Therapy should be initiated at 500 mg in order to reduce the incidence and severity of side effects, which may occur during early therapy and should not be increased by more than 500 mg in any 4-week period. The maintenance dose range is 1–2 g once a day. When combined with a statin, the statin dose should not be the maximum allowed (e.g., limit the maximum daily doses of 40 mg simvastatin and 40 mg lovastatin).[69]

When switching a patient from IR to ER niacin, the equivalent doses should not be substituted; the ER should be started at a lower total daily dose. ER niacin should be used with caution in patients with renal impairment.[68,69]

Contraindications

Active liver disease or unexplained persistent elevation in hepatic transaminase levels are contraindications to niacin use. Active peptic ulcer disease and arterial bleeding are also contraindications.[68,69]

Extended release niacin is a pregnancy category C drug. The benefit of treatment of women with hypertriglyceridemia during pregnancy should be weighed against the risk of continued therapy. Since niacin is excreted into human milk, the potential for adverse reaction in nursing infants should be taken into account.[68,69]

Adverse Effects

The most common adverse reactions are flushing, diarrhea, nausea, vomiting, increased cough, and pruritus. Flushing has been reported in as many as 88% of patients in trials. Nicotinic acid produces flushing via binding to the GPR109A receptor and mediates release of vasodilatory prostaglandins from the "Langerhans" cells in the dermis.[63,64,70] Symptoms typically last for 30–60 minutes. Skin flushing may be reduced in frequency or severity by aspirin pretreatment (up to the recommended dose of 325 mg) taken 30 minutes prior to the niacin administration. Tolerance to flushing develops rapidly over the course of several weeks. Fewer flushing episodes have been reported with ER niacin compared to IR niacin. Concomitant consumption of alcoholic drinks, hot beverages, or spicy foods may increase the side effects of flushing and pruritus and should be avoided around the time of niacin.[63,68,69]

Niacin preparations have been associated with abnormal liver tests. In clinical studies, less than 1% discontinued therapy due to transaminase elevations greater than 2 times ULN. In studies combining statin and niacin, 1% experienced reversible elevation in AST or ALT to greater than 3 times ULN; however, no patients at a dose limit of 1 g niacin had an elevation greater than 3 times ULN. Serum transaminase levels, including AST and ALT should be monitored before initiating the treatment, every 6–12 weeks for the first year, and periodically thereafter (e.g., at approximately 6-month intervals). The drug should be discontinued if the transaminase levels show evidence of progression, particularly if they rise to 3 times ULN and are persistent, or if they are associated with symptoms of nausea, fever, and/or malaise. Severe hepatic toxicity has occurred in patient substituting sustained-release niacin for IR niacin at equivalent doses. Niacin should be used with caution in patients who consume substantial quantities of alcohol and/or have a past history of liver disease.[68,69] Slow-release preparations may increase the risk for hepatotoxicity.[29,62]

The risk for myopathy and rhabdomyolysis are reported to be increased when a statin is coadministered with ER niacin, particularly in elderly patients and patients with diabetes, renal failure, or uncontrolled hypothyroidism. Caution has been recommended when prescribing niacin doses of greater than 1 g/day with a statin. However, in the absence of niacin hepatotoxicity, there is little evidence that the addition of an appropriate formulation of a moderate dose of niacin to a statin increases the risk for muscle adverse experience compared with statin therapy alone.[68,69,71]

Extended release niacin can increase serum glucose and glycosylated hemoglobin (HbA1C) levels (but generally <5 and <0.3%, respectively). Glucose levels should be monitored in diabetic or potentially diabetic patients, particularly during the first few months of use or dose adjustment, since diabetic patients may experience a dose-related increase in glucose intolerance. The insulin resistance may be related to a rebound increase in free fatty acids when nicotinic acid blood levels fall.[62,65,67,71] The majority of the increases can be treated with adjustment in the antihyperglycemic regimen. Niacin at doses less than 2 g daily are considered safe for diabetic patients when the CV benefits outweigh the risks.[63]

Elevated uric acid levels may occur with niacin therapy and, therefore, it should be used with caution in patients predisposed to gout. Elevations as high as 11% in mean uric acid levels have been reported.[68,69,71] The mechanism of the increase appears to be the competitive inhibition of the tubular secretion of uric acid by nicotinic acid.[71]

Nicotinic acid should be used with caution in patients with unstable angina or in the acute phase of an MI, particularly when such patients are also receiving vasoactive drugs since niacin may potentiate the effects of these drugs resulting in postural hypotension.[68,69]

The development or exacerbation of peptic ulcer has been described, usually in patients with high doses of regular niacin.[68,69,71]

Atrial fibrillation was more common in male patients with CAD studied in the Coronary Drug Project (CDP).[68,69] However, atrial fibrillation has not emerged as a significant adverse experience in numerous other smaller, randomized, controlled niacin trials, which mostly enrolled patients without CHD.[71]

Small decreases in phosphorous levels (i.e., 13%) have been reported with the use of 2 g niacin.

Dose-related reductions in platelet counts of about 11% may occur and caution should, therefore, be observed when niacin is administered with anticoagulants; platelet counts should be monitored in such patients. In addition, a small (i.e., 4%) increase in prothrombin time has been associated with ER niacin use.[69] However, these changes have been regarded as clinically insignificant.[71]

Clinical Evidence

Nicotinic acid produces an average 10–20% reduction in LDL-C, 30–70% reduction in triglycerides, and an average 20–35% increase in HDL. The magnitude of individual lipid and lipoprotein responses may be influenced by the severity and type of underlying lipid abnormality.[68] In a dose-escalation study, ER formulation of niacin with monthly 500 mg increases in dose, there were incremental changes in LDL-C, HDL-C, and triglycerides in the dose range of 0.5–2 g daily [69] (Table 11). When niacin is added to a statin, there may be additional LDL-C lowering of 10–20% depending on the dose of niacin.[54]

Niacin has anti-inflammatory properties with decreases in CRP by 15% and lipoprotein-associated phospholipase A2 by 20%.[72]

The CDP, completed in 1975, was designed to assess the safety and efficacy of 3 g/day of IR niacin in men 30–64 years old with a history of MI. The incidence of nonfatal, recurrent MI was reduced from 12.2% to 8.9% (a 14% RRR), although there was no difference in mortality after 5 years. A follow-up analysis performed 15 years after completion of the trial demonstrated a significant overall 11% RRR in mortality (58.2% vs 52.0%).[73]

When combined with BAS, angiographic trials demonstrated a decrease in progression of coronary lesions (*See* the heading "Clinical Evidence under BAS").

When combined with statins, several studies have used carotid intima-media thickness (CIMT) as a surrogate endpoint. In the Arterial Biology for the Investigation of the Treatment Effects of Reducing Cholesterol Study (ARBITER 2),

TABLE 11: Changes in lipoprotein levels with niacin therapy[69]

Dose	LDL (% change)	HDL (% change)	Triglycerides (% change)
Extended release niacin			
1 g	–7	14	–16
1.5 g	–13	19	–25
2 g	–16	22	–38
Lovastatin 40 mg	–32	6	–20
Extended release niacin/lovastatin			
1 g/20 mg	–30	20	–32
1 g/40 mg	–36	20	–39
1.5 g/40 mg	–37	27	–44
2 g/40 mg	–42	30	–44

LDL, low-density lipoprotein; HDL, high-density lipoprotein.

the addition of 1 g/day of niacin to baseline statin therapy prevented progression of atherosclerosis in patients with CHD and HDL less than 45 mg/dL.[74] In an extension trial, CIMT regressed and the change in CIMT was independently associated with changes in HDL but not LDL-C or triglycerides.[75] In the ARBITER-6 HDL and LDL Treatment Strategies in Atherosclerosis Trial (ARBITER-6 HALTS), the addition of 2 g ER niacin to stable statin therapy in patients with CHD or its equivalent (with LDL <100 mg/dL and HDL <50–55 mg/dL) was associated with regression by CIMT.[76]

Outcome trials demonstrating the benefit of adding niacin to statin are limited. In the HDL-Atherosclerosis Treatment Study (HATS) trial, the combination of statin and niacin was compared to placebo.[77] A RRR of 90% in the composite endpoint of nonfatal MI, revascularization, or CV death was demonstrated in the combination therapy group. In ARBITER-2, CV end-points were reduced in the statin and niacin group (3.8%) compared to statin alone (9.6%). However, the RRR of 60% was not significant (p = 0.20).[74] The addition of niacin therapy to patients with well controlled LDL-C has been shown to improve endothelial flow-mediated dilation of the brachial artery, especially in those with low baseline HDL-C.[72]

Improved outcomes when adding niacin to a statin have not been confirmed in randomized, controlled trials. In the Atherothrombosis Intervention in Metabolic Syndrome with Low HDL/High Triglycerides Impact on Global Health Outcome (AIM-HIGH) trial, ER niacin or placebo was given to patients with CAD, high triglycerides, HDL-C less than 40–50 mg/dL, and LDL-C controlled to 40–80 mg/dL with simvastatin ± ezetimibe. In patients who achieved and maintained LDL less than 70 mg/dL while receiving statin therapy treatment, ER niacin plus simvastatin did not decrease CV events over 36 months compared to patients treated with simvastatin alone.[78]

In the Heart Protection Study 2-Treatment of HDL to Reduce the Incidence of Vascular Events (HPS-THRIVE) Study, greater than 20,000 patients with coronary, cerebrovascular or peripheral arterial events were randomized to 2,000 mg ER niacin and laropiprant (a prostaglandin inhibitor to prevent flushing from niacin) or placebo (with both groups on background therapy with simvastatin 40 mg ± ezetimibe 10 mg to lower total cholesterol to target of <135 mg/dL). The primary endpoint of major vascular events was not reduced and side effects were increased with the addition of niacin. However, the mean baseline lipid values were: LDL-C 63 mg/dL, HDL-C 44 mg/dL and triglycerides 125 mg/dL, so the patients, on average, had no indication for niacin. In addition, subset analysis showed net benefit if baseline LDL-C was greater than 58 mg/dL.[79]

The clinical efficacy of combining niacin and a BAS is discussed in the section on BAS.

Choice of Therapy/Guidelines

If treatment with a statin does not achieve the selected LDL-C goal, intensification of LDL-C lowering drug therapy with niacin is reasonable as an alternative or as adjunctive therapy.[1-4] However, dietary supplemental niacin should not be used as a substitute for prescription niacin. While a recent meta-analysis suggests that simply increasing HDL does not reduce the risk of CHD events, CHD deaths, or total death, there is controversy since studies with niacin alone were not included in that meta-analysis.[80] Another meta-analysis of nicotinic acid alone or in combination demonstrated positive effects on CV events and atherosclerosis evolution.[81]

However, niacin should be used with caution in patients with low LDL-C since there was a lack of benefit in the AIM-HIGH and HPS2-THRIVE studies, although it may be used in patients with severely elevated triglycerides greater than 500 mg/dL in order to prevent pancreatitis.[1]

It remains to be established whether or not drug therapy of an isolated elevation of triglycerides influences CV disease outcome.[7]

OMEGA-3 FATTY ACIDS

Introduction

The omega-3 fatty acids (O3FAs) include the marine-derived long-chain fatty acids eicosapentaenoic acid (EPA) and docosahexaenoic acid (DHA). They may be used as monotherapy or as adjunctive therapy with fibrates and/or nicotinic acid to lower triglycerides in patients with severe hypertriglyceridemia.

Low density lipoprotein cholesterol is unchanged or variably increased with O3FA therapy that includes both EPA and DHA, and the degree of elevation is generally related to the pretreatment triglyceride level. The elevation is related to increased conversion of VLDL to LDL particles with increases in particle size. However, concurrent treatment with statins may reduce the increase in LDL-C.[82]

Drugs Under the Category

Prescription O3FAs are available as a 1 g liquid-filled gel capsule containing at least 900 mg ethyl esters of O3FAs derived from fish oils. These are predominantly a combination of ethyl esters of EPA (approximately 465 mg) and DHA (approximately 375 mg).[83]

There is also a prescription product that contains the single O3FA EPA (1 gram capsule).[84]

Mechanism of Action

The triglyceride lowering ability of O3FAs is likely mediated by their capacity to agonize and antagonize several of the same nuclear transcription factors involved in the action of fibrates[30] (Fig. 6). They also compete with other fatty acids and prevent their entry into triglyceride synthesis. Lipogenesis is suppressed by increased mitochondrial β-oxidation, and triglyceride synthesis is decreased by the inhibition of DGAT, resulting in less substrate available for synthesis of VLDL. A decrease in the concentration of APOC3 (an inhibitor of LPL activity) promotes the conversion of VLDL to LDL.[30,85]

The net effect on HDL is minimal since there are offsetting mechanisms of action. HDL is expected to increase with PPAR-α activation and enhanced RCT. However, FXR is activated, resulting in a decrease in HDL.[85]

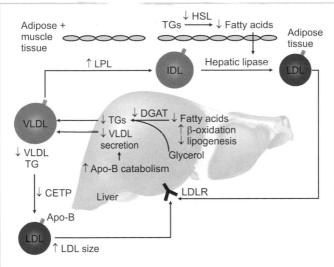

LPL, lipoprotein lipase; HSL, hormone sensitive lipase; LDL, low-density lipoprotein; LDLR, low-density lipoprotein receptor; HDL, high-density lipoprotein; CETP, cholesteryl ester transfer protein; DGAT, diacylglycerol acyltransferase; IDL, intermediate-density lipoprotein; TGs, triglycerides; VLDL, very low-density lipoprotein.

FIG. 6: Mechanism of action of omega-3 fatty acids (O3FAs). O3FAs inhibit the biosynthesis of fatty acids, decrease DGAT expression and increase apolipoprotein-B catabolism resulting in decreased VLDL secretion. A decrease in hormone sensitive lipase leads to reduced adipocyte fatty acid mobilization and release. Reduced VLDL triglyceride content leads to decreased CETP activity. This results in an increase in LDL and HDL size. With the increase in LPL activity, there is augmentation of VLDL lipolysis and increased formation of LDL.

Pharmacology

Prescription O3FA are manufactured by transesterification of fish triglycerides, which allow for the separation of individual fatty acids and selective concentrations of EPA and DHA ethyl esters while other fatty acids are discarded. After intestinal absorption and breakdown of the ethyl esters, the resulting EPA and DHA do not differ from the fatty acids produced in the body.[86]

O3FAs administered as ethyl esters induce significant, dose-dependent increases in serum phospholipid EPA content. However, the increases in DHA content are less marked and dose-dependent.[83]

Indications

Omega-3 fatty acids are indicated as an adjunct to diet for patients with severe hypertriglyceridemia and very high triglyceride levels greater than 500 mg/dL.[1,87]

Dosage

A daily dose of O3FA of 4 g/day is recommended for severe hypertriglyceridemia. The daily dose may be taken as a single 4 g dose or as two 2 g doses. The capsule should be swallowed whole and not broken open or chewed.[83] An approximate reduction of 5–10% in triglycerides is expected for each 1 g of O3FA consumed, although efficacy is greater in individuals with higher triglycerides before treatment with possibly a curvilinear relationship.[7]

Contraindications

Omega-3 fatty acid contains ethyl esters of EPA and DHA obtained from the oil of several fish source. It is not known whether patients with allergies to fish and/or shellfish are at increased risk of an allergic reaction and, therefore, should be used with caution in these patients.[83,84]

Prescription O3FAs are pregnancy category C drugs and should be used during pregnancy only if the potential benefit to the patient justifies the potential risk to the fetus. It is not known whether O3FAs are excreted in human milk, and caution should be exercised when O3FAs are administered to a nursing woman.[83,84]

Adverse Effects

Eructation, dyspepsia, and/or taste perversion have been reported in 3–4% of patients in clinical studies.[83,84] GI adverse effects, primarily eructation and taste can be minimized by highly purified, high potency formulations, that allow for much lower dosing.[88] Refrigeration of supplements and the addition of vitamin E may reduce fish oil oxidation and improve tolerance.[89]

Fasting glucose levels may rise slightly in patients with diabetes mellitus but without significant change in HbA1C.[90]

Some studies have demonstrated a prolongation of bleeding time, but the times reported have not exceeded normal limits and did not produce clinically significant bleeding episodes.[83] Clinical trials have demonstrated high dose O3FA consumption to be safe when concurrently administered with other agents, such as aspirin and warfarin that may increase bleeding. However, patients receiving treatment with high dose O3FA and an anticoagulant or other drug affecting coagulation should be monitored periodically. In the setting of an acute bleeding illness, such as during and immediately after hemorrhagic stroke, or in patients at high-risk of hemorrhagic stroke, it is prudent to discontinue high-dose fish oil consumption or supplementation. In addition, some clinicians consider discontinuing fish oil therapy 4–7 days prior to planned invasive procedures with a highest risk for bleeding complications.[89] In patients with hepatic impairment, ALT and AST levels should be monitored periodically.

In recommending the most appropriate form of fish oil to patients, clinicians should be aware of potential fish oil toxicities, and know which details of purification processes to minimize potential toxicities. This can present a challenge since no USFDA regulatory mechanisms are in place for dietary supplements. The manufacturers of dietary supplements are not required to provide excellence of efficacy, safety, or manufacturing standards before marketing products. The USFDA has determined that fish oil dietary supplements should not exceed 2 g/day of EPA and DHA. A "USP-verified" mark indicates compliance with standards set by the United States Pharmacopeia.[89]

There is a possible association between prescription EPA + DHA and more frequent recurrences of symptomatic atrial fibrillation or flutter in patients with paroxysmal or persistent atrial fibrillation, particularly within the first 2–3 months of initiating therapy.[83]

In patients with hepatic impairment, ALT and AST should be monitored since some patients may have further elevation in ALT on therapy.[83]

Finally, the combination of statins and O3FA has been shown to be safe and well-tolerated treatment for combined dyslipidemia.[88]

Clinical Evidence

In patients with severe hypertriglyceridemia (levels >500 mg/dL), 4 g prescription of O3FA (with the combination of DHA and EPA) decreased triglycerides by 45% and increased HDL by 9%. However, LDL-C may increase by up to 44%. In patients treated with simvastatin 40 mg/day and having persistently elevated triglycerides in the range of 200–499 mg/dL, the addition of 4 g prescription O3FA resulted in reductions in triglyceride levels by 23% and increases in HDL-C of 4.6% and LDL-C of 3.5%.[83] DHA use may be responsible for the increase in LDL-C since the ANCHOR (Anti-VEGF Antibody for the Treatment of Predominantly Classic Choroidal Neovascularization in AMD) study (of patients with triglyceride levels of 200 to <500 mg/dL) and the MARINE study (of patients with triglyceride levels >1,000 mg/dL) showed either no change (i.e., the MARINE study) or a decrease (i.e., the ANCHOR study) in LDL-C.[91,92] Several mechanisms for this differential effect have been proposed: (1) difference between effects of DHA and EPA on CETP activity; (2) increased conversion of VLDL to LDL by DHA via increased lipoprotein lipase activity; and (3) DHA-containing long-chain fatty acids may downregulate receptor-mediated LDL-C clearance.[93]

In the Japan EPA Lipid Intervention Study (JELIS), patients received a low dose statin plus either EPA (1.8 g) or placebo. Subgroup analysis of primary prevention patients with baseline triglyceride levels greater than 150 mg/dL and HDL less than 40 mg/dL demonstrated that combination therapy reduced CV disease risk by 53% compared with statin monotherapy.[94] However, the risk reduction was associated with only an additional 5% triglyceride reduction compared to controlled clinical trials. The effect of prescription O3FA on CV mortality and morbidity in patients with elevated triglycerides has not been determined.[83]

Whether or not triglyceride lowering results in a decrease in CV events awaits the results of the Reduction of Cardiovascular Events Outcome trial (REDUCE-IT). In this study, 8,000 patients with triglycerides greater than 150 mg/dL despite statin therapy with or at high-risk of CV disease will receive EPA or placebo and outcomes will be assessed. Completion of the study is estimated to be November, 2016.[95]

There are no outcome trials demonstrating a decreased risk of pancreatitis in patients with severe hypertriglyceridemia and treated with O3FA.[83]

Choice of Therapy/Guidelines

Prescription O3FA is indicated as initial or adjunctive treatment of patients with severe hypertriglyceridemia.

EZETIMIBE: A CHOLESTEROL ABSORPTION INHIBITOR

Introduction

Ezetimibe is in a class of lipid-lowering compounds that selectively inhibits the absorption of cholesterol by the small intestine.[54]

Ezetimibe reduces LDL-C and triglycerides and increases HDL in patients with combined hyperlipidemia. The maximal response is generally achieved within 2 weeks and maintained during chronic therapy. The addition of ezetimibe to either a statin or fenofibrate is more effective in lipid lowering than with either agent alone. However, the effect of ezetimibe as monotherapy or in addition to a statin or fenofibrate on CV morbidity and mortality has not been established.[96]

Mechanism of Action

Cholesterol entering the small intestine is derived from dietary sources or from biliary cholesterol and is emulsified by bile salts into micelles and transferred from the micelles to duodenal and jejunal enterocytes via a sterol transporter, identified as a member of the Niemann-Pick family of proteins (NPC1L1). The molecular target of ezetimibe is the NPC1L1 sterol transporter. The decrease in delivery of cholesterol to the liver causes a reduction of hepatic cholesterol stores and a compensatory increase in LDL receptors and, therefore, increased clearance of cholesterol from the blood.[96,97]

Pharmacology

Ezetimibe is primarily metabolized in the small intestine and liver via glucuronide conjugation with subsequent biliary and renal excretion. Both ezetimibe and its glucuronide metabolite have an elimination half-life of 22 hours. Excretion of the drug is 78% in feces and 11% in urine. Ezetimibe is highly (>90%) bound to plasma proteins. Ezetimibe is neither an inhibitor nor an inducer of the CYP P450 isoenzymes.[96]

Indications

Ezetimibe is indicated as monotherapy or in combination with statin therapy for the reduction of elevated LDL-C in patients with primary hyperlipidemia. It is also indicated for use in combination with fenofibrate for the reduction of elevated LDL-C and non-HDL cholesterol in patients with mixed hyperlipidemia. Ezetimibe may be administered at the same time as the statin or fenofibrate.[96]

Dosage

The recommended dose of ezetimibe is 10 mg once a day. Concomitant food administration has no effect on absorption, and ezetimibe can be administered with or without food. No dosage adjustment is necessary in patients with mild hepatic or renal impairment, or in geriatric patients. Caution should be exercised when using ezetimibe and cyclosporine concomitantly.[96]

Contraindications

Due to the unknown effects of increased exposure to ezetimibe in patients with moderate or severe hepatic impairment (i.e., Child-Pugh score >7), ezetimibe is not recommended in these patients. The combination of ezetimibe with a statin is contraindicated in patients with active liver disease or unexplained persistent elevations in hepatic transaminase levels.[96]

Ezetimibe is a pregnancy category C drug. There are no adequate and well-controlled studies of ezetimibe in pregnant women.

Adverse Effects

The most commonly reported adverse reactions in ezetimibe + statin trials were nasopharyngitis (3.7%), myalgia (3.2%), and arthralgia (2.6%).

Ezetimibe monotherapy does not cause significant elevations of hepatic transaminases.[54] While the incidence of elevations of hepatic transaminase levels ≥3 times the ULN was similar between ezetimibe and placebo, the incidence of increased transaminases is higher in patients receiving ezetimibe in combination with a statin (1.3%) compared to patients treated with a statin alone (0.4%).[96,98] The elevations are mild, transient, reversible, and without apparent clinical significance. The effect is considered to be due to statins and is dose-related. A systematic review of RCTs demonstrated that compared to ezetimibe therapy alone, combination therapy with a statin did not result in significant absolute increases in the risk of transaminase elevations, myalgia, CPK increases, rhabdomyolysis, GI adverse events, or discontinuations because of adverse events.[99]

Safety monitoring for ezetimibe monotherapy is not required; however, when used with a statin, liver function tests should be performed at the initiation of therapy and according to the recommendations of the statin.[98] Should an increase in ALT or AST to greater than equal to 3X ULN persist, withdrawal of ezetimibe and/or the statin should be considered.

Clinical Evidence

Ezetimibe produces LDL-C reductions of 14–25%.[54] Since ezetimibe monotherapy results in a decrease in hepatic cholesterol pool, there is a compensatory increase in cholesterol synthesis. However, in the presence of statin therapy, this increase in cholesterol synthesis is diminished (due to HMG-CoA reductase inhibition), resulting in the greater decrease in LDL-C (i.e., >20%) with the combination compared to ezetimibe monotherapy.[54,97] The advantage of the combination is the low incidence of side effects, but the disadvantage is the lack of clinical outcome data for ezetimibe.[54]

Ezetimibe monotherapy has not been associated with a decrease in high-sensitivity-CRP (hs-CRP) levels. However, the addition of ezetimibe to statin therapy resulted in greater hs-CRP reduction than with statin therapy alone.[97]

The ability of ezetimibe to improve measures of subclinical atherosclerosis, including CIMT, has been mixed. In the Ezetimibe and Simvastatin in Hypercholesterolemia Enhances Atherosclerosis Regression (ENHANCE) trial, the addition of ezetimibe to statin therapy did not significantly change CIMT compared to statin monotherapy, despite a greater than 50 mg/dL lowering of LDL-C in the combination therapy group.[100] The impact of ezetimibe on CV outcomes will be determined by the Improved Reduction of Outcomes: Vytorin Efficacy International Trial (IMPROVE-IT), with results expected in November, 2014.[101]

Choice of Therapy/Guidelines

If treatment with a statin does not achieve the LDL-C goal selected for a patient, intensification of LDL-C lowering drug therapy with ezetimibe may be considered.[1] However, other pharmacologic options include BAS and niacin.

CONCLUSION

Drug therapy of LDL-C begins with the identification of the patient's risk category or clinical scenario: Secondary versus primary prevention, diabetes mellitus, or familial hypercholesterolemia. Initial therapy for LDL-C reduction begins with a statin. However, the addition of niacin, a BAS, or ezetimibe, may be needed if additional LDL-C lowering beyond a statin alone is necessary (e.g., familial hypercholesterolemia or statin intolerance). If triglycerides are greater than 500 mg/dL, attention is directed at triglyceride lowering with fibrates, niacin or O3FA. When patients are on a statin and triglycerides are less than 500 mg/dL, there is residual risk of CV events, but the impact of additional therapy requires further study.

REFERENCES

1. Stone NJ, Robinson JG, Lichtenstein AH, et al. 2013 ACC/AHA guideline on the treatment of blood cholesterol to reduce atherosclerotic cardiovascular risk in adults: A report of the American College of Cardiology/American Heart Association task force on practice guidelines. Circulation. 2014;129(25 Suppl 2):S1-45.

2. Expert Panel on Detection, Evaluation, and Treatment of High Blood Cholesterol in Adults. Executive Summary of the Third Report of the National Cholesterol Education Program (NCEP) Expert Panel on Detection, Evaluation and Treatment of High Blood Cholesterol in Adults (Adult Treatment Panel III). JAMA. 2001;285(19):2486-97.

3. Grundy SM, Cleeman JI, Merz CN, et al. Implications of recent clinical trials for the National Cholesterol Education Program Adult Treatment Panel III guidelines. Circulation. 2004;110(2):227-39.

4. Expert Dyslipidemia Panel of the International Atherosclerosis Society Panel members. An International Atherosclerosis Society Position Paper: global recommendations for the management of dyslipidemia—full report. J Clin Lipidol. 2014;8(1):29-60.

5. Rader DJ, Daugherty A. Translating molecular discoveries into new therapies for atherosclerosis. Nature. 2008;451(7181):904-13.

6. Mottilo S, Filion KB, Genest J, et al.. The metabolic syndrome and cardiovascular risk: a systematic review and meta-analysis. J Am Coll Cardiol. 2010;56(14):1113-32.

7. Miller M, Stone NJ, Ballantyne C, et al. Triglycerides and cardiovascular disease: a scientific statement from the American Heart Association. Circulation. 2011;123(20):2292-333.

8. Cholesterol Treatment Trialists' (CTT) Collaboration; Baigent C, Blackwell L, et al. Efficacy and safety of more intensive lowering of LDL cholesterol: A meta-analysis of data from 170,000 participants in 26 randomized trials. Lancet. 2010; 376(9753):1670-81.

9. Lipitor (atorvastatin) prescribing information. Pfizer. New York, NY. May 2014.

10. Lescol (fluvastatin) prescribing information. Novartis Pharmaceuticals. East Hanover, NJ. Oct 2012.

11. Mevacor (lovastatin) prescribing information. Merck & Co. Whitehouse Station, NJ. Feb 2014.

12. Livalo (pitavastatin) prescribing information. Kowa Pharmaceuticals America, Inc. Montgomery, AL. Oct 2013.

13. Pravachol (pravastatin) prescribing information. Bristol-Myers Squibb Co. Princeton, NJ. Aug 2013.

14. Crestor (rosuvastatin) prescribing information. Astra Zeneca Pharmaceuticals. Wilmington, DE. July 2014.

15. Zocor (simvastatin) prescribing information. Merck Co. Whitehouse Station, NJ. Feb 2014.

16. Arnaboldi L, Corsini A. Do structural differences in statins correlate with clinical efficacy? Curr Opin Lipidol. 2010;21(4):298-304.

17. Mukhtar RY, Reid J, Reckless JP. Pitavastatin. Int J Clin Pract. 2005;59(2):239-52.

18. Corsini A, Bellosta S, Baetta R , et al. New insights into the pharmacodynamic and pharmacokinetic properties of statins. Pharmacol Ther. 1999;84(3):413-28.

19. Frishman WH, Horn J. Statin-drug interactions: Not a class effect. Cardiol Rev. 2008;16 (4):205-12.

20. Vandenberg BF, Robinson J. Management of the patient with statin intolerance. Curr Atheroscler Rep. 2010;12(1):48-57.

21. Calderon RM, Cubeddu LX, Goldberg RB, et al. Statins in the treatment of dyslipidemia in the presence of elevated liver aminotransferase levels: a therapeutic dilemma. Mayo Clin Proc. 2010;85(4):349-56.

22. FDA drug safety communication: Important safety label changes to cholesterol-lowering statin drugs. Available from: http://www.fda.gov/Drugs/DrugSafety/ucm293101.htm.

23. Weng TC, Yang YH, Lin SJ, et al. A systematic review and meta-analysis on the therapeutic equivalence of statins. J Clin Pharm Therap. 2010;35(2):139-51.

24. Gotto AM Jr, LaRosa JC. The benefits of statin therapy—what questions remain? Clin Cardiol. 2005;28(11):499-503.

25. Brugts JJ, Yetgin T, Hoeks SE, et al. The benefits of statins in people without established cardiovascular disease but with cardiovascular risk factors: meta-analysis of randomised controlled trials. BMJ. 2009;338:b2376.

26. Saha SA, Arora RR. Hyperlipidaemia and cardiovascular disease: do fibrates have a role? Curr Opin Lipidol. 2011;22(4):270-6.

27. Brinton EA. Does the addition of fibrates to statin therapy have a favorable risk to benefit ratio? Curr Atherosclerosis Rep. 2008;10(1):25-32.

28. Wierzbicki AS. Fibrates in the treatment of cardiovascular risk and atherogenic dyslipidaemia. Curr Opin Cardiol. 2009;24(4):372-9.

29. Chapman MJ, Redfern JS, McGovern ME, et al. Niacin and fibrates in atherogenic dyslipidemia: pharmacotherapy to reduce cardiovascular risk. Pharmacol Ther. 2010;126(3):314-45.

30. Toth PP, Dayspring TD, Pokrywka GS. Drug therapy for hypertriglyceridemia: fibrates and omega-3 fatty acids. Curr Atheroscler Rep. 2009;11(1):71-9.

31. Remick J, Weintraub H, Setton R, et al. Fibrate therapy: an update. Cardiol Rev. 2008;16(3):129-41..

32. Lopid (gemfibrozil) prescribing information. Pfizer. New York, NY. Sep, 2010.

33. Tricor (fenofibrate) prescribing information. AbbVie,. North Chicago, Il Feb, 2013.

34. Antara (fenofibrate) prescribing information. Lupin Pharma. Baltimore, MD. August, 2012.

35. Trilipix (fenofibric acid) prescribing information. AbbVie. North Chicago, IL. March, 2013.

36. Bezalip SR (bezafibrate) prescribing information. Tribute Pharma Canada. Milton, ON. Jul, 2013.

37. Davidson MH, Armani A, McKenney JM, et al. Safety considerations with fibrate therapy. Am J Cardiol. 2007;99(6A):3C-18C.

38. Keech A, Simes RJ, Barter P, et al. Effects of long-term fenofibrate therapy on cardiovascular events in 9795 people with type 2 diabetes mellitus (the FIELD study): randomised controlled trial. Lancet. 2005;366(9500):1849-61.

39. ACCORD Study Group; Ginsberg HN, Elam MB, et al. Effects of combination lipid therapy in type 2 diabetes mellitus. N Engl J Med. 2010;362(17):1563-74.

40. Flam M, Lovata LC, Ginsberg. Role of fibrates in cardiovascular disease prevention, the ACCORD-Lipid perspective. Curr Opin Lipidol. 2011;22(1):55 61.

41. Sica DA. Fibrate therapy and renal function. Curr Atheroscler Rep. 2009;11(5):338-42.

42. Jun M, Foote C, Lv J, et al. Effects of fibrates on cardiovascular outcomes: a systematic review and meta-analysis. Lancet. 2010; 375(9729):1875-84.

43. Frick MH, Elo O, Haapa K, et al. Helsinki Heart Study: primary prevention trial with gemfibrozil in middle-aged men with dyslipidemia. Safety of treatment, changes in risk factors, and incidence of coronary heart disease. N Engl J Med. 1987;317(20):1237-45.

44. Rubins HB, Robins SJ, Collins D, et al. Gemfibrozil for the secondary prevention of coronary heart disease in men with low levels of high-density lipoprotein cholesterol. Veterans Affairs High-density Lipoprotein Cholesterol Intervention Trial Study Group. N Engl J Med. 1999;341(6):410-8.

45. Grundy SM, Vega GL, Yuan Z, et al. Effectiveness and tolerability of simvastatin plus fenofibrate for combined hyperlipidemia (the SAFARI trial). Am J Cardiol. 2005;95(4):462-8.

46. Goldberg AC, Bays HE, Ballantyne CM, et al. Efficacy and safety of ABT-335 (fenofibric acid) in combination with atorvastatin in patients with mixed dyslipidemia. Am J Cardiol. 2009;103(4):515-22.

47. Abourbih S, Filion KB, Joseph L, et al. Effect of fibrates on lipid profiles and cardio-vascular outcomes: a systematic review. Am J Med. 2009;122(10):962.e1-8.

48. Manninen V, Tenkanen L, Koskinen P, et al. Joint effects of serum triglyceride and LDL cholesterol and HDL cholesterol concentrations on coronary heart disease risk in the Helsinki Heart Study. Implications for treatment. Circulation. 1992;85:37-45.

49. Bezafibrate Infarction Prevention (BIP) study. Secondary prevention by raising HDL cholesterol and reducing triglycerides in patient with coronary artery disease. Circulation. 2000;102(1):21-7.

50. Scott R, O'Brien R, Fulcher G, et al. Effects of fenofibrate treatment on cardiovascular disease risk in 9,795 individuals with type 2 diabetes and various components of the metabolic syndrome. The Fenofibrate Intervention and Event Lowering in Diabetes (FIELD) study. Diabetes Care. 2009;32(3):493-8.

51. Bruckert E, Labreuche J, Deplanque D, et al. Fibrates effect on cardiovascular risk is greater in patients with high triglyceride levels or atherogenic dyslipidemia profile: a systematic review and meta-analysis. J Cardiovasc Pharmacol. 2011;57(2):267-72.

52. Brunzell JD, Davidson M, Furberg CD, et al. Lipoprotein management in patients with cardiometabolic risk: consensus conference report from the American Diabetes Association and the American College of Cardiology Foundation. J Am Coll Cardiol. 2008;51(15):1512-24.

53. Goldfine AB, Kaul S, Hiatt WR. Fibrates in the treatment of dyslipidemias—time for a reassessment. N Engl J Med. 2011;365(6):481-4.

54. Hou R, Goldberg AC. Lowering low-density lipoprotein cholesterol: statins, ezetimibe, bile acid sequestrants and combination: comparative efficacy and safety. Endocrinol Metab Clin North Am. 2009;38(1):79-97.

55. Bays HE, Goldberg RB. The 'forgotten' bile acid sequestrants: Is now a good time to remember? Am J Ther. 2007;14(6):567-80.

56. Claudel T, Staels B, Kuipers F. The Farnesoid X receptor: a molecular link between bile acid and lipid and glucose metabolism. Arterioscler Thromb Vasc Biol. 2005;25(10):2020-30.

57. Davidson MH. Therapies targeting exogenous cholesterol uptake: new insights and controversies. Cur Atheroscler Rep. 2011;13(1):95-100.

58. Welchol (colesevelam) prescribing information. Daiichi Sankyo, Inc. Parsippany, NJ. Jan, 2014.

59. Colestid (colestipol) prescribing information. Pfizer, Inc. New York, NY. Jun, 2014.

60. Cholestyramine prescribing information. Par Pharmaceutical Co., Inc. Spring Valley, ND. Feb, 2013.

61. The Lipid Research Clinics Coronary Primary Prevention Trial Results. I. Reduction in incidence of coronary heart disease. JAMA. 1984;251(3):351-64.

62. Villines TC, Kim AS, Gore RS, et al. Niacin: the evidence, clinical use, and future directions. Curr Atheroscler Rep. 2012;14(1):49-59.

63. Natarajan P, Ray KK, Cannon CP. High-density lipoprotein and coronary heart disease: current and future therapies. J Am Coll Cardiol. 2010;55(13):1283-99.

64. Farmer JA. Nicotinic acid: a new look at an old drug. Curr Atheroscler Rep. 2009;11(2):87-92.

65. Wanders D, Judd RL. Future of GPR109A agonists in the treatment of dyslipidaemia. Diabetes Obes Metab. 2011;13(8):685-91.

66. Digby JE, Lee JM, Choudhury RP. Nicotinic acid and the prevention of coronary artery disease. Curr Opin Lipidol. 2009;20(4):321-6.

67. Karpe F, Chamas L. Hyperlipidaemia and cardiovascular disease: nonantilipolytic effects of nicotinic acid in adipose tissue. Curr Opin Lipid. 2010;21(3):282-3.

68. Niacor (niacin) prescribing information. Upsher-Smith Laboratories, Inc. Minneapolis, MN. Rev. 0200.

69. Niaspan (niacin extended release) prescribing information. Abbott Laboratories, North Chicago, IL. April, 2014.

70. Stern RH. The role of nicotinic acid metabolites in flushing and hepatotoxicity. J Clinical Lipid.2007;1(3):191-3.

71. Guyton JR, Bays HE. Safety considerations with niacin therapy. Am J Cardiol. 2007;99(6A):22C-31C.

72. Brooks EL, Kuvin JT, Karas RH. Niacin's role in the statin era. Expert Opin Pharmacother. 2010;11(14):2291-300.

73. Canner PL, Berge KG, Wenger NK, et al. Fifteen year mortality in Coronary Drug Project patients: long-term benefit with niacin. J Am Coll Cardiol. 1986;8(6):1245-55.

74. Taylor AJ, Sullenberger LE, Lee HJ, et al. Arterial Biology for the investigation of the Treatment Effects of Reducing Cholesterol (ARBITER) 2:a double blind, placebo-controlled study of extended-release niacin on atherosclerosis progression in secondary prevention patients treated with statins. Circulation. 2004;110(23):3512-17.

75. Taylor AJ, Lee HJ, Sullenberger LE. The effect of 24 months of combination statin and extended-release niacin on carotid intima-media thickness: ARBITER 3. Curr Med Res Opin. 2006;22(11):2243-50.

76. Taylor AJ, Villines TC, Stanek EJ, et al. Extended-release niacin or ezetimibe and carotid intima-media thickness. N Engl J Med. 2009;361(22):2113-22.

77. Brown BG, Zhao XQ, Chait A, et al. Simvastatin and niacin, antioxidant vitamins, or the combination for the prevention of coronary disease. N Eng J Med. 2001;345(22):1583-92.

78. AIM-HIGH Investigators, Boden WE, Probstfield JL, et al. Niacin in patients with low HDL cholesterol levels receiving intensive statin therapy. N Engl J Med. 2011;365(24):2255-67.

79. HPS2-THRIVE Collaborative Group, Landray MJ, Haynes R, et al. Effects of extended-release niacin with laropriprant in high-risk patients. N Engl J Med. 2014;371(3):203-12.

80. Briel M, Ferreira-Gonzalez I, You JJ, et al. Association between change in high density lipoprotein cholesterol and cardiovascular disease morbidity and mortality: systematic review and meta-regression analysis. BMJ. 2009;338:b92.

81. Bruckert E, Labreuche J, Amarenco P. Meta-analysis of the effect of nicotinic acid alone and combination on cardiovascular events and atherosclerosis. Atherosclerosis. 2010;210(2):353-61.

82. Bays HE, Tighe A, Sadovsky R, et al. Prescription omega-3 fatty acids and their lipid effects: physiologic mechanisms of action and clinical implications. Expert Rev Cardiovasc Ther. 2008;6(3):391-409.

83. Lovaza (omega-3-acid ethyl esters) prescribing information. Glaxo-Smith Kline Reserarch Triangle Park, NC. May, 2014.

84. Vascepa (eicosapentaenoic acid) prescribing information. Amarin Pharmaceuticals. Dublin, Ireland. Nov 2013.

85. Davidson MH. Mechanisms for the hypertriglyceridemic effect of marine omega-3 fatty acids. Am J Cardiol. 2006;98(4A):27i-33i.

86. Rupp H. Omacor (prescription omega-3-acid ethyl esters 90): From severe rhythm disorders to hypertriglyceridemia. Adv Ther. 2009;26(7):675-90.

87. Berglund L, Brunzell JD, Goldber AC, et al. Evaluation and treatment of hypertriglyceridemia: an Endocrine Society clinical practice guidcline. J Clin Endocrinol Metab. 2012;97(9):2969-89.

88. Nambi V, Ballantyne CM. Combination therapy with statins and omega-3 fatty acids. Am J Cardiol. 2006;98(4A):34i-38i.

89. Bays HE. Safety considerations with omega-3 fatty acid therapy. Am J Cardiol. 2007;99(6A):35C-43C.

90. Kris-Etherton PM, Harris WS, Appel LJ; American Heart Association. Nutrition Committee. Fish consumption, fish oil, omega-3 fatty acids, and cardiovascular disease. Circulation. 2002;106(21):2747-57.

91. Ballantyne CM, Bays HE, Kastelein JJ, et al. Efficacy and safety of eicosapentaenoic acid ethyl ester (AMR101) therapy in statin-treated patients with persistent high triglycerides (from the ANCHOR Study). Am J Cardiol. 2012;110(7): 984-92.

92. Bays HE, Ballantyne CM, Kastelein JJ, et al. Eicosapentaenoic acid ethyl ester (AMR101) therapy in patients with very high triglyceride levels (from the Multi-center, placebo-controlled, randomized, double-bliNd, 12-week study with an open-label Extension [MARINE] trial). Am J Cardiol. 2011;108(5):682-90.

93. Jacobson TA, Glickstein SB, Rowe JD, et al. Effects of eicosapentaenoic acid and docosahexaenoic acid on low-density lipoprotein cholesterol and other lipids: a review. J Clin Lipid. 2012;6(1):5-18.

94. Saito Y, Yokoyama M, Origasa H, et al. Effects of EPA on coronary artery disease in hypercholesterolemic patients with multiple risk factors: sub-analysis of

primary prevention cases from the Japan EPA Lipid Intervention Study (JELIS). Atherosclerosis. 2008;200(1):135-40.

95. A Study of AMR101 to evaluate its ability to reduce cardiovascular events in high risk patients with hypertriglyceridemia and on statin. (REDUCE-IT): https://clinicaltrials.gov/ct2/show/NCT0149236

96. Zetia (ezetimibe) prescribing information. Merck/Schering-Plough Pharmaceuticals, North Wales, PA. August, 2013.

97. Yatskar L, Fisher EA, Schwartzbard A. Ezetimibe: rationale and role in the management of hypercholesterolemia. Clin Cardiol. 2009;29(2):52-5.

98. Jacobson TA, Armani A, McKenney JM, et al. Safety considerations with gastrointestinally active lipid-lowering drugs. Am J Cardiol. 2007;99(6A):47C-55C.

99. Kashani A, Sallam T, Bheemreddy S, et al. Review of side-effect profile of combination ezetimibe and statin therapy in randomized clinical trials. Am J Cardiol. 2008;101(11):1606-13.

100. Kastelein JJ, Akdim F, Stroes ES, et al. Simvastatin with or without ezetimibe in familial hypercholesterolemia. New Engl J Med. 2008;358(14):1431-43.

101. IMPROVE-IT: Examining outcomes in subjects with acute coronary syndrome: Vytorin (ezetimibe/simvastatin) vs simvastatin (P04103 AM5): https://clinicaltrials.gov/ct2/show/NCT00202878.

Drugs for Diabetes and Cardiodysmetabolic Syndrome

Prakash Deedwania, Sundararajan Srikanth

INTRODUCTION

It is estimated that as much as 30–40% of the adult population in the developed countries has cardiodysmetabolic syndrome/dysmetabolic syndrome. As currently understood the epidemic of obesity is primarily responsible for preponderance of cases with cardiodysmetabolic syndrome and is an essential element in the definition of the syndrome. Obesity is associated with resistance to the effects of insulin in the muscle tissue and results in hyperinsulinemia, hyperglycemia, dyslipidemia, hypertension and endothelial dysfunction. A similar profile is seen in individuals with type 2 diabetes mellitus.[1-4] In 2001, the National Cholesterol Education Program (NCEP) defined the metabolic syndrome with a focus on the cardiovascular risk posed by the syndrome.[5] The International Diabetes Foundation (IDF) revised the adult treatment panel III (ATP III) criteria for metabolic syndrome to address disparities in waist circumference thresholds related to ethnic differences in different populations[6] (Table 1).

For the clinician, the phenotypic pattern can be recognized by a simple look at the patient and review of basic laboratory studies. In this regard, the mnemonic DROP, where D stands for dyslipidemia, R for insulin resistance, O for obesity and P for high blood pressure, helps in easier identification of the individual with this syndrome (Table 2).[7]

PREVALENCE

In the National Health and Nutrition Examination Survey (NHANES) 1999–2002 database, 34.5% of participants met ATP III criteria for the metabolic syndrome compared with 22% in NHANES III (1988–1994).[8,9] Ford reported 39% prevalence in the USA, using data from NHANES 1999–2002 participants, with IDF criteria as compared to 34.5% prevalence using the ATP III criteria.[8]

TABLE 1: International Diabetes Foundation definition of cardio-dysmetabolic syndrome

Metabolic parameter	Measurement criteria
Central obesity* (Waist circumference)	
South Asians	Men ≥90 cm; women ≥80 cm
Europids	Men ≥94 cm; women ≥80 cm
Chinese	Men ≥90 cm; women ≥80 cm
South and Central Americans	Men ≥90 cm; women ≥80 cm
Raised triglycerides	≥150 mg/dL
Reduced high-density lipoprotein	Men <40 mg/dL; women <50 mg/dL
Raised blood pressure	Systolic ≥130 mmHg
	Diastolic ≥85 mmHg
Raised fasting plasma glucose	≥100 mg/dL
	Previously diagnosed type 2 diabetes

*Central obesity according to the waist circumference plus any two of the other four risk factors.

TABLE 2: The cardiometabolic syndrome

D	Dyslipidemia
	Fasting triglycerides >140 mg/dL or
	HDL <40 mg/dL or
	LDL particle size <260 Å
R	Insulin resistance
	Fasting plasma glucose ≥110 mg/dL or
	Type 2 diabetes mellitus
O	Obesity
	Body mass index >25 kg/m^2 or
	Waist/hip ratio >0.85 or
	Waist circumference >100 cm
P	High blood pressure
	Systolic blood pressure ≥140 mmHg or
	Diastolic blood pressure ≥90 mmHg

HDL, high-density lipoprotein; LDL, low-density lipoprotein.

PATHOPHYSIOLOGY OF CARDIODYSMETABOLIC SYNDROME

The cardiodysmetabolic syndrome results from a complex interplay of insulin resistance, adiposity and endothelial dysfunction. Adipose tissue secretes many biologically active intermediaries that mediate insulin resistance (Fig. 1). Typically, in disease states associated with insulin resistance,

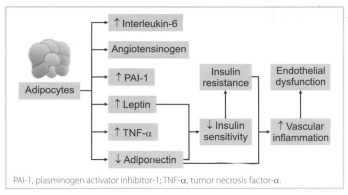

PAI-1, plasminogen activator inhibitor-1; TNF-α, tumor necrosis factor-α.

FIG. 1: Adipocyte role in insulin resistance, metabolic syndrome, and CVD.

different tissues show varying levels of insulin resistance. Thus, when plasma insulin levels increase to maintain euglycemia in the insulin resistant state, the mitogenic effects of insulin on cell growth and differentiation might become more pronounced leading to hypertriglyceridemia, hypertension and hyperandrogenism.[10]

Parallel insulin signaling pathways in metabolic and vascular tissues, cross talk between inflammatory and insulin signaling, pathway-specific insulin resistance, coupling of blood flow with glucose metabolism, cross talk between metabolic and vascular tissues and shared stressors lead to endothelial dysfunction.

CLINICAL IMPLICATIONS

There is controversy over whether cardiodysmetabolic syndrome confers incremental risk compared with risk related to the individual components of metabolic syndrome. The cardiovascular risk associated with the metabolic syndrome was found to be elevated in a recent meta-analysis of approximately 1 million patients from 87 prospective trials. NCEP and revised NCEP criteria in the general population were used to define the metabolic syndrome.[11] Overall, the metabolic syndrome was associated with a 2-fold increase in risk of cardiovascular disease (CVD), CVD mortality and stroke; and a 1.5-fold increase in the risk of all-cause mortality. There was a 2-fold increase in the risk for myocardial infarction (MI) as well. Metabolic syndrome was associated with an increased risk for cardiovascular events even after exclusion of individuals with diabetes. The estimates of cardiovascular risk were consistently higher in women as compared to men. However, there is still the need for studies to firmly establish the risk associated with cardiodysmetabolic syndrome, independent of the risk of its individual components.

THERAPY

Since visceral obesity is central to the pathophysiology of cardiodysmetabolic syndrome, therapy should be primarily directed toward this. Additionally, insulin resistance and endothelial dysfunction play an important role in the pathogenesis of the metabolic and cardiovascular perturbations as reflected by epidemiological data suggesting links between metabolic and cardiovascular disorders. Various pharmacological and nonpharmacological therapeutic interventions to treat the metabolic and cardiovascular abnormalities have been shown to improve insulin sensitivity and endothelial function. While most of the therapeutic interventions have been developed with the intention of metabolic and symptomatic control, improved long-term outcomes of any salubrious intervention appears to be predicated upon concurrent improvement in insulin sensitivity and endothelial dysfunction.

The therapeutic goals for management of metabolic syndrome have been outlined by the American Heart Association (AHA) and the Endocrine Society[12,13] (Table 3). They include reduction of abdominal obesity, increasing physical activity, dietary modification and treatment of specific cardiovascular risk factors if present.

Lifestyle Modification

Current evidence suggests that the first step in the management of patients with cardiodysmetabolic syndrome should be focused on weight loss and increased physical activity. Lifestyle modifications, including diet, weight loss and physical exercise, reduce insulin resistance, obesity and improve endothelial function. The benefit of weight management in controlling cardiodysmetabolic syndrome is highlighted by the Coronary Artery Risk Development in Young Adults (CARDIA) study.[14] In this observational study for over 15 years, more than 5,000 young individuals between the ages of 18 and 30 years, increasing body mass index (BMI) was associated with progression of components of metabolic syndrome as opposed to those in whom BMI remained stable over the same period. Obese individuals can lose up to 0.5 kg/week by restricting calories to less than 500–1,000 kcal below daily requirements.[15] Combining calorie restriction with regular exercise can lead to a weight loss of 5–10% from baseline over a 6-month period. A realistic goal for weight reduction is a target of 7–10% over a 6–12-month period. Such reductions in body weight are associated with much greater loss of visceral adiposity (the central problem in cardiodysmetabolic syndrome). This marginal weight loss results in improvement of many of the metabolic abnormalities.[16]

TABLE 3: Therapeutic goals and clinical recommendation for management of metabolic syndrome

Target	Goal	Recommendation
Abdominal obesity	10% weight loss in first year and continued weight loss thereafter	Diet control and increased physical activity
Physical inactivity	Regular moderate physical activity	30–60 minutes of exercise daily
Atherogenic diets	Reduced intake of saturated fats, trans fats and cholesterol	Total fats 25–35% of total calories, saturated fats <7% of calories
Smoking	Complete cessation	Complete cessation
High-LDL cholesterol	LDL cholesterol <100 mg/dL in moderate-risk patients and <70 mg/dL in high-risk patients	Lifestyle changes and cholesterol lowering drugs to achieve targets
High triglycerides	Insufficient data. Possibly triglycerides <100 mg/dL in high-risk patients	Lifestyle changes and triglyceride lowering drugs (fenofibrate) to achieve targets
Low-HDL cholesterol	Insufficient data	Lifestyle changes and HDL-raising drugs (nicotinic acid, CETP inhibitors) to achieve targets
High blood pressure	Blood pressure <135/85 mmHg. In diabetes and chronic kidney disease <130/80 mmHg	Lifestyle therapy and antihypertensive drugs to achieve targets
Elevated glucose	Reduction and maintenance of fasting glucose <90 mg/dL. HbA1C <7.0% for diabetics	Lifestyle therapy and hypoglycemic drugs if required
Prothrombotic state	Reduction of prothrombotic state	Low-dose aspirin in all high- and moderate-risk patients. Consider clopidogrel if aspirin not tolerated
Pro-inflammatory state	Reduction of proinflammatory state	No specific therapies. Aspirin and/or statins are being evaluated

CETP, cholesteryl ester transfer protein; HDL, high-density lipoprotein; LDL, low-density lipoprotein.

Diet Intervention

Several dietary approaches have been advocated for treatment of the metabolic syndrome. A Mediterranean diet, which is high in fruits, vegetables, nuts, whole grains and olive oil results in improved lipid profile and insulin resistance as compared to a low-fat diet.[17,18] Objective data on other weight reducing diets, such as high-protein, low-carbohydrate diet are limited. Foods with low glycemic index may be beneficial. In a cross-sectional analysis of carbohydrate-related dietary factors, insulin resistance and prevalence of metabolic syndrome in nearly 3,000 subjects from the Framingham Offspring Study; dietary glycemic index was positively associated with prevalence of the metabolic syndrome.[19]

Exercise

Current guidelines recommend practical, regular and moderate regimens for exercise. The standard exercise recommendation is a daily minimum of 30 minutes of moderate-intensity physical activity (e.g., brisk walking). The Diabetes Prevention Project (DPP) study demonstrated that multiple metabolic risk factors can be controlled and type 2 diabetes prevented or delayed by controlling weight with regular exercise. The study enrolled 3,234 normotensive subjects who were mostly obese and randomized them to intensive lifestyle modification, metformin, troglitazone, or placebo. The rate of development of diabetes or metabolic syndrome was least in the intensive lifestyle modification group, which consisted of low-fat diet and 150 minutes of walking/week.[20] Exercise may be beneficial beyond its effect on weight loss by more selectively removing abdominal fat at least in women.[21]

Pharmacological Options

Currently available pharmacologic alternatives include drugs that combat obesity and medications that address the individual components of the metabolic syndrome, including hyperglycemia, dyslipidemia, hypertension and abnormal coagulation. No specific drug has been developed that can reverse or block the fundamental abnormalities underpinning the cardiodysmetabolic syndrome, namely, insulin resistance and endothelial dysfunction.

Antiobesity Drugs

There are various medications that have been developed over the last few decades with the aim of achieving weight reductions. These medications have various mechanisms of actions. However, most of the medications that have been developed so far have all been demonstrated to have significant side effects that have ultimately led to the withdrawal of most of these medications. Metabolic benefits associated with sibutramine-induced weight loss were reported by Krejs et al.[22] Orlistat has been shown in a few studies to improve individual components of metabolic syndrome in addition to promoting weight loss and mobilizing visceral fat.[23,24] The problem with these drugs continues to be a relatively high rate of side effects leading to poor compliance. Sibutramine was recently withdrawn from the market based on postmarketing data from the Sibutramine Cardiovascular and Outcome (SCOUT) trial showing a 16% increase in the incidence of nonfatal MI and nonfatal stroke.[25] Discovery of the endocannabinoid system led to the development of cannabinoid receptor type 1 inhibitors, such as rimonabant. While manufacturer sponsored clinical trials in overweight patients demonstrated clinical benefit, the drug was subsequently withdrawn due to significant psychiatric side effects.[26-28]

Lipid Management

The ATP III guidelines emphasize that low-density lipoprotein (LDL) reduction is the primary target in lipid management even in the metabolic syndrome, with low high-density lipoprotein (HDL) and triglycerides being secondary targets.[29] The more aggressive target of LDL less than 70 mg/dL is supported by the recent Treating to New Targets (TNT) metabolic syndrome study showing greater reduction in coronary events in the group that achieved LDL levels of 70 mg/dL as opposed to the group that attained levels of less than 100 mg/dL.[30] While the efficacy of statins in reducing LDL cholesterol is well established, combination therapy has been suggested for achieving LDL targets, reducing triglycerides and apolipoprotein B, and increasing HDL cholesterol.

Antihypertensive Therapy

The value of angiotensin-converting enzyme inhibitors (ACEIs) and angiotensin receptor blockers (ARBs) in hypertensive patients with the metabolic syndrome who do not have CVD or diabetes is not clear. Animal studies have shown improvement in insulin resistance, reduction of reactive oxygen species production and increased mitochondrial biogenesis with enalapril and losartan.[31,32] Studies have also shown significant increase in adiponectin levels with inhibition of renin-angiotensin-aldosterone system, which is associated with improved insulin sensitivity.[33] ACEI and ARBs might increase peroxisome proliferators-activated receptor gamma (PPARγ) activity, which might promote adipogenesis, thus, improving metabolic perturbations.[34]

Sympathetic activation in obese hypertensive patients seems to be a contributory factor for the elevated blood pressure and cardiovascular and metabolic consequences of the metabolic syndrome. In theory, drugs inhibiting the sympathetic nervous system could be useful, but the evidence of efficacy of central imidazoline receptor binding agents and peripheral β-sympathetic blocking agents is not convincing. In fact, a diabetogenic effect has been unequivocally demonstrated with thiazide diuretics and older β-blockers, such as atenolol. Therefore, these drugs may not be suitable as first-line therapy for hypertension in subjects with metabolic syndrome.

Antithrombotic Therapy

The cardiodysmetabolic syndrome is characterized by a procoagulant state with increased levels of fibrinogen, plasminogen activator inhibitor-1 (PAI-1) and other coagulation factors. It is also a proinflammatory state that is characterized by elevated cytokines, such as the tumor necrosis factor and interleukin-6, and acute phase reactants, such as C-reactive protein and fibrinogen. In patients with the cardiodysmetabolic syndrome and a high-risk of future cardiovascular events, aspirin in a dose of 75–150 mg/day is an attractive therapeutic option for lowering the rate of cardiovascular events.[35] It is also important to note that inhibition of the renin-angiotensin system reduces PAI-1 levels and inflammatory cytokines and, thus, potentially reduces the risk of increased thrombotic events in patients with metabolic syndrome.[36]

PROGRESSION FROM METABOLIC SYNDROME TO DIABETES AND CARDIOVASCULAR DISEASE

The discussion, thus far, has been focused on the metabolic syndrome. Apart from the increased risk for CVD, the metabolic syndrome is also associated with increased risk of developing diabetes mellitus. Multiple prospective observational studies demonstrate a strong association between the metabolic syndrome and the risk for subsequent development of type 2 diabetes. The risk of diabetes appears to increase with increasing components of the metabolic syndrome.[37-39] Intuitively, it is not surprising that the risk of developing diabetes in the presence of the metabolic syndrome is higher since insulin resistance or surrogate markers of insulin resistance are generally incorporated in the definition. As noted earlier, the metabolic syndrome is characterized by insulin resistance, involving the glycogen synthetic pathway, leading to hyperglycemia and diabetes. The increased incidence of cardiovascular complications associated with the diabetic state find their explanation in varying insulin sensitivities in different tissues. Differential insulin sensitivity leads to atherogenesis via mitogen-activated protein kinase pathway, which shows normal growth promoting response to insulin and hyperglycemia from insulin resistance in the PI-3 kinase metabolic pathway.

Prevention of Hyperglycemia, Impaired Glucose Tolerance and Diabetes Mellitus

Approaching cardiodysmetabolic syndrome from the aspect of insulin resistance is conceptually reasonable. Practically, this translates into treatment of individuals with impaired fasting glucose or impaired glucose tolerance (IGT) before the development of overt hyperglycemia. Recent studies targeting individuals with IGT using aggressive lifestyle interventions or pharmacotherapy have shown reduced incidence of diabetes and the risk of cardiovascular disease. The Finnish Diabetes Prevention Study (FDPS)[40] and the United States Diabetes Prevention Program (USDPP)[20,41,42] demonstrated that diet and exercise do have a significant effect on reducing the progression from IGT to type 2 diabetes. In the Finnish study and the DPP study, personalized recommendations about diet and exercise led to a reduction in the incidence of new onset diabetes by 58% compared to the group receiving usual instructions.

Pharmacologic approaches directed at reducing insulin resistance potentially can control hyperglycemia, dyslipidemia, abnormal coagulation and possibly even hypertension. Metformin, which was first described in 1922, improves hyperglycemia primarily by suppression of hepatic glucose production. In addition, metformin increases insulin sensitivity, enhances peripheral glucose uptake, fatty acid oxidation, and decreases absorption of glucose from the gastrointestinal tract. Increased peripheral utilization of glucose may also be the result of improved insulin binding to insulin receptors. Metformin was included in one of the treatment arms along with lifestyle advice in DPP. While metformin was effective in reducing the incidence of diabetes as compared with placebo, it was not as effective as intensive lifestyle intervention.

Acarbose, an α-glucosidase inhibitor slows the digestion of carbohydrates in the intestine and reduces postprandial glucose levels. The Study to Prevent Non-Insulin Dependent Mellitus (STOP-NIDDM) was a randomized trial to evaluate whether acarbose would prevent development of type 2 in subjects with IGT.[43] The acarbose group had significantly lower incidence of diabetes compared to placebo and was likely to revert IGT to normal with concomitant decrease in cardiovascular events.

One of the first group of drugs to address all the abnormalities manifested in the insulin-resistance state is the thiazolidinediones (TZDs). TZDs are insulin-sensitizing drugs that act via the nuclear PPARγ to change activation of a plethora of genes and the levels of various expressed proteins. Rosiglitazone and pioglitazone, the currently available TZDs have been shown to improve many of the metabolic abnormalities associated with the metabolic syndrome.[44,45] However, there is as yet no strong evidence that TZDs reduce CVD end-points, and, in particular, there are no data on such risk reduction for people with metabolic syndrome. Moreover, based on cumulative data pointing toward increased risk of CV events with rosiglitazone, FDA has withdrawn its approval for this particular drug.

Cardiovascular Control with Established Type 2 Diabetes

With established diabetes mellitus, all modifiable risk factors should be addressed. These include hypertension, hyperglycemia, obesity, dyslipidemia, dietary indiscretion, physical inactivity and smoking. Intervention should start with dietary advice and advice regarding physical activity. Early initiation of a moderate exercise program may be the best strategy for reducing risk of later macrovascular complications. Dietary advice should include recommendations regarding optimal fat intake. It is recommended that intake of polyunsaturated fat should be limited to 10% of calorie intake, though there is lack of evidence to support this. Consumption of fish, high in omega-3 fatty acids (1–2 serving/week), reduced the risk of coronary death and total mortality in epidemiologic studies and randomized clinical trials, and this benefit seems to extend to the diabetic individual as well.[46] Several cohort studies have an association between dietary glycemic load and incidence of type 2 diabetes. Prospective cohort studies have also reported an inverse association between whole grain consumption and risk of diabetes and coronary heart disease (CHD). Moderate alcohol consumption (1–2 drinks or 10–20 g of alcohol per day) shows a benefit on CHD incidence in the general population. This benefit also extends to the diabetic population.

Individual interventions for CV risk factors in diabetic patients give a 15–30% risk reduction. The results of these studies have been scrutinized in detail, leading to the establishment of treatment guidelines with specific targets regarding glycemic control, desirable blood pressure and lipid levels (Table 4).

Management of Individual Risk Factors

In the following sections, recent advances in the therapeutic strategies for management of the individual risk factors associated with the diabetic state are discussed.

Hyperlipidemia

In the diabetic population, the prevalence of hyper-triglyceridemia and low HDL levels is approximately twice as high and the prevalence of high LDL level is not different

TABLE 4: Goals for risk factor management in diabetes

Risk factor	Goal of therapy	Reference**
Cigarette smoking	Complete cessation	ADA, AHA
BP	<130/80 mmHg	JNC 7, ADA
BP with proteinuria	<125/75 mmHg	JNC 7, ADA
LDL cholesterol (measured annually)	<70 mg/dL for secondary prevention*	ATP III, ADA
For age >40 years	Without CVD but >1 risk factor, LDL goal is <100. If LDL is <100 at baseline, statin is based on additional risk factors	ATP III, ADA
For age <40 years	Without CVD, but estimated to have high risk of CVD, LDL goal is <100 mg/dL	ATP III, ADA
Triglycerides 200 400 mg/dL	Non-HDL cholesterol <130 mg/dL	ATP III, AHA
Triglycerides >500 mg/dL	Fibrate/niacin before LDL lowering Non-HDL <130 mg/dL	ATP III, AHA
	Target triglycerides <150	ADA
HDL cholesterol <40 mg/dL (<50 mg/dL in women)	Raise HDL	ATP III, ADA
Prothrombotic state	Low-dose aspirin therapy (patients with CHD and other high risk factors including age >40)	ADA, AHA
Glucose	HbA1C <7%	ADA, AHA
Overweight and obesity (BMI >25 kg/m²)	Lose 5–7% of body weight	ADA, AHA
Physical inactivity	150 min moderate aerobic exercise or at least 90 min vigorous aerobic exercise/week (not more than 2 consecutive days without physical activity)	ADA, AHA
Adverse nutrition	Diets low in fat (<30%) and saturated fat <7%; lower glycemic index (when necessary with caloric restriction) 1.2–2 g sodium/day Alcohol up to 2 drinks/day (1 drink/day for women; 1 drink = 354.88 mL beer or 118.29 mL wine, or 44.36 mL distilled spirit)	ADA, AHA, ATP III, OEI, JNC 7

*NCEP.[5,29]

**ADA,[47] AHA,[47] JNC[7,48] ATP III,[5] OEI.[49]

ADA, American Diabetes Association; AHA, American Heart Association; ATP, Adult Treatment Panel; BMI, body mass index; BP, blood pressure; CHD, coronary heart disease; CVD, cardiovascular disease; HbA1C, glycosylated hemoglobin; HDL, high-density lipoprotein; JNC, Joint National Committee; LDL, low-density lipoprotein; NCEP, National Cholesterol Education Program; OEI, Obesity Education Initiative.

as compared to the nondiabetic population.[50] However, whatever the level of LDL in the diabetic individual, the LDL is atherogenic (type B small dense LDL) and, therefore, treatment with statins has been found to be highly effective in preventing macrovascular events. Initial data on benefits of statins in diabetic subjects were obtained from subgroup analyses of the major secondary intervention trials, such as the Scandinavian Simvastatin Survival Study (4S) and the cholesterol and recurrent events (CARE) trials.[51,52]

More recently, the benefits of high-dose statin use were demonstrated in the TNT study, which compared atorvastatin 10 mg to an 80 mg/day dose in patients with stable coronary artery disease (CAD).[53] A subanalysis demonstrated that major CV events were reduced by 25% in diabetic patients receiving high-dose atorvastatin, supporting the use of intensive lipid lowering regimens. Further post hoc analysis of the TNT study was done to investigate the effect of intensive lipid lowering on future CV events in patients with diabetes, with or without coexisting mild-to-moderate chronic kidney disease (CKD).[54] Compared with a 10 mg dose of atorvastatin, the 80 mg dose reduced the relative risk of major cardiovascular events by 35% in patients with diabetes and CKD and by 10% in patients with diabetes and normal epidermal growth factor receptor. The absolute risk reduction in patients with diabetes and CKD was substantial, yielding a number needed to treat of 14 to prevent one major cardiovascular event over 4.8 years. This result is very encouraging and stands in contrast to previous observations in patients with diabetes and end-stage renal disease.

These data from TNT analysis of diabetic cohort provide a strong support to the prevailing recommendations of reducing LDL to levels less than 70 mg/dL as recommended by various guidelines including American Diabetes Association (ADA). There is less evidence for interventions directed at the diabetic dyslipidemia (high triglyceride and low HDL). The Action to Control Cardiovascular Risk in Diabetes (ACCORD) lipid trial evaluated treatment with fenofibrate compared with placebo among patients with type 2 diabetes treated with an open-label statin medication.[55] Among 5,518 patients randomized into the study, the addition of fenofibrate to statin therapy was not superior to statin therapy alone. While fenofibrate reduced triglyceride levels, there was only a small difference in mean HDL and no difference in LDL between groups, which could help explain lack of benefit.

Hypertension

As regards management of hypertension, the ACCORD study demonstrated that decreasing systolic blood pressure (SBP) to a mean value of 119.3 mmHg was associated with decrease in all stroke and nonfatal stroke.[56] Results from the Action in Diabetes and Vascular Disease: Preterax and Diamicron Modified-Release Controlled Evaluation (ADVANCE) study are also instructive in the management of hypertension in the diabetic patient.[57] ADVANCE was a 2 × 2 factorial study, in which 11,140 patients were randomized to either intensive glucose control or standard glucose therapy, and fixed-dose combination of perindopril, and indapamide, or placebo. After a mean of 4.3 years of follow-up, those who received active therapy had a mean reduction in SBP of 5.6 mmHg (mean SBP of 134.7 active vs. 140.3 placebo) and diastolic blood pressure (DBP) of 2.2 mmHg (mean DBP 74.8 active vs. 77 placebo). The relative risk of death from CVD was reduced by 18% (p = 0.03) and death from any cause was reduced by 14% (p = 0.03) (Fig. 2). This benefit was attributed mostly to reduction in microvascular events.

So, the natural question that arises is what should be the target blood pressure for therapy in the diabetic patient? Although guidelines have recommended target blood pressure less than 130/80 or 120/75 in those with CKD, this target had not been supported by prospective large scale randomized controlled trial specifically designed to evaluate the benefit of targeted therapy to a goal of blood pressure less than 130/80. The ACCORD blood pressure study is the first such trial, where treatment directed to a goal of less than 120/80 was prospectively evaluated against blood pressure goal of less than 140/80. Although the findings of the ACCORD trial have not yet been incorporated into guidelines, it seems reasonable in the

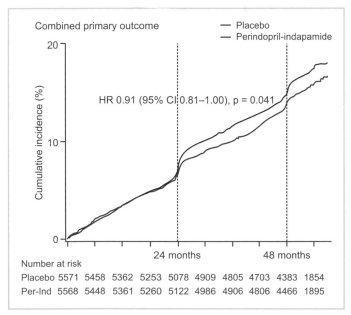

FIG. 2: Impact of therapeutic strategies on combined macro- and microvascular events.[57]

meanwhile to consider that the target blood pressure for most diabetic patients should be less than 130/85.

In choosing an antihypertensive agent, it is important to realize that the degree of blood pressure reduction obtained is more important than the specific agent, which might be selected for the purpose. Moreover, since therapy requires use of multiple antihypertensive medications at the outset, it is a moot point as to which should be the preferred initial drug. Nevertheless, ACEIs have been generally recommended as preferred initial drugs. There is persuasive data from the Heart Outcomes Prevention Evaluation (HOPE) study in support of the use of ACEIs.[58]

While ACEIs remain the cornerstone of therapy for patients with type 1 diabetes and nephropathy, the Reduction of Endpoints in NIDDM with the Angiotensin II Antagonist Losartan trial (RENAAL) and Irbesartan Type II Diabetic Nephropathy (IDNT) studies support initial therapy with angiotensin receptor blockers in type 2 diabetes. ARBs represent the only evidence-based treatment strategy for patients with type 2 diabetes mellitus and proteinuria and have been recommended as initial treatment of choice by the National Kidney Foundation.[59]

It is also important to remember that β-blockers are recommended and provide cardioprotection in patients with established CHD, and as such when additional therapy is needed, β-blockers should be considered in appropriate patients. The role of calcium channel blocker therapy was clarified by the recently published Avoiding Cardiovascular Events Through Combination Therapy in Patients Living With Systolic Hypertension (ACCOMPLISH) trial.[60] The diabetic subgroups in this study involving 6,946 subjects were randomized to treatment with benazepril plus amlodipine or benazepril plus hydrochlorothiazide. A subgroup of 2,842 high-risk diabetic patients (previous cardiovascular or stroke events) was further analyzed. While the mean achieved blood pressure was similar in both treatment groups, there were clear benefits with benazepril plus amlodipine combination in cardiovascular endpoints. The difference between the two treatment groups demonstrated that contemporary treatment with benazepril and amlodipine was better in higher risk groups, i.e., individuals with diabetes and high-risk diabetic individuals.

To conclude, pharmacologic therapy to block the renin-angiotensin-aldosterone system (RAAS) should be mandatory in patients with diabetic nephropathy (which includes patients with microalbuminuria). Since appropriate therapy of hypertension generally requires more than one agent, the initial therapy with RAAS blocking agents and amlodipine may be considered.

Hyperglycemia

While the benefit of glycemic control on delaying or preventing microvascular disease has been well documented, the relationship between hyperglycemia and macrovascular disease has been a subject of constant debate. United Kingdom Prospective Diabetes Study (UKPDS) is the largest study addressing this issue.[61,62] It was designed to answer the question as to whether intensive control of glucose compared to conventional treatment in newly diagnosed type 2 diabetics lowers the risk of complications. Over a mean follow-up duration of over 10 years in approximately 2,500 patients in each group, intensive therapy lead to a 12% reduction in any diabetes related endpoint and a significant reduction in the microvascular endpoints (25% reduction; p = 0.0099). A 16% reduction in MI (p = 0.052) and nonsignificant reduction in diabetes related and all-cause mortality was also seen in the intensively treated group. Nevertheless, the European Prospective Investigation into Cancer and Nutrition-Norfolk (EPIC-Norfolk) study found a continuous relationship between all-cause mortality and glycosylated hemoglobin (HbA1C) even for values in the nondiabetic range.[63] The increased risk of death among men with diabetes was largely explained by HbA1C concentration.

The threshold to which glycemic control needs to be pushed has probably been adequately answered by the recently published data from the ACCORD trial.[64] The goal of the trial was to evaluate intensive glycemic control through currently available means (i.e., HbA1C <6%), compared with standard glycemic control (i.e., HbA1C 7.0–7.9%), among patients with type 2 diabetes mellitus with known CVD or with additional risk factors for CVD. At 1 year, HbA1C was 6.4% versus 7.5%, respectively. The glycemic arm of the trial was stopped prematurely due to excess death that was reported in the intensive treatment group. While there was no identifiable cause for excess death in the intensively treated group in the ACCORD trial, a strategy of lowering HbA1C to a mean of less than 6.5% may not be advisable. These results were somewhat mirrored by the ADVANCE trial, which is the largest trial on diabetes treatments to date.[65] In this trial, a total of 11,140 patients with type 2 diabetes were randomly assigned to undergo either standard glucose control or intensive glucose control with gliclazide and other agents to achieve an HbA1C value ≤6.5%. At the end of 5 years, the mean HbA1C was 6.5% in the intensive control arm versus 7.3% in the standard therapy arm. The main finding of this study was that gradually implemented intensive glucose control, with a goal to achieve an HbA1C ≤6.5%, was associated with a significant reduction in some microvascular complications of diabetes but not macrovascular complications. Intensive glucose control was also associated with a higher incidence of hospitalizations and severe hypoglycemia. A recent presentation by the ADVANCE group indicated that severe hypoglycemia was associated with significant increased risk of cardiovascular and all-cause mortality.

The choice of hypoglycemic therapy should be influenced by consideration of multiple factors, including BMI, renal function, comorbidities, financial issues and patient preferences. In general, overweight individuals should preferably be initially started on metformin in the absence of contraindications. The use of TZDs noted earlier remains a topic of debate, and the decision to use them should be individualized. The 2008 ADA and the European Association for the Study of Diabetes consensus algorithm recommended against the use of rosiglitazone, owing to concern regarding safety and the availability of alternative therapies, including pioglitazone that do not have the same concerns.[66]

Recent publication of a 10-year follow-up of intensive glucose control in type 2 diabetes from the UKPDS study cohort has raised the concept of a "legacy effect". [67] In the UKPDS study, 4,209 patients with newly diagnosed type 2 diabetes were randomized to either conventional therapy (dietary restriction) or intensive therapy (either sulfonylurea, insulin, or metformin in overweight patients). In posttrial monitoring, patients returned to community or hospital-based care with no attempt to maintain their previously randomized therapies. The median follow-up was 17 years, with close to 9 years of posttrial follow-up. While between-group differences in HbA1C were lost within 1 year of cessation of assigned treatments, levels of HbA1C continued to fall in both groups over 5 years reflecting appropriate risk factor management. In the sulfonylurea or insulin group, reduction in risk persisted for microvascular disease and any diabetes-related outcome at 10 years. Additionally, reductions were also noted for diabetes-related death, MI and death from any cause. Furthermore, in the group treated with metformin, significant risk reductions persisted for any diabetes-related outcomes, MI, and death from any cause without any effect on microvascular disease. The persistence and emergence of benefits, despite early loss of within-trial differences, in HbA1C levels between the intensive-therapy group and the conventional-therapy group have been called the legacy effect.

To summarize, while glycemic control does significantly impact the incidence of microvascular complications, the effect on macrovascular cardiovascular outcomes is less obvious, especially in those with prolonged duration of diabetes or preexisting CV disease. Additionally, there appears to be a lower threshold value of glycemic control (HbA1C of 6.5%), below which the risk of therapy may outweigh the benefits. Moreover, the strategy and medications used for glycemic control may have an effect on outcomes. Based on the results of the recent trials as noted above, the American College of Cardiology (ACC), AHA, and ADA came up with a consensus statement recommending the maintenance of HbA1C levels at or less than 7% for most people with diabetes while recommending that a comprehensive risk factor reduction should be instituted for CV risk reduction in all diabetic patients.

Antithrombotic Therapy

Primary Prevention

The multiple biochemical and functional abnormalities in the platelet function in both type 1 and 2 diabetes lead to increased platelet aggregability and adhesiveness. The correction of this abnormality with antiplatelet agents, such as aspirin should logically reduce CV events in diabetics. A meta analysis of the six large trials of aspirin for primary prevention in the general population found that aspirin reduced the risk of vascular events by 12%, with the largest reduction being for nonfatal MI.[68] There was little effect on total stroke or CHD death. Three of the trials in the above meta-analysis focused on the effect of aspirin exclusively among patients with diabetes [the Early Treatment Diabetic Retinopathy Study (ETDRS) trial, the Prevention of Progression of Arterial Disease and Diabetes (POPADAD) trial and the Japanese Primary Prevention of Atherosclerosis with Aspirin for Diabetes (JPAD) trial].[69,70] None of the trials mentioned above provided definitive results.

Based on these and other studies, the US Preventive Services Task Force recently recommended encouraging aspirin use in men aged 45–79 years and women aged 55–79 years, but discouraging the use of aspirin in younger adults regardless of the presence or absence of diabetes.[71,72] Two ongoing studies with combined sample size of more than 15,000 individuals with diabetes will provide additional information on the role of low-dose aspirin for the prevention of cardiovascular events. Aspirin and Simvastatin Combination for Cardiovascular Events Prevention Trial in Diabetes (ACCEPT-D) is an open-label Italian primary prevention trial comparing aspirin 100 mg once a day to no aspirin among adults over age 50 years with diabetes who are also on simvastatin.[73] The second trial, A Study of Cardiovascular Events in Diabetes (ASCEND), will also examine the effects of 100 mg aspirin daily vs. placebo for primary prevention among men and women over age 40 years with either type 1 or type 2 diabetes.[74]

In order to provide guidelines for management, the ADA, AHA, and ACC recently published an expert consensus document recommending low-dose aspirin (75–162 mg/day) as primary prevention for adults with diabetes who are at

TABLE 5: Indications for aspirin use for primary prevention in high-risk diabetic patients

- Obesity
- Hypertension
- Cigarette smoking
- Family history of coronary heart disease
- Micro- or macroalbuminuria
- Atherogenic dyslipidemia

increased CVD risk (10-year risk of CVD events over 10%) and are not at increased risk for bleeding (prior gastrointestinal bleeding, peptic ulcer disease, or concurrent use of medication, such as nonsteroidal anti-inflammatory drugs or warfarin).[75] The accurate determination of CVD risk should be made with the use of clinical tools, such as the UKPDS risk engine, atherosclerosis risk in communities (ARIC) CHD risk calculator, or ADA risk assessment tool (Table 5).

Secondary Prevention

The efficacy of aspirin for secondary prevention of CV events is suggested by a meta-analysis of secondary prevention trials by the Antithrombotic Trialists' Collaboration (ATC). The ATC meta-analysis included 287 trials with the inclusion of 212,000 high-risk patients.[76] In more than 4,500 patients with diabetes, the incidence of vascular events was significantly reduced from 23.5% with control treatment to 19.3% with antiplatelet therapy (p < 0.01). While the overall incidence of vascular events in the diabetic subgroup was much higher, the benefit of antiplatelet therapy in the diabetic and nondiabetic patients was comparable. In the Hypertension Optimal Treatment (HOT) study, half of the 1,501 patients with diabetes included in each target group were randomized to receive aspirin. The CV event rate was reduced by 15% and MI by 36% compared to placebo. The relative effects of aspirin were similar in nondiabetic and diabetic subjects.[77]

CURRENT ISSUES AND CONTROVERSIES IN THE MANAGEMENT OF CORONARY ARTERY DISEASE IN DIABETES MELLITUS

Management of CAD in the presence of diabetes should follow current ACC/AHA guidelines, which are based on an evidence-based approach.[78] In addition, as discussed above, considerable emphasis should be placed on aggressive reduction of risk factors, and as such, strategies will yield greater benefit for a diabetic individual. Treatment of acute coronary syndrome should include measures to preserve myocardium, stabilize atherosclerotic plaques, and prevent prothrombotic activity with the goal to reduce both short-term and long-term morbidity and mortality.[79] Studies have indicated that hyperglycemia in the setting of ACS is a poor prognostic marker. The role of intensive glycemic control by means of insulin infusion in patients presenting with ACS remains controversial. Data from the Diabetes Mellitus, Insulin Glucose Infusion in Acute Myocardial Infarction (DIGAMI) trial and the Hyperglycemia: Intensive Insulin Infusion in Infarction (HI-5) trial are contradictory, and all the studies have design flaws that make their findings unreliable.[80-82] In the absence of robust clinical data, the ACC/AHA 2009 update on ST-elevation MI gives a weak recommendation for the use of an insulin-based regimen to achieve and maintain blood glucose less than 180 mg/dL while avoiding hypoglycemia.[83]

CAD should preferentially be managed with medical therapy unless revascularization is necessary for acute coronary syndrome or to mitigate intractable symptoms based on findings from the Bypass Angioplasty Revascularization Investigation in Type 2 Diabetes (BARI 2D) trial.[84] BARI 2D was designed to determine whether early use of the most appropriate revascularization intervention, combined with aggressive medical management, reduced mortality rates compared with an initial strategy of equally aggressive medical management but delayed or no revascularization. Overall, patients with diabetes mellitus have a higher mortality and morbidity after any revascularization procedure as compared to patients without diabetes mellitus.

There is considerable ongoing debate regarding the most appropriate interventional approach in the setting of diabetes mellitus. Prior data comparing percutaneous coronary intervention (PCI) to coronary artery bypass grafting (CABG) come from studies in which stenting was not practiced and contemporary dual antiplatelet therapy (DAPT) regimen was not established. Trials comparing CABG to PCI with bare-metal stents (BMS) demonstrated lower event-free survival with BMS, primarily due to higher incidence of repeat revascularization (Arterial Revascularization Therapies Study-I (ARTS-I) trial[85]). The ARTS-II study evaluating sirolimus eluting stents suggested no significant difference between drug eluting stents (DES) and CABG when outcomes were compared to the CABG arm in ARTS I trial.[86] The recently concluded Coronary Artery Revascularization in Diabetes (CARDia) trial also demonstrated no difference in all-cause mortality, MI and stroke.[87] Another trials, the synergy between PCI with taxus and cardiac surgery (SYNTAX) trial demonstrated higher event rate with DES primarily due to increased incidence of revascularization with stenting.[88] Additionally, mortality was higher with stenting in patients with complex lesions (as identified by the syntax score). In summary, until further data are available, such as from the Future Revascularization Evaluation in patients with Diabetes mellitus: Optimal management of Multivessel disease (FREEDOM) trial, current evidence supports CABG with left internal mammary artery (LIMA) graft as a better option for revascularization in patients with diabetes mellitus particularly for complex left main disease, triple vessel disease, and for two-vessel disease with a complex left anterior descending disease.

Heart Failure in Diabetes

Heart failure can occur with diabetic cardiomyopathy without coexisting hypertension or CAD. Various postulated factors seem to contribute to the development of heart failure. These include autonomic neuropathy, impaired epicardial vessel tone, microvascular dysfunction, deposition of advanced glycation end products, and insulin resistance, leading to shift toward fatty acid metabolism in the myocardium. The management of heart failure in the setting of diabetes is along the same lines as in the absence of diabetes mellitus. An additional precaution to be taken in treating diabetes in the presence of diabetes mellitus is to be aware of potential side effects of medications, including TZDs and metformin. TZDs are not recommended in patients with symptomatic heart failure particularly with New York Heart Association class III and IV heart failure.

CONCLUSION

In conclusion, cardiodysmetabolic syndrome, impaired glucose tolerance, and diabetes mellitus likely represent a spectrum of metabolic disorders associated with varying degrees of insulin resistance that lead to endothelial dysfunction. The means to prevent and treat these disorders are similar and should include a multifactorial risk reduction approach to prevent associated cardiovascular disease.

REFERENCES

1. Reaven G. Banting lecture 1988. Role of insulin resistance in human disease. Diabetes. 1988;37(12):1595-607.
2. DeFronzo RA, Ferrannini E. Insulin resistance. A multifaceted syndrome responsible for NIDDM, obesity, hypertension, dyslipidemia, and atherosclerotic cardiovascular disease. Diabetes Care. 1991;14(3):173-94.
3. Lindsay RS, Howard BV. Cardiovascular risk associated with the metabolic syndrome. Curr Diab Rep. 2004;4(1):63-8.
4. Koh KK, Han SH, Quon MJ. Inflammatory markers and the metabolic syndrome insights from therapeutic interventions. J Am Coll Cardiol. 2005;46(11): 1978-85.
5. Expert Panel on Detection, Evaluation, and Treatment of High Blood Cholesterol in Adults. Executive Summary of The Third Report of The National Cholesterol Education Program (NCEP) Expert Panel on Detection, Evaluation, And Treatment of High Blood Cholesterol In Adults (Adult Treatment Panel III). JAMA. 2001;285(19):2486-97.

6. Alberti, KG, Zimmet, P, Shaw, J; IDF Epidemiology Task Force Consensus Group. The metabolic syndrome—a new worldwide definition. Lancet. 2005; 366(9491):1059-62.

7. Fagan TC, Deedwania PC. The cardiovascular dysmetabolic syndrome. Am J Med. 1998;105(1A):77S-82S.

8. Ford ES. Prevalence of the metabolic syndrome defined by the International Diabetes Federation among adults in the US. Diabetes Care. 2005;28(11):2745-9.

9. Ford ES, Giles WH, Dietz WH. Prevalence of the metabolic syndrome among US adults: findings from the third National Health and Nutrition Examination Survey. JAMA. 2002;287(3):356-9.

10. Reaven G. The metabolic syndrome or the insulin resistance syndrome? Different names, different concepts and different goals. Endocrinol Metab Clin North Am. 2004;33(2):283-303.

11. Mottillo S, Filion KB, Genest J, et al. The metabolic syndrome and cardiovascular risk: a systematic review and meta-analysis. J Am Coll Cardiol. 2010;56(14): 1113-32.

12. Grundy SM, Cleeman JI, Daniels SR, et al. Diagnosis and management of the metabolic syndrome: an American Heart Association/National Heart, Lung, and Blood Institute Scientific Statement. Circulation. 2005;112(17):2735-52.

13. Rosenzweig JL, Ferrannini E, Grundy SM, et al. Primary prevention of cardiovascular disease and type 2 diabetes in patients at metabolic risk: an endocrine society clinical practice guideline. J Clin Endocrinol Metab. 2008;93(10):3671-89.

14. Lloyd-Jones DM, Liu K, Colangelo LA, et al. Consistently stable or decreased body mass index in young adulthood and longitudinal changes in metabolic syndrome components: the Coronary Artery Risk Development in Young Adults Study. Circulation. 2007;115(8):1004-11.

15. Yanovski SZ, Yanovski JA. Obesity. N Engl J Med. 2002;346(8):591-602.

16. Haslam DW, James WP. Obesity. Lancet. 2005;366(9492):1197-209.

17. Esposito K, Marfella R, Ciotola M, et al. Effect of a mediterranean-style diet on endothelial dysfunction and markers of vascular inflammation in the metabolic syndrome: a randomized trial. JAMA. 2004;292(12):1440-6.

18. Tortosa A, Bes-Rastrollo M, Sanchez-Villegas A, et al. Mediterranean diet inversely associated with the incidence of metabolic syndrome: the SUN prospective cohort. Diabetes Care. 2007;30(11):2957-9.

19. McKeown NM, Meigs JB, Liu S, et al. Carbohydrate nutrition, insulin resistance, and the prevalence of the metabolic syndrome in the Framingham Offspring Cohort. Diabetes Care. 2004;27(2):538-46.

20. Knowler WC, Barrett-Connor E, Fowler SE, et al. Reduction in the incidence of type 2 diabetes with lifestyle intervention or metformin. N Engl J Med. 2002;346(6): 393-403.

21. Thompson PD, Buchner D, Pina IL, et al. Exercise and physical activity in the prevention and treatment of atherosclerotic cardiovascular disease: a statement from the Council on Clinical Cardiology (Subcommittee on Exercise, Rehabilitation, and Prevention) and the Council on Nutrition, Physical Activity, and Metabolism (Subcommittee on Physical Activity). Circulation. 2003;107(24):3109-16.

22. Krejs GJ. Metabolic benefits associated with sibutramine therapy. Int J Obesity. 2002;26(4):S34-7.

23. Didangelos TP, Thanapoulou AK, Bousboulas SH, et al. The orlistat and cardiovascular risk profile in patients with metabolic syndrome and type 2 diabetes (ORLICARDIA) Study. Curr Med Res Opin. 2004;20(9):1393-401.

24. Torgerson JS, Hauptman J, Boldrin MN, et al. Xenical in the prevention of diabetes in obese subjects (XENDOS) study: a randomized study or orlistat as an adjunct to lifestyle changes for the prevention of type 2 diabetes in obese patients. Diabetes Care. 2004;27(1):155-61.

25. James WP, Caterson ID, Coutinho W, et al. Effect of sibutramine on cardiovascular outcomes in overweight and obese subjects. N Engl J Med. 2010;363(10):905-17.

26. Després JP, Golay A, Sjöström L; Rimonabant in Obesity-Lipids Study Group. Effects on metabolic risk factors in overweight patients with dyslipidemia. N Engl J Med. 2005;353(20):2121-34.

27. Pi-Sunyer FX, Aronne LJ; RIO-North America Study Group. Effect of rimonabant, a cannabinoid-1 receptor blocker, on weight and cardiometabolic risk factors in overweight or obese patients. RIO-North America: a randomized controlled trial. JAMA. 2006;295(7):761-75.

28. Rosenstock J, Iranmanesh A, Hollander PA. Improved glycemic control with weight loss plus beneficial effects on atherogenic dyslipidemia with rimonobant in drug-naïve type 2 diabetes: the SERENADE trial (Abstract). Diabetes. 2007;56(1):A49-A50.

29. Grundy SM, Cleeman JI, Merz CN, et al. Implications of recent clinical trials for the National Cholesterol Education Program Adult Treatment Panel III guidelines. Circulation. 2004;110(2):227-39.

30. Deedwania P, Barter P, Carmena R, et al. Reduction of low-density lipoprotein cholesterol in patients with coronary heart disease and metabolic syndrome: analysis of the Treating to New Targets study. Lancet. 2006;368(9539):919-28.

31. De Cavanagh EM, Piotrkowski B, Basso N, et al. Enalapril and losartan attenuate mitochondrial dysfunction in aged rats. FASEB J. 2003;17(9):1096-8.

32. De Cavanagh EM, Inserra F, Toblli J, et al. Enalapril attenuates oxidative stress in diabetic rats. Hypertension. 2001;38(5):1130-6.

33. Furuhashi M, Ura N, Higashiura K, et al. Blockade of the rennin-angiotensin system increases adiponectin concentrations in patients with essential hypertension. Hypertension. 2003;42(1):76-81.

34. Engeli S. Role of the renin-angiotensin-aldosterone system in the metabolic syndrome. Contrib Nephrol. 2006;151:122-34.

35. Patrono C, García Rodríguez LA, Landolfi R, et al. Low dose aspirin for the prevention of atherothrombosis. N Engl J Med. 2005;353(22):2373-83.

36. Deedwania PC, Fonesca VA. Diabetes, prediabetes, and cardiovascular risk: shifting the paradigm. Am J Med. 2005;118(9):939-47.

37. Sattar N, McConnachie A, Shaper AG, et al. Can metabolic syndrome usefully predict cardiovascular disease and diabetes? Outcome data from two prospective studies. Lancet. 2008;371(9628):1927-35.

38. Sattar N, Gaw A, Scherbakova O, et al. Metabolic syndrome with and without C-reactive protein as a predictor of coronary heart disease and diabetes in the West of Scotland Coronary Prevention Study. Circulation. 2003;108(4):414-9.

39. Hanson RL, Imperatore G, Bennett PH, et al. Components of the "metabolic syndrome" and incidence of type 2 diabetes. Diabetes. 2002;51(10):3120-7.

40. Tuomilehto J, Lindström J, Eriksson JG, et al. Prevention of type 2 diabetes mellitus with lifestyle intervention or metformin. N Engl J Med. 2001;344(18):1343-50.

41. Knowler WC, Hamman RF, Edelstein SL, et al. Prevention of type 2 diabetes with troglitazone in the Diabetes Prevention Program. Diabetes. 2005;54(4):1150-6.

42. Kitabchi AE, Temprosa M, Knowler WC, et al. Role of insulin sensitivity and secretion in the evolution of type 2 diabetes in the diabetes prevention program: effects of lifestyle intervention and metformin. Diabetes. 2005;54(8):2404-14.

43. Chiasson JL, Josse RG, Gomis R, et al. Acarbose for prevention of type 2 diabetes mellitus: STOP-NIDDM randomized trial. Lancet. 2002;359(9323):2072-7.

44. DREAM (Diabetes Reduction Assessment with ramipril and rosiglitazone Medication) Trial Investigators; Gerstein HC, Yusuf S, et al. Effect of rosiglitazone on the frequency of diabetes in patients with impaired glucose tolerance or impaired fasting glucose: a randomized controlled trial. Lancet. 2006;368(9541): 1096-105.

45. Rajagopalan R, Iyer S, Khan M. Effect of pioglitazone on metabolic syndrome risk factors: results of double blind, multicenter, randomized clinical trials. Curr Med Res Opin. 2005;21:163-72.

46. Mozaffarian D, Rimm EB. Fish intake, contaminants, and human health: evaluating the risks and the benefits. JAMA. 2006;296(15):1885-99.

47. Buse JB, Ginsberg HN, Bakris GL, et al. Primary prevention of cardiovascular diseases in people with diabetes mellitus: a scientific statement from the American Heart Association and the American Diabetes Association. Circulation. 2007;115(1):114-26.

48. Chobanian AV, Bakris GL, Black HR, et al. The seventh report of the Joint National Committee on detection, evaluation and treatment of high blood pressure (JNC 7). JAMA. 2003;289(19):2560-72.

49. Clinical guidelines on the identification, evaluation, and treatment of overweight and obesity in adults—the evidence report. National Institutes of Health. Obes Res. 1998;6(Suppl 2):51S-209S.

50. Garg A, Grundy SM. Management of dyslipidemia in NIDDM. Diabetes Care. 1990;13(2):153-69.

51. Pyörälä K, Pedersen TR, Kjekshus J, et al. Cholesterol lowering with simvastatin improves prognosis of diabetic patients with coronary heart disease. A subgroup analysis of the Scandinavian Simvastatin Survival Study (4S). Diabetes Care. 1997;20(4):614-20.

52. Goldberg RB, Mellies MJ, Sacks FM, et al. Cardiovascular events and their reduction with pravastatin in diabetic and glucose-intolerant myocardial infarction survivors with average cholesterol and recurrent events (CARE) trial. The CARE investigators. Circulation. 1998;98(23):2513-9.

53. Shepherd J, Barter P, Carmena R, et al. Effect of lowering LDL cholesterol substantially below currently recommended levels in patients with coronary heart disease and diabetes: the Treating to New Targets (TNT) study. Diabetes Care. 2006;29(6):1220-6.

54. Shepherd J, Kastelein JP, Bittner VA, et al. Intensive lipid lowering with atorvastatin in patients with coronary artery disease, diabetes, and chronic kidney disease. Mayo Clin Proc. 2008;83(8):870-9.

55. The ACCORD Study Group, Ginsberg HN, Elam MB, et al. Effects of combination lipid therapy in type 2 diabetes mellitus. N Engl J Med. 2010;362(17):1563-74.

56. The ACCORD study group; Cushman WC, Evans GW, Byington RP, et al. Effects of intensive blood-pressure control in type 2 diabetes mellitus. N Engl J Med. 2010;362(7):1575-85.

57. Patel A; ADVANCE Collaborative Group, MacMahon S, et al. Effects of a fixed combination of perindopril and indapamide on macrovascular and microvascular outcomes in patients with type 2 diabetes mellitus (the ADVANCE trial): a randomised controlled trial. Lancet. 2007;370(9590):829-40.

58. Effects of ramipril on cardiovascular and microvascular outcomes in people with diabetes mellitus: results of the HOPE Study and MICRO-HOPE substudy. Heart Outcomes Prevention Evaluation Study Investigators. Lancet. 2000; 355(9200):253-9.

59. National Kidney Foundation. K/DOQI clinical practice guidelines for chronic kidney disease: evaluation, classification, and stratification. Am J Kidney Dis. 2002;39(1):S1-266.

60. Weber MA, Bakris GL, Jamerson K, et al. Cardiovascular events during differing hypertension therapies in patients with diabetes. J Am Coll Cardiol. 2010;56(1):77-85.

61. Intensive blood-glucose control with sulphonylureas or insulin compared with conventional treatment and risk of complications in patients with type 2 diabetes (UKPDS 33). United Kingdom Prospective Diabetes Study Group. Lancet. 1998;352(9131):837-53.

62. Effect of intensive blood glucose control with metformin on complications in over-weight patients with type 2 diabetes (UKPDS 34). Lancet. 1998;352(9131):854-65.

63. Khaw KT, Wareham N, Luben R, et al. Glycated hemoglobin, diabetes, and mortality in men in Norfolk cohort of European prospective investigation of cancer and nutrition (EPIC-Norfolk). BMJ. 2001;322(7277):15-8.

64. The Action to Control Cardiovascular Risk in Diabetes Study Group, Gerstein HC, Miller ME, et al. Effects of intensive glucose lowering in type 2 diabetes. N Engl J Med. 2008;358(24):2545-59.

65. ADVANCE Collaborative Group, Patel A, MacMahon S, et al. Intensive blood glucose control and vascular outcomes in patients with type 2 diabetes. N Engl J Med. 2008;358(24):2560-72.

66. Nathan DM, Buse JB, Davidson MB, et al. Medical management of hyperglycemia in type 2 diabetes: a consensus algorithm for the initiation and adjustment of

therapy: a consensus statement of the American Diabetes Association and the European Association for the Study of Diabetes. Diabetes Care. 2009;32(1):193-203.

67. Holman RR, Paul SK, Bethel A, et al. 10-year follow-up of intensive glucose control in type 2 diabetes. N Engl J Med. 2008;359(15):1577-89.

68. Antithrombotic Trialists' (ATT) Collaboration; Baigent C, Blackwell L, et al. Aspirin in the primary and secondary prevention of vascular disease: collaborative meta-analysis of individual participant data from randomised trials. Lancet. 2009; 373(9678):1849-60.

69. Aspirin effects on mortality and morbidity in patients with diabetes mellitus. Early treatment diabetic retinopathy study report 14. ETDRS Investigators. JAMA. 1992; 268(10):1292-300.

70. Belch J, MacCuish A, Campbell I, et al. The prevention of progression of arterial disease and diabetes (POPADAD) trial: factorial randomized placebo controlled trial of aspirin and antioxidants in patients with diabetes and asymptomatic peripheral arterial disease. BMJ. 2008;337:a1840.

71. Wolff T, Miller T, Ko S. Aspirin for the primary prevention of cardiovascular events: an update of the evidence for the US Preventive Services Task Force. Ann Intern Med. 2009;150(6):405-10.

72. US Preventive Services Task Force. Aspirin for the prevention of cardiovascular disease: US Preventive Services Task Force recommendation statement. Ann Intern Med. 2009;150(6):396-404.

73. De Berardis G, Sacco M, Evangelista V, et al. Aspirin and Simvastatin Combination for Cardiovascular Events Prevention Trial in Diabetes (ACCEPT-D): design of a randomized study of the efficacy of low-dose aspirin in the prevention of cardiovascular events in subjects with diabetes mellitus treated with statins. Trials. 2007;8:21.

74. British Heart Foundation. ASCEND: A Study of Cardiovascular Events in Diabetes. Available from: http://clinicaltrials.gov/ct2/show/NCT00135226 (Accessed Sep 19, 2010).

75. Pignone M, Alberts MJ, Colwell JA, et al. Aspirin for primary prevention of cardiovascular events in people with diabetes. J Am Coll Cardiol. 2010;55(25): 2878-86.

76. Antithrombotic Trialists' Collaboration. Collaboration meta-analysis of randomized trials of antiplatelet therapy for prevention of death, myocardial infarction, and stroke in high risk patients. BMJ. 2002;324(7329):71-86.

77. Hansoson K, Zanchetti A, Carruthers SG, et al. Effects of intensive blood-pressure lowering and low dose aspirin on patients with hypertension: principal results of the Hypertension Optimal Treatment (HOT) randomized trial. Lancet. 1998;351(9118):1755-62.

78. Smith SC Jr, Allen J, Blair SN, Bonow RO, Brass LM, Fonarow GC, et al. AHA/ACC guidelines for secondary prevention for patient with coronary and other atherosclerotic vascular disease: 2006 update: endorsed by the National Heart, Lung and Blood Institute. Circulation. 2006;113(19):2363-72.

79. Antman EM, Anbe DT, Armstrong PW, et al. ACC/AHA guidelines for the management of patients with ST-elevation myocardial infarction: A report of the American College of Cardiology/American Heart Association Task Force on Practice Guidelines (Committee to Revise the 1999 Guidelines for the Management of patient with acute myocardial infarction). J Am Coll Cardiol. 2004;44(3):E1-E211.

80. Malmberg K. Prospective randomized study of intensive insulin treatment on long term survival after acute myocardial infarction in patients with diabetes mellitus. DIGAMI (Diabetes Mellitus, Insulin Glucose Infusion in Acute Myocardial Infarction) Study Group. BMJ. 1997;314(7093):1512-5.

81. Malmberg K, Ryden L, Wedel H, et al. Intense metabolic control by means of insulin in patients with diabetes mellitus and acute myocardial infarction (DIGAMI 2): effects on mortality and morbidity. Eur Heart J. 2005;26(7):650-61.

82. Cheung NW, Wong VW, McLean M. The Hyperglycemia: Intensive Insulin Infusion in Infarction (HI-5) study: a randomized controlled trial of insulin infusion therapy for myocardial infarction. Diabetes Care. 2006;29(4):765-70.

83. Kushner FG, Hand M, Smith SC Jr, et al. 2009 Focused Updates: ACC/AHA guidelines for the management of patients with ST-elevation myocardial infarction and ACC/AHA/SCAI guidelines on percutaneous coronary intervention: a report of the American College of Cardiology Foundation/American Heart Association Task force on practice guidelines. Circulation. 2009;120(22):2271-306.

84. BARI 2D Study Group, Frye RL, August P, et al. A randomized trial of therapies for type 2 diabetes and coronary artery disease. N Engl J Med. 2009;360(24):2503-15.

85. Serruys PW, Unger F, Sousa JE, et al. Comparison of coronary-artery bypass surgery and stenting for the treatment of multivessel disease. N Engl J Med. 2001;344(15):1117-24.

86. Daeman J, Kuck KH, Macaya C, et al. Multivessel coronary revascularization in patients with and without diabetes mellitus: 3-year follow-up of the ARTS-II (Arterial Revascularization Therapies Study-II) trial. J Am Coll Cardiol. 2008;52(24): 1957-67.

87. Kapur A, Hall RJ, Malik IS, et al. Randomized comparison of percutaneous coronary intervention with coronary artery bypass grafting in diabetic patients. 1-year results of the CANDia (Coronary Artery Revascularization in Diabetes) trial. J Am Coll Cardiol. 2010;55(5):432-40.

88. Banning AP, Westaby S, Morice MC, et al. Diabetic and nondiabetic patients with left main and/or 3-vessel coronary artery disease: comparison of outcomes with cardiac surgery and paclitaxel-eluting stents. J Am Coll Cardiol. 2010;55(11): 1067-75.

Drugs for Acute Coronary Syndromes

Krishan V Soni, Stephen W Waldo, Yerem Yeghiazarians, Kanu Chatterjee

INTRODUCTION

The formation of an atherosclerotic plaque begins with endothelial dysfunction.[1] Dysfunctional endothelial cells increase expression of adhesion molecules [vascular cell adhesion molecule 1 (VCAM-1) and intercellular adhesion molecule 1 (ICAM-1)] that promote the adherence and extravasation of monocytes into the inner surface of the arterial wall.[2] Research has demonstrated that extravasated monocytes will subsequently differentiate into macrophages in response to the surrounding cytokine environment and accumulate lipid to form a subintimal layer of foam cells.[3,4] Smooth muscle cells will then migrate from the media into the intima where they proliferate and construct a complex extracellular matrix that overlies the lipid core.[3] As the lesion progresses, ossification can occur with significant calcification of the thick fibrotic cap overlying the deposited lipid resulting in stabilization of the lesion.[5] Lipid-laden macrophages may then produce cytokines that perpetuate the inflammatory process and secrete enzymes that degrade this extracellular matrix.[6] Disruption of the extracellular matrix exposes the underlying lipid core to the vascular space, allowing it to serve as a nidus for thrombus formation.

Degradation of the extracellular matrix and exposure of the diseased vascular wall results in thrombus formation that instigates acute coronary syndromes (ACS) (Fig. 1). As the plaque becomes unstable, subendothelial tissue factor (TF) produced by macrophages and smooth muscle cells will activate the coagulation cascade.[7-9] Activated coagulation factors result in the generation of thrombin initiating the conversion of fibrinogen to fibrin.[10] Circulating platelets will subsequently adhere to the subendothelial space and become activated by the presence of von Willebrand factor (vWF), resulting in immediate aggregation and formation of

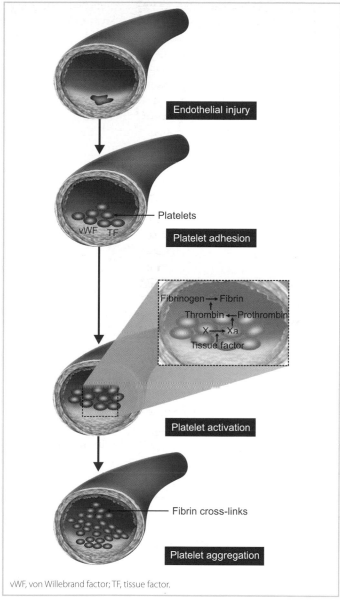

vWF, von Willebrand factor; TF, tissue factor.

FIG. 1: The pathogenesis of acute coronary syndrome. It begins with endothelial injury leading to exposure of the subendothelial space. vWF and TF lead to platelet adhesion and activation of the clotting cascade, respectively. Generation of thrombin leads to platelet degranulation and perpetuates platelet activation while also generating fibrin cross-links to facilitate platelet aggregation and complete occlusion of the arterial lumen.

the *primary platelet plug*.[11] Fibrin polymer cross-links will be attached to the adherent platelets resulting in thrombus formation. Although this thrombus is adherent to the vascular wall, there is a potential for embolization resulting in microvascular occlusion.

The clinical presentation of an epicardial thrombus encompasses unstable angina, non-ST elevation myocardial infarction (non-STEMI) and STEMI, collectively termed ACS. The pharmacologic therapy for ACS is fundamentally designed to reduce myocardial oxygen demand and increase myocardial oxygen supply to reduce the risk of myocardial infarction (MI). Decreasing myocardial oxygen demand utilizes therapies that decrease cardiac rate and inotropy. Increasing myocardial oxygen supply utilizes therapies that inhibit both the coagulation system and platelet activation to restore normal coronary blood flow. A number of anticoagulants have been used clinically to affect different aspects of the clotting cascade (Fig. 2). Similarly, a number of platelet receptors have been identified as therapeutic targets (Fig. 3 and Table 1) to reduce

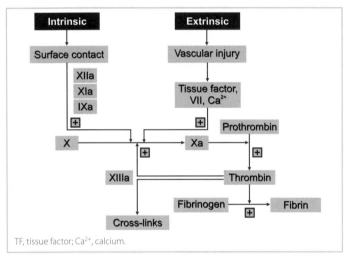

TF, tissue factor; Ca^{2+}, calcium.

FIG. 2: The intrinsic and extrinsic clotting cascade.

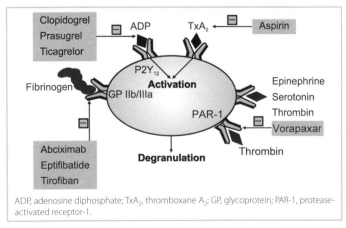

ADP, adenosine diphosphate; TxA_2, thromboxane A_2; GP, glycoprotein; PAR-1, protease-activated receptor-1.

FIG. 3: Clinical use of antiplatelet agents on various platelet receptors. Platelet activation and degranulation is mediated through ADP, TxA_2, and GP IIb/IIIa receptors. Each of these receptors is a potential target for therapeutic agents during the treatment of acute coronary syndrome.

TABLE 1: Platelet receptors identified as therapeutic targets

Receptor	Alternate Name	Function	Inhibitor
αIIbβ3	Glycoprotein IIb/IIIa	Crosslinks fibrinogen and von Willebrand factor	• Abciximab • Eptifibatide • Tirofiban
P2Y$_{12}$	ADP receptor	Platelet activation	• Clopidogrel • Prasugrel • Ticlopidine • Ticagrelor • Cangrelor
TxA$_2$	Thromboxane	Platelet activation	Aspirin
PAR-1	Thrombin	Platelet activation	Vorapaxar

PAR-1, protease-activated receptor-1; ADP, adenosine diphosphate.

the propagation of thrombus formation. In addition to these therapies, fibrinolytic agents can be used to disintegrate previously formed thrombus through destruction of fibrin cross-links. The pharmacology and clinical uses of each of these therapies will be reviewed in the following sections.

ANTI-ISCHEMIC THERAPIES

The treatment of ACS begins with therapies to reduce the ischemic burden.[12] Current guidelines suggest that patients with ACS should be initially treated with supplemental oxygen (if hypoxic) (Class I, Level C) while pharmacotherapies are being pursued. Nitroglycerin, narcotics, β-blockers and calcium-channel blockers serve as the primary anti-ischemic medications employed in the contemporary management of ACS.

Nitroglycerin

Pharmacology

Nitroglycerin degenerates *in vivo* to deliver nitric oxide throughout the vasculature. Within smooth muscle cells, nitric oxide activates guanylate cyclase resulting in an increase in guanosine 3', 5'-monophosphate (cGMP).[13] The presence of cGMP within smooth muscle cells leads to dephosphorylation of myosin light chains and results in smooth muscle relaxation. A reduction in vascular tone produces a vasodilator effect on peripheral veins and, to a lesser extent, on peripheral arteries. The dilation of the capacitance vessels increases venous pooling and decreases myocardial preload, one of the measures of myocardial demand.[12,14] Nitroglycerin also induces the dilation of the arterial vasculature resulting in a slight decline in afterload. It is important to note that this decline in afterload is often offset by a reflex increase in heart rate such that the optimal anti-ischemic effect of nitroglycerin is obtained when combined with the concomitant use of β-blockers.

Nitroglycerin also dilates normal and atherosclerotic epicardial coronary arteries. Research has suggested that endothelial dysfunction within the diseased coronary vasculature may impair the normal physiological response to changes in myocardial blood flow.[15] Because of this, patients suffering from an ACS may not achieve maximum epicardial artery dilatation without the administration of exogenous nitroglycerin. As a result, nitroglycerin has the benefit of increasing myocardial oxygen supply through the dilation of the epicardial coronary arteries.[15]

Pharmacokinetics and Doses

Nitroglycerin is available in topical, oral and intravenous (IV) formulations. To facilitate rapid absorption into the systemic circulation, oral formulations include sublingual tablets and translingual sprays (0.3–0.6 mg/dose). The oral formulations begin to take their effect on the vasculature within 1–3 minutes of administration with a peak effect occurring after approximately 5 minutes.[12,14] Because of extensive first-pass metabolism, these agents have a short half-life (1–4 minutes) and their effect has dissipated completely after 25 minutes. The IV formulation of nitroglycerin (5–400 μg/minutes) has a rapid onset of action but tolerance may develop after 8 hours of continuous therapy. The administration of nitroglycerin with phosphodiesterase inhibitors results in a profound decline in vasomotor tone resulting in recalcitrant hypotension. Because of this, nitroglycerin should not be used in patients who recently received a phosphodiesterase inhibitor, specifically within 24 hours of sildenafil or vardenafil use, or within 48 hours of tadalafil use. Nitrates should not be administered to patients with hypotension or to those in whom right ventricular infarction is suspected.

Clinical Use and Indications

There are no large randomized controlled trials (RCTs) that support the use of nitroglycerin to reduce ischemia or mortality in ACS. A meta-analysis of several small studies conducted before the reperfusion era, however, demonstrated a 35% relative risk reduction in mortality among patients that received IV nitroglycerin for ACS.[16] Clinical trials in the reperfusion era have not been able to reproduce this magnitude of benefit.[17,18] Studies have demonstrated, however, that the abrupt discontinuation of IV nitroglycerin results in worsening electrocardiographic changes.[19] Despite the lack of controlled data, nitroglycerin continues to be a widely accepted anti-ischemic agent for the treatment of ACS.

Guidelines

Current guidelines recommend the use of sublingual nitroglycerin (0.4 mg) every 5 minutes for a total of three doses to reduce ongoing ischemic discomfort in the setting of ACS (Class I, Level C). IV nitroglycerin is currently indicated in the first 48 hours after ACS for the treatment of persistent ischemia or hypertension (Class I, Level B).[12] The guidelines note that the administration of nitrates is contraindicated in the setting of hypotension [systolic blood pressure (SBP) <90 mmHg] or in patients that have recently used phosphodiesterase inhibitors because of the potential risk of cardiovascular (CV) collapse (Class III, Level B).

Narcotics

Pharmacology

Narcotics have potent analgesic and anxiolytic effects that may reduce myocardial oxygen demand in ACS. Additionally, morphine sulfate causes a reduction in vasomotor tone and a decrease in heart rate resulting in a decline in SBP. These effects are mediated through an increase in vagal tone and all result to decrease myocardial oxygen demand.[12,14]

Pharmacokinetics and Doses

Intravenous morphine sulfate (1–5 mg IV push) is the narcotic most frequently employed in ACS. The onset of action for the IV formulation is rapid (5–10 min) with a half life of 2–4 hours. Morphine sulfate is metabolized via hepatic conjugation with glucuronic acid to morphine-6-glucuronide (active analgesic) and morphine-3-glucuronide (inactive analgesic) before being excreted predominantly in the urine.

Clinical Use and Indications

There are no large RCTs that support the use of narcotics to reduce ischemia or mortality during ACS. Despite this, narcotics have been included in the clinical treatment algorithm for ACS for the last three decades. Data from a recent large observational cohort (N = 57,039) suggests that the administration of morphine may be associated with an increased risk of mortality.[20] Patients that received morphine within this registry (29.8%) had a higher risk-adjusted likelihood of all-cause in-hospital death (OR 1.48) during treatment for ACS. As an observational cohort, there are likely selection biases contributing to this finding and an RCT should be conducted to answer this question definitively. In light of this data, however, recent guidelines have tempered the enthusiasm for the widespread use of narcotics in ACS.

Guidelines

In the absence of contraindications, current guidelines suggest that it is reasonable to administer IV narcotics (morphine sulfate) to patients with ACS and persistent ischemic discomfort despite the use of nitroglycerin (Class IIb, Level B).[12] Notably, the use of nonsteroidal anti-inflammatory drugs (NSAIDs) other than aspirin for analgesia has been associated with increased CV complications and their use is contraindicated (Class III, Level B).[12]

Beta-blockers

Pharmacology

The primary benefit of β-blockers in ACS is related to their antagonism of the β1-adrenergic receptors. β1-adrenergic receptors are primarily located on the surface of the myocardium.[21] Competitive inhibition of catecholamine action on these receptors reduces myocardial contractility as well as the intrinsic sinus rate resulting in a significant decline in myocardial oxygen demand.[12,14] The decrease in ventricular rate also increases the duration of diastole allowing increased time for the epicardial coronary arteries to perfuse the ventricular myocardium, thus, increasing myocardial oxygen supply. In contrast to β1-adrenergic receptors, β2-adrenergic receptors are primarily located on the vascular and bronchial smooth muscle. Inhibition of catecholamine action at these sites produces vasoconstriction and bronchoconstriction.[14] Because of this, severe bronchospasm is a relative contra-indication to the use of β-blockers. Most β-blockers used in the contemporary management of ACS are selective β1 antagonists (Table 2).[12,14]

TABLE 2: β-blockers used in the contemporary management of acute coronary syndromes[1,24]

Drug	Selectivity	Agonist activity	Dose
Acebutolol	β1	Yes	200–600 mg BD
Atenolol	β1	No	50–200 mg daily
Betaxolol	β1	No	10–20 mg daily
Bisoprolol	β1	No	10 mg daily
Carvedilol	None	Yes	6.25–25 mg BD
Esmolol	β1	No	50–300 µg/kg/min
Labetalol	None	Yes	200–600 mg BD
Metoprolol	β1	No	50–200 mg BD
Nadolol	None	No	40–80 mg daily
Pindolol	None	Yes	2.5–7.5 mg TD
Proponalol	None	No	20–80 mg BD
Timolol	None	No	10 mg BD

BD, twice a day; TD, thrice a day.

Pharmacokinetics and Doses

Based on prior studies, metoprolol tartrate is the most commonly employed β-blocker in the immediate management of ACS.[22] The dosing regimens administered include IV metoprolol 5 mg IV push over 1 minute repeated up to three times for a total dose of 15 mg. The IV form of metoprolol reaches its peak action in 20 minutes with a duration of action of approximately 6 hours based on a half-life of 3–8 hours before being metabolized in the liver cytochrome P450 2D6 (CYP2D6) and excreted in the urine. In patients that tolerate this regimen, oral therapy (25–50 mg) can be initiated 15 minutes after the last IV dose every 6 hours. With the contemporary practice of early reperfusion, the routine administration of intravenous β-blockers has fallen out of favor due to increased risk of cardiogenic shock and lower mortality benefit.[23-25] Oral β-blockers are typically started as early as possible in patients who do not have contraindications.

Clinical Use and Indications

The initial studies of β-blockade in the treatment of ACS were conducted prior to routine anticoagulation and revascularization. A collection of these early studies suggested that routine use of β-blockade in patients with unstable angina resulted in a 13% relative risk reduction in the eventual progression to an electrocardiographically significant MI.[26] After the advent of routine percutaneous revascularization, another collection of small studies suggested that the use of β-blockers in ACS patients eventually treated with percutaneous coronary intervention (PCI) reduced the absolute risk of death at 6 months by 2%.[27]

A large randomized trial evaluating the use of IV metoprolol for ACS included 45,852 patients in Asia (COMMIT).[22] The majority of this population presented with electrocardiographic evidence of an STEMI (93%) and were randomized to receive immediate treatment with IV β-blockers (metoprolol 5 mg IVP) followed by oral metoprolol (200 mg daily) or placebo. The primary combined composite endpoint of death, reinfarction or cardiac arrest was equivalent between the two groups (9.4% vs. 9.9%). Treatment with β-blockers did result, however, in a reduction in the rate of reinfarction (2.0% vs. 2.5%) as well as an increase in the rate of cardiogenic shock (5.0% vs. 3.9%). Based on this data, β-blockers became widely employed in the immediate management of ACS.

Recent observational studies and meta-analyses have studied the effect of immediate β-blockade therapy in the treatment of ACS patients who undergo percutaneous reperfusion. An analysis of the GRACE Registry (Global Registry of Acute Coronary Events) evaluated the use of early (<24 hours) IV or oral β-blockers compared to delayed (>24 hours) oral β-blockers in 13,110 patients who presented with STEMI.[24] In this registry, 21% of patients received any early IV β-blockers, 65% received only early oral β-blockers, and 14% received delayed β-blockers. In-hospital mortality was increased with IV β-blocker use (propensity score adjusted odds ratio, 1.41) but significantly reduced with delayed β-blocker administration (propensity adjusted odds ratio, 0.44). The study concluded that oral β-blockers were associated with a decrease in the risk of cardiogenic shock, ventricular arrhythmias, and acute heart failure (HF), but early receipt of any form of β-blockers was associated with an increase in hospital mortality.

A recent meta-analysis of 60 trials including 102,000 patients with ACS demonstrated that β-blockers reduced mortality in the pre-reperfusion [incident rate ratio (IRR) 0.86] but not in the reperfusion era (IRR 0.98). In the reperfusion era, β-blockers reduced MI (IRR 0.72) and angina (IRR 0.80) at the expense of increase in HF (IRR 1.10), cardiogenic shock (IRR 1.29), and drug discontinuation (IRR 1.64), with no benefit for other outcomes. Benefits for recurrent MI and angina in the reperfusion era appeared to be short-term (30 days).[25]

Based on this and other data, greater caution is now suggested in the routine use of IV β-blockers for ACS. In particular, these agents should be avoided in patients with clinical evidence of HF or hemodynamic instability.[12]

Although the present discussion has focused on the immediate management of ACS, it is important to note that the treatment of stable coronary artery disease with left ventricular dysfunction may include the use of alternative β-blockers, particularly carvedilol.[28,29]

Guidelines

Current guidelines suggest that oral β-blocker therapy should be initiated within the first 24 hours after ACS unless there is a contraindication (Class I, Level A). Acceptable contraindications to therapy with oral β-blockers include clinical signs of HF, evidence of a low output state, increased risk for shock, or conduction abnormalities. Patients with contraindications to β-blockers in the first 24 hours should be re-evaluated to determine their subsequent eligibility (Class I, Level C). In patients with stabilized HF, it is recommended to continue β-blocker therapy with one of three drugs with proven mortality benefit (metoprolol succinate, carvedilol, or bisoprolol) (Class I, Level C). It is also reasonable to continue β-blocker therapy in patients with normal left ventricular function with ACS (Class IIA, Level C).[12]

Calcium Channel Blockers

Pharmacology

Calcium channel blockers (CCBs) reduce transmembrane inward calcium flow thus inhibiting myocardial and vascular smooth muscle contraction. Like β-blockers, this reduces myocardial contractility resulting in a reduction in myocardial oxygen demand. CCBs also dilate the epicardial coronary arteries resulting in an increase in myocardial oxygen supply.[12] Through these mechanisms, CCBs can serve as effective anti-anginal medications in certain patient populations presenting with ACS.

Pharmacokinetics and Doses

The non-dihydropyridine CCBs include diltiazem and verapamil. Most clinical studies employing these agents in ACS have used oral formulations initiated several days after the acute event. Diltiazem is available in 30 mg oral tablets with a maximum daily dose of 360 mg. The oral dose of diltiazem reaches its peak plasma levels within 1 hour with a half-life of 5 hours before being excreted in the urine and feces. Verapamil is available in 80 mg oral tablets with a maximum daily dose of 480 mg. The oral dose of verapamil reaches its peak plasma levels within 1 hour with a half-life of 3–7 hours before being excreted in the urine and feces.

Clinical Use and Indications

Several randomized trials have been performed to evaluate the utility of CCBs in ACS. The Multicenter Diltiazem Postinfarction Trial (MDPIT) randomized 2,466 patients to diltiazem (240 mg daily) or placebo 3–15 days after presenting with a MI.[30] After over 2 years of follow-up, the mortality between the two groups was identical (13.5%) with a non-significant trend toward fewer recurrent events in patients treated with diltiazem (16.4 vs. 18.3%). Similarly, the Danish Study Group on Verapamil in MI II (DAVIT II) randomized almost 1,800 patients to verapamil (360 mg daily) or placebo in the second week after admission for ACS.[31] Treatment with verapamil had a nonsignificant reduction in mortality (11.1% vs. 13.8%). A meta-analyses including 19,000 patients derived from 28 independent trials assessing the utility of CCBs has confirmed these findings.[32,33]

It is important to note that retrospective analyses of the trials incorporating CCBs suggest that caution should be used in patients with reduced left ventricular ejection fraction (LVEF). In the aforementioned MDPIT, patients with impaired LVEF (<40%) with evidence of pulmonary congestion on chest radiograph that were treated with diltiazem had an increased number of cardiac events and worsened mortality.[30] Because of this, CCBs should be avoided in patients presenting with ACS that have concomitant left ventricular systolic dysfunction.

Guidelines

Current guidelines suggest that nondihydropyridine CCBs should be given to patients presenting with ACS if they have a contraindication to β-blockers and they have absence of clinically significant left ventricular dysfunction or conduction disease (Class I, Level B). CCBs are also recommended for ACS patients with recurrent ischemic symptoms when β-blockers are not successful (Class I, Level C). Immediate release nifedipine should not be administered to ACS patients in the absence of β-blocker therapy as it increases mortality (Class III).[12]

ANTICOAGULANT THERAPIES

The treatment of ACS continues with agents designed to increase myocardial oxygen supply.[12] As previously described, ACS is characterized by the presence of a platelet plug cross-linked with fibrin polymers that obstructs an epicardial coronary artery. A variety of agents have been used to reduce the efficacy of the coagulation system and thus prevent the propagation of thrombus. Unfractionated heparin, low-molecular-weight heparin and thrombin inhibitors all have a role in the contemporary management of ACS.

Unfractionated Heparin

Pharmacology

Unfractionated heparin is a heterogeneous mucopoly-saccharide with complex effects on the coagulation cascade. A unique pentasaccharide segment of the heparin molecule will bind to endogenous antithrombin. The antithrombin-heparin molecule will then bind to and inhibit the action of thrombin preventing the formation of fibrin.[34] In addition to inhibiting the action of thrombin, the antithrombin-heparin complex also prevents the serine protease activity of a number of members of the coagulation cascade including factor Xa.

Pharmacokinetics and Doses

Because unfractionated heparin contains a heterogeneous group of molecules extracted by varying procedures, the dose-effect relationship is difficult to predict leading to strength variations among the different batches. The administration of unfractionated heparin thus requires frequent monitoring of the coagulation cascade via the activated partial thromboplastin time (aPTT). European guidelines recommend an IV bolus of 60–70 IU/kg (maximum 5,000 IU) followed by an infusion of 12–15 IU/kg-hour (maximum 1,000 IU/hour) of unfractionated heparin for the immediate management of ACS.[35,36] The IV infusion should then be titrated to obtain an aPTT that is within 1.5–2.5 times the control value, typically 50–75 seconds. The AHA/ACC guidelines recommend a lower initial bolus of 60 units/kg (maximum 4,000 units) with an initial infusion rate of 12 units/kg-hour (maximum 1,000 units/ hour) to obtain therapeutic aPTT level per hospital protocol.[12] More extreme disruption of the coagulation cascade results in an increased risk of intracranial hemorrhage (ICH) without a benefit for ACS. Nomograms are widely available for titrating IV unfractionated heparin dosing.

Regardless of the doses used, unfractionated heparin has a short onset (20–60 min) with a short half-life (60–90 min) before being metabolized in the liver and excreted in the urine. Heparin is an appropriate anticoagulant in patients with renal dysfunction. The short half-life of this anticoagulant makes it ideal for facilitating PCI. Unfractionated heparin can also be reversed with protamine sulfate (1 mg/100 units heparin), a basic compound derived from salmon that will bind to the acidic unfractionated heparin and form a stable inactive salt. Protamine sulfate also has a rapid onset (5 min) and a moderate duration of effect (2 hours). It is important to note that protamine should be used with caution in insulin-dependent diabetics as anaphylactic reactions have been reported in diabetic patients previously exposed to NPH insulin.[37]

Clinical Use and Indications

A number of small randomized trials in the prerevascularization era demonstrated the clinical benefit of unfractionated heparin for the treatment of ACS.[38-41] Taken together, these trials suggest that the rate of death or recurrent MI could be reduced by approximately 54% during the first week of therapy with the anticoagulant. Several meta-analyses have confirmed these findings suggesting a relative risk reduction of 33–56%.[42,43] Most of these trials evaluated the use of unfractionated heparin for 2–5 days. While the optimal duration of therapy continues to be undefined, guidelines suggest that therapy is continued until PCI or for a total of 48 hours for patients managed medically.[12] It is important to note that discontinuation of unfractionated heparin in ACS has led to a recurrent symptoms in some patients, particularly those not treated with aspirin.[44] Based on these findings, the administration of unfractionated heparin has become standard practice in the contemporary management of ACS and now serves as a bridge to revascularization.

Unfractionated heparin continues to be used to facilitate PCI despite the lack of randomized trials demonstrating its efficacy.

The standard regimen in the United States for unfractionated heparin is the administration of weight-adjusted boluses (70–100 IU/kg) to maintain an activated clotting time of 250–300 seconds if a glycoprotein IIb/IIIa (GpIIb/IIIa) inhibitor is not used.[12,45] If a GpIIb/IIIa inhibitor is used, then the activated clotting time goal is reduced to 200–250 seconds.[12] Heparin should be immediately discontinued after the completion of the interventional procedure unless there is another compelling clinical reason for its continuation (e.g., LV thrombus, mechanical heart valve, pulmonary embolism, use of hemodynamic support devices, etc.)

Complications

Heparin-induced thrombocytopenia (HIT) is an acquired prothrombotic disorder most commonly instigated by unfractionated heparin.[46,47] The pathophysiology underlying HIT has recently been elucidated. The administration of unfractionated heparin is thought to precipitate an antibody-mediated immune reaction after binding to platelet factor-4 (PF4), a heparin-neutralizing protein released from the α-granules of activated platelets. The heparin-PF4 complex will attract circulating antibodies (IgG) that will adhere to the platelet surface on FcãIIa receptors.[46] As these immune complexes assemble on the platelet surface, intracellular cross-linking of the FcãIIa receptors results in platelet activation and release of additional PF4 perpetuating the process and ultimately leading to platelet consumption. Ongoing platelet activation by immune complexes results in increased thrombin production and a systemic hyper-coagulable state that makes patients susceptible to both venous and arterial thrombosis.[48] Assays for the presence of antibodies to the heparin-PF4 complex identify patients at risk for this condition.[49]

According to most case series, HIT is characterized by a 50% reduction in platelet count most commonly occurring 5–10 days after the initiation of heparin therapy.[50] It is important to note that HIT can also occur after the discontinuation of therapy and has been termed *delayed-onset HIT*. Registry data suggests that HIT occurs in 3–5% of patients treated with unfractionated heparin for 5 days.[47] It is important to note that the incidence of HIT is significant lower (<1%) during treatment with low-molecular weight heparin. Because of the risk of HIT is related to the duration of exposure, current guidelines stress that IV heparin should not be administered for more than 48 hours.[51] British guidelines suggest that patients treated with heparin should receive platelet counts every 2–4 days of therapy to monitor for thrombocytopenia.[52] After there is suspicion for HIT, heparin products must be discontinued immediately and alternative anticoagulation should be initiated to mitigate the risk of thrombosis. Bivalirudin is an alternative anticoagulant used to facilitate PCI in the setting of ACS when HIT is a concern.[53]

Guidelines

The current guidelines suggest that anticoagulant therapy should be used in ACS as soon as possible after presentation for all patients, irrespective of the initial treatment strategy. Unfractionated heparin is recommended as an option for anticoagulation (Class I, Level B), and should be continued for 48 hours or until PCI (Class I, Level B).[12]

Low-molecular Weight Heparin

Pharmacology

Low molecular-weight heparins are heterogeneous in size and approximately one-third the molecular weight of unfractionated heparin. Like unfractionated heparin, low-molecular-weight heparins bind to antithrombin and inhibit the action of factor Xa with a more mild direct inhibition of thrombin. The ability of low-molecular-weight heparin to inhibit thrombin depends upon the presence of 18 or more saccharide units allowing the molecule to bind both antithrombin and thrombin. The concentration of heparins with 18 or more saccharide units varies with each agent such that enoxaparin preferentially inhibits factor Xa (2:1) more than dalteparin (4:1). Like unfractionated heparin, the effects of low-molecular-weight heparin can be reversed with the administration of protamine sulfate. Furthermore, low-molecular-weight heparin can induce HIT, although at a much lower rate than unfractionated heparin, and should be avoided when this condition is suspected.

Dalteparin

Pharmacokinetics and Doses

Dalteparin is available in a single-dose prefilled syringe or as a multi-dose vial. Each prefilled syringe contains between 2,500 IU and 10,000 IU of anti-factor Xa in the form of 16–64 mg of dalteparin. Dalteparin is designed to be administered subcutaneously, rather than intramuscularly, to ensure adequate vascular absorption and reduce the risk of local hematoma. Subcutaneous dalteparin has a rapid onset of action (1–2 hours) with a half-life of 2–5 hours leading to approximately 12 hours of therapeutic effect. The standard dose administered for treatment of ACS is 120 IU/kg subcutaneously every 12 hours with concomitant aspirin therapy for 5–8 days.

Enoxaparin

Pharmacokinetics and Doses

Enoxaparin is available in prefilled single-dose syringes or as ampules in concentrations of 100 or 150 mg/mL. Enoxaparin is designed to be administered subcutaneously to ensure adequate vascular absorption and reduce the risk of a local hematoma. Subcutaneous enoxaparin has a moderate onset of action (3–5 hours) with a half-life of 4–7 hours leading to approximately 12 hours of therapeutic effect. The standard dose administered for treatment of ACS is an initial 30 mg IV injection followed by 1 mg/kg subcutaneously every 12 hours. For patients with impaired renal function [creatinine clearance (CrCl) <30 mL/min], the dose is reduced to 1 mg/kg subcutaneously daily. Enoxaparin should be administered for the duration of the hospitalization, or until PCI is performed. PCI can be performed with enoxaparin and no additional anticoagulation is necessary if the last dose was within 8 hours. If a percutaneous intervention occurs 8–12 hours after the last dose of subcutaneous enoxaparin, a single IV dose of 0.3 mg/kg should be administered.[12,54,55]

Clinical Use and Indications

A number of randomized trials have been conducted evaluating the efficacy of low-molecular-weight heparin in the immediate management of ACS. The largest trial (FRISC) randomized 1,506 patients with unstable angina or non-Q wave MI to receive dalteparin (120 IU/kg every 12 hours) or placebo for the first 6 days of therapy followed by a reduced dose (120 IU/kg daily) for another 35–40 days.[56] Dalteparin was associated with a 63% relative risk reduction in death or recurrent MI during the first 6 days making it comparable in efficacy to unfractionated heparin.

Several heterogeneous randomized trials have compared the efficacy of low-molecular-weight heparin to unfractionated heparin in ACS.[57-64] A meta-analysis of these studies including over 49,000 patients demonstrated an equivalent number of deaths or recurrent MIs between these two therapies.[65] The bleeding risk in this population, however, was slightly higher with low-molecular-weight heparin. This analysis held true for patients with STEMI that underwent fibrinolytic therapy as well.[66] Based on these findings, low-molecular-weight heparin may be used as an alternative to unfractionated heparin for the immediate management of ACS.

Guidelines

The current guidelines suggest that anticoagulant therapy should be used in ACS as soon as possible after presentation for all patients, irrespective of the initial treatment strategy.

Low-molecular-weight heparin (enoxaparin) is recommended as an option for anticoagulation, and should be continued for the duration of hospitalization or until PCI is performed (Class I, Level A). Performance of PCI with enoxaparin may be reasonable in patients treated with upstream enoxaparin for non-STEMI (Class IIb, Level B).[12]

Thrombin Inhibitors

Pharmacology

Direct thrombin inhibitors, such as hirudin and bivalirudin, directly inhibit soluble and clot-bound thrombin without depending upon antithrombin for their anticoagulant activity. Indirect thrombin inhibitors, such as fondaparinux, inhibit thrombin through the inhibition of factor Xa greatly reducing the generation of activated thrombin. Both types of medications are highly specific and potent for thrombin inhibition. At therapeutic concentrations, these medications will inhibit 70% of circulating thrombin in contrast to only 20–40% inhibition with unfractionated heparin.

Fondaparinux

Pharmacokinetics and Doses

Fondaparinux is a synthetic pentasaccharide that is an antithrombin-dependent inhibitor of factor Xa without inhibition of the thrombin molecule itself. The agent is currently licensed for the prevention of deep venous thrombosis as well as for treatment of ACS. Most of the trials evaluating this medication utilized a fixed dose (2.5 mg) administered subcutaneously.[67] When delivered in this fashion, the agent is rapidly absorbed with a peak effect within 2 hours and a moderate half-life (17–21 hours) before being excreted in the urine. The urine excretion makes this agent contraindicated in patients with renal impairment (eGFR <30 mL/hour). Although thrombocytopenia can occur, cases of HIT have not been reported with fondaparinux.

Clinical Use and Indications

Several randomized trials have evaluated the efficacy of fondaparinux in the immediate management of ACS. The Organization for the Assessment of Strategies for Ischemic Syndromes (OASIS)-5 trial enrolled 20,078 patients with a non-STEMI to treatment with fondaparinux (2.5 mg daily) or enoxaparin (1 mg/kg BID) for 6 days.[67] The primary composite of death, MI or refractory ischemia at 9 days was similar between the two groups (5.8% vs. 5.7%). The rate of major bleeding at 9 days, however, was markedly lower with fondaparinux than with enoxaparin (2.2% vs. 4.1%) and was associated with a reduction in all-cause mortality at 30 days. The OASIS-5 study was not sufficiently powered to assess the utility of fondaparinux in patients undergoing PCI. Because of this, both the European and US guidelines recommend the addition to unfractionated heparin to fondaparinux to reduce catheter thrombosis during percutaneous interventions.[12,36] This recommendation has been supported by a post-hoc analyses of the original OASIS-5 trial.[68]

Further studies have evaluated fondaparinux in STEMI. The OASIS-6 trial included 12,092 patients with STEMI and randomized them to receive anticoagulation with fondaparinux with or without unfractionated heparin for up to 8 days. Patients treated with fondaparinux that were managed with anticoagulation or fibrinolysis alone had a 23% relative risk reduction in 30-day mortality. Patients that were managed with primary PCI, however, had an increased risk of catheter thrombosis and coronary complications.[69] Based on these results, fondaparinux should not be used in primary PCI for patients with STEMI.[51,70]

Bivalirudin

Pharmacokinetics and Doses

Bivalirudin inhibits both soluble and clot-bound thrombin resulting in prevention of thrombin-mediated platelet activation and aggregation.[71] Because of this, bivalirudin can be used for the conservative management of ACS. In this setting, a bolus is administered (0.1 mg/kg IV) followed by a continuous infusion (0.25 mg/kg/hour). This bolus dose should be increased (0.3 mg/kg) with an increased infusion (1.75 mg/kg/hour) if PCI will be performed. Patients with severe renal dysfunction (estimated glomerular filtration rate <30 mL/min) will require a reduced infusion dose (1 mg/kg/hour). Bivalirudin has an immediate onset of action and a short half-life (25 min) such that coagulation parameters will return to normal within 1 hour of discontinuing the medication. There is no antidote available for bivalirudin.

Clinical Use and Indications

A number of randomized clinical trials have compared the efficacy of bivalirudin to heparin products in the immediate management of ACS. Notably, many of these studies were conducted prior to the incorporation of novel $P2Y_{12}$ antagonists (prasugrel and ticagrelor) and radial artery PCI into routine clinical practice. The largest trial (ACUITY) enrolled 13,819 patients with ACS and randomized them to receive bivalirudin or unfractionated heparin combined with a IIb/IIIa inhibitor prior to coronary angiography. The use of bivalirudin in this setting was associated with a non-inferior rate of the composite primary endpoint which included mortality, reinfarction or revascularization.[72] There was, however, a statistically significant lower risk of major bleeding in patients treated with bivalirudin (5.3% vs. 5.7%). These findings were reinforced in a subsequent study that included 3,602 patients with a STEMI randomized to receive bivalirudin or unfractionated heparin with a IIb/IIIa inhibitor. Once again, the use of bivalirudin resulted in a relative risk reduction of 40% for major bleeding. An analysis of the secondary outcomes also demonstrated a reduced 30-day total mortality (2.1% vs. 3.1%) with bivalirudin.[73] Similar results were reported in the setting of non-urgent PCI.[74] Economic analyses have suggested that the use of bivalirudin may be more cost-effective than unfractionated heparin.[75]

The effectiveness of bivalirudin has been called into question in contemporary practice characterized by the use of new $P2Y_{12}$ inhibitors, and radial artery PCI. The EUROMAX study randomized 2,218 STEMI patients undergoing primary PCI to either bivalirudin or heparin with provisional GP IIb/IIIa inhibitors.[76] Bivalirudin was found to reduce the risk of major bleeding (2.6% vs. 6.0%) at 30 days. The risk of acute stent thrombosis was higher with bivalirudin (1.1% vs. 0.2%), but there was no significant difference in rates of death (2.9% vs. 3.1%) or reinfarction (1.7% vs. 0.9%). The HEAT-PPCI trial, an open-label RCT enrolled 1,917 STEMI patients undergoing primary PCI and randomized them to heparin or bivalirudin and followed them up for 28 days.[77] The rate of all-cause mortality, cerebrovascular accident, reinfarction, or unplanned target lesion revascularization was 8.7% in the bivalirudin group and 5.7% in the heparin group. There was no significant difference in bleeding between the two groups. The study concluded that compared with bivalirudin, heparin reduces the incidence of major adverse ischemic events in the setting of PPCI, with no increase in bleeding complications. Two recent meta-analysis have concluded that compared with the use of heparin and GP IIb/IIIa receptor antagonist in primary PCI, bivalirudin increases the risk of MI and stent thrombosis, but decreases the risk of bleeding, with the magnitude of the reduction depending on concomitant Gp IIb/IIIa inhibitor use.[78,79] Based on these data, the use of bivalirudin should be based on individual patient characteristics including the risk for bleeding.

Guidelines

The current guidelines suggest that anticoagulant therapy should be used in ACS as soon as possible after presentation for all patients, irrespective of the initial treatment strategy. In non-STEMI patients treated with an initial noninvasive strategy, fondaparinux is recommended and should be continued for the duration of hospitalization or until PCI is performed (Class I, Level B). For patients on fondaparinux undergoing PCI, unfractionated heparin or bivalirudin should be administered prior to PCI to prevent catheter thrombosis (Class I, level B). Fondaparinux should not be used as the sole anticoagulant to support PCI (Class III, Level A). Bivalirudin is useful as an anticoagulant with or without prior treatment with unfractionated heparin in both STEMI and non-STEMI patients undergoing PCI (Class I, Level B), and is currently preferred to the combination of unfractionated heparin and a GP IIa/IIIb receptor antagonist for patients at high-risk of bleeding (Class IIa, Level B).[12,51]

ANTIPLATELET THERAPIES

Antiplatelet therapies are designed to inhibit platelet activation and aggregation thus restoring patency to an occluded epicardial artery. A variety of agents with unique molecular targets are often used in concert to reduce the function of circulating platelets. Randomized trials have suggested that aspirin, adenosine 5'-diphosphate (ADP) antagonists and Gp IIb/IIIa inhibitors all have a role in the contemporary management of ACS.

Aspirin

Pharmacology

Records demonstrate that acetylsalicylic acid was isolated from willow bark and used as a pain reliever by Hippocrates over 2 millennia ago. A large pharmaceutical manufacturer synthetically produced acetylsalicylic acid for medicinal purposes in 1897 under the trade-name "Aspirin". The CV benefits of aspirin were revealed six decades later when Nobel-prize winning research demonstrated that the compound reduced the production of thromboxane, a potent mediator of platelet activation and aggregation.[80] Aspirin acetylates serine 529 on cyclooxygenase-1 irreversibly inhibiting the enzyme. This results in decreased production of an important mediator of platelet aggregation, thromboxane A_2 (TxA_2). Inhibition of cyclooxygenase-1 in vascular endothelium also leads to decreased production of prostaglandin I_2 (prostacyclin) preventing vasodilation. Because platelets do not contain protein manufacturing machinery, the inhibition of platelet cyclooxygenase-1 persists for the life of the platelets (7–10 days). In contrast, the vascular endothelium is able to transcribe and translate new unhindered cyclooxygenase-1 within hours resulting in the renewed production of prostacyclins.[80] The net effect of aspirin is thus platelet inhibition with decreased risk of thrombosis.

Pharmacokinetics and Doses

Aspirin is available in an oral and rectal formulation. Aspirin is rapidly absorbed in its oral formulation with a peak effect 1–2 hours after ingestion. For more rapid inhibition of platelet function, sublingual formulations are available and recommended in the setting of ACS. The half-life of aspirin and its functioning metabolites is approximately 5 hours but the irreversible inhibition of platelet cyclooxygenase-1 makes its therapeutic effect persist for the lifetime of the platelet.

A number of medications may limit the efficacy of aspirin. Nonsteroidal anti-inflammatory agents that reversibly inhibit cyclooxygenase-1 (ibuprofen, naproxen) interfere with the cardioprotective effects of aspirin.[81] More recent work has suggested that all nonsteroidal anti-inflammatory medications increase the risk of CV events, even when administered for short durations.[82,83]

Clinical Use and Indications

A number of studies have demonstrated the benefits of aspirin therapy in ACS. The Veterans Administration Cooperative Study included 1,266 males with unstable angina and randomized them to receive aspirin (324 mg daily × 12 weeks) or placebo. Treatment with aspirin reduced the primary composite endpoint of death or recurrent MI by 50% (5% vs. 10%).[84] A subsequent study employing higher doses of aspirin (325 mg four times a day) in a Canadian population supported these findings.[85] A meta-analysis including over 212,000 high-risk patients demonstrated that aspirin reduced the risk of nonfatal MI or death by 26% making aspirin a mainstay of therapy for unstable angina.[86]

Aspirin has also had demonstrated efficacy in the treatment of proven MI. The International Study of Infarct Survival (ISIS-2) randomized 17,187 patients admitted to 417 hospitals to receive either a placebo or aspirin (160 mg daily) with the possible addition of streptokinase. The administration of aspirin resulted in a significant reduction in vascular mortality (9.4% vs. 12%) when compared to placebo after 5 weeks of follow-up.[87] Based on subsequent analyses, the administration of aspirin (162 mg daily) for 1 month prevented 25 deaths and 10 nonfatal MIs. The survival benefit from aspirin therapy persisted over 10 years of subsequent follow-up.[88] Largely based upon this data, aspirin became a standard treatment for the immediate management of ACS.

The appropriate dosing of aspirin has been a subject of intense debate. Previous research has demonstrated that *in vitro* platelet aggregation was similar after treatment with 81 mg or 325 mg of aspirin.[89,90] Recent studies have confirmed that the initial administration of low-dose aspirin (162 mg) was as effective as higher dose aspirin (325 mg) in ACS with less bleeding risk.[91] Lower aspirin doses *in vitro* (<162 mg) result in a prolongation (~2 days) to effective therapeutic inhibition of cyclooxygenase-1.[92] A recent meta-analysis confirmed that there is no CV benefit in secondary prevention for aspirin maintenance doses greater than 81 mg each day.[93] Furthermore, a large clinical trial demonstrated that a lower aspirin dose (75–100 mg) was equivalent to a higher dose (300–325 mg) after PCI for ACS.[94] Based on these findings, most guidelines recommend an aspirin load of 162–325 mg with an indefinite maintenance dose of 75–81 mg in the treatment of ACS.[12,95]

Resistance

Aspirin resistance is a broad term that comprises biochemical resistance to the medication as well as aspirin underuse. Cellular studies suggest that some patients may have overexpression of cyclooxygenase-2 serving as a "sink" for aspirin within platelets.[96] Other work has elucidated genetic polymorphisms of other platelet proteins that may enhance their thrombogenicity despite the administration of aspirin.[97] Rather than biochemical resistance, however, a large proportion of aspirin resistance is related to aspirin underuse.[98] Epidemiological surveys suggest that as few as 60% of patients admitted to the hospital with a MI receive aspirin.[99,100] This problem is not unique to the United States as international registries report that as many as 14% of patients with coronary artery disease are not receiving any form of antiplatelet therapy.[101]

Complications

Aspirin also weakly inhibits cyclooxygenase-2, an enzyme that produces prostacyclins that protect the gastric lining from acidic irritation. Administration of aspirin may then produce gastric irritation or an increased risk of gastrointestinal (GI) hemorrhage.[102] It is important to note that the risk of GI bleeding induced by aspirin is proportional to the dose administered. Previous work has suggested that the rate of bleeding doubles when the maintenance dose is increased from 100 mg/day to 200 mg/day.[103] The risks of GI bleeding can be mitigated with the addition of a proton pump inhibitor (PPI).[104] In addition to GI bleeding, aspirin has also been associated with a small increased risk of hemorrhagic stroke.[105] This has led some individuals to suggest that a history of GI ulcers or bleeding is a relative contraindication to aspirin therapy. It is important to note that these risks are significantly lower than the reported CV benefits of aspirin described above.

Guidelines

The current guidelines suggest that non-enteric coated, chewable aspirin (162–325 mg) should be used in all ACS patients without contraindications as soon as possible after presentation (Class I, Level A). Aspirin should then be continued at a dose of 81–162 mg daily indefinitely in all patients that are not intolerant to the medication (Class I, Level A). For patients who undergo PCI, aspirin should be continued indefinitely at a dose of 81–325 mg daily (Class I, Level B), but it is considered reasonable to use the 81 mg daily dose in preference to higher maintenance doses (Class IIa, Level B).[12]

Adenosine Diphosphate Receptor Antagonists

Pharmacology

Platelet activation results in the release of ADP, a potent mediator of platelet aggregation. Circulating ADP mediates its effects primarily through the $P2Y_{12}$ receptor on the platelet surface. Activation of these receptors leads to morphologic changes in the platelet shape as well as increases in the expression in Gp IIb/IIIa that mediates platelet cross-linking within a thrombus.[106,107] Inhibition of this receptor thus hinders platelet aggregation even in the presence of TxA_2 and thrombin.[108] Thienopyridines and triazolopyrimidines are antagonists of the $P2Y_{12}$ receptor and commonly employed in the immediate management of ACS. The $P2Y_{12}$ inhibitors are described in detail below and are summarized in the accompanying Table 3.[36]

Ticlopidine

Pharmacokinetics and Doses

The oral formulation of ticlopidine has a moderate onset of action with peak platelet serum level occurring 3–5 hours after ingestion. It is important to note that the kinetics of ticlopidine are nonlinear with a markedly decreased clearance upon repeated dosing. Because of this, ticlopidine does not achieve maximum inhibition of platelet aggregation until it has been administered for 4–7 days.[109] After reaching steady state, ticlopidine undergoes extensive hepatic metabolism with a half-life of 13 hours with predominant renal excretion. The standard dosage of ticlopidine is 250 mg by mouth twice daily.

Clinical Use and Indications

One randomized multicenter trial compared ticlopidine to "conventional therapy" among patients presenting with ACS. Among the 652 patient enrolled in this trial (40% with MI), the

TABLE 3: Characteristics of P2Y$_{12}$ antagonists[2,36]

	Ticlopidine	Clopidogrel	Prasugrel	Ticagrelor	Cangrelor
Class	Thienopyridine	Thienopyridine	Thienopyridine	Triazolopyrimidine	Triazolopyrimidine
Reversibility	Irreversible	Irreversible	Irreversible	Reversible	Reversible
Activation	Prodrug, limited by metabolism	Prodrug, limited by metabolism	Prodrug, not limited by metabolism	Active drug	Active drug
Onset of effect*	3–5 hours	2–4 hours	30 minutes	30 minutes	Immediate
Duration of effect	3–5 days	3–10 days	5–10 days	3–4 days	60 minutes
Withdrawal before major surgery	NA	5 days	7 days	5 days	NA

*50% inhibition of platelet aggregation.

administration of ticlopidine reduced the risk of vascular death and nonfatal MI by over 50% (5.1% vs. 10.9%).[110] Further studies demonstrated that dual antiplatelet therapy (DAPT) with aspirin and ticlopidine produced superior outcomes during planned and unplanned PCI.[109,111] A meta-analysis of over 14,000 patients enrolled in trials or registries, however, suggests that clopidogrel results in a 50% relative risk reduction in major CV events when compared with ticlopidine.[112] Furthermore, this collection of registries identified numerous unfavorable side effects of ticlopidine. Because of this, ticlopidine has now been superseded by other thienopyridines for the immediate management of ACS.

Complications

Ticlopidine has been associated with an increased rate of neutropenia (2.4%) and thrombocytopenia purpura (0.03%).[113] The Clopidogrel Aspirin Stent International Cooperative Study (CLASSICS) demonstrated that clopidogrel was associated with a significantly lower risk of hematologic complications when compared with ticlopidine making it the standard thienopyridine used.[114]

Clopidogrel

Pharmacokinetics and Doses

Clopidogrel is an inactive prodrug that requires in vivo oxidation by hepatic CYP3A4 and 2C19 isoenzymes before becoming an irreversible inhibitor of $P2Y_{12}$. A single loading dose of clopidogrel produces detectable inhibition of platelet aggregation within 2–24 hours of its administration.[115] Studies with patients undergoing PCI, however, have demonstrated that higher loading doses (600 mg orally) achieve maximal platelet inhibition within 2 hours.[116] Clinical studies have confirmed that the higher loading dose results in improved outcomes among patients undergoing PCI.[117] The kinetics of clopidogrel are nonlinear with a markedly decreased clearance upon repeated dosing. The half-life of clopidogrel in the steady state is approximately 5 hours but the inhibition of the $P2Y_{12}$ receptor continues for the life of the platelet. Because of this, guidelines recommend cessation of clopidogrel 5 days prior to surgery to reduce the risk of perioperative bleeding.[36,118]

Clinical Use and Indications

The initial studies of clopidogrel were performed in patients with a history of vascular disease. The Clopidogrel versus Aspirin in Patients at Risk of Ischemic Events (CAPRIE) enrolled 19,185 high-risk patients and randomized them to receive clopidogrel (75 mg daily) or aspirin (325 mg daily). After a mean follow-up approaching 2 years, the administration of clopidogrel was associated with a 8.7% relative risk reduction in a composite endpoint that included vascular death, MI or ischemic stroke.[119]

Clopidogrel also has demonstrated efficacy in the immediate noninvasive management of ACS. Clopidogrel in Unstable angina to prevent Recurrent Events (CURE) randomized 12,562 patients with ACS to receive clopidogrel (300 mg once and 75 mg daily thereafter) or placebo. The average duration of clopidogrel exposure in this study was 9 months (range 3–12 months). Treatment with clopidogrel resulted in a 20% relative risk reduction and a 2.1% absolute risk reduction in the primary composite endpoint of CV death, MI or stroke after 12 months of follow-up.[120] It is important to note that this benefit was accompanied by an increased risk of major (3.7% vs. 2.7%) and minor (5.1% vs. 2.4%) bleeding. The efficacy of clopidogrel in the invasive management of ACS was evaluated in a substudy of CURE, termed PCI-CURE. Patients that received pretreatment and maintenance therapy with clopidogrel had a 44% relative risk reduction and 2.6% absolute risk reduction in CV death, MI or urgent target vessel revascularization within 30 days of their index event.[121] Subsequent results from the Clopidogrel for the Reduction of Events During Observation (CREDO) trial supported these results suggesting the importance of clopidogrel pretreatment for all patients undergoing PCI.[122]

Clopidogrel has also been investigated in the setting of STEMI. The Clopidogrel and Metoprolol in Myocardial Infarction/Second Chinese Cardiac Study (COMMIT/CCS-2) randomized 45,852 patients with an acute MI to clopidogrel (75 mg daily) or placebo in addition to aspirin (162 mg daily). The majority of these patients were managed conservatively without PCI and with only 50% receiving thrombolytics. The administration of clopidogrel for 4 weeks resulted in a 9% relative risk reduction and a 1% absolute risk reduction in the primary composite endpoint that included death, MI or stroke.[123] These findings were reinforced in the setting of thrombolysis during the Clopidogrel as Adjunctive Reperfusion Therapy Thrombolysis in Myocardial Infarction 28 (CLARITY-TIMI 28) trial. This study randomized 3,491 patients with STEMI to receive clopidogrel or placebo in addition to aspirin and thrombolysis. The addition of clopidogrel within the first 24 hours of presentation reduced the rate of death, recurrent infarction or infarct-related artery occlusion by 36% with an absolute risk reduction of 6.7%.[124] Once again, a substudy of CLARITY including 1,863 patients undergoing PCI reinforced the benefit of early clopidogrel administration.[124] Collectively, this data suggests that clopidogrel plays an integral role in the immediate management of ACS.

Surgery

Despite the demonstrated benefit of clopidogrel in ACS, some patients do not receive this medication because of the concern for increased bleeding should surgical revascularization be necessary.[122] A substudy of the CURE trial revealed that there was a trend toward benefit when clopidogrel was administered prior to surgical revascularization. This was associated, however, with a nonsignificant increased risk of bleeding primarily among patients undergoing bypass surgery within 5 days of clopidogrel administration.[125] Registry studies confirmed these findings suggesting that patients with ACS that underwent bypass surgery within 5 days of clopidogrel administration had an increased need for large blood transfusions [>4 U packed red blood cells (PRBC)] when compared to patients that waited more than 5 days.[126] Despite the increased rate of bleeding, registries have also demonstrated that the administration of clopidogrel before urgent bypass surgery resulted in a 27% relative risk reduction and a 4.6% absolute risk reduction in the rate of ischemic events (death, MI or unplanned revascularization) within 30 days of the index admission.[127] Current guidelines continue to recommend 5 days of clopidogrel abstinence prior to proceeding with elective surgery.[118] These data reveals, however, that patients benefit from clopidogrel administration even if they eventually proceed to surgical revascularization. Despite this, recent registries have demonstrated that only a fraction of patients (27%) are discharged from the hospital with clopidogrel after bypass surgery.[128] This runs counter to the current guidelines that suggest all patients presenting with ACS, including those undergoing bypass surgery, benefit from one full year of clopidogrel therapy.

Duration

The duration of clopidogrel therapy after PCI for ACS has been a controversial topic. Early registry data suggested that patients receiving drug eluting stents (DESs) had increased rates of very late stent thrombosis.[129,130] Although the overall incidence of these events was low, the results were usually catastrophic.[131,132] Numerous registries have demonstrated that premature cessation of clopidogrel therapy is a strong predictor of late stent thrombosis within the first 12 months.[133-135] In contrast, retrospective data has suggested that continuation of DAPT for greater than 1 year does not reduce mortality.[136] Several recent randomized trials have evaluated the use of $P2Y_{12}$ inhibitors (clopidogrel, prasugrel or ticagrelor) for short-term (6 months) or long-term (24–30 months) duration in the setting of new generation DESs. The ITALIC (Is There A LIfe for DES after discontinuation of Clopidogrel) trial is a prospective open-label randomized trial conducted at 70 sites in Europe and the Middle East that randomized 2,031 patients to receive 6 or

24 months of P2Y$_{12}$ inhibitor (mainly clopidogrel) plus aspirin after the placement of a new generation stent. The study was stopped prematurely due to problems with recruitment, but demonstrated that rates of bleeding and of thrombotic events were not significantly different according to 6-month versus 24-month DAPT after PCI with new generation DES in good aspirin responders.[137]

A second trial, DAPT study was an international, multicenter, randomized, placebo-controlled trial that was designed to determine the benefits and risks of continuing DAPT beyond 1 year after the placement of a coronary stent. After 12 months of treatment with a thienopyridine drug (clopidogrel or prasugrel) and aspirin, 9,961 patients were randomly assigned to continue receiving thienopyridine treatment or to receive placebo for another 18 months; all patients continued receiving aspirin. Continued treatment with thienopyridine, as compared with placebo, reduced the rates of stent thrombosis (0.4% vs. 1.4%) and major adverse CV and cerebrovascular events (4.3% vs. 5.9%). The rate of MI was lower with thienopyridine treatment than with placebo (2.1% vs. 4.1%). The rate of death from any cause was 2.0% in the group that continued thienopyridine therapy and 1.5% in the placebo group. However, the rate of moderate or severe bleeding was increased with continued thienopyridine treatment (2.5% vs. 1.6%). Overall, the trial demonstrated that longer term DAPT reduces stent thrombosis at the cost of increased bleeding.[138] Given these conflicting results, the optimal duration of DAPT remains controversial. Current guidelines recommend at least 4 weeks of clopidogrel therapy for bare metal stents and 1 year of therapy for DESs.[54]

Dosing

The initial trials investigating clopidogrel for the treatment of ACS employed a standard loading dose (300 mg) and maintenance dose (75 mg). Further research demonstrated that an elevated loading dose (600 mg) resulted in a more rapid inhibition of platelet function.[115] Furthermore, clinical studies have confirmed that the higher loading dose results in improved outcomes among patients undergoing PCI.[117,139] Additional studies have not demonstrated additional benefit from even higher loading doses of clopidogrel (900 mg) in the setting of ACS.[140,141] Current guidelines for PCI now reflect this data and recommend the higher loading dose (600 mg).[54] Clinical trials have also explored alternative maintenance doses for clopidogrel therapy. The CURRENT-OASIS 7 trial randomized 25,086 patients to receive double-dose clopidogrel (600 mg followed by 150 mg × 6 days) or standard dose clopidogrel (300 mg followed by 75 mg daily). The rate of CV death, MI or stroke was equivalent between the two treatment groups.[94] A subgroup of these 17,263 patients that received early invasive therapy with PCI, however, did demonstrate a relative risk reduction of 14% and an absolute risk reduction of 0.6% in these outcomes.[121] This was associated with a 0.5% increased risk of major bleeding. The use of the increased clopidogrel maintenance dose for 7 days in patients without increased bleeding risk now carries a Class IIa (Level B) recommendation in the European guidelines.[36]

Resistance

Like aspirin resistance, patients that have had a recurrent event on clopidogrel have been denoted as suffering from clopidogrel resistance. As mentioned previously, clopidogrel is a prodrug that requires activation from the CYP system. Research has demonstrated that patients with reduced function alleles of CYP isoform C19 that are treated with clopidogrel have significantly higher risk of in-stent thrombosis.[142] Functional assays have noted that reduced platelet inhibition by clopidogrel is also associated with worse outcomes.[143,144] Attempts to modulate clopidogrel dosing to functional assays as in the Gauging Responsiveness with a VerifyNow Assay-Impact on Thrombosis and Safety (GRAVITAS) trial, however, has not yet proved fruitful.[145]

The administration of other medications may also interfere with the CYP system and thus prevent the formation of active clopidogrel metabolites. Initial studies suggested that patients treated with omeprazole and clopidogrel had significantly reduced platelet inhibition.[146] A retrospective analysis of 8,205 veterans treated with clopidogrel and omeprazole had a 25% greater risk of death or recurrent ACS than those treated with clopidogrel alone.[147] The Food and Drug Administration (FDA) subsequently released a black-box warning regarding the interaction between clopidogrel and omeprazole. A recent randomized trial designed to assess the safety of a combined omeprazole-clopidogrel formulation, however, refuted these findings. The Clopidogrel and the Optimization of Gastrointestinal Events (COGENT) trial enrolled and analyzed 3,761 patients randomized to receive clopidogrel with or without omeprazole in a single pill before being prematurely discontinued due to lack of funding. After 180 days of follow-up, the two groups had similar rates of CV events (4.9% vs. 5.7%) suggesting that omeprazole administration did not reduce the efficacy of clopidogrel in most patients.[148] The latest European guidelines recommend using a PPI (preferably not omeprazole) for patients on DAPT with risk factors for GI bleeding (including a history of GI hemorrhage, peptic ulcer or multiple, *Helicobacter pylori* infection, older age or concurrent use of steroids or anticoagulants) (Class I, Level A).[36] The American guidelines are more conservative and recommend the use of a PPI only in the setting of triple antithrombotic therapy with a vitamin K antagonist, aspirin and a $P2Y_{12}$ inhibitor (Class I, Level C for patients with a history of GI bleeding; Class IIa, Level C for patients without a known history of GI bleeding).[12]

Prasugrel

Pharmacokinetics and Doses

Prasugrel is an inactive prodrug that requires in vivo oxidation by hepatic CYP before becoming an irreversible inhibitor of $P2Y_{12}$. Unlike clopidogrel, however, prasugrel is converted to its active metabolite rapidly resulting in maximal serum concentrations within 30 minutes of administration.[149,150] Studies have also demonstrated that there is significantly less inter-patient variability in platelet inhibition when compared to standard doses of clopidogrel.[151] The half-life of the active prasugrel metabolites is approximately 7 hours but the clinical effect persists for the lifetime of the treated platelets. The standard dose of prasugrel was established in the Joint Utilization of Medications to Block Platelets Optimally-Thrombolysis In Myocardial Infarction 26 (JUMBO-TIMI 26) trial with a loading dose of 60 mg followed by a maintenance dose of 10 mg daily.[152] Clinical studies have confirmed that this dosing strategy results in earlier and more potent platelet inhibition than standard loading doses of clopidogrel.[153]

Clinical Use and Indications

A large multicenter randomized trial demonstrated the clinical efficacy of prasugrel in the treatment of ACS. The Trial to Assess Improvement in Therapeutic Outcomes by Optimizing Platelet Inhibition with Prasugrel (TRITON-TIMI 38) randomized 13,608 patients with ACS (26% STEMI) to receive prasugrel or clopidogrel for 6–15 months.[154] The primary endpoint of CV death, recurrent MI or stroke was reduced from 12.1% to 9.9% in the patients that received prasugrel. The difference in primary endpoint was primarily driven by recurrent MI. A post-hoc analysis demonstrated that prasugrel was also independently associated with a lower risk of in-stent thrombosis (2.4% vs. 1.1%).[155] It is important to note that the CV benefits of prasugrel were accompanied by an increased risk of major bleeding (2.4% vs. 1.8%).[154] Because of the concern for increased intracranial bleeding, prasugrel is not recommended for patients with a history of cerebrovascular disease or pathological bleeding. Patients over the age of 75 years or under 60 kg also have an increased bleeding risk and thus should not be given prasugrel.

A subgroup analysis of patients presenting with STEMI also demonstrated benefit. Of these 3,534 patients, the vast majority (>90%) were treated with PCI and followed for up to 15 months. Patients treated with prasugrel had a 2.4% absolute risk reduction in CV death, recurrent MI or stroke when compared to standard doses of clopidogrel.[156] It is important to note that this study did not demonstrate overall differences in major bleeding among the two groups. The subgroup of patients who underwent bypass surgery, however, did have a significant increase in major bleeding (18.8% vs. 2.7%). Collectively, this data suggests a decrease in CV events with an increased risk of major bleeding for prasugrel.

Ticagrelor

Pharmacokinetics and Doses

Ticagrelor is a potent oral reversible inhibitor of the $P2Y_{12}$ receptors. Unlike the thienopyridines, ticagrelor is a modification of adenosine triphosphate to cyclopentyl-triazolo-pyrimidine that does not require metabolic conversion prior to inhibiting its target. Ticagrelor is rapidly absorbed reaching its peak plasma levels within 2 hours of ingestion and providing approximately 12 hours of platelet inhibition. Dose finding studies demonstrated that ticagrelor is effective when administered as 90 mg or 180 mg twice a day.[157] These doses provide more rapid maximal platelet inhibition than standard doses of clopidogrel.[158] It is important to note that post-hoc analyses have demonstrated a rebound in platelet aggregation in those patients that only take the medication once a day.[149]

Clinical Use and Indications

A large multicenter trial has demonstrated the promise of ticagrelor in the treatment of ACS. The PLATelet inhibition and patient Outcomes (PLATO) trial randomized 18,624 patients with ACS (38% STEMI) to receive ticagrelor (180 mg loading dose and 90 mg BID maintenance) or clopidogrel (300–600 mg loading dose and 75 mg daily maintenance). After 12 months of follow-up, the primary composite endpoint including vascular death, recurrent MI or stroke was reduced among the ticagrelor group (9.8% vs. 11.7%) with similar rates of major bleeding (11.6% vs. 11.2%).[159] Patients treated with ticagrelor did have, however, a slightly higher rate of fatal intracranial bleeding as well as a higher rate of dyspnea and bradycardia than those treated with clopidogrel. A regional analysis has suggested that the benefit of ticagrelor was not present in patients recruited from North America.[160] Some have suggested that the benefit was reduced in this population because of the concomitant use of higher aspirin doses (>100 mg/day). Based on this, regulatory agencies have recommended that low dose aspirin (81 mg/day) be used in conjunction with ticagrelor.[12] The ongoing PEGASUS-TIMI 54 trial (Prevention of Cardiovascular Events in Patients with Prior Heart Attack Using Ticagrelor Compared to Placebo on a Background of Aspirin) is investigating whether the addition of intensive antiplatelet therapy with ticagrelor to low-dose aspirin reduces major adverse CV events in high-risk patients with a history of MI.[161]

Cangrelor

Pharmacokinetics

Cangrelor is a potent IV reversible inhibitor of the $P2Y_{12}$ receptors created from a chemical modification to ticagrelor. Like ticagrelor, cangrelor does not require conversion to an active metabolite and serves to immediately inhibit platelet aggregation upon its administration. After its discontinuation, normal platelet function returns within 60 minutes and is not dependent upon renal or liver function.[162]

Clinical Use and Indications

Cangrelor has been studied in several large multicenter trials. The Cangrelor Versus Standard Therapy to Achieve Optimal Management of Platelet Inhibition (CHAMPION) study randomized 5,362 patients with ACS to cangrelor with clopidogrel (600 mg) at the time of PCI or clopidogrel (600 mg) alone. The trial failed to demonstrate superiority of cangrelor over clopidogrel as the primary endpoint of death, recurrent MI or revascularization at 48 hours was similar between the two groups (7% vs. 8%).[162] These results were confirmed in a similar study that included patients with STEMI.[163]

The most recent randomized study to evaluate cangrelor is the (CHAMPION) PHOENIX (Cangrelor versus Standard Therapy to Achieve Optimal Management of Platelet Inhibition) trial. In this double-blind, placebo-controlled trial 11,145 patients who were undergoing either urgent or elective PCI and were receiving guideline recommended therapy were randomly assigned to receive a bolus and infusion of cangrelor or to receive a loading dose of 600 mg or 300 mg of clopidogrel.[164] The primary efficacy end point (a composite of death, MI, ischemia-driven revascularization, or stent thrombosis at 48 hours) was met (4.7% in the cangrelor group and 5.9% in the clopidogrel group) and stent thrombosis developed in 0.8% of the patients in the cangrelor group versus 1.4% in the clopidogrel group with no increases in severe bleeding. In 2014, however, citing flawed methodology,[165] the FDA did not recommend approval of cangrelor for use in any indication in the United States.

Guidelines

The current guidelines suggest that clopidogrel should be used in ACS for all patients who are unable to tolerate aspirin (Class I, Level B). A loading dose of a $P2Y_{12}$ inhibitor (either clopidogrel or ticagrelor) and a maintenance dose for up to 12 months should be administered in addition to aspirin to all patients with ACS without contraindications who are managed in a noninvasive fashion (Class I, Level B). For ACS patients who are treated invasively with coronary stents, a loading dose of clopidogrel, prasugrel, or ticagrelor should be given before PCI and a maintenance dose should be continued for at least 12 months (Class I, Level B). Prasugrel is not currently recommended for ACS patients who are treated noninvasively (without PCI). In patients that have had a prior stroke or transient ischemic attack (TIA), prasugrel is not recommended as a part of DAPT (Class III, Level B). Patients over the age of 75 years or under 60 kg weight should also avoid this medication.[12]

It is considered reasonable to choose ticagrelor in preference to clopidogrel for $P2Y_{12}$ treatment in all patients with ACS (Class IIa, Level B). If ticagrelor is used, the aspirin dose should not exceed 81 mg daily. It is also considered reasonable to choose prasugrel over clopidogrel in patients with ACS who undergo PCI and are not at high-risk for bleeding (Class IIa, Level B).[12]

The duration of therapy with a $P2Y_{12}$ antagonist should be at least 12 months for patients receiving PCI in the setting of ACS (Class I, Level B). Early discontinuation of DAPT can be considered if the risks of bleeding outweigh the benefits (Class IIa, Level C). Continuation of DAPT beyond 12 months may be considered in patients who undergo PCI (Class IIb, Level C). Current guidelines recommend the discontinuation of clopidogrel and ticagrelor 5 days prior, and prasugrel 7 days prior to planned surgical revascularization (Class I, Level C).[12]

If triple antithrombotic therapy with a vitamin K antagonist, aspirin, and a $P2Y_{12}$ inhibitor is required, the duration should be minimized to the extent possible to limit the risk of bleeding (Class I, Level C), a lower international normalized ratio (INR) target of 2.0–2.5 may be reasonable (Class IIb, Level C), and a PPI should be prescribed in patients with a history of GI bleeding (Class I, Level C). Use of PPIs in patients requiring triple antithrombotic therapy without a known history of GI bleeding is considered reasonable (Class IIa, Level C).[12]

Clopidogrel remains the $P2Y_{12}$ antagonist of choice for patients with ACS treated with fibrinolytic therapy (Class I, Level A).[51,166]

IIb/IIIa Antagonists

Pharmacology

Glycoprotein IIb/IIIa is a platelet adhesion receptor that facilitates the final steps of platelet activation and aggregation. After platelet activation, Gp IIb/IIIa receptors crosslink fibrinogen to form a platelet-rich thrombus.[167] Inhibition of this receptor thus hinders platelet aggregation in a unique fashion that is independent of the mechanisms of aspirin and ADP antagonists. Initial studies demonstrated that oral Gp IIb/IIIa antagonists were unsuccessful.[168] Because of this, there are currently only three IV Gp IIb/IIIa antagonists available for clinical use: abciximab, eptifibatide and tirofiban. It is important to note that the majority of the Gp IIb/IIIa antagonists were developed and tested prior to the widespread use of $P2Y_{12}$ receptor antagonists.[169,170] Because of this, previous trials may have overestimated the benefit of these agents in the contemporary management of ACS.[171]

Abciximab

Pharmacokinetics and Doses

Abciximab is a chimeric monoclonal antibody directed against the Gp IIb/IIIa receptor. This agent is administered intravenously with a loading dose (0.25 mg/kg) followed by a maintenance infusion (0.125 µg/kg-hour) for up to 12 hours. Abciximab has a half-life of approximately 10–30 minutes but remains platelet bound in the circulation for up to 15 days after administration. The monoclonal antibody can generate immunological side effects including severe thrombocytopenia in approximately 1% of patients. This thrombocytopenia may be effectively treated with platelet transfusions.[172,173]

Clinical Use and Indications

Abciximab was initially evaluated in the conservative management of ACS. The Global Utilization of Streptokinase and Tissue Plasminogen Activator for Occluded Coronary Arteries-IV (GUSTO IV) randomized 7,800 patients with ACS to receive abciximab bolus and maintenance infusions (24 hours or 48 hours) or placebo. Patients that eventually underwent percutaneous or surgical revascularization were excluded. There was no significant difference in the primary composite endpoint of death or recurrent MI within 30 days between the two groups. There were, however, higher rates of thrombocytopenia and bleeding in the patients treated with abciximab.[174] In contrast, abciximab has been demonstrated to have benefit in patients undergoing PCI. The C7e3 Fab Anti-Platelet Therapy in Unstable Refractory Angina (CAPTURE) trial enrolled 1,265 patients with ACS refractory to treatment with anticoagulation and nitrates. Patients were randomized to receive abciximab or placebo 2 hours prior to a planned PCI. The patients treated with abciximab had a significantly lower rate of death, MI or urgent intervention compared to placebo (11.3% vs. 15.9%).[175] A subgroup analysis of this study demonstrated that patients that had positive cardiac biomarkers derived the greatest benefit from abciximab. Further studies have corroborated these findings.[176]

Abciximab has also been investigated in patients presenting with STEMI. The Abciximab before direct angioplasty and stenting in Myocardial Infarction Regarding Acute and Long term follow-up (ADMIRAL) trial randomized 300 patients with STEMI treated with aspirin, heparin and a thienopyridine to receive either abciximab or placebo prior to PCI. The administration of abciximab reduced the composite primary endpoint of death, recurrent MI or urgent target vessel revascularization by over 50% (7.4 vs. 15.9%).[177] Further investigations of patients with STEMI undergoing PCI in the Controlled Abciximab Device Investigation to Lower Late Angioplasty Complications (CADILLAC) trial support these findings.[178] The role of abciximab in STEMI treated with fibrinolytics is not as clear. The GUSTO-V and Assessment of the Safety and Efficacy of a New Thrombolytic trials compared abciximab with half-dose thrombolytics to thrombolytics alone in patients presenting with STEMIs. Both of these trials demonstrated a reduction in the secondary endpoint of MI without differences in mortality.[179,180] There was, however, an increased risk of bleeding particularly in patients over the age of 75 years. Based on this data, abciximab use is currently limited to patients with ACS that will undergo PCI.

Eptifibatide

Pharmacokinetics and Doses

Eptifibatide is a synthetic cyclic heptapeptide considered to be a small molecule inhibitor of the Gp IIb/IIIa receptor. Like other small molecules in this class, eptifibatide has lower binding affinity for the receptor than abciximab but is significantly more specific. Because of this, eptifibatide does not produce the same degree of immunological side effects with a lower rate of thrombocytopenia.[181] Platelet transfusions are not helpful to reverse the effects of eptifibatide as the circulating small molecule is equally likely to bind to new platelets. Eptifibatide is administered as a bolus (180 µg/kg) and a maintenance infusion (2 µg/kg/min) that should be adjusted for renal function. The agent has a clearance half-life of 2.5 hours and effectively inhibits platelet aggregation for 4 hours after discontinuation.

Clinical Use and Indications

The initial studies of eptifibatide demonstrated a benefit to patients presenting with ACS. The Platelet Glycoprotein IIb/IIIa in Unstable Angina: Receptor Suppression Using Integrilin Therapy (PURSUIT) randomized 10,948 patients to eptifibatide (180 µg/kg followed by 1.3 µg/kg/min or 2.0 µg/kg/min) or placebo. Approximately 60% of the patients enrolled eventually underwent PCI. The administration of eptifibatide resulted in a 2.2% absolute risk reduction in death or recurrent MI after

30 days of follow-up.[182] A double-bolus of eptifibatide (180 µg/kg twice separated by 10 minutes) has been demonstrated to be equally effective in reducing mortality and recurrent MI at 1 year (8% vs. 12.4%) for patients undergoing PCI.[183] A large Swedish registry (Swedish Coronary Angiography and Angioplasty Registry) reviewed 11,479 STEMI patients who underwent primary PCI with either eptifibatide or abciximab and found eptifibatide to be non-inferior in the primary endpoint of death or MI at 1 year of follow-up.[184] Because of this, double-bolus eptifibatide has become the standard dosing regimen for many interventions and can be used during primary PCI for STEMI.

Recent studies have evaluated the use of eptifibatide prior to PCI, termed upstream. The EARLY Glycoprotein IIb/IIIa inhibition in non-ST-segment elevation Acute Coronary Syndrome (EARLY-ACS) trial randomized 9,492 patients with ACS and positive cardiac biomarkers (84%) or ischemic electrocardiographic changes to a double-bolus of eptifibatide upon presentation or a delayed administration after angiography if PCI was going to be pursued. The early administration of eptifibatide did not reduce death, recurrent MI or thrombotic complications during intervention. It did, however, significantly increase the risk of major bleeding.[171] Further trials to evaluate upstream administration of eptifibatide with thrombolysis or PCI for STEMI have not been powered to address clinical endpoints.[185-188] A meta-analysis of 12 clinical trials including eptifibatide and tirofiban did find that treatment with upstream small-molecule GP IIb/IIIa inhibitors for patients with non-STEMI provides a significant but modest ischemic benefit when compared with initial placebo and a trend toward fewer ischemic events when compared with delayed, selective use at PCI. However, these modest benefits were again associated with an increased risk of bleeding.[189]

It is important to note that the addition of eptifibatide to a regimen that includes bivalirudin leads to increased bleeding risk without a mortality benefit and thus is not currently recommended.[73] Eptifibatide is thus now primarily employed in patients with ACS refractory to other medical management or prior to PCI.

Tirofiban

Pharmacokinetics and Doses

Tirofiban is a highly specific nonpeptide derivative of tyrosine that selectively inhibits the Gp IIb/IIIa receptor. As a small molecule, tirofiban has a higher specificity for the receptor with a lower affinity than abciximab. Unlike other agents in this class, tirofiban can be stored at room temperature without significant degradation. Tirofiban is administered in a "high bolus" loading dose (25 µg/kg IV infused over 3 minutes) and maintenance dose (0.15 μg/kg/min) up to 18 hours with adjustments for impaired renal function. The half-life of the medication is approximately 2 hours but platelet inhibition will continue for up to 4 hours after discontinuation.[172,173]

Clinical Use and Indications

Early studies demonstrated the benefit of tirofiban compared to heparin alone, or in addition to heparin for the management of ACS patients. The Platelet Receptor Inhibition in Ischemic Syndrome Management (PRISM) trial suggested that tirofiban was superior to heparin for the conservative management of patients with unstable angina.[190] The PRISM-PLUS study randomized 1,915 patients with non-STEMI to tirofiban alone, heparin alone or tirofiban with heparin. Coronary angiography was performed in the vast majority of these patients (90%) but PCI was performed in a minority (30.5%). The tirofiban alone arm was associated with an increased risk of death leading to its early termination. When combined with heparin, however, tirofiban significantly reduced the rate of death, recurrent MI or refractory ischemia over 7 days when compared to heparin alone (12.9% vs. 17.9%). This benefit was similar for patients treated non-invasively or invasively.[191] Studies comparing tirofiban with other Gp IIb/IIIa inhibitors have had conflicting results. The Do Tirofiban and ReoPro Give Similar Efficacy Trial (TARGET) randomized 4,809 patients undergoing percutaneous intervention to either tirofiban or abciximab before the procedure. Patients receiving tirofiban had higher rates of death MI or urgent target revascularization at 30 days compared to abciximab (7.6% vs. 6%).[192] Subsequent trials and meta-analyses comparing tirofiban to abciximab and eptifibatide and found to have similar efficacy among the three agents.[193-195] Notably, the initial studies with tirofiban used a lower loading dose; when the "high bolus dose" (25 μg/kg IV over 3 minutes) was tested, tirofiban performed similarly to other Gp IIb/IIIa inhibitors. Based on this data, "high bolus" dose tirofiban can be employed for the immediate management of ACS in the same settings as eptifibatide.

Guidelines

The current guidelines suggest that DAPT with a $P2Y_{12}$ inhibitor and aspirin should be initiated for patients with ACS. For intermediate- and high-risk patients with non-STEMI and unstable angina treated with an early invasive strategy and DAPT (ASA and $P2Y_{12}$ inhibitor), it is considered reasonable to add a Gp IIb/IIIa inhibitor as part of the initial antiplatelet therapy; eptifibatide and tirofiban are preferred options (Class IIb, Level B). High-risk non-STEMI patients who are not adequately pretreated with clopidogrel or ticagrelor should receive a Gp IIb/IIIa inhibitor (abciximab, double bolus eptifibatide, or high bolus dose tirofiban) at the time of PCI (Class I, Level A). For high-risk non-STEMI patients who are treated with heparin and adequately treated with clopidogrel, it is considered reasonable to add a Gp IIb/IIIa inhibitor at the time of PCI (Class IIa, Level B).[12] For STEMI patients who are treated with heparin, it is reasonable to start a Gp IIb/IIIa inhibitor at the time of primary PCI (Class IIa, Level A for abciximab, Level B for tirofiban and eptifibatide).[51] Abciximab should generally be administered only to patients that will undergo PCI. For patients at high-risk of bleeding, bivalirudin is preferred to the use of heparin and Gp IIb/IIIa inhibitors (Class IIa, Level B).[12]

Early administration of Gp IIb/IIIa inhibitors in the pre-catheterization setting (in the ambulance or in the emergency department) for STEMI patients in whom primary PCI is intended may be considered (Class IIb, Level B).[51] The European guidelines recommend against the routine use of Gp IIb/IIIa inhibitors before angiography or in patients who are treated conservatively (Class III, Level A).[36] Short-acting Gp IIb/IIIa inhibitors (eptifibatide and tirofiban) should be discontinued at least 2–4 hours before urgent coronary artery bypass grafting (CABG) surgery (Class I, level B). Abciximab should be discontinued at least 12 hours before urgent CABG surgery (Class I, Level B).[51]

THROMBIN RECEPTOR ANTAGONISTS

Vorapaxar

Pharmacology

The protease-activated receptor-1 (PAR-1) is the predominant thrombin receptor on human platelets.[196] After an ACS, intravascular thrombin levels are elevated and induce platelet activation via the PAR-1 receptor despite the use of other antiplatelet agents. Vorapaxar is a novel competitive and selective antagonist of the PAR-1 receptor and thrombin receptor agonist peptide (TRAP) induced platelet aggregation, blocking thrombin mediated platelet activation. The PAR-1 receptor provides an additional target for platelet suppression beyond the receptors for ADP, Gp IIb/IIIa, and TxA_2, which have already been discussed above.[197,198]

Pharmacokinetics and Doses

The oral formulation of vorapaxar has effective half-life of 3–4 days and a terminal elimination half-life of 8 days (range 5–13 days). Steady state is achieved by 21 days following daily dosing. While vorapaxar is a competitive reversible antagonist of PAR-1, its long half-life makes it effectively irreversible. Vorapaxar achieves ≥80% inhibition of TRAP-induced platelet aggregation within 1 week of initiation and inhibition at a level of 50% can be expected at 4 weeks after discontinuation. Peak serum concentrations of vorapaxar occur 1 hour after oral administration. The drug is metabolized via the CYP3A4 and CYP2J2 systems and is excreted primarily in the feces. The standard dosage of vorapaxar is 2.08 mg (equivalent to 2.5 mg vorapaxar sulfate) by mouth daily.[199,200]

Clinical Use and Indications

Vorapaxar was approved by the US FDA in May 2014 based on the Results of the Thrombin Receptor Antagonist in Secondary Prevention of Atherothrombotic Ischemic Events—Thrombolysis in Myocardial Infarction 50 (TRA 2P-TIMI 50) trial.[197] In this study, 26,449 patients with a history of MI, ischemic stroke, or peripheral arterial disease (PAD) were randomly assigned to receive vorapaxar 2.5 mg daily or placebo and were followed for a median of 30 months.[201] Most patients with previous MI were on DAPT with aspirin and clopidogrel. The primary efficacy endpoint of death from CV causes, MI, or stroke occurred in 9.3% of the vorapaxar patients versus 10.5% in the placebo patients (HR 0.87, p <0.001). The primary safety endpoint of moderate or severe bleeding was 4.2% versus 2.5% in the groups, respectively (HR 1.66, p <0.001). Although not powered for subgroup analysis, the trial did detect a significant increase in ICH in the vorapaxar group among patients with a history of stroke (2.4% compared with 0.9%, P <0.001.) Given the excess bleeding risk in patients with stroke, the Data Safety Monitoring Board prematurely discontinued vorapaxar use in patients with a history of stroke or ICH.

The Thrombin Receptor Antagonist for Clinical Event Reduction in Acute Coronary Syndrome (TRACER) trial evaluated the use of vorapaxar in patients with ACS. Approximately, 12,944 patients with ACS without ST-segment elevation were randomized to a 40 mg loading dose of vorapaxar followed by a 2.5 mg daily dose or placebo.[202] After a median follow-up of 502 days, the trial was terminated prematurely due to safety concerns. The primary end point was a composite of death from CV causes, MI, stroke, recurrent ischemia with re-hospitalization, or urgent coronary revascularization, and was not significantly different between the two groups (vorapaxar 18.5% vs. placebo 19.9%, HR 0.92, P 0.07). Rates of moderate and severe bleeding were 7.2% in the vorapaxar group and 5.2% in the placebo group (HR 1.35, P <0.001). ICH rates were 1.1% and 0.2%, respectively (HR 3.39, P <0.001).

Given the results of these two studies, vorapaxar is now indicated for secondary prevention of thrombotic CV events in patients with a history of MI or with PAD. It is contraindicated in patients with a history of stroke, TIA, or ICH because of an increased risk of ICH in this population. It is also contraindicated in patients with active pathological bleeding including peptic ulcer. Patients with ACS undergoing coronary intervention and receiving aggressive antithrombotic therapy should not receive vorapaxar because of the increased bleeding risk.[200] Vorapaxar has only been studied in combination with aspirin and/or clopidogrel. There is limited clinical experience using vorapaxar as a sole antiplatelet agent or with agents other than aspirin and clopidogrel.

Guidelines

Clinical guidelines do not currently address the use of vorapaxar.

FIBRINOLYTIC AGENTS

The definitive management of ACS requires restoration of cardiac perfusion. Numerous studies have demonstrated that PCI improves morbidity and mortality in STEMI.[203] There are many regions of the world, however, that do not have access to PCI facilities. Fibrinolytic agents can be used in these cases to degrade epicardial coronary artery thrombus to preserve left ventricular function and decrease mortality.[204,205] It is important to note that these agents have a significant risk of hemorrhage and are not indicated in other forms of ACS, including unstable angina and non-STEMI.

Pharmacology

All thrombolytic agents are designed to facilitate the conversion of plasminogen to plasmin (Fig. 4). Active plasmin will then degrade fibrinogen resulting in the dissolution of the thrombus. Four agents are currently available to facilitate this process through different mechanisms.

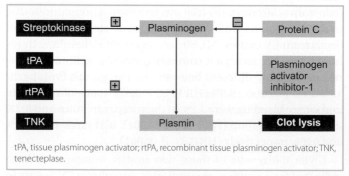

tPA, tissue plasminogen activator; rtPA, recombinant tissue plasminogen activator; TNK, tenecteplase.

FIG. 4: Thrombolytic agents. Most mechanisms of therapeutic thrombolysis accelerate the conversion of plasminogen to plasmin, thus, facilitating clot destruction.

Alteplase

Pharmacokinetics and Doses

Alteplase is a naturally occurring enzyme that binds to fibrin and converts entrapped plasminogen to plasmin. The medication has a rapid onset of action and undergoes hepatic metabolism before leaving the blood stream within 10 minutes of infusion discontinuation. Because of this short half-life, anticoagulation should be administered with alteplase to prevent reocclusion. The standard IV regimen uses a bolus (15 mg) than a fast maintenance infusion (50 mg over 30 min) followed by a slower maintenance infusion (35 mg over 60 minutes). This dosing should be reduced for individuals weighing less than 68 kg. The major side effect of alteplase is the risk of major bleeding including ICH.

Reteplase

Pharmacokinetics and Doses

The removal of two nonactive domains from alteplase produces the mutant protein reteplase. Like its parent compound, reteplase initiates local fibrinolysis by binding to fibrin in a thrombus and converting entrapped plasminogen to plasmin. Changes to the protein structure result in the prolongation of its half-life to 13-16 minutes before being excreted in the feces and urine. The longer half-life allows reteplase to be administered in a double bolus regimen (10 units over 10 minutes twice 30 minutes apart). The major side effect of reteplase remains major bleeding including ICH.

Streptokinase

Pharmacokinetics and Doses

Streptokinase is a single-chain protein released by β-hemolytic streptococci that binds with human plasminogen. The streptokinase-plasminogen complex then becomes an active enzyme capable of converting plasminogen to plasmin to facilitate thrombolysis (Fig. 4). Streptokinase was the original thrombolytic agent and continues to be used around the world because of its low cost. As a bacterial product, the administration of streptokinase can precipitate an immune response that includes anaphylaxis.[206] Repeated administration of streptokinase may result in the formation of antibodies to the agent which would neutralize its efficacy. Streptokinase is administered as a slow infusion (1.5 million IU over 60 minutes) with an immediate effect. It is important to note that some generic formulations of streptokinase may have decreased efficacy ranging from 21% to 81% of the activity claimed.[207]

Tenecteplase

Pharmacokinetics and Doses

Tenecteplase is a genetically engineered mutant of tissue plasminogen activator. The resulting compound has three amino acid substitutions that result in decreased plasma clearance and a longer half-life (20 minutes). These mutations may also increase the specificity of the compound to binding fibrin and increase its efficacy. A single-bolus of tenecteplase (0.5 mg/kg) is administered for the treatment of STEMI.

Clinical Use and Indications

Fibrinolytic agents are most beneficial in the early stages of STEMI. The Myocardial Infarction Triage and Intervention (MITI) trial randomized 360 patients with STEMI to receive alteplase and aspirin before or after reaching the hospital. The early administration of thrombolytics (<70 minutes since symptom onset) resulted in a 7.5% absolute risk reduction in mortality (8.7–1.2%) while also decreasing infarct size when compared to those that received late thrombolytics (<180 minutes since symptom onset).[208] These findings were confirmed in the FTT Collaborative Overview of 58,000 randomized patients in fibrinolytic trials.[209] Mortality was reduced by 25% in patients receiving fibrinolysis within 3 hours of symptom onset and 18% within 6 hours. Late administration of fibrinolytics is less efficacious as the thrombus matures and is less prone to pharmacological degradation. Because of this, fibrinolytic therapies administered 12 hours after symptom onset have a minimal reduction in a mortality with a persistent risk of hemorrhage.[210] Current guidelines thus recommend that fibrinolytic agents be administered within 30 minutes if PCI cannot be performed within 120 minutes of first medical contact (Class I, Level B).[211] Patients that present over 12 hours after symptom onset should only be considered for mechanical revascularization.

Several large randomized trials have compared different fibrinolytic regimens for the treatment of ACS. The GUSTO-I trial demonstrated that alteplase produced a 14% relative risk reduction and a 1% absolute risk reduction compared to streptokinase in patients with STEMI.[212] However, the administration of alteplase also resulted in an increased risk of hemorrhagic stroke. The Assessment of the Safety and Efficacy of a New Thrombolytic Regimen-2 (ASSENT-2) trial demonstrated that tenecteplase was equivalent to alteplase with a decreased rate of major bleeding.[213] Each of the fibrinolytic agents was assessed with the concomitant use of anticoagulation.[214] Based on this data, all four agents are used for thrombolysis when primary PCI is not available. The absolute and relative contraindications of systemic lytic therapy are listed in the accompanying Table 4.[211]

TABLE 4: Contraindications to thrombolysis[211]

Absolute contraindications
• Intracranial process
– Prior hemorrhage
– Prior malignant neoplasm
– Prior cerebral vascular lesion
– Prior trauma (within 3 months)
– Prior ischemic stroke (within 3 months)
– Prior intracranial or intraspinal surgery (within 2 months)
• Suspected aortic dissection
• Active bleeding

Relative contraindications
• Cardiovascular comorbidities
– Hypertension (SBP >180/DBP >110)
– Prior ischemic stroke (>3 months)
• Recent bleeding
– Internal bleeding (within 2–4 weeks)
– Noncompressible vascular punctures
– Active peptic ulcer
– Current use of anticoagulants
• Other intracranial pathology
– Pregnancy
– Traumatic or prolonged (>10 minutes) CPR
– Major surgery (<3 weeks)
– Active peptic ulcer
– Oral anticoagulant therapy

Facilitation

A number of trials have evaluated the clinical utility in the administration of half-dose or full-dose thrombolytics prior to proceeding to planned PCI, previously termed facilitated PCI. The majority of these studies demonstrated no mortality benefit with an increased bleeding risk.[215,216] However, there are increasing data suggesting that a strategy of early routine catheterization after fibrinolysis improves clinical outcomes, most notably in higher-risk patients. In the GRACIA (Grupo de Analisis de la Cardiopatia Isquemica Aguda) study, early catheterization within 6–24 hours of successful fibrinolysis in stable patients was compared with an ischemia guided approach. It resulted in improved outcomes, including a significantly lower rate of death, reinfarction, or ischemia driven revascularization at 1 year.[217] The TRANSFER-AMI (Trial of Routine Angioplasty and Stenting after Fibrinolysis to Enhance Reperfusion in Acute Myocardial Infarction) study was the largest (n = 1,059) of the RCTs evaluating transfer for coronary angiography and revascularization among high-risk patients and showed a significant reduction in the combined primary endpoint of death, recurrent MI, recurrent ischemia, new or worsening HF, or shock at 30 days with immediate transfer for the angiography group compared with conservative care.[218] The findings from this and other studies indicate that high-risk patients with STEMI appear to benefit from immediate transfer for early catheterization, compared with either an ischemia-guided approach or delayed routine catheterization.[219]

The use of rescue PCI after failed fibrinolysis has demonstrated clinical benefit in patients with persistent ischemia or cardiogenic shock.[220] PCI in these patients is more effective than repeat thrombolysis or no treatment for failed reperfusion.[221]

Guidelines

The current guidelines suggest that patients presenting with STEMI should be treated with primary PCI within 90 minutes (Class I, Level A). If a patient presents to a facility without this capability, they should be transferred to a center with PCIs if they can then undergo the procedure within 120 minutes of their first medical contact (Class I, Level B). For STEMI patients that cannot be transferred to a PCI facility, treatment with fibrinolytic therapy within 30 minutes of hospital presentation is recommended (Class I, Level B).[211]

Patients receiving fibrinolytic therapy should be given a loading dose of aspirin (162–325 mg) and clopidogrel (300 mg if age ≤75 years, 75 mg if age >75 years) (Class I, Level A). Aspirin (81–325 mg daily) should be continued indefinitely (Class 1, Level A) with 81 mg daily as the preferred dose (Class IIa, Level B). Clopidogrel should be continued for at least 14 days (Class I, Level A), and up to 1 year (Class I, Level C). Other $P2Y_{12}$ agents have not been studied in this context. STEMI patients treated with fibrinolysis should be also treated with concomitant anticoagulation for a minimum of 48 hours and preferably for the duration of the index hospitalization up to 8 days or until revascularization is performed (Class I, Level A). Enoxaparin is preferred to unfractionated heparin if anticoagulation is to be given for longer than 48 hours, given the risk of heparin induced thrombocytopenia.[211]

Coronary angiography with possible PCI (rescue PCI) can be pursued in patients that have received fibrinolytic therapy if they have persistent cardiogenic shock or acute severe congestive HF (Class I, Level B). Urgent transfer to a PCI-capable hospital for coronary angiography is reasonable for patients with STEMI who demonstrate evidence of failed reperfusion or reocclusion after fibrinolytic therapy (Class IIa, Level B). Transfer to a PCI-capable hospital for coronary angiography is also reasonable for patients with STEMI who have received fibrinolytic therapy even when hemodynamically stable and with clinical evidence of successful reperfusion (Class IIa, Level B). In this case, angiography can be performed as soon as logistically feasible at the receiving hospital, and ideally within 24 hours, but should not be performed within the first 2–3 hours after administration of fibrinolytic therapy.[211]

LONG-TERM DRUG THERAPY FOR PATIENTS WITH ACUTE CORONARY SYNDROMES

Introduction

The patients with ACS, whether STEMI, non-STEMI, or unstable angina, require long-term treatments to decrease the risks of adverse CV events. Both pharmacotherapy and nonpharmacologic treatments should be considered for these patients.

The pharmacologic agents that have been documented to decrease the risks of adverse CV events are:
- Antiplatelet agents
- Angiotensin inhibitors
- β-adrenergic antagonists
- Aldosterone antagonists
- Lipid-lowering agents.

ANTIPLATELET DRUGS

Introduction

The antiplatelet drugs are employed not only during the initial management of patients with ACS but also for their long-term management. Nonparenteral aspirin, clopidogrel, ticagrelor or prasugrel are used as antiplatelet drugs during long-term treatment of patients with ACS. The Gp IIb/IIIa inhibitors are used only for patients requiring percutaneous coronary artery interventions.

Aspirin

Mechanism of Action and Dosage

Aspirin is the most commonly used antiplatelet drug in patients with CV disorders. Its mechanism of action, dosage, and metabolism have been discussed earlier. It attenuates aggregations of platelets by inhibiting the enzyme cyclooxygenase and blocking the TxA_2 receptors. It has a relatively long half-life. The dose is between 75 mg and 325 mg daily. Because of its long half-life, it can be used, if necessary, 2–3 times weekly. However, it is preferable to use lower dose of aspirin daily, which is associated with lower risk of complications and appears to be equally effective to larger dose.[86]

Long-term use of aspirin has been reported to reduce the risk of nonfatal MI by 32%, nonfatal stroke by 27%, total vascular event by 25%, and total CV death by 15%.[222]

It has been observed that aspirin in combination with angiotensin-converting enzyme inhibitors (ACEIs) and statins significantly decrease mortality and morbidity of patients with ACS.[223]

Adverse Effects

The GI complications are most frequent adverse effects of the long-term use of aspirin. Indigestion, symptoms of gastric erosions, and ulcerations are the usual manifestations. Frank hematemesis is a rare manifestation. Upper GI endoscopy may be required to establish the diagnosis. The concomitant use of antacids and/or H_2-blockers is preferable to discontinuation of aspirin.

Slow GI blood loss may cause anemia during long-term use of aspirin. If anemia develops, appropriate investigations, including upper endoscopy should be undertaken. After gastric complications are treated, aspirin treatment should be reinstated along with antacids and/or H_2-blockers. In patients intolerant to oral aspirin, it can be administered as a suppository. ICH is a rare complication of aspirin.

Contraindications

Aspirin may cause exacerbation of allergic sinusitis. Recurrent exacerbations with nasal bleedings are a relative contraindication for long-term use of aspirin. Recurrent gastric ulcerations, or erosions with or without blood loss, and unresponsive to antacids and H_2-blocker therapies is also a relative contraindication for the long-term use of aspirin. Severe bronchospastic disease, such as bronchial asthma is a contraindication for the use of aspirin. The Samter's triad, which consists of sensitivity to salicylates, asthma, and nasal polyps is regarded as an absolute contraindication to the long-term use of aspirin. Aspirin is also contraindicated in patients with retinal hemorrhage, urogenital bleeding, hemophilia, and untreated severe hypertension.

CLOPIDOGREL

Introduction

Clopidogrel is a thienopyridine derivative that exerts its antiplatelet effects by blocking the activity of the ADP receptors on the surface of the platelets.

Indications

The major indication for the long-term use of clopidogrel is to reduce the risk of stent thrombosis after percutaneous coronary artery intervention. It is being increasingly used because PCI with the use of stents is recommended therapy for patients with ACS. Clopidogrel is used along with aspirin (DAPT). Ideally, clopidogrel should be continued for at least 1 year after stent placement in the setting of ACS,[12] but the duration of therapy can potentially be shortened depending on the type of coronary artery stent placed. When the bare metal stents are used, it is recommended that clopidogrel be continued for at least 1 month. If DESs are used, clopidogrel should be continued for at least 12 months.[54] The usual dose of clopidogrel is 75 mg daily.

Adverse Effects

Gastrointestinal upset and skin rash may occur with clopidogrel. Thrombocytopenia is a rare complication of clopidogrel.

Contraindications

Severe thrombocytopenia is a contraindication for the long-term use of clopidogrel.

PRASUGREL

Introduction

Like clopidogrel, prasugrel exerts its antiplatelet activity by inhibiting platelet ADP receptors. The half-life of its active metabolites is approximately 7 hours. For the long-term use, the standard dose of prasugrel is 10 mg daily.[152]

Indications

The principal indication for the long-term use of prasugrel is to reduce the risk of stent thrombosis after PCI. In a large randomized trial of STEMI, it was reported that prasugrel resulted in a 2.4% absolute risk reduction in CV death, recurrent MI, or stroke compared to standard doses of clopidogrel.[156]

Adverse Effects

The use of prasugrel is associated with increased risk of major bleeding compared to clopidogrel.[154]

Contraindications

Prasugrel is contraindicated in patients with history of cerebrovascular disease and pathological bleeding. It is also relatively contraindicated in patients over the age of 75 years or weight under 60 kg.

TICAGRELOR

Introduction

Like clopidogrel and prasugrel, ticagrelor exerts its antiplatelet activity by inhibiting platelet ADP receptors. However, unlike the thienopyridines, ticagrelor is a modification of adenosine triphosphate to cyclopentyl-triazolo-pyrimidine that does not require metabolic conversion prior to inhibiting its target. Ticagrelor is rapidly absorbed reaching its peak plasma levels within 2 hours of ingestion and providing approximately 12 hours of platelet inhibition. The standard dose of ticagrelor is 90 mg twice a day.[157] At this dose, ticagrelor provides more rapid maximal platelet inhibition than standard doses of clopidogrel.[158] It is important to note that post-hoc analyses have demonstrated a rebound in platelet aggregation in those patients that only take the medication once a day.[149]

Indications

The principal indication for the long-term use of ticagrelor is to reduce the risk of stent thrombosis after primary coronary artery intervention. A large multicenter trial comparing ticagrelor with clopidogrel use in patients after ACS demonstrated a 1.9% absolute risk reduction in vascular death, recurrent MI or stroke in the ticagrelor group (9.8% vs. 11.7%) with similar rates of major bleeding (11.6% vs. 11.2%).[159] Ticagrelor is currently indicated only for patients who have had ACS, but can be used both for patients who undergo conservative medical management or invasive management with stent placement. Guidelines also suggest that ticagrelor should be used in preference to clopidogrel in ACS patients.[12] Aspirin doses higher than 100 mg/day can reduce the efficacy of ticagrelor. Therefore, the recommended maintenance dose of aspirin is 81 mg daily when used with ticagrelor.[12]

Adverse Effects

Patients treated with ticagrelor have a slightly higher rate of fatal intracranial bleeding as well as a higher rate of dyspnea and bradycardia than those treated with clopidogrel.[159]

Contraindications

Ticagrelor is contraindicated in patients with history of ICH, active pathological bleeding, or severe hepatic impairment.

ANGIOTENSIN INHIBITORS

Introduction

Angiotensin-converting enzyme inhibitors or angiotensin receptor blocking (ARB) agents have been demonstrated to decrease mortality and morbidity of patients with acute coronary artery syndromes.[17,18,223-230] The ACEIs—captopril, lisinopril, ramipril, trandolapril, and zofenopril—have been used in various studies. With the use of these ACEIs, in general, there was a substantial reduction in all-cause mortality, incidence of fatal and nonfatal MI, and development of overt HF. It is of interest that the beneficial effects of the ACEIs were observed in patients with depressed left ventricular systolic function. ARB agents exert similar beneficial effects in patients with reduced LVEF (Fig. 5).[229] In contrast, no beneficial effects

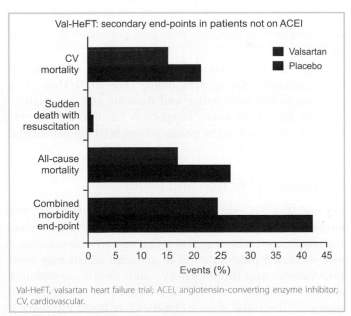

Val-HeFT, valsartan heart failure trial; ACEI, angiotensin-converting enzyme inhibitor; CV, cardiovascular.

FIG. 5: Effects of angiotensin receptor blocking agent valsartan in post-myocardial infarction patients showing decreased risk of all-cause mortality, sudden death with resuscitation, and combined morbidity.

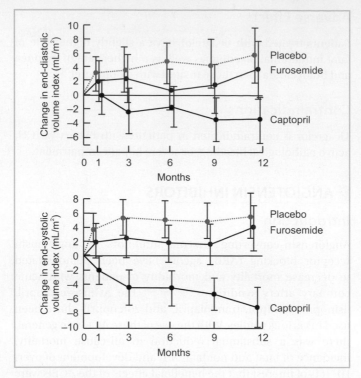

FIG. 6: The effects of angiotensin-converting enzyme inhibitors on left ventricular remodeling showing a decrease in end systolic and end diastolic volumes. Values shown are least squares means with upper and lower least significant difference intervals (p <0.05).[231]

were observed in patients who had preserved LVEF after ACS.[230]

Angiotensin-converting enzyme inhibitors can produce left ventricular reverse remodeling (Fig. 6).[231] There is a decrease in left ventricular end-diastolic and end-systolic volumes and an increase in ejection fraction. ARB agents also have the potential to produce beneficial left ventricular reverse remodeling.

Mechanism of Action and Doses

Angiotensin-converting enzyme inhibitors reduce the formation of angiotensin by blocking the converting enzyme. The inhibitions of the converting enzymes are also associated with increased production of bradykinins which may exert vasodilatory, anti-inflammatory, and reverse remodeling effects. Commonly used ACEIs are enalapril, lisinopril, and captopril. The usual dose of enalapril is 10–20 mg twice a day. After oral dose of enalapril, the peak concentration of its active metabolite enalaprilat occurs at 3–4 hours and the half-life of enalaprilat is about 11 hours. Lisinopril has a half-life of about 12 hours. Doses of 10–80 mg once a day are effective in majority of patients. The half-life of captopril is 2.2 hours, and the dose is 25–50 mg three times a day.

Angiotensin receptor blocking agents directly block the angiotensin II receptors and attenuate the deleterious effects of angiotensin. Angiotensin promotes vasoconstriction, vascular smooth muscle cells hypertrophy, myocyte hypertrophy, and extracellular matrix degradation and myocardial fibrosis. Furthermore, angiotensin promotes atherothrombosis. The ARB agents counteract these deleterious effects of angiotensin. ARB agents do not exert any effect on bradykinin metabolism.

Valsartan is the most commonly used ARB agent in patients with acute coronary artery syndrome. It has a relatively long half-life. The usual dose of valsartan is 40–160 mg twice a day. Losartan has also been used in patients with ACS. The half-life of losartan is 1–2 hours but that of its active metabolite is 3–4 hours. The usual dose of losartan is 25–50 mg twice a day.

Adverse Effects

A marked fall in blood pressure may occur after the first dose of ACEIs, in patients with relative hypovolemia due to diuretic therapy. Acute renal failure is a serious adverse effect which occurs more frequently in patients with bilateral renal artery stenosis. During long-term treatment with ACEIs, worsening renal function due to hypotension may be observed in a few patients. Hyperkalemia tends to occur more frequently in patients with renal failure or diabetes.

The most frequent side effect of ACEIs is nonproductive paroxysms of cough. However, intractable cough is uncommon. Another uncommon complication is angioedema. Skin rash and altered taste are also uncommon complications. With high doses of ACEIs, neutropenia, or proteinuria may occur. The major side effects of the ARB agents are hypotension and worsening renal function. Hyperkalemia may also occur along with renal failure. The use of ARB agents is not usually associated with intractable cough or angioedema.

Contraindications

Intractable cough and angioedema are contraindications for the use of ACEIs. Hypotension, worsening renal function, and hyperkalemia are contraindications for the use of both ACEIs and ARB agents. Cardiogenic shock is a contraindication for the use of ACEIs or ARB agents. These agents are also contraindicated during second and third trimesters of pregnancy, as irreversible fetal renal failure can develop. There is also increased risk of teratogenicity.

β-ADRENERGIC ANTAGONISTS

Introduction

β-blockers should be considered for long-term treatment of patients with ACS. In post-MI patients with reduced LVEF, long-term use of carvedilol is associated with decreased mortality and morbidity.[28] There is also decreased risk of development of overt HF. β-blockers have been shown to decrease the risk of mortality and nonfatal CV events in post-MI patients already on angiotensin inhibition therapy.[229] In patients with chronic systolic HF due to ischemic cardiomyopathy, β-blocker therapy has been shown to reduce mortality and morbidity.[232] There is also reverse remodeling of the left ventricle. There is a reduction in left ventricular end-systolic and end-diastolic volumes and an increase in ejection fraction.

Indications

For the long-term use in chronic systolic HF, carvedilol, bisoprolol, or long-acting slow release metoprolol are used. Carvedilol is a nonselective β-blocking agent with also α-blocking property. It also has an antioxidant property. Compared to short-acting immediate release metoprolol, carvedilol has been reported to be more effective to decrease the risk of mortality and morbidity.[29] The half-life of carvedilol is about 7–10 hours. The optimal dose of carvedilol for systolic HF is 25 mg twice a day. The initiating dose is between 3.125 mg and 12.5 mg twice a day.

Bisoprolol is a selective β-receptor blocking agent with a direct vasodilating property. It has a relatively long half-life and can be administered once a day. The optimal dose of bisoprolol is 10 mg daily, but the initiating dose is 2.5–5 mg once a day.

Long-acting slow release metoprolol is a selective β1-receptor blocking agent. Short-acting metoprolol has a half-life of 3–4 hours, while the slow release metoprolol has a much longer half-life and can be administered once daily. The optimal dose of slow release metoprolol is 100–200 mg daily. The initiating dose is between 25 mg and 50 mg daily.

Adverse Effects

Hypotension, bradycardia, and exacerbation of HF are adverse effects that usually occur at the initiation of therapy. Worsening lower extremity claudication, depression, and bronchospasm are other adverse effects of β-blocker therapy.

Contraindications

Extreme bradycardia, heart block, and severe bronchospasm are contraindications for the use of β-blockers. Cardiogenic shock and pulmonary edema are also contraindications for the use of β-adrenergic antagonists.

ALDOSTERONE ANTAGONISTS

Introduction

Aldosterone exerts adverse effects on ventricular function and promotes ventricular remodeling. It causes myocyte hypertrophy, and induces collagen synthesis and myocardial fibrosis. In addition, it can cause fluid retention and exacerbate HF. Aldosterone antagonists have the potential to reverse the adverse effects of aldosterone.

Indications

In post-MI patients with reduced LVEF, aldosterone antagonist, eplerenone decreases mortality and morbidity, reduces the risk of developing congestive HF, and has the potential of reducing myocardial fibrosis and to promote beneficial left ventricular reverse remodeling. The EPHESUS trial (Eplerenone Post–Acute Myocardial Infarction Heart Failure Efficacy and Survival Study) randomized 3,634 patients with acute MI complicated by left ventricular dysfunction and HF to receive eplerenone 25 mg titrated to a maximum of 50 mg once per day versus placebo.[233] During the mean follow-up of 16 months, the relative risk of death was reduced by 15% (relative risk, 0.85). The rate of the second primary end point, death from CV causes or hospitalization for CV events, was also reduced by eplerenone (relative risk, 0.87). The rate of serious hyperkalemia was 5.5% in the eplerenone group and 3.9% in the placebo group (P = 0.002), whereas the rate of hypokalemia was 8.4% in the eplerenone group and 13.1% in the placebo group (P <0.001). As a result of this trial, eplerenone is now recommended in post-MI patients without significant renal dysfunction (creatinine >2.5 mg/dL in men or >2.0 mg/dL in women) or hyperkalemia (K >5.0 mEq/L) who are receiving therapeutic doses of ACE inhibitor and β-blocker and have an LVEF 40% or less, diabetes mellitus, or HF (Class I, Level A).[12]

Mechanism of Action and Doses

Eplerenone is a competitive antagonist to aldosterone. It is a more selective aldosterone antagonist than spironolactone. It does not exert antiandrogenic effects and does not cause gynecomastia and breast enlargement. In the kidney, its major site of action is on the distal tubule and collecting ducts. The optimal dose of eplerenone is between 25 mg and 50 mg twice a day. The initiating dose is between 12.5 mg and 25 mg once a day.

Adverse Effects

Hyperkalemia and worsening renal failure are the major adverse effects of aldosterone antagonists. When used with loop diuretics, it may exacerbate hyponatremia. Gynecomastia and breast enlargements are other side effects of spironolactone.

Contraindications

Renal failure with creatinine more than 2.5 mg/dL and/or serum potassium level ≥5 mEq/L are contraindications for the use of aldosterone antagonists.

STATINS

Introduction

In patients with ACS, intensive lipid-lowering therapy with 3-hydroxy-3-methylglutaryl coenzyme-A reductase inhibitors (statins) decreases the risks of mortality and recurrent adverse CV events.[234,235] Based on the results of these studies, ACC/AHA guidelines recommended early and intensive lipid lowering therapy with statins in patients with ACS.[12,211,236]

Mechanism of Action and Doses of Statins in Acute Coronary Syndrome

As the treatment with statins is associated with the beneficial effects which occur early and irrespective of the baseline levels of low-density lipoprotein (LDL), lipid-lowering effects do not appear to be the primary mechanism. Statins can improve endothelial function and decrease inflammation and myocardial ischemia. These beneficial effects which are independent of its lipid lowering effects are referred as its "pleiotropic" effect. The dose of atorvastatin used in these trials was 80 mg/daily.

Clinical Trials

In the Myocardial Ischemia Reduction with Aggressive Cholesterol Lowering (MIRACL) trial, 3,038 patients with ACS were randomized to receive either 80 mg of atorvastatin or placebo. The composite primary end-point in this trial was—death, non-fatal MI, cardiac arrest, or recurrent unstable myocardial ischemia. There was a relative risk reduction of the primary end-point by 50% in the treated group.[234]

In the Pravastatin or Atorvastatin Evaluation and Infection Therapy-TIMI 22 Trial (PROVE IT), 4,162 patients were randomized to receive either 40 mg of pravastatin or 80 mg of atorvastatin. The composite primary end-point was all-cause mortality, MI, unstable angina requiring hospitalizations, need for revascularization, and stroke. During a mean follow-up period of 24 months, the incidence of primary end-point in the pravastatin group was 26.3% and that of in the atorvastatin group, 22.4%. There was a statistically significant 16% reduction in the relative risk of incidence of primary endpoint with atorvastatin compared to pravastatin.[235] There was also a reduction in the rate of hospitalization for HF.[237] Intensive lipid-lowering treatment with large dose of atorvastatin (80 mg) appears to reduce the risk of major CV events by a greater magnitude compared to treatment with 40 mg of pravastatin in patients undergoing PCI for ACS.[238] It has been also reported that early intervention with statin reduces the lipid components of the atherothrombotic plaques in patients with ACS which may produce beneficial effect in plaque stabilization.[239]

Current guidelines recommend that "high-intensity statin therapy" be initiated for ACS patients below the age of 75 years and have no safety concerns. For patients above 75 years, or with safety concerns, "moderate-intensity statin therapy" should be prescribed. High-intensity statin therapy reduces LDL cholesterol on average by 50%, and includes atorvastatin 40–80 mg daily and rosuvastatin 40 mg daily. Moderate-intensity statin therapy reduces LDL-C on average by 30–50% and includes atorvastatin 10–20 mg, rosuvastatin 5–10 mg, simvastatin 20–40 mg, pravastatin 40–80 mg, lovastatin 40 mg (all at daily dosing), and fluvastatin 40 mg twice daily.[236]

Pharmacokinetics

Atorvastatin is a metabolically active agent and its absorption after oral therapy varies between 40% and 75%. The half-life of atorvastatin is approximately 14 hours. In ACS, 80 mg of atorvastatin is employed.

Rosuvastatin is also a metabolically active agent and its absorption after oral therapy is approximately 20%, with peak plasma concentrations reached in 3–5 hours. The half-life of rosuvastatin is approximately 19 hours. In ACS, rosuvastatin is dosed at 40 mg daily.

Adverse Effects

The skeletal muscle "aches and pains" are common complaints during statin therapy. Until these symptoms are intolerable in patients with coronary artery disease, it should be continued indefinitely. The benefits of statin therapy are more than the risks, and the risk-benefits should be explained to the patients.

Slight elevation of muscle creatine kinase is common, but it is not a contraindication for discontinuing statin therapy.

Similarly, slight or modest elevation of hepatic enzymes is frequent but not a contraindication for statin therapy.

Contraindications

Severe myopathy with a marked elevation of skeletal muscle creatine kinase enzyme, renal failure, obvious skeletal muscle wasting are contraindications for statin therapy. Progressive hepatic failure manifested by a marked elevation of hepatic enzymes is also a contraindication for statin therapy.

CONCLUSION

Several drugs are used both for immediate treatment and for long-term management of patients with ACS. Antiplatelet drugs, thrombin inhibitors, anticoagulants, and thrombolytic drugs are used during the acute phase in patients undergoing either catheter based or pharmacologic reperfusion therapy. β-adrenergic blocking agents and angiotensin inhibitors are adjunctive therapy in patients with ACS during the acute phase management. In patients with ACS, large doses of statins are used. In patients with reduced LVEF, who have already received reperfusion therapy, aldosterone antagonists are indicated.

For long-term management of patients with ACS, antiplatelet drugs, angiotensin inhibitors, β-blockers, and statins should be used indefinitely in absence of contraindications. It should be appreciated that all drugs can produce complications. Some complications are minor and others are more severe. The major complications are usually contraindications for continued therapy.

REFERENCES

1. Libby P, Theroux P. Pathophysiology of coronary artery disease. Circulation. 2005;111(25):3481-8.
2. Kinlay S, Ganz P. Role of endothelial dysfunction in coronary artery disease and implications for therapy. Am J Cardiol. 1997;80(9A):11I-6I.
3. Ross R. The pathogenesis of atherosclerosis: a perspective for the 1990s. Nature. 1993;362(6423):801-9.
4. Waldo SW, Li Y, Buono C, et al. Heterogeneity of human macrophages in culture and in atherosclerotic plaques. Am J Pathol. 2008;172(4):1112-26.
5. Demer LL. Vascular calcification and osteoporosis: inflammatory responses to oxidized lipids. Int J Epidemiol. 2002;31(4):737-41.
6. Shah PK, Falk E, Badimon JJ, et al. Human monocyte-derived macrophages induce collagen breakdown in fibrous caps of atherosclerotic plaques. Potential role of matrix-degrading metalloproteinases and implications for plaque rupture. Circulation. 1995;92(6):1565-9.
7. Toschi V, Gallo R, Lettino M, et al. Tissue factor modulates the thrombogenicity of human atherosclerotic plaques. Circulation. 1997;95(3):594-9.
8. Hoffman M, Monroe DM 3rd. A cell-based model of hemostasis. Thromb Haemost. 2001;85(6):958-65.
9. Steffel J, Lüscher TF, Tanner FC. Tissue factor in cardiovascular diseases: molecular mechanisms and clinical implications. Circulation. 2006;113(5):722-31.

10. Mackman N, Tilley RE, Key NS. Role of the extrinsic pathway of blood coagulation in hemostasis and thrombosis. Arterioscler Thromb Vasc Biol. 2007;27(8):1687-93.

11. Ruggeri ZM, Mendolicchio GL. Adhesion mechanisms in platelet function. Circ Res. 2007;100(12):1673-85.

12. Amsterdam EA, Wenger NK, Brindis RG, et al. 2014 AHA/ACC Guideline for the Management of Patients With Non-ST-Elevation Acute Coronary Syndromes: A Report of the American College of Cardiology/American Heart Association Task Force on Practice Guidelines. Circulation. 2014;130(25):2354-94.

13. Francis SH, Busch JL, Corbin JD, et al. cGMP-dependent protein kinases and cGMP phosphodiesterases in nitric oxide and cGMP action. Pharmacol Rev. 2010; 62:525-63.

14. Anderson JL, Adams CD, Antman EM, et al. ACC/AHA 2007 guidelines for the management of patients with unstable angina/non-ST-Elevation myocardial infarction: a report of the American College of Cardiology/American Heart Association Task Force on Practice Guidelines (Writing Committee to Revise the 2002 Guidelines for the Management of Patients With Unstable Angina/Non-ST-Elevation Myocardial Infarction) developed in collaboration with the American College of Emergency Physicians, the Society for Cardiovascular Angiography and Interventions, and the Society of Thoracic Surgeons endorsed by the American Association of Cardiovascular and Pulmonary Rehabilitation and the Society for Academic Emergency Medicine. J Am Coll Cardiol. 2007;50(7):e1-e157.

15. Feldman RL, Pepine CJ, Conti CR. Magnitude of dilatation of large and small coronary arteries of nitroglycerin. Circulation. 1981;64(2):324-33.

16. Yusuf S, Collins R, MacMahon S, et al. Effect of intravenous nitrates on mortality in acute myocardial infarction: an overview of the randomised trials. Lancet. 1988;1(8594):1088-92.

17. GISSI-3: effects of lisinopril and transdermal glyceryl trinitrate singly and together on 6-week mortality and ventricular function after acute myocardial infarction. Gruppo Italiano per lo Studio della Sopravvivenza nell'infarto Miocardico. Lancet. 1994;343(8906):1115-22.

18. ISIS-4: a randomised factorial trial assessing early oral captopril, oral mononitrate, and intravenous magnesium sulphate in 58,050 patients with suspected acute myocardial infarction. ISIS-4 (Fourth International Study of Infarct Survival) Collaborative Group. Lancet. 1995;345(8951):669-85.

19. Figueras J, Lidon R, Cortadellas J. Rebound myocardial ischaemia following abrupt interruption of intravenous nitroglycerin infusion in patients with unstable angina at rest. Eur Heart J. 1991;12:405-11.

20. Meine TJ, Roe MT, Chen AY, et al. Association of intravenous morphine use and outcomes in acute coronary syndromes: results from the CRUSADE Quality Improvement Initiative. Am Heart J. 2005;149(6):1043-9.

21. Bristow MR, Ginsburg R, Umans V, et al. β1- and β2-adrenergic-receptor subpopulations in nonfailing and failing human ventricular myocardium: coupling of both receptor subtypes to muscle contraction and selective β1-receptor down-regulation in heart failure. Circ Res. 1986;59(3):297-309.

22. Chen ZM, Pan HC, Chen YP, et al. Early intravenous then oral metoprolol in 45,852 patients with acute myocardial infarction: randomised placebo-controlled trial. Lancet. 2005;366(9497):1622-32.

23. Nakatani D, Sakata Y, Suna S, et al. Impact of b blockade therapy on long-term mortality after ST-segment elevation acute myocardial infarction in the percutaneous coronary intervention era. Am J Cardiol. 2013;111(4):457-64.

24. Park KL, Goldberg RJ, Anderson FA, et al. β-blocker use in ST-segment elevation myocardial infarction in the reperfusion era (GRACE). Am J Med. 2014;127(6): 503-11

25. Bangalore S, Makani H, Radford M, et al. Clinical Outcomes with β-Blockers for myocardial infarction: a meta-analysis of randomized trials. Am J Med. 2014; 127(10):939-53.

26. Yusuf S, Wittes J, Friedman L. Overview of results of randomized clinical trials in heart disease. I. Treatments following myocardial infarction. JAMA. 1988;260(14): 2088-93.

27. Ellis K, Tcheng JE, Sapp S, et al. Mortality benefit of beta blockade in patients with acute coronary syndromes undergoing coronary intervention: pooled results from the Epic, Epilog, Epistent, Capture and Rapport Trials. J Interv Cardiol. 2003;16(4):299-305.

28. Dargie HJ. Effect of carvedilol on outcome after myocardial infarction in patients with left-ventricular dysfunction: the CAPRICORN randomised trial. Lancet. 2001;357(9266):1385-90.

29. Poole-Wilson PA, Swedberg K, Cleland JG, et al. Comparison of carvedilol and metoprolol on clinical outcomes in patients with chronic heart failure in the Carvedilol Or Metoprolol European Trial (COMET): randomised controlled trial. Lancet. 2003;362(9377):7-13

30. The effect of diltiazem on mortality and reinfarction after myocardial infarction. The Multicenter Diltiazem Postinfarction Trial Research Group. N Engl J Med. 1988;319(7):385-92.

31. Effect of verapamil on mortality and major events after acute myocardial infarction (the Danish Verapamil Infarction Trial II—DAVIT II). Am J Cardiol. 1990;66(10):779-85.

32. Held PH, Yusuf S, Furberg CD. Calcium channel blockers in acute myocardial infarction and unstable angina: an overview. BMJ. 1989;299(6709):1187-92.

33. Yusuf S, Wittes J, Friedman L. Overview of results of randomized clinical trials in heart disease. II. Unstable angina, heart failure, primary prevention with aspirin, and risk factor modification. JAMA. 1988;260(15):2259-63.

34. Hirsh J, O'Donnell M, Eikelboom JW. Beyond unfractionated heparin and warfarin: current and future advances. Circulation. 2007;116(5):552-60.

35. Harrington RA, Becker RC, Cannon CP, et al. Antithrombotic therapy for non-ST-segment elevation acute coronary syndromes: American College of Chest Physicians Evidence-Based Clinical Practice Guidelines (8th Edition). Chest. 2008;133(6 Suppl):670S-707S.

36. Hamm CW, Bassand JP, Agewall S, et al. ESC Guidelines for the management of acute coronary syndromes in patients presenting without persistent ST-segment elevation: The Task Force for the management of acute coronary syndromes (ACS) in patients presenting without persistent ST-segment elevation of the European Society of Cardiology (ESC). Eur Heart J. 2011;32(23):2999-3054.

37. Gupta SK, Veith FJ, Ascer E, et al. Anaphylactoid reactions to protamine: An often lethal complication in insulin-dependent diabetic patients undergoing vascular surgery. J Vasc Surg. 1989;9(2):342-50.

38. Telford AM, Wilson C. Trial of heparin versus atenolol in prevention of myocardial infarction in intermediate coronary syndrome. Lancet. 1981;1(8232):1225-8.

39. Theroux P, Waters D, Qiu S, et al. Aspirin versus heparin to prevent myocardial infarction during the acute phase of unstable angina. Circulation. 1993;88 (5 Pt 1): 2045-8.

40. Cohen M, Adams PC, Hawkins L, et al. Usefulness of antithrombotic therapy in resting angina pectoris or non-Q-wave myocardial infarction in preventing death and myocardial infarction (a pilot study from the Antithrombotic Therapy in Acute Coronary Syndromes Study Group). Am J Cardiol. 1990;66(19):1287-92.

41. Holdright D, Patel D, Cunningham D, et al. Comparison of the effect of heparin and aspirin versus aspirin alone on transient myocardial ischemia and in-hospital prognosis in patients with unstable angina. J Am Coll Cardiol. 1994;24(1):39-45.

42. Cohen M, Adams PC, Parry G, et al. Combination antithrombotic therapy in unstable rest angina and non-Q-wave infarction in nonprior aspirin users. Primary end points analysis from the ATACS trial. Antithrombotic Therapy in Acute Coronary Syndromes Research Group. Circulation. 1994;89(1):81-8.

43. Oler A, Whooley MA, Oler J, et al. Adding heparin to aspirin reduces the incidence of myocardial infarction and death in patients with unstable angina. A meta-analysis. JAMA. 1996;276(10):811-5.

44. Théroux P, Waters D, Lam J, et al. Reactivation of unstable angina after the discontinuation of heparin. N Engl J Med. 1992;327(3):141-5.

45. Kastrati A, Mehilli J, Schühlen H, et al. A clinical trial of abciximab in elective percutaneous coronary intervention after pretreatment with clopidogrel. N Engl J Med. 2004;350(3):232-8.

46. Otis SA, Zehnder JL. Heparin-induced thrombocytopenia: current status and diagnostic challenges. Am J Hematol. 2010;85(9):700-6.

47. Davoren A, Aster RH. Heparin-induced thrombocytopenia and thrombosis. Am J Hematol. 2006;81(1):36-44.

48. Tardy-Poncet B, Piot M, Chapelle C, et al. Thrombin generation and heparin-induced thrombocytopenia. J Thromb Haemost. 2009;7(9):1474-81.

49. Pouplard C, Gueret P, Fouassier M, et al. Prospective evaluation of the '4Ts' score and particle gel immunoassay specific to heparin/PF4 for the diagnosis of heparin-induced thrombocytopenia. J Thromb Haemost. 2007;5(7):1373-9.

50. Lo GK, Juhl D, Warkentin TE, et al. Evaluation of pretest clinical score (4 T's) for the diagnosis of heparin-induced thrombocytopenia in two clinical settings. J Thromb Haemost. 2006;4(4):759-65.

51. O'Gara PT, Kushner FG, Ascheim DD, et al. 2013 ACCF/AHA guideline for the management of ST-elevation myocardial infarction: executive summary: a report of the American College of Cardiology Foundation/American Heart Association Task Force on Practice Guidelines. Circulation. 2013;127(4):529-55.

52. Keeling D. Universal or selected screening for thrombophilia. Br J Haematol. 2006,133(1):106-7.

53. Cruz-Gonzalez I, Sanchez-Ledesma M, Baron SJ, et al. Efficacy and safety of argatroban with or without glycoprotein IIb/IIIa inhibitor in patients with heparin induced thrombocytopenia undergoing percutaneous coronary intervention for acute coronary syndrome. J Thromb Thrombolysis. 2008;25(2):214-8.

54. Levine GN, Bates ER, Blankenship JC, et al. 2011 ACCF/AHA/SCAI Guideline for Percutaneous Coronary Intervention: executive summary: a report of the American College of Cardiology Foundation/American Heart Association Task Force on Practice Guidelines and the Society for Cardiovascular Angiography and Interventions. Circulation 2011;124(23):2574-609.

55. Hirsh J, Guyatt G, Albers GW, et al. Executive summary: American College of Chest Physicians Evidence-based Clinical Practice Guidelines (8th Edition). Chest. 2008;133(6 Suppl):71S-109S.

56. Low-molecular-weight heparin during instability in coronary artery disease, Fragmin during Instability in Coronary Artery Disease (FRISC) study group. Lancet. 1996;347(9001):561-8.

57. Antman EM, Cohen M, Radley D, et al. Assessment of the treatment effect of enoxaparin for unstable angina/non-Q-wave myocardial infarction. TIMI 11B ESSENCE meta-analysis. Circulation. 1999;100(15):1602-8.

58. Comparison of two treatment durations (6 days and 14 days) of a low molecular weight heparin with a 6-day treatment of unfractionated heparin in the initial management of unstable angina or non-Q wave myocardial infarction: FRAX.I.S. (FRAxiparine in Ischaemic Syndrome). Eur Heart J. 1999;20(21):1553-62.

59. Cohen M, Demers C, Gurfinkel EP, et al. A comparison of low-molecular-weight heparin with unfractionated heparin for unstable coronary artery disease. Efficacy and Safety of Subcutaneous Enoxaparin in Non-Q-Wave Coronary Events Study Group. N Engl J Med. 1997;337(7):447-52.

60. Klein W, Buchwald A, Hillis SE, et al. Comparison of low-molecular-weight heparin with unfractionated heparin acutely and with placebo for 6 weeks in the management of unstable coronary artery disease. Fragmin in unstable coronary artery disease study (FRIC). Circulation. 1997;96(1):61-8.

61. Blazing MA, de Lemos JA, White HD, et al. Safety and efficacy of enoxaparin vs unfractionated heparin in patients with non-ST-segment elevation acute coronary syndromes who receive tirofiban and aspirin: a randomized controlled trial. JAMA. 2004;292(1):55-64.

62. Cohen M, Theroux P, Borzak S, et al. Randomized double-blind safety study of enoxaparin versus unfractionated heparin in patients with non-ST-segment elevation acute coronary syndromes treated with tirofiban and aspirin: the ACUTE

ll study. The Antithrombotic Combination Using Tirofiban and Enoxaparin. Am Heart J. 2002;144(3):470-7.

63. Ferguson JJ, Califf RM, Antman EM, et al. Enoxaparin vs unfractionated heparin in high-risk patients with non-ST-segment elevation acute coronary syndromes managed with an intended early invasive strategy: primary results of the SYNERGY randomized trial. JAMA. 2004;292(1):45-54.

64. Goodman SG, Fitchett D, Armstrong PW, et al. Randomized evaluation of the safety and efficacy of enoxaparin versus unfractionated heparin in high-risk patients with non-ST-segment elevation acute coronary syndromes receiving the glycoprotein IIb/IIIa inhibitor eptifibatide. Circulation. 2003;107(2):238-44.

65. Murphy SA, Gibson CM, Morrow DA, et al. Efficacy and safety of the low-molecular weight heparin enoxaparin compared with unfractionated heparin across the acute coronary syndrome spectrum: a meta-analysis. Eur Heart J. 2007;28(17):2077-86.

66. Sosnowski C. [Commentary to the article: Antman EM, Morrow DA, McCabe CH, et al. ExTRACT-TIMI 25 Investigators. Enoxaparin versus unfractionated heparin with fibrinolysis for ST-elevation myocardial infarction. N Engl J Med 2006; 354: 1477-88]. Kardiol Pol. 2006 Nov;64(11):1321-4.

67. Fifth Organization to Assess Strategies in Acute Ischemic Syndromes Investigators1, Yusuf S, Mehta SR, et al. Comparison of fondaparinux and enoxaparin in acute coronary syndromes. N Engl J Med. 2006;354(14):1464-76.

68. Mehta SR, Granger CB, Eikelboom JW, et al. Efficacy and safety of fondaparinux versus enoxaparin in patients with acute coronary syndromes undergoing percutaneous coronary intervention: results from the OASIS-5 trial. J Am Coll Cardiol. 2007;50(18):1742-51.

69. Yusuf S, Mehta SR, Chrolavicius S, et al. Effects of fondaparinux on mortality and reinfarction in patients with acute ST-segment elevation myocardial infarction: the OASIS-6 randomized trial. JAMA. 2006;295(13):1519-30.

70. Task Force on the management of ST-segment elevation acute myocardial infarction of the European Society of Cardiology (ESC), Steg PG, James SK, et al. ESC Guidelines for the management of acute myocardial infarction in patients presenting with ST-segment elevation. Eur Heart J. 2012;33(20):2569-619.

71. Reed MD, Bell D. Clinical pharmacology of bivalirudin. Pharmacotherapy. 2002;22 (6 Pt 2):105S-11S.

72. Stone GW, McLaurin BT, Cox DA, et al. Bivalirudin for patients with acute coronary syndromes. N Engl J Med. 2006;355(21):2203-16.

73. Stone GW, Witzenbichler B, Guagliumi G, et al. Bivalirudin during primary PCI in acute myocardial infarction. N Engl J Med. 2008;358(21):2218-30.

74. Lincoff AM, Kleiman NS, Kereiakes DJ, et al. Long-term efficacy of bivalirudin and provisional glycoprotein IIb/IIIa blockade vs heparin and planned glycoprotein IIb/IIIa blockade during percutaneous coronary revascularization: REPLACE-2 randomized trial. JAMA. 2004;292(6):696-703.

75. Stone GW, White HD, Ohman EM, et al. Bivalirudin in patients with acute coronary syndromes undergoing percutaneous coronary intervention: a subgroup analysis from the Acute Catheterization and Urgent Intervention Triage strategy (ACUITY) trial. Lancet. 2007;369(9565):907-19.

76. Steg PG, van't Hof A, Hamm CW, et al. Bivalirudin started during emergency transport for primary PCI. N Engl J Med. 2013;369(23):2207-17.

77. Shahzad A, Kemp I, Mars C, et al. Unfractionated heparin versus bivalirudin in primary percutaneous coronary intervention (HEAT-PPCI): an open-label, single centre, randomised controlled trial. Lancet. 2014;384(9957):1849-58.

78. Cavender MA, Sabatine MS. Bivalirudin versus heparin in patients planned for percutaneous coronary intervention: a meta-analysis of randomised controlled trials. Lancet. 2014;384(9943):599-606.

79. Bangalore S, Toklu B, Kotwal A, et al. Anticoagulant therapy during primary percutaneous coronary intervention for acute myocardial infarction: a meta-analysis of randomized trials in the era of stents and $P2Y_{12}$ inhibitors. BMJ. 2014;349:g6419.

80. Vane JR. Inhibition of prostaglandin synthesis as a mechanism of action for aspirin-like drugs. Nat New Biol. 1971;231(25):232-5.

81. MacDonald TM, Wei L. Effect of ibuprofen on cardioprotective effect of aspirin. Lancet. 2003;361(9357):573-4.

82. Andersohn F, Suissa S, Garbe E. Use of first- and second-generation cyclooxygenase-2-selective nonsteroidal antiinflammatory drugs and risk of acute myocardial infarction. Circulation. 2006;113(16):1950-7.

83. Helin-Salmivaara A, Virtanen A, Vesalainen R, et al. NSAID use and the risk of hospitalization for first myocardial infarction in the general population: a nationwide case-control study from Finland. Eur Heart J. 2006;27(14):1657-63.

84. Lewis HD Jr., Davis JW, Archibald DG, et al. Protective effects of aspirin against acute myocardial infarction and death in men with unstable angina. Results of a Veterans Administration Cooperative Study. N Engl J Med. 1983;309(7):396-403.

85. Cairns JA, Gent M, Singer J, et al. Aspirin, sulfinpyrazone, or both in unstable angina. Results of a Canadian multicenter trial. N Engl J Med. 1985;313(22):1369-75.

86. Collaborative meta-analysis of randomised trials of antiplatelet therapy for prevention of death, myocardial infarction, and stroke in high risk patients. BMJ. 2002;324(7329):71-86.

87. Randomised trial of intravenous streptokinase, oral aspirin, both, or neither among 17,187 cases of suspected acute myocardial infarction: ISIS-2. ISIS-2 (Second International Study of Infarct Survival) Collaborative Group. Lancet. 1988;2(8607):349-60.

88. Baigent C, Collins R, Appleby P, et al. ISIS-2: 10 year survival among patients with suspected acute myocardial infarction in randomised comparison of intravenous streptokinase, oral aspirin, both, or neither. The ISIS-2 (Second International Study of Infarct Survival) Collaborative Group. BMJ. 1998;316(7141):1337-43.

89. Garcia-Dorado D, Theroux P, Tornos P, et al. Previous aspirin use may attenuate the severity of the manifestation of acute ischemic syndromes. Circulation. 1995;92(7):1743-8.

90. Fuster V, Dyken ML, Vokonas PS, et al. Aspirin as a therapeutic agent in cardiovascular disease. Special Writing Group. Circulation. 1993;87(2):659-75.

91. Berger JS, Stebbins A, Granger CB, et al. Initial aspirin dose and outcome among ST-elevation myocardial infarction patients treated with fibrinolytic therapy. Circulation. 2008;117(2):192-9.

92. Reilly IA, FitzGerald GA. Inhibition of thromboxane formation in vivo and ex vivo: implications for therapy with platelet inhibitory drugs. Blood. 1987;69(1):180-6.

93. Campbell CL, Smyth S, Montalescot G, et al. Aspirin dose for the prevention of cardiovascular disease: a systematic review. JAMA. 2007;297(18):2018-24.

94. Mehta SR, Bassand JP, Chrolavicius S, et al. Dose comparisons of clopidogrel and aspirin in acute coronary syndromes. N Engl J Med. 2010;363(10):930-42.

95. Smith SC Jr., Blair SN, Criqui MH, et al. Preventing heart attack and death in patients with coronary disease. Circulation. 1995;92(1):2-4.

96. Weber AA, Zimmermann KC, Meyer-Kirchrath J, et al. Cyclooxygenase-2 in human platelets as a possible factor in aspirin resistance. Lancet. 1999;353(9156):900.

97. Jefferson BK, Foster JH, McCarthy JJ, et al. Aspirin resistance and a single gene. Am J Cardiol. 2005;95(6):805-8.

98. Tantry US, Bliden KP, Gurbel PA. Overestimation of platelet aspirin resistance detection by thrombelastograph platelet mapping and validation by conventional aggregometry using arachidonic acid stimulation. J Am Coll Cardiol. 2005;46(9):1705-9.

99. Ayanian JZ, Guadagnoli E, McNeil BJ, et al. Treatment and outcomes of acute myocardial infarction among patients of cardiologists and generalist physicians. Arch Intern Med. 1997;157(22):2570-6.

100. Krumholz HM, Radford MJ, Ellerbeck EF, et al. Aspirin in the treatment of acute myocardial infarction in elderly Medicare beneficiaries. Patterns of use and outcomes. Circulation. 1995;92(10):2841-7.

101. Bhatt DL, Steg PG, Ohman EM, et al. International prevalence, recognition, and treatment of cardiovascular risk factors in outpatients with atherothrombosis. JAMA. 2006;295(2):180-9.

102. Ridker PM, Manson JE, Gaziano JM, et al. Low-dose aspirin therapy for chronic stable angina. A randomized, placebo-controlled clinical trial. Ann Intern Med. 1991;114(10):835-9.

103. Peters RJ, Mehta SR, Fox KA, et al. Effects of aspirin dose when used alone or in combination with clopidogrel in patients with acute coronary syndromes: observations from the Clopidogrel in Unstable angina to prevent Recurrent Events (CURE) study. Circulation. 2003;108(14):1682-7.

104. Chan FK, Ching JY, Hung LC, et al. Clopidogrel versus aspirin and esomeprazole to prevent recurrent ulcer bleeding. N Engl J Med. 2005;352(3):238-44.

105. Farrell B, Godwin J, Richards S, et al. The United Kingdom transient ischaemic attack (UK-TIA) aspirin trial: final results. J Neurol Neurosurg Psychiatry. 1991;54(12):1044-54.

106. Maree AO, Fitzgerald DJ. Variable platelet response to aspirin and clopidogrel in atherothrombotic disease. Circulation. 2007;115(16):2196-207.

107. Bhatt DL, Topol EJ. Scientific and therapeutic advances in antiplatelet therapy. Nat Rev Drug Discov. 2003;2(1):15-28.

108. Angiolillo DJ, Fernandez-Ortiz A, Bernardo E, et al. Variability in individual responsiveness to clopidogrel: clinical implications, management, and future perspectives. J Am Coll Cardiol. 2007;49(14):1505-16.

109. Steinhubl SR, Ellis SG, Wolski K, et al. Ticlopidine pretreatment before coronary stenting is associated with sustained decrease in adverse cardiac events: data from the Evaluation of Platelet IIb/IIIa Inhibitor for Stenting (EPISTENT) Trial. Circulation. 2001;103(10):1403-9.

110. Balsano F, Rizzon P, Violi F, et al. Antiplatelet treatment with ticlopidine in unstable angina. A controlled multicenter clinical trial. The Studio della Ticlopidina nell'Angina Instabile Group. Circulation. 1990;82(1):17-26.

111. Schomig A, Neumann FJ, Kastrati A, et al. A randomized comparison of antiplatelet and anticoagulant therapy after the placement of coronary-artery stents. N Engl J Med. 1996;334(17):1084-9.

112. Bhatt DL, Bertrand ME, Berger PB, et al. Meta-analysis of randomized and registry comparisons of ticlopidine with clopidogrel after stenting. J Am Coll Cardiol. 2002;39(1):9-14.

113. Steinhubl SR, Tan WA, Foody JM, et al. Incidence and clinical course of thrombotic thrombocytopenic purpura due to ticlopidine following coronary stenting. EPISTENT Investigators. Evaluation of Platelet IIb/IIIa Inhibitor for Stenting. JAMA. 1999;281(9):806-10.

114. Bertrand ME, Rupprecht HJ, Urban P, et al. Double-blind study of the safety of clopidogrel with and without a loading dose in combination with aspirin compared with ticlopidine in combination with aspirin after coronary stenting: the clopidogrel aspirin stent international cooperative study (CLASSICS). Circulation. 2000;102(6):624-9.

115. Hochholzer W, Trenk D, Bestehorn HP, et al. Impact of the degree of peri-interventional platelet inhibition after loading with clopidogrel on early clinical outcome of elective coronary stent placement. J Am Coll Cardiol. 2006;48(9):1742-50.

116. Muller I, Seyfarth M, Rudiger S, et al. Effect of a high loading dose of clopidogrel on platelet function in patients undergoing coronary stent placement. Heart. 2001;85(1):92-3.

117. Dangas G, Mehran R, Guagliumi G, et al. Role of clopidogrel loading dose in patients with ST-segment elevation myocardial infarction undergoing primary angioplasty: results from the HORIZONS-AMI (harmonizing outcomes with revascularization and stents in acute myocardial infarction) trial. J Am Coll Cardiol. 2009;54(15):1438-46.

118. Amsterdam EA, Wenger NK, Brindis RG, et al. 2014 AHA/ACC Guideline for the Management of Patients With Non-ST-Elevation Acute Coronary Syndromes: Executive Summary: A Report of the American College of Cardiology/American Heart Association Task Force on Practice Guidelines. Circulation. 2014;130(25):2354-94.

119. CAPRIE Steering Committee. A randomised, blinded, trial of clopidogrel versus aspirin in patients at risk of ischaemic events (CAPRIE). Lancet. 1996;348(9038):1329-39.

120. Yusuf S, Zhao F, Mehta SR, et al. Effects of clopidogrel in addition to aspirin in patients with acute coronary syndromes without ST-segment elevation. N Engl J Med. 2001;345(7):494-502.

121. Mehta SR, Yusuf S, Peters RJ, et al. Effects of pretreatment with clopidogrel and aspirin followed by long-term therapy in patients undergoing percutaneous coronary intervention: the PCI-CURE study. Lancet. 2001;358(9281):527-33.

122. Steinhubl SR, Berger PB, Mann JT 3rd, et al. Early and sustained dual oral antiplatelet therapy following percutaneous coronary intervention: a randomized controlled trial. JAMA. 2002;288(19):2411-20.

123. Chen ZM, Jiang LX, Chen YP, et al. Addition of clopidogrel to aspirin in 45,852 patients with acute myocardial infarction: randomised placebo-controlled trial. Lancet. 2005;366(9497):1607-21.

124. Sabatine MS, Cannon CP, Gibson CM, et al. Effect of clopidogrel pretreatment before percutaneous coronary intervention in patients with ST-elevation myocardial infarction treated with fibrinolytics: the PCI-CLARITY study. JAMA. 2005;294(10):1224-32.

125. Fox KA, Mehta SR, Peters R, et al. Benefits and risks of the combination of clopidogrel and aspirin in patients undergoing surgical revascularization for non-ST-elevation acute coronary syndrome: the Clopidogrel in Unstable angina to prevent Recurrent ischemic Events (CURE) Trial. Circulation. 2004;110(10): 1202-0.

126. Mehta RH, Roe MT, Mulgund J, et al. Acute clopidogrel use and outcomes in patients with non-ST-segment elevation acute coronary syndromes undergoing coronary artery bypass surgery. J Am Coll Cardiol. 2006;48(2):281-6.

127. Ebrahimi R, Dyke C, Mehran R, et al. Outcomes following pre-operative clopidogrel administration in patients with acute coronary syndromes undergoing coronary artery bypass surgery: the ACUITY (Acute Catheterization and Urgent Intervention Triage strategY) trial. J Am Coll Cardiol. 2009;53(21):1965-72.

128. Sorensen R, Abildstrom SZ, Hansen PR, et al. Efficacy of post-operative clopidogrel treatment in patients revascularized with coronary artery bypass grafting after myocardial infarction. J Am Coll Cardiol. 2011;57(10):1202-9.

129. Jensen LO, Maeng M, Kaltoft A, et al. Stent thrombosis, myocardial infarction, and death after drug-eluting and bare-metal stent coronary interventions. J Am Coll Cardiol. 2007;50(5):463-70.

130. Alfonso F, Perez-Vizcayno MJ, Hernandez R, et al. Long-term clinical benefit of sirolimus-eluting stents in patients with in-stent restenosis results of the RIBS-II (Restenosis Intra-stent: Balloon angioplasty vs. elective sirolimus-eluting Stenting) study. J Am Coll Cardiol. 2008;52(20):1621-7.

131. Chechi T, Vecchio S, Vittori G, et al. ST-segment elevation myocardial infarction due to early and late stent thrombosis a new group of high-risk patients. J Am Coll Cardiol 2008;51(25):2396-402.

132. Iakovou I, Schmidt T, Bonizzoni E, et al. Incidence, predictors, and outcome of thrombosis after successful implantation of drug-eluting stents. JAMA. 2005;293(17):2126-30.

133. Ho PM, Peterson ED, Wang L, et al. Incidence of death and acute myocardial infarction associated with stopping clopidogrel after acute coronary syndrome. JAMA. 2008;299(5):532-9.

134. Pfisterer M, Brunner-La Rocca HP, et al. Late clinical events after clopidogrel discontinuation may limit the benefit of drug-eluting stents: an observational study of drug-eluting versus bare-metal stents. J Am Coll Cardiol. 2006;48(12):2584-91.

135. Spertus JA, Kettelkamp R, Vance C, et al. Prevalence, predictors, and outcomes of premature discontinuation of thienopyridine therapy after drug-eluting stent placement: results from the PREMIER registry. Circulation. 2006;113(24):2803-9.

136. Park SJ, Park DW, Kim YH, et al. Duration of dual antiplatelet therapy after implantation of drug-eluting stents. N Engl J Med. 2010;362(15):1374-82.

137. Gilard M, Barragan P, Noryani AAL, et al. Six-month versus 24-month dual antiplatelet therapy after implantation of drug eluting stents in patients non-resistant to aspirin: ITALIC, a randomized multicenter trial. J Am Coll Cardiol. 2014 pii: S0735-1097(14)06970-8.

138. Mauri L, Kereiakes DJ, Yeh RW, et al. Twelve or 30 Months of Dual Antiplatelet Therapy after Drug-Eluting Stents. N Engl J Med. 2014;371(23):2155-66.

139. Patti G, Colonna G, Pasceri V, et al. Randomized trial of high loading dose of clopidogrel for reduction of periprocedural myocardial infarction in patients undergoing coronary intervention: results from the ARMYDA-2 (Antiplatelet therapy for Reduction of MYocardial Damage during Angioplasty) study. Circulation. 2005;111(16):2099-106.

140. Montalescot G, Sideris G, Meuleman C, et al. A randomized comparison of high clopidogrel loading doses in patients with non-ST-segment elevation acute coronary syndromes: the ALBION (Assessment of the Best Loading Dose of Clopidogrel to Blunt Platelet Activation, Inflammation and Ongoing Necrosis) trial. J Am Coll Cardiol. 2006;48(5):931-8.

141. von Beckerath N, Taubert D, Pogatsa-Murray G, Schomig E, Kastrati A, Schomig A. Absorption, metabolization, and antiplatelet effects of 300-, 600-, and 900-mg loading doses of clopidogrel: results of the ISAR-CHOICE (Intracoronary Stenting and Antithrombotic Regimen: Choose Between 3 High Oral Doses for Immediate Clopidogrel Effect) Trial. Circulation. 2005;112(19):2946-50.

142. Mega JL, Close SL, Wiviott SD, et al. Cytochrome p-450 polymorphisms and response to clopidogrel. N Engl J Med. 2009;360(4):354-62.

143. Cuisset T, Frere C, Quilici J, et al. Benefit of a 600-mg loading dose of clopidogrel on platelet reactivity and clinical outcomes in patients with non-ST-segment elevation acute coronary syndrome undergoing coronary stenting. J Am Coll Cardiol. 2006;48(7):1339-45.

144. Matetzky S, Shenkman B, Guetta V, et al. Clopidogrel resistance is associated with increased risk of recurrent atherothrombotic events in patients with acute myocardial infarction. Circulation. 2004;109(25):3171-5.

145. Price MJ, Berger PB, Teirstein PS, et al. Standard- vs high-dose clopidogrel based on platelet function testing after percutaneous coronary intervention: the GRAVITAS randomized trial. JAMA. 2011;305(11):1097-105.

146. Gilard M, Arnaud B, Cornily JC, et al. Influence of omeprazole on the antiplatelet action of clopidogrel associated with aspirin: the randomized, double-blind OCLA (Omeprazole CLopidogrel Aspirin) study. J Am Coll Cardiol. 2008;51(3):256-60.

147. Ho PM, Maddox TM, Wang L, et al. Risk of adverse outcomes associated with concomitant use of clopidogrel and proton pump inhibitors following acute coronary syndrome. JAMA. 2009;301(9):937-44.

148. Bhatt DL, Cryer BL, Contant CF, et al. Clopidogrel with or without omeprazole in coronary artery disease. N Engl J Med. 2010;363(20):1909-17.

149. Angiolillo DJ, Capranzano P. Pharmacology of emerging novel platelet inhibitors. Am Heart J. 2008;156 (2 Suppl):S10-5.

150. Farid NA, Smith RL, Gillespie TA, et al. The disposition of prasugrel, a novel thienopyridine, in humans. Drug Metab Dispos. 2007;35(7):1096-104.

151. Brandt JT, Payne CD, Wiviott SD, et al. A comparison of prasugrel and clopidogrel loading doses on platelet function: magnitude of platelet inhibition is related to active metabolite formation. Am Heart J. 2007;153(1):66.

152. Wiviott SD, Antman EM, Winters KJ, et al. Randomized comparison of prasugrel (CS-747, LY640315), a novel thienopyridine $P2Y_{12}$ antagonist, with clopidogrel in percutaneous coronary intervention: results of the Joint Utilization of Medications to Block Platelets Optimally (JUMBO)-TIMI 26 trial. Circulation. 2005;111(25):3366-73.

153. Wiviott SD, Trenk D, Frelinger AL, et al. Prasugrel compared with high loading- and maintenance-dose clopidogrel in patients with planned percutaneous coronary intervention: the Prasugrel in Comparison to Clopidogrel for Inhibition of Platelet Activation and Aggregation-Thrombolysis in Myocardial Infarction 44 trial. Circulation. 2007;116(25):2923-32.

154. Wiviott SD, Braunwald E, McCabe CH, et al. Prasugrel versus clopidogrel in patients with acute coronary syndromes. N Engl J Med. 2007;357(20):2001-15.

155. Murphy SA, Antman EM, Wiviott SD, et al. Reduction in recurrent cardiovascular events with prasugrel compared with clopidogrel in patients with acute coronary syndromes from the TRITON-TIMI 38 trial. Eur Heart J. 2008;29(20):2473-9.

156. Montalescot G, Wiviott SD, Braunwald E, et al. Prasugrel compared with clopidogrel in patients undergoing percutaneous coronary intervention for ST-elevation myocardial infarction (TRITON-TIMI 38): double-blind, randomised controlled trial. Lancet. 2009;373(9665):723-31.

157. Cannon CP, Husted S, Harrington RA, et al. Safety, tolerability, and initial efficacy of AZD6140, the first reversible oral adenosine diphosphate receptor antagonist, compared with clopidogrel, in patients with non-ST-segment elevation acute coronary syndrome: primary results of the DISPERSE-2 trial. J Am Coll Cardiol. 2007;50(19):1844-51.

158. Storey RF, Husted S, Harrington RA, et al. Inhibition of platelet aggregation by AZD6140, a reversible oral P2Y$_{12}$ receptor antagonist, compared with clopidogrel in patients with acute coronary syndromes. J Am Coll Cardiol. 2007;50(19):1852-6.

159. Wallentin L, Becker RC, Budaj A, et al. Ticagrelor versus clopidogrel in patients with acute coronary syndromes. N Engl J Med. 2009;361(11):1045-57.

160. Mahaffey KW, Wojdyla DM, Carroll K, et al. Ticagrelor Compared With Clopidogrel by Geographic Region in the Platelet Inhibition and Patient Outcomes (PLATO) Trial. Circulation. 2011;124(5):544-54.

161. Bonaca MP, Bhatt DL, Braunwald E, et al. Design and rationale for the Prevention of Cardiovascular Events in Patients With Prior Heart Attack Using Ticagrelor Compared to Placebo on a Background of Aspirin-Thrombolysis in Myocardial Infarction 54 (PEGASUS TIMI 54) trial. Am Heart J. 2014;107(4):437-44.

162. Bhatt DL, Lincoff AM, Gibson CM, et al. Intravenous platelet blockade with cangrelor during PCI. N Engl J Med. 2009;361(24):2330-41.

163. Harrington RA, Stone GW, McNulty S, et al. Platelet inhibition with cangrelor in patients undergoing PCI. N Engl J Med. 2009;361(24):2318-29.

164. Bhatt DL, Stone GW, Mahaffey KW, et al. Effect of platelet inhibition with cangrelor during PCI on ischemic events. N Engl J Med. 2013;368(14):1303-13.

165. Lange RA, Hillis LD. The duel between dual antiplatelet therapies. N Engl J Med. 2013;368(14):1356-7.

166. Kushner FG, Hand M, Smith SC Jr., et al. 2009 Focused Updates: ACC/AHA Guidelines for the Management of Patients With ST-Elevation Myocardial Infarction (updating the 2004 Guideline and 2007 Focused Update) and ACC/AHA/SCAI Guidelines on Percutaneous Coronary Intervention (updating the 2005 Guideline and 2007 Focused Update): a report of the American College of Cardiology Foundation/American Heart Association Task Force on Practice Guidelines. Circulation. 2009;120(22):2271-306.

167. Meadows TA, Bhatt DL. Clinical aspects of platelet inhibitors and thrombus formation. Circ Res. 2007;100(9):1261-75.

168. Chew DP, Bhatt DL, Sapp S, et al. Increased mortality with oral platelet glycoprotein IIb/IIIa antagonists: a meta-analysis of phase III multicenter randomized trials. Circulation. 2001;103(2):201-6.

169. Lefkovits J, Plow EF, Topol EJ. Platelet glycoprotein IIb/IIIa receptors in cardio-vascular medicine. N Engl J Med. 1995;332(23):1553-9.

170. Bhatt DL, Topol EJ. Current role of platelet glycoprotein IIb/IIIa inhibitors in acute coronary syndromes. JAMA. 2000;284(12):1549-58.

171. Giugliano RP, White JA, Bode C, et al. Early versus delayed, provisional eptifibatide in acute coronary syndromes. N Engl J Med. 2009;360(21):2176-90.

172. Kereiakes DJ, Broderick TM, Roth EM, et al. Time course, magnitude, and consistency of platelet inhibition by abciximab, tirofiban, or eptifibatide in patients with unstable angina pectoris undergoing percutaneous coronary intervention. Am J Cardiol. 1999;84(4):391-5.

173. Proimos G. Platelet aggregation inhibition with glycoprotein IIb—IIIa inhibitors. J Thromb Thrombolysis. 2001;11(2):99-110.

174. Simoons ML. Effect of glycoprotein IIb/IIIa receptor blocker abciximab on outcome in patients with acute coronary syndromes without early coronary revascularisation: the GUSTO IV-ACS randomised trial. Lancet. 2001;357(9272):1915-24.

175. Randomised placebo-controlled trial of abciximab before and during coronary intervention in refractory unstable angina: the CAPTURE Study. Lancet. 1997; 349(9063):1429-35.

176. Topol EJ, Byzova TV, Plow EF. Platelet GPIIb-IIIa blockers. Lancet. 1999;353(9148): 227-31.

177. Montalescot G, Barragan P, Wittenberg O, et al. Platelet glycoprotein IIb/IIIa inhibition with coronary stenting for acute myocardial infarction. N Engl J Med. 2001;344(25):1895-903.

178. Stone GW, Grines CL, Cox DA, et al. Comparison of angioplasty with stenting, with or without abciximab, in acute myocardial infarction. N Engl J Med. 2002;346(13):957-66.

179. Assessment of the Safety and Efficacy of a New Thrombolytic Regimen (ASSENT)-3 Investigators. Efficacy and safety of tenecteplase in combination with enoxaparin, abciximab, or unfractionated heparin: the ASSENT-3 randomised trial in acute myocardial infarction. Lancet. 2001;358(9282):605-13.

180. Topol EJ, GUSTO V Investigators. Reperfusion therapy for acute myocardial infarction with fibrinolytic therapy or combination reduced fibrinolytic therapy and platelet glycoprotein IIb/IIIa inhibition: the GUSTO V randomised trial. Lancet. 2001;357(9272):1905-14.

181. Phillips DR, Scarborough RM. Clinical pharmacology of eptifibatide. Am J Cardiol. 1997;80(4A):11B-20B.

182. Inhibition of platelet glycoprotein IIb/IIIa with eptifibatide in patients with acute coronary syndromes. The PURSUIT Trial Investigators. Platelet Glycoprotein IIb/IIIa in Unstable Angina: Receptor Suppression Using Integrilin Therapy. N Engl J Med. 1998;339(7):436-43.

183. O'Shea JC, Buller CE, Cantor WJ, et al. Long-term efficacy of platelet glycoprotein IIb/IIIa integrin blockade with eptifibatide in coronary stent intervention. JAMA. 2002;287(5):618-21.

184. Akerblom A, James SK, Koutouzis M, et al. Eptifibatide is noninferior to abciximab in primary percutaneous coronary intervention: results from the SCAAR (Swedish Coronary Angiography and Angioplasty Registry). J Am Coll Cardiol. 2010;56(6):470-5.

185. Ohman EM, Kleiman NS, Gacioch G, et al. Combined accelerated tissue-plasminogen activator and platelet glycoprotein IIb/IIIa integrin receptor blockade with Integrilin in acute myocardial infarction. Results of a randomized, placebo-controlled, dose-ranging trial. IMPACT-AMI Investigators. Circulation. 1997;95(4):846-54.

186. Brener SJ, Zeymer U, Adgey AA, et al. Eptifibatide and low-dose tissue plasminogen activator in acute myocardial infarction: the integrilin and low-dose thrombolysis in acute myocardial infarction (INTRO AMI) trial. J Am Coll Cardiol. 2002;39(3):377-86.

187. Giugliano RP, Roe MT, Harrington RA, et al. Combination reperfusion therapy with eptifibatide and reduced-dose tenecteplase for ST-elevation myocardial infarction: results of the integrilin and tenecteplase in acute myocardial infarction (INTEGRITI) Phase II Angiographic Trial. J Am Coll Cardiol. 2003;41(8):1251-60.

188. Gibson CM, Kirtane AJ, Murphy SA, et al. Early initiation of eptifibatide in the emergency department before primary percutaneous coronary intervention for ST-segment elevation myocardial infarction: results of the Time to Integrilin Therapy in Acute Myocardial Infarction (TITAN)-TIMI 34 trial. Am Heart J. 2006;152(4):668-75.

189. Tricoci P, Newby LK, Hasselblad V, et al. Upstream use of small-molecule glycoprotein iib/iiia inhibitors in patients with non-ST-segment elevation acute coronary syndromes: a systematic overview of randomized clinical trials. Circ Cardiovasc Qual Outcomes. 2011;4(4):448-58.

190. A comparison of aspirin plus tirofiban with aspirin plus heparin for unstable angina. Platelet Receptor Inhibition in Ischemic Syndrome Management (PRISM) Study Investigators. N Engl J Med. 1998;338(21):1498-505.

191. Inhibition of the platelet glycoprotein IIb/IIIa receptor with tirofiban in unstable angina and non-Q-wave myocardial infarction. Platelet Receptor Inhibition in Ischemic Syndrome Management in Patients Limited by Unstable Signs and Symptoms (PRISM-PLUS) Study Investigators. N Engl J Med. 1998;338(21):1488-97.

192. Topol EJ, Moliterno DJ, Herrmann HC, et al. Comparison of two platelet glycoprotein IIb/IIIa inhibitors, tirofiban and abciximab, for the prevention of ischemic events with percutaneous coronary revascularization. N Engl J Med. 2001;344(25):1888-94.

193. Valgimigli M, Campo G, Percoco G, et al. Comparison of angioplasty with infusion of tirofiban or abciximab and with implantation of sirolimus-eluting or uncoated stents for acute myocardial infarction: the MULTISTRATEGY randomized trial. JAMA. 2008;299(15):1788-99.

194. Valgimigli M, Biondi-Zoccai G, Tebaldi M, et al. Tirofiban as adjunctive therapy for acute coronary syndromes and percutaneous coronary intervention: a meta-analysis of randomized trials. Eur Heart J. 2010;31(1):35-49.

195. De Luca G, Ucci G, Cassetti E, et al. Benefits from small molecule administration as compared with abciximab among patients with ST-segment elevation myocardial infarction treated with primary angioplasty: a meta-analysis. J Am Coll Cardiol. 2009;53(18):1668-73.

196. Davi G, Patrono C. Platelet activation and atherothrombosis. N Engl J Med. 2007;357(24):2482-94.

197. Krantz MJ, Kaul S. Secondary prevention of cardiovascular disease with vorapaxar: a new era of 3-drug antiplatelet therapy? JAMA Intern Med. 2015;175(1):9-10

198. Goto S, Yamaguchi T, Ikeda Y, et al. Safety and exploratory efficacy of the novel thrombin receptor (PAR-1) antagonist SCH530348 for non-ST-segment elevation acute coronary syndrome. J Atheroscler Thromb. 2010;17(2):156-64.

199. Kosoglou T, Reyderman L, Tiessen RG, et al. Pharmacodynamics and pharmaco-kinetics of the novel PAR-1 antagonist vorapaxar (formerly SCH 530348) in healthy subjects. Eur J Clin Pharmacol. 2012;68(3):249-58.

200. Voraxapar: FULL PRESCRIBING INFORMATION. 2014. (Accessed 12/21/2014, 2014, at http://www.merck.com/product/usa/pi_circulars/z/zontivity/zontivity_pi.pdf.)

201. Morrow DA, Braunwald E, Bonaca MP, et al. Vorapaxar in the secondary prevention of atherothrombotic events. N Engl J Med. 2012;366(15):1404-13.

202. Tricoci P, Huang Z, Held C, et al. Thrombin-receptor antagonist vorapaxar in acute coronary syndromes. N Engl J Med. 2012;366(1):20-33.

203. Keeley EC, Boura JA, Grines CL. Primary angioplasty versus intravenous thrombolytic therapy for acute myocardial infarction: a quantitative review of 23 randomised trials. Lancet. 2003;361(9351):13-20.

204. Gersh BJ, Anderson JL. Thrombolysis and myocardial salvage. Results of clinical trials and the animal paradigm—paradoxic or predictable? Circulation. 1993;88(1):296-306.

205. White HD, Van de Werf FJ. Thrombolysis for acute myocardial infarction. Circulation. 1998;97(16):1632-46.

206. Tsang TS, Califf RM, Stebbins AL, et al. Incidence and impact on outcome of streptokinase allergy in the GUSTO-I trial. Global Utilization of Streptokinase and t-PA in Occluded Coronary Arteries. Am J Cardiol. 1997;79(9):1232-5.

207. Hermentin P, Cuesta-Linker T, Weisse J, et al. Comparative analysis of the activity and content of different streptokinase preparations. Eur Heart J. 2005;26(9): 933-40.

208. Weaver WD, Cerqueira M, Hallstrom AP, et al. Prehospital-initiated vs hospital-initiated thrombolytic therapy. The Myocardial Infarction Triage and Intervention Trial. JAMA. 1993;270(10):1211-6.

209. Indications for fibrinolytic therapy in suspected acute myocardial infarction: collaborative overview of early mortality and major morbidity results from all randomised trials of more than 1000 patients. Fibrinolytic Therapy Trialists' (FTT) Collaborative Group. Lancet. 1994;343(8893):311-22.

210. Steg PG, Bonnefoy E, Chabaud S, et al. Impact of time to treatment on mortality after prehospital fibrinolysis or primary angioplasty: data from the CAPTIM randomized clinical trial. Circulation. 2003;108(23):2851-6.

211. American College of Emergency Physicians; Society for Cardiovascular Angiography and Interventions, O'Gara PT, et al. 2013 ACCF/AHA guideline for the management of ST-elevation myocardial infarction: a report of the American College of Cardiology Foundation/American Heart Association Task Force on Practice Guidelines. J Am Coll Cardiol. 2013;61(4):e78-140.

212. An international randomized trial comparing four thrombolytic strategies for acute myocardial infarction. The GUSTO investigators. N Engl J Med. 1993;329(10): 673-82.

213. Assessment of the Safety and Efficacy of a New Thrombolytic (ASSENT-2) Investigators, Van De Werf F, Adgey J, et al. Single-bolus tenecteplase compared with front-loaded alteplase in acute myocardial infarction: the ASSENT-2 double-blind randomised trial. Lancet. 1999;354(9180):716-22.

214. Collins R, MacMahon S, Flather M, et al. Clinical effects of anticoagulant therapy in suspected acute myocardial infarction: systematic overview of randomised trials. BMJ. 1996;313(7058):652-9.

215. Ellis SG, Tendera M, de Belder MA, et al. Facilitated PCI in patients with ST-elevation myocardial infarction. N Engl J Med. 2008;358(21):2205-17.

216. Primary versus tenecteplase-facilitated percutaneous coronary intervention in patients with ST-segment elevation acute myocardial infarction (ASSENT-4 PCI): randomised trial. Lancet. 2006;367(9510):569-78.

217. Fernandez-Avilés F, Alonso JJ, Castro-Beiras A, et al. Routine invasive strategy within 24 hours of thrombolysis versus ischaemia-guided conservative approach for acute myocardial infarction with ST-segment elevation (GRACIA-1): a randomised controlled trial. The Lancet 2004;364(9439):1045-53.

218. Cantor WJ, Fitchett D, Borgundvaag B, et al. Routine early angioplasty after fibrinolysis for acute myocardial infarction. N Engl J Med. 2009;360(26):2705-18.

219. Borgia F, Goodman SG, Halvorsen S, et al. Early routine percutaneous coronary intervention after fibrinolysis vs. standard therapy in ST-segment elevation myocardial infarction: a meta-analysis. Eur Heart J. 2010;31(17):2156-69.

220. Bonnefoy E, Lapostolle F, Leizorovicz A, et al. Primary angioplasty versus prehospital fibrinolysis in acute myocardial infarction: a randomised study. Lancet. 2002;360(9336):825-9.

221. Gershlick AH, Stephens-Lloyd A, Hughes S, et al. Rescue angioplasty after failed thrombolytic therapy for acute myocardial infarction. N Engl J Med. 2005;353(26):2758-68.

222. Secondary prevention of vascular disease by prolonged antiplatelet treatment. Antiplatelet Trialists' Collaboration. Br Med J (Clin Res Ed). 1988;296(6618):320-31.

223. Zeymer U, Jünger C, Zahn R, et al. Effects of a secondary prevention combination therapy with an aspirin, an ACE inhibitor and a statin on 1-year mortality of patients with acute myocardial infarction treated with a b-blocker. Support for a polypill approach. Curr Med Res Opin. 2011 Aug;27(8):1563-70.

224. Pfeffer MA, Braunwald E, Moye LA, et al. Effect of captopril on mortality and morbidity in patients with left ventricular dysfunction after myocardial infarction. Results of the survival and ventricular enlargement trial. The SAVE Investigators. N Engl J Med. 1992;327(10):669-77.

225. Effect of ramipril on mortality and morbidity of survivors of acute myocardial infarction with clinical evidence of heart failure. The Acute Infarction Ramipril Efficacy (AIRE) Study Investigators. Lancet. 1993;342(8875):821-8.

226. Kober L, Torp-Pedersen C, Carlsen JE, et al. A clinical trial of the angiotensin-converting-enzyme inhibitor trandolapril in patients with left ventricular dysfunction after myocardial infarction. Trandolapril Cardiac Evaluation (TRACE) Study Group. N Engl J Med. 1995;333(25):1670-6.

227. Ambrosioni E, Borghi C, Magnani B. The effect of the angiotensin-converting-enzyme inhibitor zofenopril on mortality and morbidity after anterior myocardial infarction. The Survival of Myocardial Infarction Long-Term Evaluation (SMILE) Study Investigators. N Engl J Med. 1995;332(2):80-5.

228. Dickstein K, Kjekshus J, OPTIMAAL Steering Committee of the OPTIMAAL Study Group. Effects of losartan and captopril on mortality and morbidity in high-risk patients after acute myocardial infarction: the OPTIMAAL randomised trial. Optimal Trial in Myocardial Infarction with Angiotensin II Antagonist Losartan. Lancet. 2002;360(9335):752-60.

229. Pfeffer MA, McMurray JJ, Velazquez EJ, et al. Valsartan, captopril, or both in myocardial infarction complicated by heart failure, left ventricular dysfunction, or both. N Engl J Med. 2003;349:1893-906.

230. Scirica BM, Morrow DA, Bode C, et al. Patients with acute coronary syndromes and elevated levels of natriuretic peptides: the results of the AVANT GARDE-TIMI 43 Trial. Eur Heart J. 2010;31(16):1993-2005.

231. Sharpe N, Murphy J, Smith H, et al. Treatment of patients with symptomless left ventricular dysfunction after myocardial infarction. Lancet. 1988;1(8580):255-9.

232. Packer M. Effects of b-adrenergic blockade on survival of patients with chronic heart failure. Am J Cardiol. 1997;80(11A):46L-54L.

233. Pitt B, Remme W, Zannad F, et al. Eplerenone, a selective aldosterone blocker, in patients with left ventricular dysfunction after myocardial infarction. N Engl J Med. 2003;348(14):1309-21.

234. Schwartz GG, Olsson AG, Ezekowitz MD, et al. Effects of atorvastatin on early recurrent ischemic events in acute coronary syndromes: the MIRACL study: a randomized controlled trial. JAMA. 2001;285(13):1711-8.

235. Cannon CP, Braunwald E, McCabe CH, et al. Intensive versus moderate lipid lowering with statins after acute coronary syndromes. N Engl J Med. 2004;350(15):1495-504.

236. Stone NJ, Robinson JG, Lichtenstein AH, et al. 2013 ACC/AHA guideline on the treatment of blood cholesterol to reduce atherosclerotic cardiovascular risk in adults: a report of the American College of Cardiology/American Heart Association Task Force on Practice Guidelines. Circulation. 2014;129(25 Suppl 2):S1-45.

237. Scirica BM, Morrow DA, Cannon CP, et al. Intensive statin therapy and the risk of hospitalization for heart failure after an acute coronary syndrome in the PROVE IT-TIMI 22 study. J Am Coll Cardiol. 2006;47(11):2326-31.

238. Gibson CM, Pride YB, Hochberg CP, et al. Effect of intensive statin therapy on clinical outcomes among patients undergoing percutaneous coronary intervention for acute coronary syndrome. PCI-PROVE IT: A PROVE IT-TIMI 22 (Pravastatin or Atorvastatin Evaluation and Infection Therapy-Thrombolysis In Myocardial Infarction 22) Substudy. J Am Coll Cardiol. 2009;54(24):2290-5.

239. Otagiri K, Tsutsui H, Kumazaki S, et al. Early intervention with rosuvastatin decreases the lipid components of the plaque in acute coronary syndrome: analysis using integrated backscatter IVUS (ELAN study). Circ J. 2011;75(3):633-41.

Drugs for Dysrhythmias

Rakesh Gopinathannair, Brian Olshansky

INTRODUCTION

Antiarrhythmic drugs (AADs) suppress cardiac arrhythmias through their effects on various cardiac ion channels and receptors. Although originally developed with the goal of improving survival in patients with structural heart disease and arrhythmias, large randomized clinical trials demonstrated that AADs have been a disappointment in this regard. The role of AAD therapy has undergone constant evolution over the years, as new therapies have emerged and the risk-benefit profile of these drugs on major clinical endpoints are better understood. AAD therapy continues to have a critical role in the management of patients with both atrial and ventricular arrhythmias but, for the most part, is used as an adjunct to curative therapies, such as catheter ablation as well as those targeted at improving the underlying substrate. For primary and secondary prevention of sudden cardiac death, AADs have been surpassed by implantable cardioverter defibrillators (ICDs). Many older AADs have been taken off the market, and newer, perhaps, safer AADs have taken their place.

The biggest concern a clinician faces upon deciding to initiate and maintain AAD therapy is the risk of proarrhythmia as well as systemic toxicity with AADs. Very few classes of medications exist where the initiation of therapy is guided by a "safety first" approach. Proarrhythmia may have offset the efficacy of the AADs, resulting in failure to impact hard clinical endpoints in large, randomized trials. Safety concerns also make AADs, as a class, the most complex to prescribe and monitor.

Compared to years past, a better understanding of the benefits and risks of specific AADs have led them to be used in a more selective and regulated fashion. Careful considerations of the proarrhythmic and toxic effects have led to elimination of several AADs from the market (oral procainamide, tocainide, and bretylium) and marked reduction in use of several others (quinidine, phenytoin, mexiletine, and disopyramide). At the same time, research in this arena has been strong, leading to the development and marketing of several new AADs.

AADs continue to play an important role in treatment of a wide variety of atrial and ventricular ectopy as well as tachyarrhythmias. This, plus the fact that there has been constant evolution in the risk profile as well as indications for AADs, makes it extremely important that clinicians who use these drugs be familiar with their pharmacology, mechanisms of action, indications, dosing, adverse effects, including proarrhythmic effects and drug interactions.

This chapter will describe the classification schema, clinical pharmacology, adverse effects and interactions of individual drugs. A significant portion of the chapter will be devoted to discuss the clinical role of these agents in the modern era. We will also focus on the clinical applicability of the individual agents based on available clinical data. Available data on emerging and investigational AADs will also be discussed. β-blockers and calcium-channel blockers, given their pleiotropic properties, will be discussed in detail in separate chapters.

ARRHYTHMIA MECHANISMS AND ANTIARRHYTHMIC DRUGS

Three major mechanisms contribute to development of cardiac arrhythmias: automaticity, reentry and triggered activity. AADs primarily affect ion channels (and/or receptors) in the heart and can affect various arrhythmia mechanisms by altering cardiac excitability, conduction and refractoriness. Some AADs can affect more than one cardiac ion channel (and/or receptors) and so can affect more than one arrhythmia mechanism, whereas some newer AADs can have novel mechanisms of action altogether. Some AADs are specific for certain cardiac tissue, such as atrial, ventricular, or atrioventricular (AV) nodal, whereas others have more generalized effects.

INDICATIONS FOR ANTIARRHYTHMIC DRUG THERAPY

In the modern era, the most common indication for AAD therapy is atrial fibrillation (AF).[1] Secondary prevention of ventricular arrhythmias as well as treatment of other supraventricular arrhythmias constitutes other important indications. Occasionally, AADs are used to suppress ventricular and atrial ectopy, including nonsustained ventricular tachycardia (VT). The main goal of AAD therapy in AF is to reduce symptoms and improve quality-of-life, although expectations have been raised by recent data on class III AAD dronedarone, which demonstrated mortality benefit in low-risk patients with paroxysmal AF.[2]

PROARRHYTHMIA

All AADs can be proarrhythmic, which further underlines the fact that these agents should be used judiciously. The same mechanisms that contribute to their antiarrhythmic effects can also induce arrhythmias that range from atrial or ventricular ectopy to QT prolongation and torsades de pointes. This makes it difficult to assess efficacy of the drug. Depending on drug properties, interactions with concomitant drugs, as well as patient factors, the following proarrhythmic effects are seen: (i) sinus bradycardia, (ii) atrioventricular (AV) block, (iii) increased ventricular or atrial ectopy, (iv) VT (monomorphic and polymorphic), including torsades de pointes related to QT interval prolongation, (v) ventricular fibrillation (VF) and (vi) slowing of atrial tachyarrhythmias allowing one to one AV conduction when this was not present before the drug.

CLASSIFICATION

Two major classification schemes exist. The Vaughan Williams classification classifies AADs based on their most prominent electrophysiological property and is the most clinically relevant (Table 1).[3] The "Sicilian Gambit" scheme classifies AADs based on their cellular mechanism of action, is complex, and is mostly utilized for research and drug development.[4] Neither classification is perfect. Most AADs and their active metabolites have multiple pharmacological effects, some of which are not well understood, and therefore, a "one scheme fits all" approach may be overly simplistic.

Pharmacokinetic properties and dosing of currently available oral AADs are shown in Table 2. The common uses and adverse effects of AADs are shown in Table 3, whereas the major drug interactions are listed in Table 4.

Class I Antiarrhythmic Drugs

The class I AADs act primarily by blocking the cardiac sodium (Na^+) channel. These drugs, therefore, cause significant conduction slowing by interfering with the depolarization phase of the cardiac action potential ("phase 0") and also decrease excitability (reduction in V_{max}). The magnitude of Na^+ channel blockade is determined by specific drug properties, heart rate, membrane potential and autonomic (parasympathetic and sympathetic) activation, among others.

TABLE 1: The Vaughan Williams classification of antiarrhythmic drugs

	Drug	Mechanism (Ion channel effect)	Electrophysiological effect
Class I Sodium channel blockers			
IA	■ Quinidine ■ Procainamide ■ Disopyramide	Combined sodium and potassium channel blockade, intermediate kinetics of binding and dissociation	Moderate conduction slowing (predominant effect) and increase refractoriness
IB	■ Lidocaine ■ Mexiletine	Sodium channel blockade, rapid kinetics of binding and dissociation	Shorten APD, especially in depolarized cells
IC	■ Flecainide ■ Propafenone	Sodium channel blockade, slow kinetics of binding and dissociation	Marked conduction slowing (minimal effect on refractoriness)
Class II β-blockers: β-adrenoceptor blockade			
β1-selective	■ Acebutolol (membrane stabilizing) ■ Atenolol ■ Bisoprolol ■ Esmolol (IV only) ■ Metoprolol	—	—
Non-β1-selective	■ Nadolol ■ Propranolol	—	—
Non-β-selective and α-receptor blockers	■ Carvedilol ■ Labetalol	—	—

(continued)

Table 1 (*continued*)

Drug	Mechanism (Ion channel effect)	Electrophysiological effect
Class III Potassium channel blockers		
▪ Sotalol	Block IKr and β-receptors	Prolong APD and refractoriness
▪ Amiodarone	Blocks multiple potassium channels, Na$^+$ channels, Ca^{2+} channels, β-receptors	Prolong APD and refractoriness
▪ Dronedarone	Blocks multiple potassium channels, Na$^+$ channels, Ca^{2+} channels, β-receptors	Prolong APD and refractoriness
▪ Ibutilide	Blocks IKr and late Na$^+$ current	Prolong refractoriness and APD
▪ Dofetilide	Blocks IKr	Prolong refractoriness and APD
▪ Azimilide	Blocks IKr and IKs	Prolong refractoriness and APD
Class IV Calcium channel blockers	Blocks L-type Ca^{2+} channels	Negative chronotropic and inotropic effects

APD, action potential duration; Na$^+$, sodium; Ca^{2+}, calcium; IV, intravenous; IKr, rapid delayed potassium rectifier current; IKs, slow delayed potassium rectifier current.

TABLE 2: Pharmacokinetic properties of common antiarrhythmic drugs

Drug	Daily dose (mg/day)	Route of administration	Oral bio-availability (%)	Protein binding (%)	Major elimination route	Elimination half-life	Active metabolite
Quinidine	600–1,600	Oral	80	80	Hepatic	6–12 hours	3-hydroxyquinidine
Procainamide	—	IV	—	15–20	Hepatic and renal	3–4 hours	N-acetyl procainamide
Disopyramide	400–600	Oral	80	50–65 (saturable)	Renal and hepatic	6–9 hours	Mono-N-dealkyldisopyramide
Lidocaine	—	IV, IM	—	60–80	Hepatic	2 hours	Monoethylglycinexylidide and glycinexylidide
Mexiletine	450–900	Oral	90–100	50–60	Hepatic	9–12 hours	None
Flecainide	200–400	Oral	95	40	Hepatic and renal	10–17 hours	None
Propafenone	450–675	Oral	5–50	85–97	Hepatic	2–10 hours	5-hydroxy propafenone
Metoprolol	25–200	Oral, IV	95	5–15	Hepatic	3–7.5 hours	None
Sotalol	160–320	Oral	100	0	Renal	12–16 hours	None
Dofetilide	0.5–1	Oral	90	60–70	Renal	8–10 hours	None
Ibutilide	1 mg over 10 minutes	IV	—	—	Hepatic and renal	6–9 hours	None
Amiodarone	200–400	Oral, IV	35–50	95	Hepatic	13–103 days	Desethylamiodarone

(continued)

Table 2 (continued)

Drug	Daily dose (mg/day)	Route of administration	Oral bio-availability (%)	Protein binding (%)	Major elimination route	Elimination half-life	Active metabolite
Dronedarone	800	Oral	15–20	98	Hepatic	24 hours	N-debutyl metabolite
Azimilide	75–125	Oral, IV	95	94	Hepatic and renal	4–5 days	None measurable
Verapamil	120–480	Oral, IV	20–35	90	Hepatic	3–7 hours	Norverapamil
Diltiazem	120–360	Oral, IV	40	70–80	Hepatic	4 hours	Desacetyl diltiazem; desmethyl diltiazem
Ranolazine	1,000–2,000	Oral	35–50	61–65	Hepatic and renal	1.4–1.9 hours	—
Vernakalant	3 mg/kg body weight	IV	—	—	Hepatic	1.7–5.4 hours	None

IV, intravenous; IM, intramuscular.

TABLE 3: Uses and side effects of orally available antiarrhythmic agents

Drug	Adverse effects	Uses
Class IA		
Quinidine	• Gastrointestinal • Tinnitus, hearing loss, visual disturbance, and confusion (cinchonism) • Thrombocytopenia and hemolytic anemia • Hypotension and anaphylaxis • QRS prolongation, QT prolongation, and torsades de pointes	• Secondary prevention of VT and VF (in ICD patients) • Short QT syndrome • Brugada syndrome
Procainamide	• Rash, myalgia, and vasculitis • Drug-induced lupus • Fever and agranulocytosis • Hypotension, bradycardia, QT prolongation, and torsades de pointes	• Sustained VT • Unmasking Brugada syndrome • Brugada syndrome • AF in WPW syndrome
Disopyramide	• Urinary retention, constipation, glaucoma, and xerostomia • QT prolongation and torsades de pointes • Negative inotropic effects	• Symptomatic hypertrophic cardiomyopathy • Vagally mediated AF
Class IB		
Mexiletine	• Tremor, anxiety, dysarthria, dizziness, and nystagmus • Gastrointestinal • Hypotension and bradycardia	• VT • Reduction of ICD shocks • LQT3

(continued)

Table 3 (continued)

Drug	Adverse effects	Uses
Class IC		
Flecainide	- Negative inotropy, AV block, and bradycardia - Decreases pacing threshold	- Paroxysmal AF - SVT - PVCs and idiopathic VT
Propafenone	- Confusion and irritability - Dizziness and blurred vision - Bronchospasm (in slow metabolizers) - AV block, bradycardia, and heart failure exacerbation - Decreases pacing threshold	- Paroxysmal AF - SVT - PVCs and idiopathic VT
Class II		
β-blockers	- Hypotension, bradycardia, heart block, and heart failure exacerbation - Bronchospasm - Depression - Impairment of sexual function	- Atrial arrhythmias - Rate control in AF - SVTs - PVCs - VT
Class III		
Amiodarone	- Pulmonary fibrosis - Abnormal liver function tests - Hyper or hypothyroidism - Bradycardia and heart failure exacerbation - Tremor and paresthesia	- VT - VF - Reduction of ICD shocks - AF - Atrial flutter

(continued)

Table 3 (continued)

Drug	Adverse effects	Uses
Sotalol	▪ Photosensitivity ▪ Corneal deposits ▪ Bradycardia and torsades de pointes	▪ AF in WPW syndrome ▪ Other SVTs ▪ VT in ARVD ▪ Reduction of ICD shocks ▪ AF ▪ Atrial flutter
Dofetilide	▪ Torsades de pointes	▪ Rhythm control in AF
Dronedarone	▪ Gastrointestinal side effects ▪ Fulminant hepatic failure (rare) ▪ Heart failure exacerbation (in patients with severe left ventricular dysfunction)	▪ To reduce the risk of cardiovascular hospitalization in patients with paroxysmal and persistent AF and low cardiovascular risk ▪ Rhythm control in low risk AF patients
Class IV		
Calcium channel blocker (verapamil)	▪ Hypotension, bradycardia, and AV block	▪ Idiopathic VT ▪ PVCs ▪ Rate control in AF ▪ SVTs

VT, ventricular tachycardia; VF, ventricular fibrillation; ICD, implantable cardioverter defibrillator; AF, atrial fibrillation; WPW, Wolff-Parkinson-White; ARVD, arrhythmogenic right ventricular dysplasia; LQT3, long-QT syndrome type 3; SVT, supraventricular tachycardia; PVC, premature ventricular contraction.

TABLE 4: Major drug interactions of antiarrhythmic drugs

Drug	Interacting drug	Interaction
Quinidine	Phenytoin	↓ Quinidine levels
	Phenobarbital	↓ Quinidine levels
	Rifampicin	↓ Quinidine levels
	Ketoconazole	↑ Quinidine levels
	Verapamil	↑ Quinidine levels
	Propafenone	↑ Propafenone level
	β-blockers	↑ β-blockade
	Digoxin	↑ Digoxin concentration
Mexiletine	Phenytoin	↓ Mexiletine levels
	Phenobarbital	↓ Mexiletine levels
	Rifampicin	↓ Mexiletine levels
	Ketoconazole	↑ Mexiletine levels
	Isoniazid	↑ Mexiletine levels
	Theophylline	↑ Theophylline levels
Flecainide	Digoxin	↑ Digoxin levels
	Amiodarone	↑ Flecainide levels
	Quinidine	↑ Flecainide levels
Propafenone	Digoxin	↑ Digoxin levels
	Warfarin	↓ Warfarin clearance
	Cyclosporine	↑ Cyclosporine levels
	Quinidine	↑ Propafenone levels
Amiodarone	Digoxin	↑ Digoxin effect
	Warfarin	↑ Warfarin effect
	QT prolonging drugs	↑ Risk of torsades de pointes
	β-blockers	Bradycardia and AV block
	Diltiazem and verapamil	Bradycardia and AV block
	Anesthetic drugs	Hypotension and bradycardia
	Cyclosporine	↑ Cyclosporine concentration
Sotalol	QT prolonging drugs	↑ Risk of torsades de pointes
Dofetilide	QT prolonging drugs	↑ Risk of torsades de pointes
Dronedarone	Digoxin	↑ Digoxin effect
	Cyclosporine	↑ Cyclosporine concentration
	Simvastatin	↑ Risk of myopathy
β-blockers	Quinidine	↑ β-blockade
	Amiodarone, digoxin, diltiazem, verapamil	Bradycardia
CCBs (verapamil)	Digoxin	↑ Digoxin levels

AV, atrioventricular; CCBs, calcium-channel blockers.

Based on their affinity for the cardiac sodium channel, class I drugs are further classified into IA (quinidine, procainamide, and disopyramide), IB (mexiletine and lidocaine) and IC (flecainide and propafenone).[5] The specific pharmacodynamic properties of class I AADs are shown in Table 5. The pioneering works of Hodgkin and Huxley demonstrated that sodium channels normally transit through three distinct conformational states during the action potential: open, inactivated and closed.[6]

Only open channels conduct sodium current. Sodium-channel blockers interact with open as well as inactivated channel states but not usually bind to closed channels. Thus, sodium channel blockade is phasic and depends on the conformational state of the channel. The extent of sodium channel blockers depends on the recovery rate of the sodium channel. Class IC AADs (flecainide and propafenone) cause significant conduction slowing secondary to very slow recovery from the sodium channel blockade. Alternatively, disease states, such as ischemia can slow sodium channel recovery and can increase sodium-channel blockade.

Class I drugs exhibit use-dependence. Tachycardia increases the number of sodium channels in the open and inactivated states, and since sodium-channel blockers have greater affinity for the open and inactivated channels, the extent of sodium-channel blockade and consequent conduction slowing is greater during faster heart rates. This phenomenon is called use-dependence.

Class IA drugs exhibit moderate conduction slowing and have effects in both atrial and ventricular myocardium. As listed in Table 5, they have potassium channel blocking properties and can prolong repolarization. Disopyramide, in particular, can have a marked anticholinergic effect.

A variety of serious side effects has limited the use of class IA AADs. Most importantly, they are all rapid delayed rectifier potassium current (IKr) blockers, which can result in dose-independent QT prolongation, and have the potential to cause torsades de pointes. Given modest efficacy for atrial and ventricular arrhythmias[7] and potential for serious toxicity, these agents are not used as first-line therapy anymore.

Class IA Antiarrhythmic Drugs

Quinidine

Quinidine is derived from the parent compound quinine, an antimalarial agent extracted from the bark of the cinchona tree. Quinidine blocks the rapid sodium current as well as multiple potassium currents including rapid (IKr) and slow (IKs) components of the delayed potassium rectifier current, the inward potassium rectifier current (IKI), the adenosine

TABLE 5: Pharmacodynamic properties of class I antiarrhythmic drugs

Drug class	Recovery from sodium channel	Other ion channel blockade	Other properties
Class IA			
Quinidine	Intermediate	Ito, IKr, IKs, IKATP, IKI	• Vasodilator • Anticholinergic
Procainamide	Intermediate	IKr	• Active metabolite, N-acetyl procainamide is a pure class III agent • β-blocking and anticholinergic properties • Vasodilator (intravenous procainamide)
Disopyramide	Intermediate	Ito, IKr, IKACh	• Anticholinergic • Negative inotropy
Class IB			
Lidocaine	Fast	—	—
Mexiletine	Fast	—	—
Class IC			
Flecainide	Slow	IKr, IKur	• β-blocking properties
Propafenone	Slow	IKr, IKur	• β-blocking properties

Ito, transient outward current; IKr, rapid delayed potassium rectifier current; IKs, slow delayed potassium rectifier current; IKATP, adenosine triphosphate-sensitive potassium current; IKI, inward potassium rectifier current; IKACh, acetylcholine-dependent cardiac and adenosine sensitive potassium current; IKur, ultrarapid potassium current.

triphosphate (ATP)-sensitive potassium channel (IKATP) and transient outward current (Ito). Effects of quinidine on the sodium channel result in moderate conduction slowing. Quinidine can block IKr at very low concentrations with resultant action potential prolongation and potential for torsade de pointes that is nondose dependent. Thus, quinidine is best initiated in the hospital. The IKr blockade effect is blunted at higher doses, as the sodium-channel blockade becomes prominent.[8]

Ito blockade by quinidine is believed to reduce the heterogeneity of repolarization in the right ventricular outflow tract and thereby attenuates anterior precordial ST-segment elevation in the Brugada syndrome. Quinidine has been shown to decrease ventricular arrhythmias and suppress electrical storm in small studies of Brugada syndrome patients.[9,10] Quinidine has, therefore, been used as an adjunct but not an alternative to ICD therapy in high-risk patients with Brugada syndrome.[11] Quinidine is also effective for short QT syndrome[12-15] and for idiopathic VF.[16] Quinidine has also been used to suppress ventricular arrhythmias in structural heart disease when other AADs have been tried and failed. Overall, the proarrhythmic and other adverse effects of quinidine have severely limited the role of quinidine in the management of atrial and ventricular arrhythmias.

Quinidine is an α-blocker and can result in hypotension when administered intravenously, but it is not a negative inotrope. Vagolytic effects of quinidine enhance AV conduction. Upon oral absorption, quinidine is 80% bound to plasma proteins as well as to α1 acid glycoprotein. Therefore, higher than normal dosing may be needed to keep quinidine at therapeutic levels during depolarized states, such as acute myocardial infarction. Quinidine is metabolized predominantly by the cytochrome P450 3A4 (CYP3A4) system in the liver with an elimination half-life of 6–12 hours and approximately 20% is excreted unchanged by the kidneys. The major active metabolite of quinidine, 3-hydroxyquinidine, has marked sodium channel and IKr blocking properties and is partially responsible for the clinical effects of quinidine.[17] Quinidine is also a potent inhibitor of CYP2D6, decreasing clearance of drugs, such as propafenone.[18] It also inhibits p-glycoprotein, resulting in increased serum digoxin levels.[19] Effective therapeutic plasma concentrations of quinidine are between 2 μg/mL and 5 μg/mL and no dosage adjustment is needed for renal failure or congestive heart failure.

Diarrhea is by far the most common adverse effect, happening in 30–50% of patients, and the mechanism is not well elucidated. In years past, Amphojel was used to offset this common problem, but now it is not used often due to concerns of toxicity. Thrombocytopenia can occur and is immunologic.

Headache and tinnitus are dose-dependent side effects that are part of the symptom complex known as cinchonism. Quinidine can cause idiosyncratic QT prolongation and torsades de pointes, the incidence of which is estimated to be approximately 2–4%. High plasma levels of quinidine can result in monomorphic VT secondary to sodium channel blockade. Quinidine can increase and even double the digoxin levels. The dose of quinidine is generally 200–400 mg four times a day, but long-acting preparations are available to a limited extent. There has been recent serious talk about taking quinidine off the market despite the vital role it plays in the management of select channelopathies.[20-23]

Procainamide

Procainamide is currently only available in the intravenous form in the USA. Procainamide blocks open sodium channels and has an intermediate recovery from channel block. It also blocks IKr, prolonging action potential duration. Like quinidine, procainamide slows atrial and ventricular myocardial conduction, suppresses automaticity and increases refractoriness. The major metabolite of procainamide, N-acetyl procainamide (NAPA), a class III AAD, prolongs refractoriness but lacks sodium channel blocking properties. Procainamide has negligible negative inotropic properties but is a ganglionic blocker, resulting in hypotension on intravenous use.

Procainamide is metabolized by both hepatic and renal routes, with an elimination half-life of 3–4 hours, and its elimination is in part dependent upon the rapidity of acetylation. NAPA is eliminated completely by renal excretion and, with its IKr blocking properties, can result in dose-dependent QT prolongation and torsade de pointes in patients with renal insufficiency.[24]

Like quinidine, the adverse effects as well as the proarrhythmic effects of procainamide outweigh the potential benefits in many cases, and, therefore, this drug is rarely used. Marked conduction slowing with infra-Hisian block (particularly in the presence of conduction system disease), QT prolongation, monomorphic VT, and hypotension can occur with intravenous administration. Nausea, lupus-like syndrome (positive ANA with anti-histone antibodies), and agranulocytosis are uncommon, since the oral form is not used anymore.

Intravenous procainamide is very useful in the acute management of supraventricular tachycardia, in particular, rapidly conducted AF and atrial flutter in patients with Wolff-Parkinson-White syndrome. Procainamide can help facilitate pace termination of atrial arrhythmias.[25] Intravenous procainamide is used commonly in the electrophysiology laboratory to unmask Brugada syndrome in patients with resuscitated cardiac arrest or unexplained syncope who have an abnormal baseline electrocardiogram. Procainamide may occasionally have a role in treating monomorphic VT, but this role has been generally supplanted by amiodarone.

Disopyramide

Disopyramide blocks the sodium channel resulting in moderate conduction slowing and has prominent anticholinergic and negative inotropic properties. Disopyramide is available in oral form but is hardly used.

Disopyramide is well absorbed orally (80–90% bioavailable) and undergoes hepatic metabolism, possibly utilizing the CYP3A4 system, to its major metabolite, mono-N-dealkyldisopyramide, and is excreted renally. The drug undergoes variable plasma protein binding (50–65%) which is saturable, and, therefore, measurement of disopyramide plasma concentrations is not useful clinically. The elimination half-life of disopyramide is 6–9 hours. Disopyramide can be removed by hemodialysis.

The primary use of disopyramide is in patients with hypertrophic cardiomyopathy and symptomatic left ventricular outflow tract obstruction as well as to treat vagally-mediated AF. A multicenter study of disopyramide in symptomatic hypertrophic obstructive cardiomyopathy demonstrated that 66% of patients remained asymptomatic at 3 years with a 50% reduction in outflow gradient. No mortality benefit was seen; nevertheless, disopyramide, if tolerated, should be considered before invasive options, such as surgical myectomy.[26]

Long-term use of disopyramide, however, is limited due to its severe anticholinergic effects (constipation, dry mouth and urinary retention). It cannot be used in elderly males due to the problem of urinary retention. It can prolong QT interval and cause torsades de pointes. Disopyramide is contraindicated in patients with heart failure due to marked negative inotropic properties. Disopyramide is usually used in a long-acting preparation with dosing between 400 mg/day and 600 mg/day.

Class IB Antiarrhythmic Drugs

The only currently available and utilized class IB drugs are lidocaine and mexiletine. As a group, class IB drugs block sodium channels in both open and inactivated states but have a "fast offset" in terms of channel recovery. They slow conduction primarily in ventricular myocardium and have little, if any, effect on atrial myocardium or on AV conduction. The result is shortening of action potential duration and refractoriness. They exhibit use-dependence and have marked effects in depolarized tissues, making them effective in suppression of VT in ischemic myocardium.

Lidocaine

Lidocaine, available intravenously, may be useful to treat patients who have had recurrent VT or VF (especially in the face of acute ischemia).[27] However, it has not been shown to be effective or beneficial (and may be harmful) as a prophylactic drug for patients who have had myocardial infarction.[28-30] It has negligible effects on atrial myocardium, likely attributable to very short atrial action potential duration leaving the atrial sodium channels in the open and inactivated states briefly. Lidocaine slows conduction preferentially in ischemic myocardium and can suppress reentrant arrhythmias. It can alter the excitability threshold and reduce the slope of phase-4 depolarization, thereby, reducing automaticity. Action potential duration is unaffected or shortened and no significant effects on PR interval and QRS duration are seen, whereas QT interval can shorten.

Its pharmacokinetics and dosing are complex. Since it undergoes extensive first pass metabolism in the liver, it can only be administered parenterally. Lidocaine has a rapid initial distribution (a half-life of 8 minutes) and so should be administered with multiple loading doses followed by a maintenance infusion to maintain levels in therapeutic range. The drug has two active metabolites, i.e., mono-ethylglycinexylidide and glycinexylidide that exert modest sodium channel blocking properties. Up to 70% of the drug is protein bound, and this number increases in the acute phase of a myocardial infarction when the acute phase reactant α-1-acid glycoprotein increases. As such, lidocaine levels tend to rise slowly after myocardial infarction. In congestive heart failure, where the central volume of distribution is reduced, lidocaine achieves higher than normal initial concentration and so reduction in loading dose is required to avoid toxicity. Similarly, active binding of lidocaine to α-1-acid glycoprotein, whose levels are increased in heart failure, can result in reduced drug availability in heart failure.

Lidocaine has an elimination (b) half-life of about 2 hours and steady state plasma concentrations are reached in 8–10 hours (4–5 hours half-lives). Steady state concentration is determined by hepatic blood flow.[31] Thus, maintenance dose of lidocaine should be reduced in both hepatic failure and congestive heart failure, where hepatic blood flow is decreased. No dosage adjustment is needed in renal dysfunction.

Lidocaine is usually administered as a loading dose followed by a maintenance infusion. A commonly used regimen employs an initial bolus of 75 mg, followed by 50 mg three doses at 5 minutes interval for a total loading dose of 225 mg.[32] This method usually achieves and maintains plasma concentrations in the therapeutic range of 1.55 µg/mL. This is followed by a maintenance infusion at 1–4 mg/min. Wide interindividual variability in peak plasma concentration exists and, therefore, patients should be monitored closely for evidence of toxicity during loading.

Lidocaine is most commonly used for acute suppression of potentially life-threatening ventricular arrhythmias, especially in the setting of coronary ischemia. Lidocaine administration in this setting is based more on anecdotal experience than randomized controlled clinical trials. Lidocaine is frequently ineffective, has a narrow therapeutic range, and is frequently associated with neurological toxicity. A review of the randomized trials demonstrated no mortality benefit for lidocaine in this setting.[33] Lidocaine has little effect on atrial tissue, is not useful in treating supraventricular tachycardias, and has little role in treating Wolff-Parkinson-White syndrome.[34]

The most frequent adverse effects of lidocaine are related to the central nervous system and include paresthesias, confusion, drowsiness, perioral numbness, diplopia, dysarthria, nystagmus and hallucinations. Toxic levels can result in seizures and coma. Lidocaine can worsen conduction in patients with known infranodal conduction abnormalities. Propranolol, metoprolol, and cimetidine can reduce hepatic blood flow, decrease lidocaine clearance, and concomitant administration can potentially result in lidocaine toxicity.[35,36]

Mexiletine

Mexiletine is an oral congener of lidocaine, with little effects on atrial electrophysiology, hemodynamics and ventricular function.[37] Mexiletine, almost completely absorbed orally, is primarily metabolized (90%) in the liver by the CYP2D6 system to inactive metabolites and excreted in urine. Renal excretion is pH dependent with increased renal clearance in the presence of acidic urine. Clearance is decreased in the presence of cirrhosis. Mexiletine has a plasma half-life of 9–12 hours and is only available in oral form in the USA.

Mexiletine is used primarily to suppress ventricular arrhythmias and ICD shocks in patients with structural heart disease, either as monotherapy or in combination with another AAD, such as amiodarone. Mexiletine has not been shown to improve survival in high-risk patients,[38] and effectiveness of mexiletine in suppressing ventricular arrhythmias varies widely and ranges from 6% to 60%, with majority of studies suggesting a success rate around 20%.[39] Mexiletine may shorten the QT interval and has been used to suppress arrhythmias in patients with the congenital long QT syndrome type III and in those with history of drug-induced torsades de pointes.[40]

Mexiletine is usually initiated at a dose of 150 mg every 8 hours, with slow escalation to maximally effective or maximally tolerated doses. Maximum suggested dose for maintenance is

300 mg 3–4 times a day. Patients with renal failure should be initiated at a lower dose. Dosage adjustment is also advised in patients with hepatic failure. Mexiletine has been combined with quinidine. The combination was once touted as highly effective and less proarrhythmic.[41-46] Sometimes, mexiletine is combined with amiodarone as a synergistic drug in patients who have recurrent VT, but data supporting this approach are scant.[47]

The most common adverse events with mexiletine are gastrointestinal and neurologic, and the side effects can be severe. Tremor, nausea and vomiting are common, and dizziness, confusion, blurred vision and ataxia are also seen. Mexiletine-induced tremor may respond to β-blockers. Thrombocytopenia is an uncommon side effect.[48] Neurologic side effects are dose-dependent. Gastrointestinal side effects can be ameliorated by administering the drug with food. Severe bradycardia and abnormal sinus node recovery times have been reported.

The major drug interactions of mexiletine are listed in Table 4. Inducers and inhibitors of the CYP2D6 system can influence mexiletine metabolism and can affect effectiveness and/or toxicity. Plasma theophylline concentrations are increased with coadministration secondary to decrease in theophylline clearance.[49] Digoxin and warfarin levels are unaffected.

Class IC Antiarrhythmic Drugs

Flecainide and propafenone, the currently available class IC drugs, are potent sodium-channel blockers with "slow offset" from the sodium channel, resulting in marked conduction slowing in cardiac tissues. Both drugs exhibit marked dose dependency, making them desirable agents in restoration and management of sinus rhythm in AF. At therapeutic doses, class IC drugs prolong PR and QRS intervals without having any significant effects on the QTc interval. In addition, they exhibit negative inotropic effects and can worsen heart failure in patients with left ventricular dysfunction. The use of these drugs is contraindicated in patients with left ventricular dysfunction, marked left ventricular hypertrophy, or any evidence for ischemic heart disease.[50]

Flecainide

Oral flecainide is well absorbed and is predominantly metabolized by CYP2D6 in the liver to inactive metabolites. Flecainide is also excreted renally to some extent and because of this, genetic variations in CYP2D6 do not significantly affect its pharmacological actions. Elimination half-life of flecainide ranges from 10 hours to 17 hours, permitting twice a day dosing. Flecainide absorption is delayed by milk products. Removal of milk or milk products from diet can result in higher serum levels and toxicity.[51]

Flecainide is highly effective in suppressing a variety of ventricular and supraventricular tachycardias[52] and is one of the most potent drugs to suppress ventricular ectopy.[50] At present, flecainide is most commonly used for restoration and maintenance of sinus rhythm in patients with paroxysmal AF and structurally normal hearts. It appears to be effective for vagally-mediated AF. Flecainide is also effective as a "pill-in-the-pocket" drug for AF termination.[53,54] The drug is also used to suppress symptomatic right and left ventricular outflow tract arrhythmias[55] and to treat supraventricular arrhythmias in patients with Wolff-Parkinson-White syndrome.

Flecainide was recently shown to be effective in suppression of polymorphic ectopy and VT in catecholaminergic polymorphic VT (CPVT), an inherited, potentially lethal arrhythmic syndrome resulting from mutations in the ryanodine and calsequestrin receptors, causing abnormal calcium handling. Experimental work demonstrated that flecainide has direct inhibitory effects on the defective ryanodine receptor-mediated calcium release.[56] Sodium channel blocking effects further reduced triggered activity.

In a multicenter prospective study of 29 symptomatic CPVT patients who received flecainide in addition to conventional therapy, 22 patients (76%) had partial (n = 8) or complete (n = 14) suppression of exercise-induced polymorphic ectopy and/or VT. The mean daily dose of flecainide was 150 mg in those who responded. One patient who had recurrent ICD shocks while on flecainide was found to have a low serum flecainide level. Although not randomized, these results support the utility of flecainide in CPVT.[57] Flecainide may also be beneficial for patients with long QT interval syndrome type III with a specific SCN5A (D1790G) mutation.[58] It is also used in the electrophysiology laboratory to unmask electrocardiographic conduction abnormalities in patients suspected of having Brugada syndrome.[59]

The Cardiac Arrhythmia Suppression Trial I (CAST I) demonstrated that flecainide, when used in postmyocardial infarction patients, increased mortality compared to placebo. Similar results were noted with another, now obsolete, class IC AAD—encainide.[50] In the CAST II trial, moricizine, another class I AAD, was shown to have an early proarrhythmic effect.[60] Based on these findings, class IC drugs are contraindicated in patients with ischemic and structural heart disease.

Several unique forms of proarrhythmias can occur with flecainide. In patients with monomorphic VT, especially if structural heart disease is present, flecainide can result in development of a persistent form of VT that can be impossible to cardiovert. For patients with AF, the AF can "organize" into atrial flutter, and as the flutter is rather slow, there can be one-to-one conduction in the form of a rapid wide-complex tachycardia from bundle branch aberrancy. To prevent this concerning form of "IC" flutter, rate controlling drugs, such as β-blockers or calcium channel blockers are recommended in patients with AF who are started on flecainide.

Oral flecainide is usually initiated at a dose of 50–100 mg twice a day, and slowly titrated to a maximum recommended dose of 300 mg daily. Up to 25% increase in QRS duration is seen at effective doses and is usually evaluated by exercise treadmill testing at high heart rates.[61] A single dose of 300 or 600 mg flecainide is used as a "pill-in-the-pocket" dosing.[62] Serum flecainide levels can be measured, and there is little issue with regard to active metabolites. Lower initial dosing and slow up titration is advised in patients with hepatic and renal dysfunction. Table 4 lists the major drug interactions of flecainide.

Flecainide is generally well tolerated. Common adverse effects are dose-dependent and include headache, ataxia and blurred vision. Negative inotropic effects can precipitate heart failure in patients with left ventricular dysfunction.[63] The drug can significantly increase pacing and defibrillation thresholds and so should be used with caution.[64,65] Flecainide is contraindicated in patients with suspected sodium channelopathies like Brugada syndrome, as it can worsen this condition. Additionally, caution should be exercised in patients with advanced His-Purkinje conduction system disease, as infra-Hisian block can result. The American College of Cardiology/American Heart Association/Heart Rhythm Society (ACC/AHA/HRS) AF guidelines recommend not to use flecainide in patients with substantial left ventricular hypertrophy.[53] Flecainide may also increase pacing thresholds.

Propafenone

Propafenone is structurally similar to propranolol but has electrophysiological effects that are similar to flecainide. In addition to being a potent sodium-channel blocker, propafenone has β-adrenergic blocking (about 1/30th of the potency of propranolol) and calcium channel blocking properties. Significant β-blocking property is seen in patients who are slow metabolizers of propafenone.[66]

Propafenone is metabolized through the hepatic CYP2D6 pathway into 5-hydroxypropafenone, which blocks sodium channels to a similar degree as the parent compound but lacks significant β-blocking properties. This process, however, is largely genetically determined. Approximately 7% of the USA population is deficient in CYP2D6, resulting in very slow conversion of propafenone to 5-hydroxypropafenone, with consequent accumulation of high concentrations of propafenone and significant β-antagonism in poor metabolizers.[67,68] The genetic phenotype, while determining the degree of β-blockade, does not seem to alter the antiarrhythmic effects of propafenone for most patients.

Propafenone is most commonly used to maintain sinus rhythm in patients with paroxysmal or persistent AF who have no underlying structural heart disease. Oral dosing ranges from 150 mg to 300 mg 2–3 times a day (a long-acting form is available). Peak plasma concentrations are achieved in 1–3 hours following an oral dose and, like flecainide, propafenone increases the PR and the QRS intervals without prolonging the QT interval.

The most common side effects of propafenone are nausea, dizziness and metallic taste. Neurological side effects like paresthesias and blurred vision are dose-dependent and are more common in poor metabolizers. Enhanced β-blockade resulting from poor metabolism can result in bronchospasm and asthma exacerbations. Sustained VT as a proarrhythmic effect of sodium channel blockade has been reported to occur in patients with structural heart disease and a history of VT. This is uncommon, as the drug is not used in this setting anymore. Propafenone can result in conversion of AF into slow atrial flutter with accelerated, at times 1:1 AV conduction. Therefore, when used for AF, administration of an AV nodal blocking drug along with propafenone is recommended. Propafenone is contraindicated in patients with prior myocardial infarction, known ischemic heart disease, severe ventricular hypertrophy and history of sustained VT or severe structural heart disease.[53]

Propafenone, by inhibiting CYP2C9, increases the anti-coagulant effect of warfarin by decreasing clearance. Propafenone markedly increases digoxin levels by decreasing nonrenal clearance of digoxin, and concomitant administration is not recommended. Levels of metoprolol[69] and propranolol, which are also metabolized by CYP2D6, are increased in the presence of propafenone. Quinidine, cimetidine, and antidepressants like fluoxetine and paroxetine can all inhibit CYP2D6, thereby, increasing propafenone levels.

Class II Antiarrhythmic Drugs

β-adrenergic blocking drugs are one of the most commonly used drugs in clinical cardiology. β-blockers have anti-arrhythmic properties and can reduce the risk of sudden cardiac death and ventricular arrhythmias in selected patients, inhibit sympathetically-mediated AF, prevent paroxysmal supraventricular tachyarrhythmias of various types, and have additive effects to other AADs. Specifically, β-blockers are efficacious in postoperative AF,[70] arrhythmias in the setting of thyrotoxicosis, suppression of catecholamine-mediated arrhythmias[71] that occur in CPVT, suppress delayed after depolarization-mediated idiopathic outflow tract tachycardias, and polymorphic VT in patients with long QT interval syndrome type 1.[40] They are also used to slow AV nodal conduction in patients with rapid atrial tachyarrhythmias, including AF and atrial flutter.[72] In addition, β-blockers exhibit pleiotropic effects, which are translated into survival benefits in patients with heart failure, myocardial infarction and ischemic heart disease.

By facilitating AV nodal block, β-blockers interfere with the reentry circuit in patients with AV node reentry and with AV reentry tachycardia.[73] They can suppress automaticity and trigger for atrial tachycardias, AF and VF. β-blockers can facilitate effectiveness of class I AADs. Furthermore, combination of the class III AAD amiodarone and β-blockers was most effective at preventing potentially life-threatening arrhythmias in an ICD population,[74] although the mechanism by which this occurs is not completely known.

Several β-blockers have central nervous system effects, and this effect depends on lipid solubility. Water-soluble and renally excreted β-blockers (atenolol, nadolol, sotalol and pindolol) rarely cross the blood-brain barrier, whereas lipid soluble β-blockers (propranolol, metoprolol, acebutolol and carvedilol) cross the blood-brain barrier easily. Additionally, agents, such as carvedilol, in addition to β-blocking properties and α1 antagonism, can inhibit IKr, IKs, Ito and the L-type calcium current.[75] Pharmacology and properties of specific β-blockers will be discussed in detail in a separate chapter.

Class III Antiarrhythmic Drugs

Class III AADs prolong repolarization. As a class, they predominantly block cardiac potassium channels [mainly the rapid component of the delayed-rectifier potassium channel (IKr), and to a lesser extent, the slow component of the delayed-rectifier potassium channel (IKs)], resulting in an increase in action potential duration and refractoriness in various cardiac tissues. This makes these agents very useful in interruption of reentrant circuits, whose maintenance is dependent on a critical balance between conduction velocity and refractoriness. Class III agents, such as d,l-sotalol (equimolar amounts of dextro and levo isomers) and NAPA, exhibit reverse use-dependence, where the AAD effect is most pronounced during slow heart rates. Quinidine, although classified as a class I AAD, can show reverse use-dependence for the potassium channel but use-dependence for the sodium channel.

Amiodarone, on the other hand, is a class III agent that does not demonstrate reverse use-dependence. In the current era, class III AADs are being used more and more to combat atrial and ventricular arrhythmias, whereas class I AAD use has faded.

Sotalol

Sotalol is a class III AAD with nonselective β-blocking properties. The currently available form is a racemic mixture of d- and l-stereoisomers. The dextro isomer of sotalol is a pure class III agent whereas the levo isomer is responsible for the β-blocking properties. This combination thus results in sinus slowing, decrease in AV nodal conduction [prolongs PR and Atrial-His (AH) interval], and increased refractoriness in atria, AV node, ventricle (prolongs QT interval) and accessory pathways. Sotalol is a competitive β-blocker and the β-blocking properties are pronounced at lower doses. Sotalol exhibits a modest negative inotropic effect.

Oral bioavailability of sotalol is almost 100%. Peak concentrations are seen in 2.5–4 hours following a dose. The elimination half-life is 12–16 hours and the drug is excreted unchanged by the kidneys. Renal insufficiency results in drug accumulation, increasing the risk of torsades de pointes.

Sotalol is available in the USA only in oral form. Usual starting dose of sotalol is 80 mg twice a day with gradual increase up to 240–320 mg daily, provided the QTc is within accepted limits [<500 milliseconds (ms)]. The effects on repolarization are dose-dependent and tend to occur at doses exceeding 80 mg twice a day in patients with normal renal function. Given the potential for torsades de pointes, sotalol should be started in the hospital, and the following proposed dosing algorithm is employed in patients with renal insufficiency (Table 6). Hepatic insufficiency does not require dosage adjustment. Substantial β-blocking effects make the drug unsuitable in patients with heart failure and severe left ventricular dysfunction, with approximately 3.3% incidence of heart failure or pulmonary edema.[76]

The combined class III and β-blocking properties make sotalol effective for a wide range of supraventricular and ventricular arrhythmias.[77] Sotalol is most commonly used as a rhythm control agent to maintain sinus rhythm in AF and to suppress VT in patients with ICDs. Sotalol, unlike amiodarone, tends to decrease defibrillation thresholds modestly.

TABLE 6: Dose of sotalol with respect to creatinine clearance

Creatinine clearance (mL/min) (Measured by Cockroft-Gault method)	Dosing frequency
>60	Every 12 hours
30–60	Every 24 hours
10–30	Every 36–48 hours
<10	Individualize

The Survival With Oral d-Sotalol (SWORD) trial tested the effect of d-sotalol, a pure class III drug and one that is no longer available versus placebo, on mortality in patients with previous myocardial infarction and a left ventricular ejection fraction ≤40%. The trial was stopped prematurely due to increased mortality, primarily from arrhythmic death in the d-sotalol arm.[78] In another multicenter, double-blind study of 1,456 patients with recent myocardial infarction randomized to d,l-sotalol 320 mg once a day versus placebo, the mortality rate at 1-year follow-up was not statistically different (8.9% in the sotalol group versus 7.3% in the placebo group). The reinfarction rate, however, was 41% lower in the sotalol group (p <0.05) and was attributed to the β-blocking properties of d,l-sotalol.[79]

In the Electrophysiologic Study Versus Electrocardiographic Monitoring (ESVEM) trial, a randomized, multicenter trial, primarily designed to determine the best method to guide AAD therapy for patients who had malignant ventricular arrhythmias, sotalol was effective in 31% of the patients, which was the best among the different AADs tested.[80] ESVEM, however, did not test amiodarone or ICDs. Sotalol has been shown to be effective in an ICD population where, when compared to placebo, it significantly reduced the number of both appropriate and inappropriate ICD shocks and remains one of the commonly used agents for secondary prevention of VT in the ICD population.[81]

The Sotalol Amiodarone AF Efficacy Trial (SAFE-T), a randomized, double-blind, placebo-controlled trial that compared sotalol versus amiodarone in restoration and maintenance of sinus rhythm in patients with persistent AF, randomized 665 patients to sotalol (n = 261), amiodarone (n = 261), and placebo (n = 137) who were followed for 1–4.5 years with weekly monitoring. Sotalol and amiodarone were equally efficacious in converting AF to sinus rhythm (24% in sotalol group vs. 27% in amiodarone group), and both were superior to placebo. The median time to AF recurrence, the primary endpoint was 487 days in the amiodarone group when compared to 74 days in the sotalol group and 6 days in the placebo group. Amiodarone was clearly superior to sotalol and placebo for maintenance of sinus rhythm, except in the subgroup of patients with ischemic heart disease, where sotalol was equally effective as amiodarone. Major adverse events were comparable among the three groups.[82]

Sotalol can result in QTc prolongation of 10–40 ms at doses ranging from 160 mg to 240 mg/day. In the real world, sotalol toxicity is of particular concern in a situation where patients receive concomitant diuretics with frequent dose changes and inadequate potassium replacement. The overall incidence of torsades de pointes appears to be 2% and is more common in females, structural heart disease, and is exacerbated by hypokalemia, renal insufficiency, doses more than 320 mg/day, recent cardioversion, bradycardia, and concomitant use of other AADs or QT-prolonging agents. β-blocker induced adverse effects, such as bronchospasm, masking of hypoglycemia, and rebound tachycardia and hypertension on drug withdrawal may be seen with sotalol.

Dofetilide

Dofetilide is a potent and selective oral IKr blocker that prolongs action potential duration and refractoriness, more so in the atrium than in the ventricle.[83] IKr blockade by dofetilide exhibits reverse use-dependence. Dofetilide does not exhibit any negative inotropic properties and has no effect on conduction velocity or hemodynamics.

Oral bioavailability of dofetilide exceeds 90%. Peak plasma concentrations are attained in 2-3 hours following a dose and slightly longer if the drug is taken with food. Dofetilide is excreted predominantly (80%) in the urine with an elimination half-life of 8–10 hours and partially metabolized by hepatic CYP3A4 to inactive metabolites. Drug accumulation results in renal failure, necessitating dosage adjustment and/or discontinuation. Similarly, drug that inhibits CYP3A4 can increase dofetilide concentrations and can potentially lead to adverse effects.[84]

Dofetilide is used primarily for the restoration and maintenance of sinus rhythm in AF, especially in patients with structural heart disease. Dofetilide, like amiodarone has a neutral effect on mortality when used in patients with structural heart disease and left ventricular dysfunction. The Danish Investigations of Arrhythmia and Mortality on Dofetilide (DIAMOND) trial, which evaluated dofetilide versus placebo on all-cause mortality in 1,518 patients with symptomatic congestive heart failure and severe left ventricular dysfunction, demonstrated no difference in all-cause mortality between the two arms. A significant decrease in the risk of heart failure hospitalization was observed in the dofetilide group. In patients with AF, dofetilide was significantly more effective in maintaining sinus rhythm than placebo [hazard ratio (HR) 0.35; 95% confidence interval (CI) 0.22–0.57; p <0.001]. There was a high incidence of torsades de pointes in the dofetilide group (3.3%; n = 25) when compared to the placebo group.[85]

Given the risk of torsades de pointes, dofetilide prescribing is highly regulated[86] and physicians are required to receive special training prior to prescribing dofetilide. The recommended dosage of dofetilide is 500 μg twice a day, but this is determined by baseline renal function. The drug has to be initiated in the hospital with continuous electro-cardiographic monitoring for either 3 days or 12 hours after

TABLE 7: Dose of dofetilide with respect to creatinine clearance

Creatinine clearance (mL/min) (measured by Cockcroft-Gault method)	Dosing frequency
>60	500 μg twice a day
40–60	250 μg twice a day
20–39	125 μg twice a day
<20	Contraindicated
Hemodialysis	Contraindicated

conversion to sinus rhythm, whichever is greater. Creatinine clearance needs to be measured (using the Cockcroft-Gault formula) prior to initiation. A 500 μg twice a day dosing is initiated only in patients with creatinine clearance more than 60 mL/min. The renal dosing algorithm for dofetilide is shown in Table 7. Once initiated, if the QTc at 2–3 hours following the first dose is more than 15% from baseline or more than 500 ms (>550 ms for bundle branch block or intraventricular conduction delay), then the dose needs to be cut in half. If the QTc is more than 500 ms (>550 ms for bundle branch block or intraventricular conduction delay) at any time during doses 2–6 hours, dofetilide needs to be discontinued and an alternative agent sought.

The major adverse effect of dofetilide is torsades de pointes, the incidence of which is dose-dependent and is also influenced by structural heart disease, renal insufficiency and concomitant use of QT-prolonging medications.[85,87] The overall incidence during maintenance therapy at 500 μg twice a day is around 1.7%.[88] Verapamil, trimethoprim, thiazides, azole antifungals, and cimetidine should be discontinued prior to dofetilide initiation, as concomitant administration results in markedly elevated plasma concentrations of dofetilide and increases risk of torsades de pointes.[84] Inducers of CYP3A4, such as phenobarbital and rifampicin, can enhance dofetilide metabolism and decrease its efficacy. Dofetilide does not interact with digoxin or warfarin.

Ibutilide

Ibutilide is a methane sulfonamide analog of sotalol that is a potent IKr blocker, resulting in prolongation of action potential duration and refractoriness. Experimental studies have also shown ibutilide to be an inducer of the slow inward sodium current.[89] No significant effect on heart rate, PR interval, or QRS duration is noted. Ibutilide is currently approved for rapid conversion of recent-onset AF and atrial flutter and is only available for intravenous use.

The Ibutilide Repeat Dose Study, a multicenter trial that randomized 266 patients with AF or atrial flutter of recent onset (3–45 days) to ibutilide or matching placebo, demonstrated a conversion rate of 47% with ibutilide versus 2% with placebo (p < 0.0001), with the drug being more efficacious in atrial flutter than in AF (63% vs. 31%; p < 0.0001). Following infusion, the mean time to cardioversion was 27 minutes. Of concern was the high incidence (8.3%) of torsades de pointes in the ibutilide arm.[90] Ibutilide is useful in improving the success of subsequent cardioversion when the initial attempt is followed by immediate return of AF.[91] Ibutilide is also effective in patients with AF and rapid conduction down an accessory pathway, by virtue of conversion of AF to sinus rhythm as well as by increasing accessory pathway refractoriness.[92]

Recommended intravenous dose is 1 mg to be given over 10 minutes. A second 1 mg dose, separated from the first dose by 10 minutes, can be given if the atrial arrhythmia persists. The elimination half-life is approximately 6 hours (range 2–12 hours) and the drug is primarily metabolized by the liver. No dosage adjustments are recommended for hepatic or renal dysfunction.

The major side effect of ibutilide is QTc prolongation and torsades de pointes, which developed in 8.3% of patients in the Ibutilide Repeat Dose Study.[90] Because of this, patients receiving ibutilide must have continuous electrocardiographic monitoring for at least 4–6 hours following treatment, with skilled personnel and resuscitation equipment on standby. Given higher risk of torsade de pointes, ibutilide should be avoided in patients with prolonged baseline QTc (>440 ms), advanced structural heart disease and marked hypokalemia or hypomagnesemia.

Use of ibutilide for pharmacological cardioversion of AF or atrial flutter was never popular, given the modest efficacy, risk of torsades de pointes, and the need for close monitoring following drug administration. Concurrent administration of intravenous magnesium appears to improve efficacy and safety of ibutilide.[93-97] A better method to improve the safety and efficacy of ibutilide was addressed in a recent randomized trial that assigned patients with recent onset AF to receive ibutilide alone or a combination of ibutilide and esmolol. The study demonstrated that intravenous β-blockade significantly improved the conversion rate (67% for the combination vs. 46% for ibutilide alone) with marked improvement in the safety profile (no cases of polymorphic VT in the combination group vs. 6.5% in the ibutilide group).[98] This combination of ibutilide and esmolol, along with newer agents like vernakalant, may result in an expanded role for pharmacological agents in acute conversion of rapid AF.[99]

Amiodarone

Amiodarone is structurally similar to thyroxine. It is an iodinated benzofuran derivative that was initially identified during work on the *Ammi visnaga* plant and became popular as an antianginal agent in Europe in the 1960s.[100]

Although classified as a class III AAD, amiodarone is a complex drug that is essentially in a "class of its own" due to electrophysiologic properties spanning all four Vaughan Williams classes. In addition to its multichannel blocking properties, amiodarone interacts with and can block cell surface receptors and various other molecules. To date, the exact mechanism responsible for the antiarrhythmic actions of amiodarone remains unclear. Animal experiments have shown amiodarone to prolong action potential duration and refractoriness in the atria, ventricles, AV node and His-Purkinje system.[101] Amiodarone tends to have a potent effect on prolongation of the action potential and repolarization uniformly, and perhaps for this reason, the risk of torsades de pointes is low. It also blocks inactivated sodium channels, slows phase 4 depolarization in sinus node, and delays AV nodal conduction.[102] Amiodarone blocks α- and β-receptors in a noncompetitive fashion, blocks L-type calcium channels and blocks conversion of thyroxine to triiodothyronine. Intravenous administration can result in coronary and peripheral vasodilatation.

Amiodarone is available in oral and intravenous forms with each formulation exhibiting differing electrophysiological properties. During intravenous use, amiodarone exhibits sodium and calcium channel blocking properties, exhibits use-dependence, and has a greater effect in depolarized tissues, making it very useful in treatment of ischemic ventricular arrhythmias. Oral maintenance therapy with amiodarone predominantly prolongs action potential duration and refractoriness but does not exhibit reverse use-dependence.

Amiodarone is highly lipophilic with a large volume of distribution that averages 60 L/kg (range: 20–200 L/kg).[103] Oral bioavailability is highly variable and is approximately between 35% and 65% and peak plasma concentrations are achieved 3–7 hours after an oral dose. A dose of more than 10 g, which is usually needed to saturate the fat stores, requiring weeks before a steady state is reached. Elimination is by hepatic excretion into bile. Amiodarone is metabolized by the liver to its major metabolite, desethylamiodarone. The plasma half-life after intravenous administration ranges from 4.8 hours to 68.2 hours.[104] Therapeutic plasma levels range from 1 μg/mL to 2.5 μg/mL, can be measured but do not correlate well with clinical efficacy. Elimination is slow and extremely variable with a half-life ranging from 13 days to 103 days. There is negligible renal excretion and so no dosage adjustment is needed in renal disease. Amiodarone and desethylamiodarone cannot be removed by peritoneal or hemodialysis. It is a potent inhibitor of CYP3A4, CYP2C9 and P-glycoprotein, resulting in significant drug-drug interactions.

Amiodarone is widely used for the management of both atrial and ventricular arrhythmias despite the fact that the drug is currently FDA approved only for refractory, life-threatening ventricular arrhythmias. Clinical data supporting the use of amiodarone for both atrial and ventricular arrhythmias as well as for primary and secondary prevention of sudden cardiac death are discussed below.

The impact of amiodarone in outcomes postmyocardial infarction was evaluated in the European Myocardial Infarction Amiodarone Trial (EMIAT)[105] and Canadian Amiodarone Myocardial Infarction Arrhythmia Trial (CAMIAT).[106] EMIAT randomized 1,486 postmyocardial infarction patients with a left ventricular ejection fraction less than 40% to receive either amiodarone (n = 743) or matching placebo (n = 743). Presence of ventricular arrhythmia was not needed for inclusion. After a mean follow-up of 21 months, a 35% risk reduction (p <0.05) in arrhythmic death was seen in the amiodarone group but no difference in all-cause or cardiovascular death was seen.[105]

In CAMIAT, 1,202 patients who were 6–45 days after a myocardial infarction and had a mean of at least 10 premature ventricular contractions (PVCs)/hour were randomly assigned to amiodarone (n = 606) or placebo (n = 596) and followed for a mean of 1.8 years. When compared to placebo, patients in the amiodarone group had a 48.5% reduction (p = 0.016) in the combined endpoint of resuscitation from VF or arrhythmic death (3.3% in the amiodarone group vs. 6.6% in the placebo group). Like EMIAT, there was no significant difference in all-cause mortality (p = 0.13) between the two groups.[106]

EMIAT and CAMIAT demonstrated that amiodarone given postmyocardial infarction can reduce arrhythmic death and had a neutral effect on total mortality. A pooled post-hoc analysis of EMIAT and CAMIAT demonstrated that the combination of amiodarone with a β-blocker significantly improved arrhythmic death or resuscitated cardiac arrest when compared to β-blockers alone, amiodarone alone, or placebo. Nonsignificant reductions in total mortality were noted with the combination when compared to those not receiving β-blockers.[107]

Estudio Piloto Argentino de Muerte Súbita y Amiodarone (EPAMSA), Grupo de Estudio de la Sobrevida en la Insuficiencia Cardiaca en Argentina (GESICA) and Congestive Heart Failure Survival Trial of Antiarrhythmic Therapy (CHF-STAT) were randomized trials that evaluated the role of amiodarone in patients with congestive heart failure.[108-110] EPAMSA randomized patients with a left ventricular ejection fraction ≤35% and asymptomatic ventricular arrhythmias to receive either amiodarone (n = 66) or placebo (n = 61) and demonstrated a significant reduction in total mortality (10.6 vs. 28.8%, p = 0.02) and sudden death (7 vs. 20.4%, p = 0.04) in patients receiving amiodarone compared to placebo.[108]

GESICA was a multicenter, randomized trial of 516 patients in Argentina with congestive heart failure and left ventricular systolic function ≤35% but no history of symptomatic ventricular arrhythmias. Only 39% of the patient population had ischemic cardiomyopathy. Compared to placebo, amiodarone resulted in a 28% reduced risk of death and a 31% reduced risk of heart failure hospitalizations.[109]

In CHF-STAT, 647 patients with congestive heart failure, a left ventricular ejection fraction ≤40%, and at least 10 PVCs/hour, were randomized to amiodarone (n = 336) or placebo (n = 338). Over a median follow-up of 45 months, amiodarone was associated with PVC suppression and improved left ventricular function, but no significant difference in total mortality or sudden death was found between the two groups.[110] Discontinuation rates for amiodarone in these studies ranged from 20% to 40%. The higher percentage of ischemic cardiomyopathy in CHF-STAT is a potential reason for differences in outcomes in CHF-STAT versus EPAMSA and GESICA.

A meta-analysis of 15 randomized controlled trials (n = 8,522) of amiodarone versus placebo for prevention of sudden cardiac death demonstrated that amiodarone was associated with a 29% reduced risk of sudden cardiac death (7.1 vs. 9.7%; OR 0.72, p < 0.001) and an 18% reduced risk of cardiovascular death (14.0 vs. 16.3%; OR 0.82, p = 0.004). No significant difference in all-cause mortality was demonstrated. The modest improvement in cardiac and arrhythmic death came at a cost as patients who received amiodarone had a significantly higher incidence of thyroid problems (OR 5.68; p <0.0001), hepatotoxicity (OR 2.1; p = 0.015), lung toxicity (OR 1.97; p = 0.002), and bradyarrhythmias (OR 1.78; p = 0.008) when compared to the control group.[111]

In summary, amiodarone is beneficial to treat ventricular arrhythmias in patients with structural heart disease and is a reasonable option for secondary prevention of sudden cardiac death in patients who either refuse or are not otherwise candidates for an ICD. Currently, however, the most common use for amiodarone in patients with structural heart disease is to suppress recurrent episodes of VT and VF leading to ICD shocks. Amiodarone can increase the defibrillation threshold in ICD patients, but the effects may be modest.[64,74] Amiodarone can also slow VT rates to below the programmed detection limits for the ICD.[64]

Amiodarone remains the most potent AAD to maintain sinus rhythm in patients with AF. This was shown clearly in the Canadian Trial of AF (CTAF), a prospective, multicenter trial that randomized 403 patients with at least one episode of AF in the past 6 months to receive amiodarone or either, sotalol or propafenone. Patients were followed for a mean of 16 months with the primary endpoint being first recurrence of AF. The primary endpoint was reached in 35% of patients in the amiodarone group versus 63% in the sotalol or propafenone groups (p < 0.001). Adverse reactions were higher in the amiodarone group (18 vs. 11% in the sotalol/propafenone group) but were not statistically significant.[112]

Amiodarone was equally efficacious as sotalol in restoring sinus rhythm but was vastly superior to sotalol in maintaining sinus rhythm, with major adverse events comparable to placebo.[82] A Cochrane database review of 45 randomized controlled studies (n = 12,559) that evaluated the different AADs used for rhythm control of AF demonstrated that class IA, class IC, and class III drugs all demonstrated a significant reduction in AF recurrence (odds ratio 0.19–0.60, number needed to treat; 2–9) compared to placebo, but none improved mortality. Class IA drugs actually increased mortality and all drugs, except propafenone and amiodarone, increased proarrhythmic risk.[7]

Given huge volume of distribution, a loading dose regimen is essential to ensure onset of therapeutic action within a reasonable time frame. Loading can be via the intravenous or oral route. The manufacturer recommended intravenous infusion regimen follows three phases over 24 hours: 150 mg over 10 min (with an additional bolus dose of 150 mg for patients with recurrent VT), followed by 1 mg/min over the next 6 hours, followed by 0.5 mg/min over next 18 hours.

Even with intravenous loading, the actual class III electrophysiological effects do not necessarily take place for several days. Alternatively, if possible, oral loading with high dosages can be useful for patients with recurrent VT and those patients for whom AF is highly problematic. In the hospital, oral loading can be initiated with doses as high as 600 mg thrice a day for up to 7–10 days. At this high dose, various neurological and gastrointestinal side effects may be observed.

For outpatient initiation, we routinely employ a loading regimen (400 mg three to four times a day) that ensures a 10–15 g loads within 7–10 days after initiation. Following completion of the loading period, the patient is switched to a maintenance dose of 200 mg/day for AF and 400 mg/day for secondary prevention of VT.

Intravenous amiodarone infusion should preferably be through a central line to avoid risk of phlebitis and cellulitis in the event of extravasation. Hypotension is common with intravenous use and should be monitored closely. Chronic oral therapy with amiodarone is reasonably well tolerated, provided close attention is paid to screen for and recognize adverse events.[113]

Side effects are common and can range from 15% in the first year to 50% with long-term use. Amiodarone prolongs PR, QRS and QT intervals, but the incidence of torsades de pointes is extremely rare, perhaps, resulting from multichannel and β-blocking properties.[114] No significant negative inotropic effects are seen at maintenance doses. Sinus bradycardia and AV block can occur.[113]

Amiodarone has significant extracardiac side effects, with the most serious one being interstitial pneumonitis leading to pulmonary fibrosis.[115] The incidence of pulmonary fibrosis ranges from 1% to 7% and is very difficult to predict and challenging to detect with reduction in diffusion capacity for carbon monoxide (DLCO) being the best screening test.[115,116] Thyroid problems are common, and both hyperthyroidism and hypothyroidism can occur. Hepatotoxicity can occur but rarely progresses to cirrhosis. Other significant extracardiac side effects include hypersensitivity to the sun, bluish skin discoloration, central and peripheral neurological effects (weakness, walking difficulty especially in the elderly), and rarely, optic neuritis resulting in vision loss. Almost all patients on chronic amiodarone therapy develop corneal microdeposits, but these are of little clinical importance.[113]

Majority of the adverse reactions secondary to amiodarone can be easily managed and do not necessitate drug discontinuation. Since most side effects of amiodarone depend, in part, on the dose and the duration of therapy, the lowest possible effective dose should be used for chronic maintenance therapy. Despite this, regular screening for adverse events is essential. At initiation of therapy, all patients should have a 12-lead electrocardiogram, chest X-ray, pulmonary function test with DLCO, laboratory evaluation for electrolytes and renal function, liver function and thyroid function. An ophthalmological evaluation is recommended at baseline if there is visual impairment and a follow-up evaluation should be done for new eye-related symptoms. Liver function and thyroid function tests are assessed every 6 months. An electrocardiogram and a chest X-ray should be repeated yearly. Follow-up pulmonary function tests should be done for new or unexplained dyspnea or if there are abnormalities in the chest X-ray compared to baseline.[113]

Amiodarone increases serum levels of digoxin, quinidine, procainamide, flecainide, cyclosporine and warfarin. It also decreases statin metabolism through CYP3A4, resulting in increased statin levels and increasing risk of myopathy. Warfarin as well as statin dose should be reduced in half and digoxin should be discontinued if a patient is started on amiodarone. The major drug interactions of amiodarone are listed in Table 4.

Dronedarone

Dronedarone is structurally similar to amiodarone except that it lacks the iodine moiety and was developed with idea of maintaining potency while eliminating amiodarone-induced systemic toxicity attributable to the iodine moiety. Although it has multichannel blocking properties similar to amiodarone, it is far less potent in maintenance of sinus rhythm in AF. For clinical purposes, dronedarone is classified as a Vaughan Williams class III AAD, but exhibits myriad electrophysiological properties including inhibitory effects on the rapid delayed rectifier, slow delayed rectifier, acetylcholine-activated, inward rectifier potassium channels, inward sodium current, T- and L-type calcium channels and α- and β-adrenoceptors.[117,118] Suppressed sinus node automaticity and alteration of the slope of phase 4 depolarization in the sinus node results in sinus slowing.[119] Dronedarone also slows AV conduction, increases AV nodal and ventricular effective refractory period and has been shown to reduce VT and PVCs in ischemic animal models.[117,120]

Dronedarone has negligible proarrhythmic effect but has been shown to increase mortality and heart failure hospitalization in patients with acute heart failure, severe left ventricular dysfunction and high-risk patients with permanent AF.[121,122] When compared to amiodarone, dronedarone appears devoid of pulmonary, hepatic, thyroid and neurological toxicity. Like amiodarone, dronedarone causes mild increase in serum creatinine without affecting the glomerular filtration rate. This is secondary to inhibition of the renal tubular cation transport.[123]

Dronedarone is metabolized by the hepatic CYP3A4 system. Dronedarone, in turn, is an inhibitor of the CYP3A4, CYP2D6 and P-glycoprotein systems. These inhibitory properties can result in increased levels of drugs like cyclosporine, digoxin, and some statins when coadministered with dronedarone.[123] No drug interactions with warfarin have been reported.

Several randomized trials have evaluated the role of dronedarone in AF and heart failure.[2,121,122,124-127] These are listed in Table 8 and the recent major trials are summarized below.

The ATHENA (A Placebo-Controlled, Double-Blind, Parallel Arm Trial to Assess the Efficacy of Dronedarone 400 mg BD for the Prevention of Cardiovascular Hospitalization or Death from Any Cause in Patients with Atrial Fibrillation/Atrial Flutter) trial assessed the effect of dronedarone in reducing a composite endpoint of death or cardiovascular hospitalizations in 4,628 paroxysmal or persistent AF patients who had risk factors for stroke and/death.[2] Patients were randomized to dronedarone or placebo and were followed for a median of

TABLE 8: Summary of randomized clinical trials that assessed the efficacy and safety of dronedarone in patients with atrial fibrillation and heart failure

Clinical trial	Patient profile	Number of patients	Intervention (mg)	Primary end-point	Follow up (month)	Results
DAFNE[124]	Persistent AF post-cardioversion	199	Dronedarone (400–800 BD) vs. placebo	Time to first recurrence of AF	6	Use of dronedarone associated with longer median time to AF recurrence (60 vs. 5.3 days for dronedarone and placebo, respectively; p = 0.026; 55% relative risk reduction, p = 0.001); likewise, patients receiving dronedarone, 400 mg orally twice a day, more likely to maintain sinus rhythm compared with patients receiving placebo
EURIDIS[127]/ADONIS[127]	Paroxysmal AF	1,237	Dronedarone (400 BD) vs. placebo	Time to first recurrence of AF	12	Dronedarone significantly lengthened the time to AF recurrence (41 vs. 96 days [EURIDIS] and 59 vs. 158 days [ADONIS] for dronedarone and placebo, respectively), as well as symptoms associated with atrial fibrillation, compared with placebo. Ventricular rates during AF recurrence were significantly lower with dronedarone
DIONYSOS[125]	Persistent AF for >3 days	504	Dronedarone (400 BD) vs. amiodarone (600 and then 200/day)	AF recurrence or drug intolerance resulting in discontinuation	7	More patients on dronedarone had AF recurrence or stopped the drug due to intolerance or lack of efficacy compared with patients receiving amiodarone (75.1 vs. 58.8% for dronedarone and amiodarone, respectively, HR 1.59)
ERATO[126]	Permanent AF with ventricular rates >80 bpm on rate-controlling agents	630	Dronedarone (400 BD) vs. placebo	Mean ventricular rate at 2 weeks	1	Dronedarone use associated with decrease in ventricular rate, at rest (12.3 bpm with dronedarone vs. 0.2 bpm with placebo) and with exercise (25.6 bpm with dronedarone vs. 2.2 bpm with placebo)

(continued)

Table 8 (continued)

Clinical trial	Patient profile	Number of patients	Intervention (mg)	Primary end-point	Follow up (month)	Results
ATHENA[2]	Paroxysmal or persistent AF or atrial flutter with one or more associated risk factors	4,628	Dronedarone (400 BD) vs. placebo	Composite of all-cause mortality and cardiovascular hospitalization	21 ± 5	The use of dronedarone was associated with decreased cardiovascular deaths and arrhythmic deaths compared with placebo (31.9% in dronedarone arm vs. 39.8% in placebo arm, HR 0.76). There was also a decrease in hospitalizations for AF and acute coronary syndrome in patients receiving dronedarone compared with placebo
ANDROMEDA[122]	Congestive heart failure (NYHA Class III-IV); left ventricular ejection fraction <35%	627	Dronedarone (400 BD) vs. placebo	All-cause mortality or heart failure hospitalization	2	Trial stopped early. Dronedarone associated with increase in all-cause mortality (8.1% in the dronedarone arm vs. ≥8% in placebo arm, HR 2.13)
PALLAS[121]	Permanent AF with high risk for vascular events	3,236	Dronedarone (400 BD) vs. placebo	Composite of stroke, myocardial infarction systemic embolism, or death from cardiovascular causes	~1 year	Trial stopped early due to safety concerns. Primary outcome occurred in 43 patients in the dronedarone arm when compared to 19 in the placebo arm (HR 2.29; 95% CI 1.34–3.94; p = 0.002). Cardiovascular deaths, arrhythmic deaths, stroke, and heart failure hospitalizations were higher in the dronedarone arm when compared to placebo

DAFNE, the phase II Dronedarone Atrial Fibrillatio N study after Electrical cardioversion; EURIDIS/ADONIS, European Trial In Atrial Fibrillation Or Flutter Patients Receiving Dronedarone For The Maintenance of Sinus Rhythm/American-Australian-African Trial With Dronedarone In Atrial Fibrillation/flutter Patients For The Maintenance of Sinus Rhythm studies; DIONYSOS, the Efficacy & Safety of Dronedarone vs. Amiodarone for the Maintenance of Sinus Rhythm in Patients With Atrial Fibrillat on study; ERATO, the Efficacy and safety of dRonedarone for the cOntrol of ventricular rate during atrial fibrillation study; ATHENA, A Placebo-Controlled, Double-Blind, Parallel Arm Trial to Assess the Efficacy of Dronedarone 400 mg BD for the Prevention of Cardiovascular Hospitalization or Death from Any Cause in Patients with Atrial Fibrillation/Atrial Flutter trial; ANDROMEDA, Antiarrhythmic Trial with Dronedarone in Mode ate to Severe Congestive Heart Failure Evaluating Morbidity Decrease; PALLAS, the Permanent Atrial Fibrillation Outcome Study Using Dronedarone on Top of Standard Therapy trial; NYHA, New York Heart Association; BD, twice a day; AF, atrial fibrillation; HR, hazard ratio; CI, confidence interval.

In summary, although it is fair to say that dronedarone has definitely expanded the horizon in terms of management options for AF, more studies are needed to understand the mechanisms underlying the diametrically opposite effects of this drug in low-risk versus high-risk AF patients.

Azimilide

Azimilide dihydrochloride is a class III AAD that blocks both the rapid (IKr) and the slow (IKs) delayed rectifier potassium channels.[132] Unlike other class III drugs, azimilide does not exhibit reverse use-dependence and this is presumed to be secondary to IKs blockade.

Azimilide prolongs the action potential duration and refractoriness in atrial and ventricular myocardium and has been shown to cause dose-dependent QTc prolongation.[132] In a randomized study of 3,713 patients, 1–3 weeks after a myocardial infarction and with a left ventricular ejection fraction of 15–35%; azimilide did not show any survival advantage when compared to placebo. The incidence of torsades de pointes and severe neutropenia were 0.3% and 0.9%, respectively, and were slightly higher than in that placebo group.[133]

The effectiveness of azimilide in reducing ICD therapies was evaluated in the international Shock Inhibition Evaluation with azimilide (SHIELD) trial. SHIELD randomized 633 patients to azimilide, either 75 mg (n = 220) or 125 mg (n = 199) daily, or matching placebo (n = 214). All enrolled patients had an ICD implanted and had either a documented episode of cardiac arrest or spontaneous sustained VT with left ventricular ejection fraction ≤0.40 during 42 days prior to the first ICD implantation or an ICD shock for spontaneous VT or VF within the previous 180 days. Patients were followed for a median of 1 year and the primary endpoint was all-cause shocks and symptomatic tachycardia terminated by antitachycardia pacing and appropriate ICD therapies.[134] Azimilide at 75 mg/day demonstrated a 57% reduction in the primary endpoint compared to placebo (HR = 0.43; CI 0.26–0.69; p = 0.0006), whereas a 47% reduction was seen in the azimilide 125 mg/day group (HR = 0.53; CI 0.34–0.83; p = 0.0053). When compared to placebo, azimilide 75 and 125 mg/day reduced appropriate ICD shocks and ATP by 48% (p = 0.017) and 62% (p = 0.0004), respectively. Drug discontinuation rates were high (35–40%) but comparable in both the drug and placebo groups. Four patients in the azimilide group and one in the placebo group had torsades de pointes. Thus, it appears that azimilide has beneficial effects in prevention of ventricular arrhythmias in ICD patients and is currently approved for this clinical use in Europe but not in the USA. A multicenter placebo-controlled randomized trial (SHIELD 2) to assess the efficacy of azimilide in reducing cardiovascular hospitalizations/emergency visits was prematurely stopped by the sponsor.

Two trials evaluated the effectiveness of azimilide in maintenance of sinus rhythm in AF. The North American Azimilide Cardioversion Maintenance Trial (A-COMET II) study compared azimilide (125 mg once a day) with sotalol (160 mg twice a day) or placebo for maintaining sinus rhythm in 658 patients with persistent AF who were undergoing electrical cardioversion.[135] Azimilide was found to be superior to placebo in preventing recurrence of AF but was significantly inferior to sotalol in this regard.

The Azimilide Supraventricular Tachyarrhythmia Reduction (A-STAR) trial[136] randomized 220 patients to azimilide (125 mg once a day) versus matching placebo. There was no significant difference between the azimilide and placebo groups in terms of time to first recurrence of AF. A dose-dependent increase in torsades de pointes was noted with the incidence rates ranging from 0.3% for the 75 mg dose to 1.2% for the 100 mg dose.[137] Thus, in terms of AF rhythm control, the risk-benefit ratio has not been in favor of azimilide and the drug, therefore, has faded from the AF scene.

Class IV Antiarrhythmic Drugs

Verapamil and diltiazem are the most commonly employed calcium-channel blockers to combat arrhythmias. Both verapamil and diltiazem block the slow calcium channel and decrease the L-type calcium current in all cardiac myocytes. Electrophysiological effects include reduction in the plateau height of the action potential without significant changes in action potential amplitude or rate of rise of phase 0. Verapamil and diltiazem suppress sinus and AV nodal conduction and, therefore, are used to control the ventricular response rate in atrial flutter and AF as well as to suppress AV-node dependent supraventricular arrhythmias. Furthermore, these drugs can prevent delayed after depolarization-mediated triggered activity and can inhibit idiopathic ventricular outflow tract tachycardias as well as certain focal atrial tachycardias by this mechanism. A specific reentrant form of VT, the idiopathic left septal VT, is exquisitely sensitive to verapamil. The dose of verapamil is 120–480 mg/day in single or divided doses and diltiazem 120–360 mg/day in divided doses. Both verapamil and diltiazem are available in oral and intravenous formulations.

Other Drugs

Adenosine

Adenosine is an ultrashort acting endogenous purine nucleoside agonist that is approved for the acute termination of symptomatic supraventricular arrhythmias and certain idiopathic VT. It is also vagotonic. Adenosine exerts its cardiac actions by binding to the adenosine A1 receptor on the extracellular surface of the cardiac myocytes, in turn, activating the acetylcholine-dependent cardiac and adenosine-sensitive potassium channels (IKACh/IKAdo). This results in increased outward potassium current, which leads to shortening of atrial action potential duration and membrane hyperpolarization and transient AV nodal block and sinus node depression.[138] IKAdo channels are absent in the ventricular myocytes and so adenosine has not much of an effect in the ventricular myocardium.

Indirectly, adenosine has an antiadrenergic action due to inhibition of adenylate cyclase, resulting in a decrease in cyclic AMP and subsequent decrease in L-type calcium current. This property accounts for its suppressive effect on outflow tract VT as well subgroup of focal atrial tachycardias, which are delayed after depolarization-mediated triggered rhythms resulting from intracellular calcium overload. Adenosine also decreases the funny channel (I_f) current in the sinus node cells, resulting in a reduction in V_{max}. Similar actions are seen in the AV node, resulting in increase in AH interval, and high degree, transient, AV block. His-Purkinje conduction is not usually affected.

Adenosine is administered commonly as an intravenous bolus of 6 or 12 mg followed by a flush. If given by a central venous route, a smaller dose (3 mg) is recommended. Pediatric dose is 0.1–0.3 mg/kg administered intravenously. Adenosine is eliminated rapidly from the extracellular space by various mechanisms, including enzymatic degradation, phosphorylation, or cellular reuptake with an elimination half-life of a few seconds. Adenosine has a rapid onset of action following intravenous administration and results in almost immediate sinus node slowing and transient AV block, making this as an excellent choice to terminate AV node-dependent supraventricular tachycardias, such as AV node reentry and orthodromic AV reentry tachycardias. Adenosine can terminate idiopathic VT originating from the ventricular outflow tract location[139] as well as some focal atrial tachycardias mediated by triggered activity.[140] Adenosine normally does not affect accessory pathway conduction, and this property is made use of in the electrophysiology laboratory to diagnose the presence of a concealed accessory pathway. The vasodilatory properties of adenosine make it a suitable agent for pharmacological stress testing in the diagnosis of myocardial ischemia.

Adverse effects of adenosine typically include dyspnea, flushing and bronchospasm. These are short-lasting and resolve quickly. Adenosine should be used cautiously in patients with reactive airway disease. Shortening of atrial refractory periods can result in AF in 10–15% of patients and the drug is sometimes used to test the efficacy of pulmonary vein isolation procedure for AF. Transplanted hearts are exquisitely sensitive to adenosine and dose reduction up to 1 mg is recommended.[141] Methylxanthines (caffeine and theophylline) block adenosine receptors and counteract the effects of adenosine. Dipyridamole reduces the reuptake of adenosine, thereby prolonging the effect of adenosine and so people on oral dipyridamole who are undergoing pharmacologic stress testing should not receive adenosine but should instead receive intravenous dipyridamole as the stressing agent.

FUTURE OF ANTIARRHYTHMIC THERAPY

Throughout this discussion, there is an underlying theme that AADs are by no means perfect in terms of arrhythmia treatment and those substantial side effects and proarrhythmia have changed their use. Results from the controlled clinical trials [International Mexiletine and Placebo Antiarrhythmic Coronary Trial (IMPACT),[142] CAST,[60] SWORD,[78] Acute Lung Injury Ventilator Evaluation (ALIVE), DIAMOND, CHF-STAT, Sudden Cardiac Death in Heart Failure Trial (SCD-HeFT), CAMIAT, EMIAT, SHIELD, Atrial Fibrillation Follow-up Investigation of Rhythm Management (AFFIRM) and PALLAS] do not suggest a brilliant future but, instead, a jaded past. In fact, many of the drugs, such as procainamide, phenytoin, bretylium, encainide, moricizine, tocainide, quinidine, etc. are disappearing. Optimism over dronedarone has also faded. So where does that leave us? The future of AADs in many ways remains bright and includes atrial selective ion channel blockers, I_f blockers, ranolazine, sarcoendoplasmic reticulum ATPase (SERCA) modifiers, ion channel modification by gene therapy, stem cells and therapy for genetic disorders.

NEWER ANTIARRHYTHMIC AGENTS

Vernakalant

Vernakalant is the first in the new generation of AADs that demonstrate electrophysiological effects preferentially in the atrium and not in the ventricle. Atrial-selective agents are currently being developed to restore and maintain sinus rhythm in AF while avoiding adverse ventricular events, such as QTc prolongation and torsades de pointes.[143]

Vernakalant acts selectively in the atrium, targeting multiple ion channels including the ultrarapid potassium current IKur, acetylcholine-mediated potassium current IKACh, IKATP, Ito and late sodium current (INa).[144] These actions result in prolongation of atrial refractoriness as well as atrial conduction slowing. The recommended dose is a single intravenous infusion of 3 mg/kg administered over 10 minutes. No dose adjustment is necessarily based on patient characteristics and concomitant drugs.[145]

Three randomized, placebo-controlled, double-blind Atrial Arrhythmia Conversion (ACT) trials[146-148] tested the efficacy and safety of intravenous vernakalant (administered as a 10-minute intravenous infusion at a dose of 3 mg/kg followed by a second 10-minute infusion at a dose of 2 mg/kg 15 minutes later if AF had not been terminated) for treatment of AF. The ACT I and ACT III trials investigated vernakalant in the treatment of patients with sustained AF (duration >3 hours, but not more than 45 days). These two trials enrolled 612 patients and found that vernakalant was significantly more efficacious than placebo for conversion of AF to sinus rhythm. In ACT I, sinus rhythm was achieved in 62% of patients receiving vernakalant compared with 4.9% of patients receiving placebo for AF of 3–48 hours duration.[146] In ACT III, 51.2% of patients receiving vernakalant converted to sinus rhythm compared with 3.6% of patients receiving placebo for AF of 3 hours to 7 days.[148] The median time conversion was 10 minutes from the start of infusion and sinus rhythm was maintained more than 24 hours in 97% of patients. The ACT II trial evaluated the efficacy of intravenous vernakalant in 150 patients with sustained AF (3–72 hours duration) that occurred between 24 hours and 7 days after coronary artery bypass graft and/ or valvular surgery and showed that vernakalant resulted in a 47% conversion rate of AF to sinus rhythm compared to 14% for placebo.[147]

The AVRO (A Phase III Superiority Study of Vernakalant vs. Amiodarone in Subjects With Recent Onset Atrial Fibrillation) trial randomized 254 patients with recent onset of AF (3–48 hours duration) to intravenous vernakalant or intravenous amiodarone and demonstrated that vernakalant achieved a superior conversion rate (51.7% of patients to sinus rhythm at 90 minutes) compared to amiodarone (5.2%).[149]

Available data show that vernakalant does not appear to be effective in atrial flutter or AF of longer duration (>7 days).[148] Studies are ongoing to determine efficacy and safety of an oral formulation (5 mg/kg). Vernakalant is well tolerated with common side effects being nausea, dysgeusia, paresthesias and hypotension.[148] No episodes of drug-induced torsades de pointes were reported in the ACT trials.

Intravenous vernakalant is currently approved in Europe for rapid conversion of recent-onset AF (≤7 days duration for nonsurgery patients and ≤3 days duration for postcardiac surgery patients) to sinus rhythm in adults.[150] In the USA, although the FDA recommended approval of vernakalant in 2007, the drug is not currently available for clinical use as more safety and efficacy data are being collected.[151] The study, called the ACT 5, is currently suspended as one patient developed cardiogenic shock. The study has not been restarted. Thus, vernakalant, by virtue of its atrial selectivity, good conversion rate, and excellent safety profile, appears to be an important agent for pharmacological conversion of AF, although it is not clear whether it is time yet to "get into the ACT" even if oral vernakalant becomes available.[152]

Tedisamil

Tedisamil blocks multiple potassium channels, including IKr, IKs, IKur, Ito and IKATP, and is classified as a Vaughan Williams class III AAD.[153] These ion channels effect prolong atrial and ventricular action potential duration and refractoriness. The effects of tedisamil, however, appear to be more pronounced in the atrial tissue. Tedisamil also causes sinus node slowing and appears to have antianginal properties.[137] The elimination half-life of tedisamil is 8–13 hours. The drug is not metabolized and is renally excreted.

A small, randomized, placebo-controlled dose-response study of 175 patients demonstrated that tedisamil at doses of 0.4 and 0.6 mg/kg was superior to placebo in converting new-onset AF to sinus rhythm, with a 41% conversion rate for 0.4 mg/kg and 51% conversion rate for the 0.6 mg/kg group. Two patients in the tedisamil group had ventricular arrhythmias (one case of torsades de pointes and one case of monomorphic VT).[153] Tedisamil appears promising, but more studies are needed to further evaluate its safety and efficacy.

Ivabradine

High resting sinus heart rates have been independently associated with mortality and major adverse cardiovascular outcomes.[154-157] Ivabradine is a selective I_f current blocker in the sinus node, resulting in sinus slowing, independent of autonomic tone.[158]

Results from the prospective, randomized, double-blind, placebo-controlled parallel group Systolic Heart Failure Treatment with I_f Inhibitor Ivabradine Trial (SHIFT)[159] of patients with congestive heart failure (left ventricular ejection fraction ≤0.35 and heart rate ≥70 despite standard medical therapy) indicated that ivabradine (titrated to a maximum of 7.5 mg twice a day) can consistently lower the heart rate over long-term when compared to matching placebo and can significantly improve the primary endpoint of cardiovascular death or hospitalization for worsening heart failure.

In this rather large study (n = 6,558), hospitalizations for worsening heart failure (672 placebo vs. 514 ivabradine; HR 0.74; 0.66–0.83; p < 0.0001) and mortality due to heart failure (151 vs. 113; HR 0.74; 0.58–0.94; p = 0.014) was clearly better in the ivabradine group and with few serious side effects, but more patients in the ivabradine group (5%) had symptomatic bradycardia versus the placebo group (1%), p < 0.0001.

Ivabradine, to lower heart rate, may not be beneficial for all patients at risk. In the randomized, prospective, double-blind, placebo-controlled BEAUTIFUL (morbidity-mortality Evaluation of the I_f inhibitor ivabradine in patients with coronary disease and left ventricular dysfunction) trial[160] of 10,917 eligible patients who had coronary artery disease and a left-ventricular ejection fraction of less than 40%, outcomes were not clearly improved by ivabradine. Considering the primary composite endpoint of cardiovascular death, admission to hospital for acute myocardial infarction, and admission to hospital for new onset or worsening heart failure, ivabradine did not affect the primary composite endpoint but in patients with a heart rate ≥70 beats per minute (bpm), ivabradine treatment did reduce secondary endpoints: admission to hospital for fatal and nonfatal myocardial infarction (0.64; 95% CI 0.49–0.84; p = 0.001) and coronary revascularization (0.70; 95% CI 0.52–0.93; p = 0.016).

Ivabradine, in combination with a β-blocker, can be effective to prevent angina.[161]

Ivabradine has emerged as a promising treatment for inappropriate sinus tachycardia (IST), which, at times, can be debilitating and refractory to medical therapy. In a prospective, randomized, cross-over study of 21 patients with highly symptomatic IST, use of ivabradine (5 mg twice daily) resulted in significant decline in HR at rest, with standing and with moderate exercise, and was associated with more than 70% symptom resolution in all patients and complete elimination of symptoms in 47% of patients.[162] In patients already on well-tolerated doses of metoprolol, adding ivabradine had a synergistic role in HR reduction and associated significant reduction in symptoms and improvement in exercise capacity.[163] When compared with metoprolol, ivabradine resulted in similar heart rate reduction but patients on ivabradine had significant reduction in symptoms,[164] ivabradine has also been shown to be beneficial in postural orthostatic tachycardia syndrome (POTS).[165]

While the exact role for heart rate reduction with ivabradine remains somewhat uncertain, for select individuals, it may be time to redefine tachycardia.[157] Usual dose for ivabradine is 5–7.5 mg twice a day. This drug is currently not available for use in the USA.

Ranolazine

Ranolazine is an antianginal drug approved for the treatment of chronic angina in patients who have not responded to standard antianginal medications.[166] The antianginal mechanism of ranolazine was believed to result from the drug's ability to block the late sodium current, thereby, suppressing calcium and sodium overload in response to ischemia. This selective affinity for the late sodium current has resulted in ranolazine being investigated as a novel AAD.[167]

In ventricular myocardium, ranolazine inhibits the late sodium channel (late INa) and the rapidly activating component of the IKr.[167,168] In atrial myocardium, in addition to late INa and IKr, ranolazine also inhibits the peak INa.[169,170] Ranolazine does not seem to have any effect on IK1 and Ito.[168] Ranolazine has no effect on resting membrane potential in the atria as well as in the ventricle. In therapeutic concentrations, action potential amplitude and duration in the ventricle is not affected, but the rate of rise of action potential upstroke (V_{max}) in the atria is significantly depressed and action potential duration prolonged. The drug prolongs effective refractory period, increases the diastolic excitation threshold and reduces conduction velocity in the atrial myocardium.[168]

In the Metabolic Efficiency With Ranolazine for Less Ischemia in Non-ST-Elevation Acute Coronary Syndrome Thrombolysis in Myocardial Infarction 36 (MERLIN-TIMI 36) trial, ranolazine significantly lowered nonsustained VT and supraventricular tachyarrhythmias in patients with non-ST elevation myocardial infarction when compared to placebo.[171] Recent data from a canine model suggest that ranolazine in combination with dronedarone may be a potent combination to reduce AF.[172] Early clinical studies have shown that a single dose of 2 g of ranolazine was highly effective as a "pill-in-the-pocket" approach to AF, converting 77% of patients, without any significant side effects.[173] These included patients with structural heart disease, a contraindication for current class IC agents, and could potentially expand the use of ranolazine.

Available data show that ranolazine is associated with a good safety profile, even in patients with structural heart disease.[171] Although it can block IKr and prolong QT interval, torsade de pointes has not been reported, possibly secondary to late INa inhibition.[168,174] What is sorely lacking, despite encouraging animal and early clinical data, is a randomized placebo-controlled trial evaluating antiarrhythmic efficacy of ranolazine in both atrial and ventricular arrhythmias. One such study, the Ranolazine Implantable Cardioverter-Defibrillator Trial (RAID), where ranolazine is compared to standard medical therapy for reducing ventricular arrhythmias and death in ICD patients is currently enrolling and is expected to complete in 2015 (ClinicalTrials.gov identifier NCT01215253).[168]

ON THE HORIZON

Cellular Calcium Handling

Sarcoendoplasmic reticulum ATPase (SERCA) appears to be potentially critical in the regulation of intracellular calcium along with stabilization by the ryanodine (RyR2) receptor.[175,176] There is a dynamic interplay between the sarcolemmal transport of calcium, the intracellular transport of calcium and sodium, the autonomic nervous system and morphological and ultrastructural remodeling. The ryanodine receptor has been implicated as causal for the development for CPVT. Additionally, the ryanodine receptor, affecting intracellular calcium handling has been implicated as a cause for ventricular arrhythmias in heart failure. Furthermore, calcium modulated-dependent protein kinase (CaMKII) has been considered an effector of the ryanodine receptor. This may also influence the presence of ventricular arrhythmias. SERCA may also be a cause for ventricular arrhythmias that lead to sudden cardiac death. Therefore, therapies that affect these potential targets may be valuable to reduce the risk of potentially life-threatening ventricular arrhythmias. To date, the data are rather sketchy that therapy can be developed in this regard.

The ryanodine receptor (RyR2) stabilizer, JTV-519 enhances the binding of the protein calstabin-2 to the ryanodine receptor, thereby, correcting abnormal calcium handling.[177,178] The common form of the disease CPVT is due to a gain of function ryanodine receptor mutation, resulting in increased intracellular calcium leading to delayed after depolarization-mediated triggered VT. JTV-519 can attenuate increased diastolic sarcoplasmic reticulum calcium leak of the mutant ryanodine receptor. One problem, however, is that JTV-519 may bind to other ryanodine receptor regions under other specific conditions. Other drugs are being developed to affect this potential target.

Another approach is to consider gene transfer. In experimental models, it is possible to affect SERCA2 and prevent triggered activity leading to VF.[179] The risk of developing alternans in the action potential and the incidence of VF is markedly reduced. This would suggest that perhaps gene transfer is a new approach to be considered.

Gene Therapies—Potential ("Near Practical") Applications

There are a variety of exciting possibilities with regard to the use of gene therapies as antiarrhythmic therapy.[180] Consideration has been given to use gene therapy to enhance automaticity in patients with bradycardia (a biological pacemaker), gene therapy to affect AV conduction and slow conduction in AF, and gene therapy to affect the presence of VT by affecting repolarization and accelerating conduction.

With regard to attempts to create a biopacemaker, genes only can be transferred into cells. In this way, there would be episomal overexpression of ion channels (Adv-Kir2.1AAA, NCN and SPC). Another approach is to have a hybrid of genes and cells that can lead to either cell fusion [hyperpolarization-activated cyclic nucleotide-gated (HCN) in a fibroblast] or spontaneous junctional coupling (HCN in mesenchymal stem cells). Another approach that has been considered is to use stem cells to "entrain" and pace cells.[180]

Gene therapy has also been considered to reduce the ventricular rate in AF.[181] In one report, gene therapy was performed using wild type GEM gene transfer in swine hearts. After 7 days, the AH and PR intervals increased, and the ventricular rate in AF decreased with or without atropine or isoproterenol compared with baseline controls. The ventricular refractory period can also be extended using gene therapy. In rats, Kv1.3 fibroblast transplants can be shown to almost double the ventricular effective refractory period.[182] Additionally, in an animal model of inducible VT, use of a viral vector to transfect the KCNH2-G628S channel completely eliminated VT and markedly prolonged action potential duration when compared to controls.[183]

To date, there is a long list of potential gene therapies to affect electrical dysfunction, including therapies and targets for atrial arrhythmias and ventricular arrhythmias as well as for biopacemaker development.[184] There are various gene targets and various vectors to deliver the gene. The methodology is rather complex and the target tissue quite variable. All of the studies have been performed in animals. Nevertheless, the data are intriguing and suggestive that there may be potent ways to affect arrhythmias using gene transfer.

One major concern, however, is that stem cells could be proarrhythmic and, therefore, a double-edged sword.[185] Nevertheless, stem cell technology is progressing rapidly and further developments and refinement may indeed bring about the dawn of "personalized medicine".

OLD DRUGS WILL BE NEW AGAIN

There still may be a role for old drugs, which can affect clinical syndromes and channelopathies that are only now being understood. For example, while rather uncommon, the short QT interval syndrome (SQTS) cannot be well treated by standard AAD therapy. Nevertheless, for SQTS1, quinidine (or disopyramide) may be the only drug(s) that could be effective.[12,15] For SQTS2, 3, class III AADs may be effective and for SQTS4, 5, quinidine due to its Ito blocking effects may be helpful.[12-15] Due to its effect on the Ito channel, quinidine may be effective for the Brugada syndrome.[9] Furthermore, propafenone appears to have unique benefits to treat AF in patients with SQTS.[15] For patients with long QT interval syndrome (LQTS 3), mexiletine, flecainide, or ranolazine may be effective therapy.[15]

DRUGS WITH NOVEL ANTIARRHYTHMIC MECHANISMS

Several novel agents with antiarrhythmic properties are under various stages of preclinical research. These include nifekalant, an IKr blocker, for use in ventricular arrhythmias, several IKur (and multichannel) blockers (AVE0118, AZD7009 and NIP-141/142), sodium current blockers (pilsicainide), amiodarone analogs (celivarone, ATI-2042 and PM 101), selective IKs blockers (HMR1556) and Kv1.5 blockers (XEN-D0101).[186]

Other drugs, which work by novel mechanisms, are also being developed and include tertiapin-Q, a specific inhibitor of the atrial acetylcholine regulated potassium current (IKACh), KB-R7943 that acts as a sodium/calcium exchange inhibitor, GsMTx-4 as a SAC (stretch channel) blocker, those that are gap junction modifiers (rotigaptide, GAP-134), those that antagonize the serotonin 5-hydroxytryptamine receptors (RS-100-302), and those that are long-acting adenosine A1 receptors (tecadenoson and selodenoson).[186]

ANTIARRHYTHMIC DRUG SELECTION IN ATRIAL FIBRILLATION

The primary principle that guides AAD selection in AF is "safety over efficacy." This principle is reflected in the 2014 ACC/AHA/HRS guidelines for management of AF that provide recommendations regarding AAD selection if rhythm control is planned for AF.[187] For patients with no evidence of structural heart disease or who have hypertension without substantial left ventricular hypertrophy, flecainide, propafenone, sotalol, dofetilide or dronedarone is first-line therapy, followed by amiodarone or catheter ablation. In patients with coronary artery disease, dofetilide, dronedarone or sotalol is first-line therapy followed by amiodarone or catheter ablation. For heart failure patients, amiodarone or dofetilide is first-line therapy, followed by catheter ablation. The guidelines state that dronedarone may be considered for rhythm control in AF patients who do not have heart failure. Dronedarone is contraindicated in patients with NYHA III-IV heart failure or if they have had a decompensated heart failure episode within the last 4 weeks. Dronedarone is also contraindicated in permanent AF.[187]

OUTPATIENT VS. IN-HOSPITAL INITIATION FOR ANTIARRHYTHMIC DRUG THERAPY

The severity of the arrhythmia and the proarrhythmic risk of the AAD determine whether the drug should be initiated in the hospital. All class IA AADs should be started in the hospital given the potential risk of idiosyncratic, nondose dependent torsades de pointes. Mexiletine, the only orally available class IB AAD, can be started and titrated as an outpatient treatment, as the risk of proarrhythmia is low. Class IC AADs have a very low risk of proarrhythmia and can be started as an outpatient treatment, provided structural heart disease and severe left ventricular hypertrophy are ruled out. If initiated for AF, it is recommended to add an AV blocking drug along with the class IC agent to reduce the risk of atrial flutter with rapid ventricular rates. Sotalol and dofetilide should be initiated in the hospital due to the risk of developing dose-dependent QT prolongation and torsades de pointes. Dofetilide must be started in the hospital and strict regulations govern its initiation and titration. Amiodarone can be started as an outpatient for patients who have AF and atrial flutter, as the proarrhythmic risk is low. On the other hand, if used for secondary prevention of VT, it is preferable to initiate amiodarone in the hospital. Although amiodarone prolongs QT interval, incidence of torsades de pointes with amiodarone is extremely low. Dronedarone is generally not proarrhythmic and can be started outside the hospital.

ANTIARRHYTHMIC DRUGS IN PREGNANCY AND LACTATION

An overview of the effect of various AADs in pregnancy and lactation is presented in Table 9. Sotalol is the only pregnancy

TABLE 9: Antiarrhythmic drugs in pregnancy and lactation

Agent	Pregnancy	Lactation
Quinidine	C	Excreted
Procainamide	C	Excreted
Disopyramide	C	Excreted
Mexiletine	C	Excreted
Flecainide	C	Excreted
Propafenone	C	?
Sotalol	B	Excreted
Dofetilide	C	?
Dronedarone	X	?
Amiodarone	D	Excreted

category B [either animal-reproduction studies have not demonstrated a fetal risk, but there are no controlled studies in pregnant women, or animal-reproduction studies have shown an adverse effect (other than a decrease in fertility) that was not confirmed in controlled studies in women in the first trimester (and there is no evidence of a risk in later trimesters)] agent, while amiodarone is classified as pregnancy category D [there is positive evidence of human fetal risk, but the benefits from use in pregnant women may be acceptable despite the risk (e.g., if the drug is needed in a life-threatening situation or for a serious disease for which safer drugs cannot be used or are ineffective)]. Dronedarone is a pregnancy category X drug (studies in animals or human beings have demonstrated fetal abnormalities, or there is evidence of fetal risk based on human experience or both, and the risk of the use of the drug in pregnant women clearly outweighs any possible benefit) and so is contraindicated in women who are or may become pregnant. The rest of the AADs are considered pregnancy category C [either studies in animals have revealed adverse effects on the fetus (teratogenic or embryocidal or other), and there are no controlled studies in women, or studies in women and animals are not available. Drugs should be given only if the potential benefit justifies the potential risk to the fetus]. β-blockers can be safely used in pregnancy except atenolol, which is a pregnancy category D drug.

ANTIARRHYTHMIC DRUG-DEVICE INTERACTIONS

AADs, especially amiodarone and sotalol, are commonly used in an ICD population to suppress VT and prevent ICD shocks. When used in this setting, AADs can affect pacemaker and defibrillation thresholds. In addition, AADs can slow VT rate to below the programmable limits, can cause sinus node dysfunction and AV block, and, occasionally, can be proarrhythmic. The effects of various AADs on pacing and defibrillation thresholds are listed in Table 10.

The Optimal Pharmacologic Therapy in cardioverter Defibrillator Patients (OPTIC) trial was a prospective, randomized study that compared the effects of β-blockers, β-blocker and amiodarone, and sotalol on defibrillation energy requirements in 94 ICD patients. The study found that changes in defibrillation threshold with amiodarone and sotalol are at best modest and argues against repeat defibrillation threshold testing after initiating therapy with either drug.[188] The combination of amiodarone and a β-blocker was most effective in preventing ICD shocks at 1 year and was more effective than sotalol (10.3 vs. 24.3% for sotalol; HR 0.43; p = 0.02).[74]

TABLE 10: Effect of antiarrhythmic drugs on defibrillation and pacing thresholds

Drug	Pacing threshold	Defibrillation threshold
Quinidine	Increases	Increases
Procainamide	Increases	No change/increases
Lidocaine	No change	Increases
Flecainide	Increases	Increases
β-blockers	Increases	Decreases
Digoxin	Decreases	Decrease or no change
Ibutilide	Not known	Decreases
Sotalol	No effect	Decreases
Amiodarone	No effect	Increases
Dofetilide	No change	Decreases
Verapamil	Increases	Not known

CONCLUSION

AADs therapy continues to play an important role in the management of a wide variety of atrial and ventricular arrhythmias. Their role has changed over time, as newer and better therapies aimed at curing arrhythmias and modifying underlying disease process have taken center stage. While the future of AAD therapy may not necessarily be as bright as it once was, many enticing possibilities exist, and the field is by no means without future. Translating therapeutic possibility into clinical reality remains the challenge. Several currently available drugs have found new indications for use. Novel therapeutic targets for patients with arrhythmias are far from over, but, as we have learned, innovation will require extensive clinical testing in lieu of important hard endpoints.

REFERENCES

1. Gopinathannair R, Sullivan RM, Olshansky B. Update on medical management of atrial fibrillation in the modern era. Heart Rhythm. 2009;6(8 Suppl):S17-22.
2. Hohnloser SH, Crijns HJ, van Eickels M, et al. Effect of dronedarone on cardiovascular events in atrial fibrillation. N Engl J Med. 2009;360(7):668-78.
3. Vaughan Williams EM. A classification of antiarrhythmic actions reassessed after a decade of new drugs. J Clin Pharmacol. 1984;24(4):129-47.
4. The Sicilian gambit. A new approach to the classification of antiarrhythmic drugs based on their actions on arrhythmogenic mechanisms. Task Force of the Working Group on Arrhythmias of the European Society of Cardiology. Circulation. 1991;84(4):1831-51.
5. Harrison DC. Antiarrhythmic drug classification: new science and practical applications. Am J Cardiol. 1985;56(1):185-7.
6. Hodgkin AL, Huxley AF. A quantitative description of membrane current and its application to conduction and excitation in nerve. J Physiol. 1952;117(4):500-44.
7. Lafuente-Lafuente C, Mouly S, Longás-Tejero MA, et al. Antiarrhythmic drugs for maintaining sinus rhythm after cardioversion of atrial fibrillation: a systematic review of randomized controlled trials. Arch Intern Med. 2006;166(7):719-28.

8. Antzelevitch C, Shimizu W, Yan GX, et al. The M cell: its contribution to the ECG and to normal and abnormal electrical function of the heart. J Cardiovasc Electrophysiol. 1999;10(8):1124-52.

9. Belhassen B, Glick A, Viskin S. Efficacy of quinidine in high-risk patients with Brugada syndrome. Circulation. 2004;110(13):1731-7.

10. Mok NS, Chan NY, Chiu AC. Successful use of quinidine in treatment of electrical storm in Brugada syndrome. Pacing Clin Electrophysiol. 2004;27(6 Pt 1):821-3.

11. Mizusawa Y, Sakurada H, Nishizaki M, et al. Effects of low-dose quinidine on ventricular tachyarrhythmias in patients with Brugada syndrome: low-dose quinidine therapy as an adjunctive treatment. J Cardiovasc Pharmacol. 2006;47(3): 359-64.

12. Kaufman ES. Quinidine in short QT syndrome: an old drug for a new disease. J Cardiovasc Electrophysiol. 2007;18(6):665-6.

13. Milberg P, Tegelkamp R, Osada N, et al. Reduction of dispersion of repolarization and prolongation of postrepolarization refractoriness explain the antiarrhythmic effects of quinidine in a model of short QT syndrome. J Cardiovasc Electrophysiol. 2007;18(6):658-64.

14. Wolpert C, Schimpf R, Giustetto C, et al. Further insights into the effect of quinidine in short QT syndrome caused by a mutation in HERG. J Cardiovasc Electrophysiol. 2005;16(1):54-8.

15. Kaufman ES. Mechanisms and clinical management of inherited channelopathies: long QT syndrome, Brugada syndrome, catecholaminergic polymorphic ventricular tachycardia, and short QT syndrome. Heart Rhythm. 2009;6(8 Suppl):S51-5.

16. Belhassen B, Glick A, Viskin S. Excellent long-term reproducibility of the electrophysiologic efficacy of quinidine in patients with idiopathic ventricular fibrillation and Brugada syndrome. Pacing Clin Electrophysiol. 2009;32(3):294-301.

17. Thompson KA, Murray JJ, Blair IA, et al. Plasma concentrations of quinidine, its major metabolites, and dihydroquinidine in patients with torsades de pointes. Clin Pharmacol Ther. 1988;43(6):636-42.

18. Caporaso NE, Shaw GL. Clinical implications of the competitive inhibition of the debrisoquin-metabolizing isozyme by quinidine. Arch Intern Med. 1991;151(10): 1985-92.

19. Fromm MF, Kim RB, Stein CM, et al. Inhibition of P-glycoprotein-mediated drug transport: a unifying mechanism to explain the interaction between digoxin and quinidine [see comments]. Circulation. 1999;99(4):552-7.

20. Estes NA 3rd, Page RL. To the editor: response—Irreplaceable antiarrhythmic medications are disappearing: the case of quinidine. Heart Rhythm. 2010;7(6):863-4.

21. Olsson G. To the editor: Market withdrawal of quinidine bisulfate (Kinidin Durules) in 2006. Heart Rhythm. 2010;7(6):864.

22. Viskin S, Belhassen B, Wilde AA. To the editor: Irreplaceable antiarrhythmic medications are disappearing: the case of quinidine. Heart Rhythm. 2010;7(6):863.

23. Inama G, Durin O, Pedrinazzi C, et al. 'Orphan drugs' in cardiology: nadolol and quinidine. J Cardiovasc Med (Hagerstown). 2010;11(2):143-4.

24. Olshansky B, Martins J, Hunt S. N-acetyl procainamide causing torsades de pointes. Am J Cardiol. 1982;50(6):1439-41.

25. Olshansky B, Okumura K, Hess PG, et al. Use of procainamide with rapid atrial pacing for successful conversion of atrial flutter to sinus rhythm. J Am Coll Cardiol. 1988;11(2):359-64.

26. Sherrid MV, Barac I, McKenna WJ, et al. Multicenter study of the efficacy and safety of disopyramide in obstructive hypertrophic cardiomyopathy. J Am Coll Cardiol. 2005;45(8):1251-8.

27. Lie KI, Wellens HJ, van Capelle FJ, et al. Lidocaine in the prevention of primary ventricular fibrillation. A double-blind, randomized study of 212 consecutive patients. N Engl J Med. 1974;291(25):1324-6.

28. Alexander JH, Granger CB, Sadowski Z, et al. Prophylactic lidocaine use in acute myocardial infarction: incidence and outcomes from two international trials. The GUSTO-I and GUSTO-IIb Investigators. Am Heart J. 1999;137(5):799-805.

29. Singh BN. Routine prophylactic lidocaine administration in acute myocardial infarction. An idea whose time is all but gone? Circulation. 1992;86(3):1033-5.

30. Hine LK, Laird N, Hewitt P, et al. Meta-analytic evidence against prophylactic use of lidocaine in acute myocardial infarction. Arch Intern Med. 1989;149(12): 2694-8.

31. Stenson RE, Constantino RT, Harrison DC. Interrelationships of hepatic blood flow, cardiac output, and blood levels of lidocaine in man. Circulation. 1971;43(2):205-11.

32. Wyman MG, Slaughter RL, Farolino DA, et al. Multiple bolus technique for lidocaine administration in acute ischemic heart disease. II. Treatment of refractory ventricular arrhythmias and the pharmacokinetic significance of severe left ventricular failure. J Am Coll Cardiol. 1983;2(4):764-9.

33. MacMahon S, Collins R, Peto R, et al. Effects of prophylactic lidocaine in suspected acute myocardial infarction. An overview of results from the randomized, controlled trials. JAMA. 1988;260(13):1910-6.

34. Josephson ME, Kastor JA, Kitchen JG 3rd. Lidocaine in Wolff-Parkinson-White syndrome with atrial fibrillation. Ann Intern Med. 1976;84(1):44-5.

35. Ochs HR, Carstens G, Greenblatt DJ. Reduction in lidocaine clearance during continuous infusion and by coadministration of propranolol. N Engl J Med. 1980;303(7):373-7.

36. Feely J, Wilkinson GR, McAllister CB, et al. Increased toxicity and reduced clearance of lidocaine by cimetidine. Ann Intern Med. 1982;96(5):592-4.

37. Stein J, Podrid P, Lown B. Effects of oral mexiletine on left and right ventricular function. Am J Cardiol. 1984;54(6):575-8.

38. International mexiletine and placebo antiarrhythmic coronary trial: I. Report on arrhythmia and other findings. Impact Research Group. J Am Coll Cardiol. 1984;4(6):1148-63.

39. Campbell RW. Mexiletine. N Engl J Med. 1987;316(1):29-34.

40. Shimizu W, Aiba T, Antzelevitch C. Specific therapy based on the genotype and cellular mechanism in inherited cardiac arrhythmias. Long QT syndrome and Brugada syndrome. Curr Pharm Des. 2005;11(12):1561-72.

41. Bonavita GJ, Pires LA, Wagshal AB, et al. Usefulness of oral quinidine-mexiletine combination therapy for sustained ventricular tachyarrhythmias as assessed by programmed electrical stimulation when quinidine monotherapy has failed. Am Heart J. 1994;127(4 Pt 1):847-51.

42. Duff HJ, Mitchell LB, Wyse DG, et al. Mexiletine/quinidine combination therapy: electrophysiologic correlates of anti-arrhythmic efficacy. Clin Invest Med. 1991;14(5):476-83.

43. Frank MJ, Watkins LO, Prisant LM, et al. Mexiletine versus quinidine as first-line antiarrhythmia therapy: results from consecutive trials. J Clin Pharmacol. 1991;31(3):222-8.

44. Duff HJ, Rahmberg M, Sheldon RS. Role of quinidine in the mexiletine-quinidine interaction: electrophysiologic correlates of enhanced antiarrhythmic efficacy. J Cardiovasc Pharmacol. 1990;16(5):685-92.

45. Roden DM, Iansmith DH, Woosley RL. Frequency-dependent interactions of mexiletine and quinidine on depolarization and repolarization in canine Purkinje fibers. J Pharmacol Exp Ther. 1987;243(3):1218-24.

46. Duff HJ, Gault NJ. Mexiletine and quinidine in combination in an ischemic model: supra-additive antiarrhythmic and electrophysiologic actions. J Cardiovasc Pharmacol. 1986;8(4):847-57.

47. Waleffe A, Mary-Rabine L, Legrand V, et al. Combined mexiletine and amiodarone treatment of refractory recurrent ventricular tachycardia. Am Heart J. 1980;100(6 Pt 1):788-93.

48. Fasola GP, D'Osualdo F, de Pangher V, et al. Thrombocytopenia and mexiletine. Ann Intern Med. 1984;100(1):162.

49. Bigger JT Jr. The interaction of mexiletine with other cardiovascular drugs. Am Heart J. 1984;107(5 Pt 2):1079-85.

50. Preliminary report: effect of encainide and flecainide on mortality in a randomized trial of arrhythmia suppression after myocardial infarction. The Cardiac Arrhythmia Suppression Trial (CAST) Investigators. N Engl J Med. 1989;321(6):406-12.

51. Perry JC, Garson A Jr. Flecainide acetate for treatment of tachyarrhythmias in children: review of world literature on efficacy, safety, and dosing. Am Heart J. 1992;124(6):1614-21.

52. Roden DM, Woosley RL. Drug therapy. Flecainide. N Engl J Med. 1986;315(1):36-41.

53. Wann LS, Curtis AB, January CT, et al. 2011 ACCF/AHA/HRS focused update on the management of patients with atrial fibrillation (updating the 2006 guideline): a report of the American College of Cardiology Foundation/American Heart Association Task Force on Practice Guidelines. Circulation. 2011;123(1):104-23.

54. Konety SH, Olshansky B. The "pill-in-the-pocket" approach to atrial fibrillation. N Engl J Med. 2005;352(11):1150-1.

55. Buxton AE, Waxman HL, Marchlinski FE, et al. Right ventricular tachycardia: clinical and electrophysiologic characteristics. Circulation. 1983;68(8):917-27.

56. Watanabe H, Chopra N, Laver D, et al. Flecainide prevents catecholaminergic polymorphic ventricular tachycardia in mice and humans. Nat Med. 2009;15(4):380-3.

57. van der Werf C, Kannankeril PJ, Sacher F, et al. Flecainide therapy reduces exercise-induced ventricular arrhythmias in patients with catecholaminergic polymorphic ventricular tachycardia. J Am Coll Cardiol. 2011;57(22):2244-54.

58. Benhorin J, Taub R, Goldmit M, et al. Effects of flecainide in patients with new SCN5A mutation: mutation-specific therapy for long-QT syndrome? Circulation. 2000;101(14):1698-706.

59. Rossenbacker T, Priori SG. The Brugada syndrome. Curr Opin Cardiol. 2007;22(3): 163-70.

60. Effect of the antiarrhythmic agent moricizine on survival after myocardial infarction. The Cardiac Arrhythmia Suppression Trial II Investigators. N Engl J Med. 1992;327(4):227-33.

61. Vik-Mo H, Ohm OJ, Lund-Johansen P. Electrophysiologic effects of flecainide acetate in patients with sinus nodal dysfunction. Am J Cardiol. 1982;50(5):1090-4.

62. Alboni P, Botto GL, Baldi N, et al. Outpatient treatment of recent-onset atrial fibrillation with the "pill-in-the-pocket" approach. N Engl J Med. 2004;351(23):2384-91.

63. Muhiddin KA, Turner P, Blackett A. Effect of flecainide on cardiac output. Clin Pharmacol Ther. 1985;37(3):260-3.

64. Rajawat YS, Dias D, Gerstenfeld EP, et al. Interactions of antiarrhythmic drugs and implantable devices in controlling ventricular tachycardia and fibrillation. Curr Cardiol Rep. 2002;4(5):434-40.

65. Hellestrand KJ, Burnett PJ, Milne JR, et al. Effect of the antiarrhythmic agent flecainide acetate on acute and chronic pacing thresholds. Pacing Clin Electrophysiol. 1983;6(5 Pt 1):892-9.

66. McLeod AA, Stiles GL, Shand DG. Demonstration of beta adrenoceptor blockade by propafenone hydrochloride: clinical pharmacologic, radioligand binding and adenylate cyclase activation studies. J Pharmacol Exp Ther. 1984;228(2):461-6.

67. Siddoway LA, Thompson KA, McAllister CB, et al. Polymorphism of propafenone metabolism and disposition in man: clinical and pharmacokinetic consequences. Circulation. 1987;75(4):785-91.

68. Lee JT, Kroemer HK, Silberstein DJ, et al. The role of genetically determined polymorphic drug metabolism in the beta-blockade produced by propafenone. N Engl J Med. 1990;322(25):1764-8.

69. Wagner F, Kalusche D, Trenk D, et al. Drug interaction between propafenone and metoprolol. Br J Clin Pharmacol. 1987;24(2):213-20.

70. Olshansky B. Management of atrial fibrillation after coronary artery bypass graft. Am J Cardiol. 1996;78(8A):27-34.

71. Olshansky B, Martins JB. Usefulness of isoproterenol facilitation of ventricular tachycardia induction during extrastimulus testing in predicting effective chronic therapy with beta-adrenergic blockade. Am J Cardiol. 1987;59(6):573-7.

72. Olshansky B, Rosenfeld LE, Warner AL, et al. The Atrial Fibrillation Follow-up Investigation of Rhythm Management (AFFIRM) study: approaches to control rate in atrial fibrillation. J Am Coll Cardiol. 2004;43(7):1201-8.

73. Zicha S, Tsuji Y, Shiroshita-Takeshita A, et al. Beta-blockers as antiarrhythmic agents. Handb Exp Pharmacol. 2006;(171):235-66.

74. Connolly SJ, Dorian P, Roberts RS, et al. Comparison of beta-blockers, amiodarone plus beta-blockers, or sotalol for prevention of shocks from implantable cardioverter defibrillators: the OPTIC Study: a randomized trial. JAMA. 2006;295(2):165-71.

75. Cheng J, Niwa R, Kamiya K, et al. Carvedilol blocks the repolarizing K+ currents and the L-type Ca2+ current in rabbit ventricular myocytes. Eur J Pharmacol. 1999;376(1-2):189-201.

76. MacNeil DJ. The side effect profile of class III antiarrhythmic drugs: focus on d,l-sotalol. Am J Cardiol. 1997;80(8A):90G-8G.

77. Hohnloser SH, Woosley RL. Sotalol. N Engl J Med. 1994;331(1):31-8.

78. Waldo AL, Camm AJ, deRuyter H, et al. Effect of d-sotalol on mortality in patients with left ventricular dysfunction after recent and remote myocardial infarction. The SWORD Investigators. Survival with Oral d-Sotalol. Lancet. 1996;348(9019):7-12.

79. Julian DG, Prescott RJ, Jackson FS, et al. Controlled trial of sotalol for one year after myocardial infarction. Lancet. 1982;1(8282):1142-7.

80. Mason JW. A comparison of seven antiarrhythmic drugs in patients with ventricular tachyarrhythmias. Electrophysiologic Study versus Electrocardiographic Monitoring Investigators. N Eng J Med. 1993;329(7):452-8.

81. Pacifico A, Hohnloser SH, Williams JH, et al. Prevention of implantable-defibrillator shocks by treatment with sotalol. d,l-Sotalol Implantable Cardioverter-Defibrillator Study Group. N Engl J Med. 1999;340(24):1855-62.

82. Singh BN, Singh SN, Reda DJ, et al. Amiodarone versus sotalol for atrial fibrillation. N Engl J Med. 2005;352(18):1861-72.

83. Baskin EP, Lynch JJ Jr. Differential atrial versus ventricular activities of class III potassium channel blockers. J Pharmacol Exp Ther. 1998;285(1):135-42.

84. Abel S, Nichols DJ, Brearley CJ, et al. Effect of cimetidine and ranitidine on pharmacokinetics and pharmacodynamics of a single dose of dofetilide. Br J Clin Pharmacol . 2000;49(1):64-71.

85. Torp-Pedersen C, Moller M, Bloch-Thomsen PE, et al. Dofetilide in patients with congestive heart failure and left ventricular dysfunction. Danish Investigations of Arrhythmia and Mortality on Dofetilide Study Group. N Engl J Med. 1999;341(12):857-65.

86. Olshansky B. Dofetilide versus quinidine for atrial flutter: viva la difference!? J Cardiovasc Electrophysiol. 1996;7(9):828-32.

87. Yap YG, Camm AJ. Drug induced QT prolongation and torsades de pointes. Heart. 2003;89(11):1363-72.

88. Elming H, Brendorp B, Pedersen OD, et al. Dofetilide: a new drug to control cardiac arrhythmia. Expert Opin Pharmacother. 2003;4(6):973-85.

89. Murray KT. Ibutilide. Circulation. 1998;97(5):493-7.

90. Stambler BS, Wood MA, Ellenbogen KA, et al. Efficacy and safety of repeated intravenous doses of ibutilide for rapid conversion of atrial flutter or fibrillation. Ibutilide Repeat Dose Study Investigators. Circulation. 1996;94(7):1613-21.

91. Oral H, Souza JJ, Michaud GF, et al. Facilitating transthoracic cardioversion of atrial fibrillation with ibutilide pretreatment. N Engl J Med. 1999;340(24):1849-54.

92. Glatter KA, Dorostkar PC, Yang Y, et al. Electrophysiological effects of ibutilide in patients with accessory pathways. Circulation. 2001;104(16):1933-9.

93. Tercius AJ, Kluger J, Coleman CI, et al. Intravenous magnesium sulfate enhances the ability of intravenous ibutilide to successfully convert atrial fibrillation or flutter. Pacing Clin Electrophysiol. 2007;30(11):1331-5.

94. Patsilinakos S, Christou A, Kafkas N, et al. Effect of high doses of magnesium on converting ibutilide to a safe and more effective agent. Am J Cardiol. 2010;106(5):673-6.

95. Coleman CI, Sood N, Chawla D, et al. Intravenous magnesium sulfate enhances the ability of dofetilide to successfully cardiovert atrial fibrillation or flutter: results of the dofetilide and intravenous magnesium evaluation. Europace. 2009;11(7):892-5.

96. Steinwender C, Hönig S, Kypta A, et al. Pre-injection of magnesium sulfate enhances the efficacy of ibutilide for the conversion of typical but not of atypical persistent atrial flutter. Int J Cardiol. 2010;141(3): 260-5.

97. Coleman CI, Kalus JS, Caron MF, et al. Model of effect of magnesium prophylaxis on frequency of torsades de pointes in ibutilide-treated patients. Am J Health Syst Pharm. 2004;61(7):685-8.

98. Fragakis N, Bikias A, Delithanasis I, et al. Acute beta-adrenoceptor blockade improves efficacy of ibutilide in conversion of atrial fibrillation with a rapid ventricular rate. Europace. 2009;11(1):70-4.

99. Gopinathannair R, Olshansky B. Ibutilide revisited: stronger and safer than ever. Europace. 2009;11(1):9-10.

100. Deltour G, Binon F, Tondeur R, et al. Studies in the benzofuran series. VI. Coronary-dilating activity of alkylated and aminoalkylated derivatives of 3-benzoylbenzofuran. Arch Int Pharmacodyn Ther. 1962;139:247-54.

101. Mason JW. Amiodarone. N Engl J Med. 1987;316(8):455-66.

102. Mason JW, Hondeghem LM, Katzung BG. Amiodarone blocks inactivated cardiac sodium channels. Pflugers Arch. 1983;396(1):79-81.

103. Holt DW, Tucker GT, Jackson PR, et al. Amiodarone pharmacokinetics. Br J Clin Pract Suppl. 1986;44:109-14.

104. Plomp TA, van Rossum JM, Robles de Medina EO, et al. Pharmacokinetics and body distribution of amiodarone in man. Arzneimittelforschung. 1984;34(4):513-20.

105. Julian DG, Camm AJ, Frangin G, et al. Randomised trial of effect of amiodarone on mortality in patients with left-ventricular dysfunction after recent myocardial infarction: EMIAT. European Myocardial Infarct Amiodarone Trial Investigators. Lancet. 1997;349(9053):667-74.

106. Cairns JA, Connolly SJ, Roberts R, et al. Randomised trial of outcome after myocardial infarction in patients with frequent or repetitive ventricular premature depolarisations: CAMIAT. Canadian Amiodarone Myocardial Infarction Arrhythmia Trial Investigators. Lancet. 1997;349(9053):675-82.

107. Boutitie F, Boissel JP, Connolly SJ, et al. Amiodarone interaction with beta-blockers: analysis of the merged EMIAT (European Myocardial Infarct Amiodarone Trial) and CAMIAT (Canadian Amiodarone Myocardial Infarction Trial) databases. The EMIAT and CAMIAT Investigators. Circulation. 1999;99(17):2268-75.

108. Garguichevich JJ, Ramos JL, Gambarte A, et al. Effect of amiodarone therapy on mortality in patients with left ventricular dysfunction and asymptomatic complex ventricular arrhythmias: Argentine Pilot Study of Sudden Death and Amiodarone (EPAMSA). Am Heart J. 1995;130(3 Pt 1):494-500.

109. Doval HC, Nul DR, Grancelli HO, et al. Randomised trial of low-dose amiodarone in severe congestive heart failure. Grupo de Estudio de la Sobrevida en la Insuficiencia Cardiaca en Argentina (GESICA). Lancet. 1994;344(8921):493-8.

110. Singh SN, Fletcher RD, Fisher SG, et al. Amiodarone in patients with congestive heart failure and asymptomatic ventricular arrhythmia. Survival Trial of Antiarrhythmic Therapy in Congestive Heart Failure. N Engl J Med. 1995;333(2):77-82.

111. Piccini JP, Berger JS, O'Connor CM. Amiodarone for the prevention of sudden cardiac death: a meta-analysis of randomized controlled trials. Eur Heart J. 2009;30(10):1245-53.

112. Roy D, Talajic M, Dorian P, et al. Amiodarone to prevent recurrence of atrial fibrillation. Canadian Trial of Atrial Fibrillation Investigators. N Engl J Med. 2000;342(13):913-20.

113. Goldschlager N, Epstein AE, Naccarelli GV, et al. A practical guide for clinicians who treat patients with amiodarone: 2007. Heart Rhythm. 2007;4(9):1250-9.

114. Vorperian VR, Havighurst TC, Miller S, et al. Adverse effects of low dose amiodarone: a meta-analysis. J Am Coll Cardiol. 1997;30(3):791-8.

115. Olshansky B, Sami M, Rubin A, et al. Use of amiodarone for atrial fibrillation in patients with preexisting pulmonary disease in the AFFIRM study. Am J Cardiol. 2005;95(3):404-5.

116. Olshansky B. Images in clinical medicine. Amiodarone-induced pulmonary toxicity. N Engl J Med. 1997;337(25):1814.

117. Manning AS, Bruyninckx C, Ramboux J, et al. SR 33589, a new amiodarone-like agent: effect on ischemia- and reperfusion-induced arrhythmias in anesthetized rats. J Cardiovasc Pharmacol. 1995;26(3):453-61.

118. Djandjighian L, Planchenault J, Finance O, et al. Hemodynamic and antiadrenergic effects of dronedarone and amiodarone in animals with a healed myocardial infarction. J Cardiovasc Pharmacol. 2000;36(3):376-83.

119. Sun W, Sarma JS, Singh BN. Electrophysiological effects of dronedarone (SR33589), a noniodinated benzofuran derivative, in the rabbit heart: comparison with amiodarone. Circulation. 1999;100(22):2276-81.

120. Finance O, Manning A, Chatelain P. Effects of a new amiodarone-like agent, SR 33589, in comparison to amiodarone, D,L-sotalol, and lignocaine, on ischemia-induced ventricular arrhythmias in anesthetized pigs. J Cardiovasc Pharmacol. 1995;26(4):570-6.

121. Connolly SJ, Camm AJ, Halperin JL, et al. Dronedarone in high-risk permanent atrial fibrillation. N Engl J Med. 2011;365(24):2268-76.

122. Køber L, Torp-Pedersen C, McMurray JJ, et al. Increased mortality after dronedarone therapy for severe heart failure. N Engl J Med. 2008;358(25):2678-87.

123. Dronedarone prescribing information. 2011. [online] Available from http://www.multaq.com/docs/consumer_pdf/pi.aspx. 2011.

124. Touboul P, Brugada J, Capucci A, et al. Dronedarone for prevention of atrial fibrillation: a dose-ranging study. Eur Heart J. 2003;24:1481-7.

125. Piccini JP, Hasselblad V, Peterson ED, et al. Comparative efficacy of dronedarone and amiodarone for the maintenance of sinus rhythm in patients with atrial fibrillation. J Am Coll Cardiol. 2009;54:1089-95.

126. Davy JM, Herold M, Hoglund C, et al. Dronedarone for the control of ventricular rate in permanent atrial fibrillation: the efficacy and safety of dronedarone for the control of ventricular rate during atrial fibrillation (ERATO) study. Am Heart J. 2008;156:527. e1-9.

127. Singh BN, Connolly SJ, Crijns HJ, et al. Dronedarone for maintenance of sinus rhythm in atrial fibrillation or flutter. N Engl J Med. 2007;357:987-99.

128. Connolly SJ, Crijns HJ, Torp-Pedersen C, et al. Analysis of stroke in ATHENA: a placebo-controlled, double-blind, parallel-arm trial to assess the efficacy of dronedarone 400 mg BID for the prevention of cardiovascular hospitalization or death from any cause in patients with atrial fibrillation/atrial flutter. Circulation. 2009;120:1174-80.

129. Sanofi Aventis. Important drug warning on hepatic failure in patients treated with Multaq: Letter to Healthcare Provider- Jan 14, 2011. [online] Available from http://www.multaq.com/docs/pdf/MultaqDHCPLetterJan2011.pdf.

130. FDA Drug Safety Communication: Multaq (dronedarone) and increased risk of death and serious cardiovascular adverse events. [online] Available from http://www.fda.gov/Drugs/DrugSafety/ucm264059.htm [Accessed July 2011].

131. Nattel S. Dronedarone in atrial fibrillation—Jekyll and Hyde? N Engl J Med. 2011;365(24):2321-2.

132. Lombardi F, Terranova P. Pharmacological treatment of atrial fibrillation: mechanisms of action and efficacy of class III drugs. Curr Med Chem. 2006;13(14):1635-53.

133. Camm AJ, Pratt CM, Schwartz PJ, et al. Mortality in patients after a recent myocardial infarction: a randomized, placebo-controlled trial of azimilide using heart rate variability for risk stratification. Circulation. 2004;109(8):990-6.

134. Dorian P, Borggrefe M, Al-Khalidi HR, et al. Placebo-controlled, randomized clinical trial of azimilide for prevention of ventricular tachyarrhythmias in patients with an implantable cardioverter defibrillator. Circulation. 2004;110(24):3646-54.

135. Lombardi F, Borggrefe M, Ruzyllo W, et al. A-COMET-II Investigators. Azimilide vs. placebo and sotalol for persistent atrial fibrillation: the A-COMET-II (Azimilide-CardiOversion MaintEnance Trial-II) trial. Eur Heart J. 2006;27(18): 2224-31.

136. Kerr CR, Connolly SJ, Kowey P, et al. Efficacy of azimilide for the maintenance of sinus rhythm in patients with paroxysmal atrial fibrillation in the presence and absence of structural heart disease. Am J Cardiol. 2006;98(2):215-8.

137. Conway E, Musco S, Kowey PR. New horizons in antiarrhythmic therapy: will novel agents overcome current deficits? Am J Cardiol. 2008;102(6A):12H-19H.

138. Lerman BB, Belardinelli L. Cardiac electrophysiology of adenosine. Basic and clinical concepts. Circulation. 1991;83(5):1499-509.

139. Wilber DJ, Baerman J, Olshansky B, et al. Adenosine-sensitive ventricular tachycardia. Clinical characteristics and response to catheter ablation. Circulation. 1993;87(1):126-34.

140. Kall JG, Kopp D, Olshansky B, et al. Adenosine-sensitive atrial tachycardia. Pacing Clin Electrophysiol. 1995;18(2):300-6.

141. Ellenbogen KA, Thames MD, DiMarco JP, et al. Electrophysiological effects of adenosine in the transplanted human heart. Evidence of supersensitivity. Circulation. 1990;81(3):821-8.

142. Alamercery Y, Wilkins P, Karrison T. Functional equality of coordinating centers in a multicenter clinical trial. Experience of the International Mexiletine and Placebo Antiarrhythmic Coronary Trial (IMPACT). Control Clin Trials. 1986;7(1):38-52.

143. Wijffels MC, Crijns HJ. Recent advances in drug therapy for atrial fibrillation. J Cardiovasc Electrophysiol. 2003;14(9 Suppl):S40-7.

144. Naccarelli GV, Wolbrette DL, Samii S, et al. Vernakalant—a promising therapy for conversion of recent-onset atrial fibrillation. Expert Opin Investig Drugs. 2008;17(5):805-10.

145. Mao ZL, Townsend RW, Gao C, et al. Population pharmacokinetics of vernakalant hydrochloride injection (RSD1235) in patients with atrial fibrillation or atrial flutter. J Clin Pharmacol. 2012;52(7):1042-53.

146. Roy D, Pratt CM, Torp-Pedersen C, et al. Vernakalant hydrochloride for rapid conversion of atrial fibrillation: a phase 3, randomized, placebo-controlled trial. Circulation. 2008;117(12):1518-25.

147. Kowey PR, Dorian P, Mitchell LB, et al. Vernakalant hydrochloride for the rapid conversion of atrial fibrillation after cardiac surgery: a randomized, double-blind, placebo-controlled trial. Circ Arrhythm Electrophysiol. 2009;2(6):652-9.

148. Pratt CM, Roy D, Torp-Pedersen C, et al.. Usefulness of vernakalant hydrochloride injection for rapid conversion of atrial fibrillation. Am J Cardiol. 2010;106(9):1277-83.

149. Camm AJ, Capucci A, Hohnloser SH, et al. A randomized active-controlled study comparing the efficacy and safety of vernakalant to amiodarone in recent-onset atrial fibrillation. J Am Coll Cardiol. 2011;57(3):313-21.

150. European Medicines Agency. Assessment Report for Brinavess. 2011.

151. US Food and Drug Administration, Center for Drug Evaluation and Research. Minutes of the meeting of the Cardio-Renal Advisory Committee, 14 Nov, 2007.

152. Torp-Pedersen C, Raev DH, Dickinson G, et al. A randomized, placebo-controlled study of vernakalant (oral) for the prevention of atrial fibrillation recurrence after cardioversion. Circ Arrhythm Electrophysiol. 2011;4(5):637-43.

153. Hohnloser SH, Dorian P, Straub M, et al. Safety and efficacy of intravenously administered tedisamil for rapid conversion of recent-onset atrial fibrillation or atrial flutter. J Am Coll Cardiol. 2004;44(1):99-104.

154. Ahmadi-Kashani M, Kessler DJ, Day J, et al. Heart rate predicts outcomes in an implantable cardioverter-defibrillator population. Circulation. 2009;120(21): 2040-5.

155. Gopinathannair R, Sullivan R, Olshansky B. Tachycardia-mediated cardiomyopathy: recognition and management. Curr Heart Fail Rep. 2009;6(4):257-64.

156. Fox K, Borer JS, Camm AJ, et al. Resting heart rate in cardiovascular disease. J Am Coll Cardiol. 2007;50(9):823-30.

157. Gopinathannair R, Sullivan RM, Olshansky B. Slower heart rates for healthy hearts: time to redefine tachycardia? Circ Arrhythm Electrophysiol. 2008;1(5):321-3.

158. DiFrancesco D, Camm JA. Heart rate lowering by specific and selective I(f) current inhibition with ivabradine: a new therapeutic perspective in cardiovascular disease. Drugs . 2004;64(16):1757-65.

159. Swedberg K, Komajda M, Böhm M, et al. Ivabradine and outcomes in chronic heart failure (SHIFT): a randomised placebo-controlled study. Lancet. 2010;376(9744):875-85.

160. Fox K, Ford I, Steg PG, et al. BEAUTIFUL Investigators. Ivabradine for patients with stable coronary artery disease and left-ventricular systolic dysfunction (BEAUTIFUL): a randomised, double-blind, placebo-controlled trial. Lancet. 2008;372(9641):807-16.

161. Tardif JC, Ponikowski P, Kahan T; ASSOCIATE Study Investigators. Efficacy of the I(f) current inhibitor ivabradine in patients with chronic stable angina receiving beta-blocker therapy: a 4-month, randomized, placebo-controlled trial. Eur Heart J. 2009;30(5):540-8.

162. Cappato R1, Castelvecchio S, Ricci C, et al. Clinical efficacy of ivabradine in patients with inappropriate sinus tachycardia: a prospective, randomized, placebo-controlled, double-blind, crossover evaluation. J Am Coll Cardiol. 2012;60(15):1323-9.

163. Ptaszynski P1, Kaczmarek K, Ruta J, et al. Ivabradine in combination with metoprolol succinate in the treatment of inappropriate sinus tachycardia. J Cardiovasc Pharmacol Ther. 2013;18:338-44.

164. Ptaszynski P, Kaczmarek K, Ruta J, et al. Metoprolol succinate vs. ivabradine in the treatment of inappropriate sinus tachycardia in patients unresponsive to previous pharmacological therapy. Europace. 2013;15:116-21.

165. Khan S, Hamid S, Rinaldi C. Treatment of inappropriate sinus tachycardia with ivabradine in a patient with postural orthostatic tachycardia syndrome and a dual chamber pacemaker. Pacing Clin Electrophysiol. 2009;32(1):131-3.

166. Administration UFaD. FDA approves new treatment for chest pain. 2006.

167. Antzelevitch C, Belardinelli L, Zygmunt AC, et al. Electrophysiological effects of ranolazine, a novel antianginal agent with antiarrhythmic properties. Circulation. 2004;110(8):904-10.

168. Antzelevitch C, Burashnikov A, Sicouri S, et al. Electrophysiologic basis for the antiarrhythmic actions of ranolazine. Heart Rhythm. 2011;8(8):1281-90.

169. Burashnikov A, Di Diego JM, Zygmunt AC, et al. Atrium-selective sodium channel block as a strategy for suppression of atrial fibrillation: differences in sodium channel inactivation between atria and ventricles and the role of ranolazine. Circulation. 2007;116(13):1449-57.

170. Undrovinas AI, Belardinelli L, Undrovinas NA, et al. Ranolazine improves abnormal repolarization and contraction in left ventricular myocytes of dogs with heart failure by inhibiting late sodium current. J Cardiovasc Electrophysiol. 2006;17 Suppl 1:S169-S77.

171. Scirica BM, Morrow DA, Hod H, et al. Effect of ranolazine, an antianginal agent with novel electrophysiological properties, on the incidence of arrhythmias in patients with non ST-segment elevation acute coronary syndrome: results from the metabolic efficiency with ranolazine for less ischemia in non ST-elevation acute coronary syndrome thrombolysis in myocardial infarction 36 (MERLIN-TIMI 36) randomized controlled trial. Circulation. 2007;116(15):1647-52.

172. Burashnikov A, Sicouri S, Di Diego JM, et al. Synergistic effect of the combination of ranolazine and dronedarone to suppress atrial fibrillation. J Am Coll Cardiol. 2010;56(15):1216-24.

173. Murdock DK, Kersten M, Kaliebe J, et al. The use of oral ranolazine to convert new or paroxysmal atrial fibrillation: a review of experience with implications for possible "pill in the pocket" approach to atrial fibrillation. Indian Pacing Electrophysiol J. 2009;9(5):260-7.

174. Antzelevitch C, Belardinelli L, Wu L, et al. Electrophysiologic properties and antiarrhythmic actions of a novel antianginal agent. J Cardiovasc Pharmacol Ther. 2004;9 Suppl 1:S65-83.

175. Thireau J, Pasquié JL, Martel E, et al. New drugs vs. old concepts: a fresh look at antiarrhythmics. Pharmacol Ther. 2011;132(2):125-45.

176. Nattel S, Carlsson L. Innovative approaches to anti-arrhythmic drug therapy. Nat Rev Drug Discov. 2006;5(12):1034-49.

177. Liu N, Colombi B, Memmi M, et al. Arrhythmogenesis in catecholaminergic polymorphic ventricular tachycardia: insights from a RyR2 R4496C knock-in mouse model. Circ Res. 2006;99(33):292-8.

178. Brette F. Calcium polymorphic ventricular tachycardia: a new name for CPVT? Cardiovasc Res. 2010;87(1):10-1.

179. Cutler MJ, Wan X, Laurita KR, et al. Targeted SERCA2a gene expression identifies molecular mechanism and therapeutic target for arrhythmogenic cardiac alternans. Circ Arrhythm Electrophysiol. 2009;2(6):686-94.

180. Cho HC, Marbán E. Biological therapies for cardiac arrhythmias: can genes and cells replace drugs and devices? Circ Res. 2010;106(4):674-85.

181. Murata M, Cingolani E, McDonald AD, et al. Creation of a genetic calcium channel blocker by targeted gem gene transfer in the heart. Circ Res. 2004;95(4):398-405.

182. Yankelson L, Feld Y, Bressler-Stramer T, et al. Cell therapy for modification of the myocardial electrophysiological substrate. Circulation. 2008;117(6):720-31.

183. Sasano T, McDonald AD, Kikuchi K, et al. Molecular ablation of ventricular tachycardia after myocardial infarction. Nat Med. 2006;12(11):1256-8.

184. Greener I, Donahue JK. Gene therapy strategies for cardiac electrical dysfunction. J Mol Cell Cardiol. 2011;50(5):759-65.

185. Makkar RR, Lill M, Chen PS. Stem cell therapy for myocardial repair: is it arrhythmogenic? J Am Coll Cardiol. 2003;42(12):2070-2.

186. Savelieva I, Camm J. Anti-arrhythmic drug therapy for atrial fibrillation: current anti-arrhythmic drugs, investigational agents, and innovative approaches. Europace. 2008;10(6):647-65.

187. January CT, Wann LS, Alpert JS, et al. 2014 AHA/ACC/HRS guideline for the management of patients with atrial fibrillation: executive summary: a report of the American College of Cardiology/American Heart Association Task Force on practice guidelines and the heart rhythm society. Circulation. 2014;130(23):2071-104.

188. Hohnloser SH, Dorian P, Roberts R, et al. Effect of amiodarone and sotalol on ventricular defibrillation threshold: the optimal pharmacological therapy in cardioverter defibrillator patients (OPTIC) trial. Circulation. 2006;114(2):104-9.

Drugs for Heart Failure

Lee Joseph, Kanu Chatterjee

INTRODUCTION

Heart failure (HF) is a common complex clinical syndrome resulting from structural or functional impairment of ventricular filling or ejection of blood.[1] It can be caused by disorders of the endocardium, myocardium, pericardium, heart valves, great vessels and certain metabolic abnormalities. It can be acute and of recent onset or chronic and may be present for months or years. Based on left ventricular ejection fraction (EF), patients with clinical HF are classified into HF with preserved EF (HFpEF) if EF ≥50% and HF with reduced EF (HFrEF) if EF ≤40%. HFpEF also includes two subsets, HFpEF (borderline) that refers to patients with clinical HF and EF 41–49% and HFpEF (improved) that refers to patients who previously had HFrEF and EF consequently improved to more than 40%. HFrEF is also called systolic HF and HFpEF, diastolic HF.

EPIDEMIOLOGY

The incidence of HF resulting primarily from myocardial disease is high. The lifetime risk of developing HF is estimated at about 20% for all adults older than 40 years.[2] Presently, the worldwide prevalence of HF is approximately 23 million.[3] Based on data from National Health and Nutrition Examination Survey (NHANES) 2007 to 2010, an estimated 5.1 million Americans aged 20 years or above (2.1%) have HF.[4] It has been estimated that by the year 2030, more than 8 million people, aged 18 years or above, will have HF in the USA.[5] The prevalence of HF increases with age irrespective of gender.

Management of HF is expensive. In many developed countries, the cost of management of HF is about 1–2% of the total healthcare budget. In 2012, total cost for HF was estimated to be $30.7 billion in the USA and is estimated to increase to $70 billion by 2030.[5] This enormous cost is primarily due to recurrent admissions to hospital for treatment of HF. Thus, one of the major goals of management of patients with HF is to reduce the rate of hospital admissions.

The prevalence of HFrEF and HFpEF is similar. Approximately 50% of patients with HF have HFpEF.[6] The risk factors for developing HFpEF are similar to those of HFrEF.[7] In both HFrEF and HFpEF, advancing age, hypertension, diabetes and obesity are the major risk factors. The incidence of coronary artery disease (CAD) is higher in HFrEF than in HFpEF. The incidence of CAD in HFpEF is about 54% as compared to 63% in HFrEF. The patients with HFrEF are younger than patients with HFpEF. The average age of patients with HFrEF and HFpEF is 69.9 years and 74.2 years, respectively.[7] HFpEF is more frequent in women than in men. In the Cardiovascular Health Study, the prevalence of HFpEF was 67% in women and only 42% in men.[8]

DIAGNOSIS

Diagnosis of HF is based on the analysis of signs and symptoms. Paroxysmal nocturnal dyspnea, orthopnea, elevated jugular venous pressure, a positive hepatojugular reflux and presence of an S3 gallop or gallop rhythm are almost diagnostic of HF.[9] Significantly, elevated B-type natriuretic peptide (BNP) or N terminal of the prohormone BNP (NT-proBNP) confirms the diagnosis of HF. It should be appreciated that BNP and NT-proBNP levels are typically elevated in both HFpEF and HFrEF.[9]

Noninvasive tests, such as echocardiography, electro-cardiography and chest radiography are routinely performed. Echocardiography is essential to distinguish between HFpEF and HFrEF. Cardiac magnetic resonance imaging and radionuclide ventriculography are alternate methods to assess EF. Invasive tests, such as coronary angiography is also performed to establish presence or absence of CAD. A stress test (exercise or pharmacologic) or contrast cardiac computed tomography can also be performed to detect CAD.

PATHOPHYSIOLOGY

There have been considerable advances in the understanding of pathophysiology of both HFrEF and HFpEF. In HFrEF, the primary hemodynamic abnormality is reduced left ventricular EF (LVEF). Reduced EF is associated with reduced stroke volume and increased left ventricular end-diastolic and end-systolic volumes. Increased left ventricular diastolic volume is associated with increased left ventricular diastolic pressures, a passive increase in left atrial and pulmonary venous pressure. There is also an obligatory increase in pulmonary artery pressure, which is right ventricular afterload. A substantial increase in pulmonary artery pressure (increased right ventricular afterload) may cause right ventricular failure.

In HFpEF, the primary functional abnormality is increased left ventricular stiffness and impaired left ventricular relaxation. Increased left ventricular stiffness is associated with an increase in left ventricular diastolic pressure, a passive increase in left atrial and pulmonary venous pressure. There is an obligatory increase in pulmonary artery pressure, which may precipitate right ventricular failure. It is apparent that the hemodynamic abnormalities of both HFrEF and HFpEF are similar.

It should be appreciated that left ventricular contractile function is reduced in HFrEF and is preserved in HFpEF (Fig. 1). In both HFrEF and HFpEF, there is myocyte hypertrophy. In HFrEF, myocyte is thinner but longer, whereas in HFpEF, the myocyte is thicker. Calcium regulation is abnormal in both HFrEF and HFpEF. The collagen crosslinks are decreased in HFrEF but increased in HFpEF (Table 1).

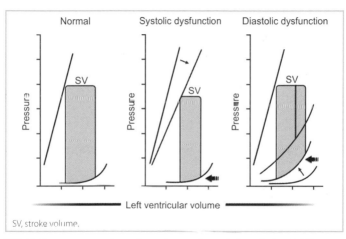

SV, stroke volume.

FIG. 1: The pressure volume loops in systolic and diastolic heart failure are illustrated. In systolic heart failure, contractile function is impaired as evident from the downward shift of the isovolumic pressure line. In diastolic heart failure, diastolic compliance is decreased as evident from upward and leftward shift of the diastolic pressure-volume curve.

TABLE 1: Morphologic differences in heart failure with reduced ejection fraction (HFrEF) and heart failure with preserved ejection fraction (HFpEF)

	HFrEF	HFpEF
Myocyte hypertrophy	+	+
Myocyte necrosis	+	+
Myocyte apoptosis	+	+
Fibrosis	+	+
Collagen cross-links	–	+
Calcium regulation	–	–

+, increased; –, decreased.

In HFrEF, left ventricle is dilated. As discussed before, there is an increase in end-diastolic and end-systolic volumes. The magnitude of increase in end-systolic volume is greater than that of the increase in end-diastolic volume; as a result, LVEF is decreased. Left ventricular wall is thinner or remains unchanged in HFrEF. Left ventricular wall stress, therefore, is increased in HFrEF. The mechanism of decreased EF is not only due to impaired contractile function but also due to increased wall stress.

There is a considerable change in the geometry and shape of the left ventricle in HFrEF. Left ventricle is spherical and globular. Synchronous contraction of left ventricular walls is frequently absent in HFrEF. The lateral wall contracts earlier than the interventricular septum. This mechanical dyssynchrony occurs most frequently in the presence of left bundle branch block. However, it may occur in the absence of conduction abnormality. The altered shape, geometry and dyssynchrony are the principal mechanisms for secondary mitral regurgitation in HFrEF. The morphologic and functional changes in HFrEF are summarized in Table 2.

In HFpEF, there is little or no increase in left ventricular end-diastolic or end-systolic volumes. LVEF remains unchanged. Left ventricular wall thickness, in general, is increased and left ventricular wall stress is decreased. Decreased wall stress is associated with increased EF. The morphologic and functional changes in HFpEF are summarized in Table 3.

TABLE 2: Morphologic and functional changes in heart failure with reduced ejection fraction

- Usually eccentric hypertrophy
- Disproportionate increase in ventricular cavity size
- Increased ventricular mass
- Wall thickness—decreased or unchanged
- Increased wall stress
- Reduced ejection fraction
- Altered ventricular shape and geometry
- Frequent mechanical dyssynchrony with or without electrical dyssynchrony

TABLE 3: Morphologic and functional changes in heart failure with preserved ejection fraction

- Ventricular hypertrophy is usually concentric
- Increased left ventricular mass
- Increased left ventricular wall thickness
- Little or no change in left ventricular volumes
- Decreased left ventricular wall stress
- Maintained ejection fraction
- Little or no change in ventricular shape
- Mechanical dyssynchrony with or without electrical dyssynchrony is present in approximately 30% of patients

Based on pathophysiology, the clinical subset, whether compensated or decompensated and acute or chronic, several pharmacologic therapeutic strategies have evolved. In this chapter, the drugs that are used for management of HF will be discussed.

MANAGEMENT OF HEART FAILURE WITH REDUCED EJECTION FRACTION

The severity of HF is classified by New York Heart Association (NYHA) functional class. The class I patients are asymptomatic, class II are symptomatic with ordinary physical activity, class III are symptomatic with less than ordinary physical activity and the class IV patients are symptomatic at rest.

There is another classification of HF, which is based on the presence of risk factors for developing HF, presence or absence of symptomatic or asymptomatic systolic dysfunction and response to therapy. There are four stages of HF. Stage A patients are those who have only the risk factors for developing HF but do not have structural heart disease. The risk factors are hypertension, diabetes, obesity, hyperlipidemia and smoking. Patients in stage B have structural heart disease but are asymptomatic. Patients in stage C have current or prior symptoms of HF and are being treated with recommended treatments. Patients in stage D are refractory to standard therapy and are awaiting cardiac transplant or requiring ventricular assist devices.

In all patients, irrespective of whether they are symptomatic or asymptomatic (stages A–D), modifications of risk factors for developing HF are essential. Adequate treatment of hypertension, diabetes and obesity should be undertaken. In patients with suspected or established CAD, treatment for dyslipidemia is indicated.

In stage B-D patients, in addition to risk factor modification, the pharmacologic treatments with proven benefit to decrease mortality and morbidity are recommended. The pharmacologic treatments that have been clearly documented to improve prognosis of patients with HFrEF are:

- Angiotensin inhibitors
- Beta-blockers
- Aldosterone antagonists
- Combination of hydralazine and isosorbide dinitrate (nitric oxide donors).

The treatment strategies based on the stages of HF and the effects of various drug classes that are used are summarized in Tables 4 and 5, respectively.

TABLE 4: Treatment strategies based on stage of heart failure with reduced ejection fraction

Stage A	• Treat hypertension
	• Encourage smoking cessation
	• Treat lipid disorders
	• Encourage regular exercise
	• Discourage alcohol abuse
	• Discourage illicit drug use
	• Angiotensin inhibition in appropriate patients
Stage B	• Treatment for stage A
	• Angiotensin inhibition in appropriate patients
	• β-blockers in appropriate patients
Stage C	• Treatment for stage A
	• Angiotensin inhibition therapy
	• Adrenergic blocking agents
	• Aldosterone antagonists in appropriate patients
	• Hydralazine-isosorbide dinitrate combination in appropriate patients
	• Diuretics to relieve congestive symptoms
	• Cardiac resynchronization therapy
	• Implantable cardioverter defibrillator
	• Cardiac resynchronization treatment-implantable cardioverter defibrillator
	• Digitalis in selected patients
Stage D	• Treatments for stage A
	• Those who have failed or have become refractory to recommended therapy
	• Those who are waiting for cardiac transplantation or for assist devices treatment
	• Treatment strategies for stages A–C with modifications

TABLE 5: Effects of various drug classes in chronic heart failure

Reduce mortality	• ACEIs of ARBs
	• Aldosterone antagonists
	• Beta-blockers
Symptom relief	• Diuretics
	• Low-dose digoxin
	• Nitrates
	• Iron for anemia
	• Inotropes and inodilators
May have deleterious effects	• Antiarrhythmics
	• Calcium channel blockers
	• High-dose digoxin

ACEIs, angiotensin-converting enzyme inhibitors; ARBs, angiotensin II receptor blockers.

Neurohormonal Modulation

Introduction of neurohormonal modulators has been a major advance in the management of HFrEF. The rationale for the use of neurohormonal modulators is to attenuate the adverse effects of neurohormones. Neurohormones, such as angiotensin, norepinephrine and aldosterone produce a number of adverse effects on myocardial morphology, structure and function. The adverse hemodynamic effects include increased systemic and pulmonary vascular resistance resulting from systemic and pulmonary vascular vasoconstriction. This may result in low cardiac output, pulmonary hypertension and right ventricular failure.

Neurohormonal activation also causes vascular remodeling. There is hyperplasia of vascular smooth muscle cells and intimal thickening There is also vascular endothelial dysfunction.

The neurohormonal activation also causes ventricular myocardial adverse remodeling. There is myocyte hypertrophy with dysregulation of myosin metabolism. There are also changes in extracellular matrix. There is increased synthesis of collagen with increased collagen volume and fibrosis along with disruption of collagen architecture. Neurohormones promote atherothrombosis partly due to endothelial dysfunction. There is also abnormal lipid metabolism. The risk of vascular thrombosis resulting from enhanced coagulopathy is increased by elevated neurohormones. The adverse effects of neurohormones are summarized in Table 6.

In patients with HF, plasma levels of several neuro-hormones are elevated (Fig. 2).[10] Plasma-renin activity is increased. There is also an increase in aldosterone plasma level. Plasma catecholamines including norepinephrine, dopamine and epinephrine are increased (Fig. 3). Plasma-arginine-vasopressin levels are also elevated. The neurohormonal activation is higher in symptomatic patients compared to asymptomatic ones with systolic left ventricular dysfunction

TABLE 6: Adverse effects of neurohormonal activation

- Adverse hemodynamic effects
- Vascular remodeling
- Ventricular remodeling
  - Myocyte hypertrophy
  - Extracellular matrix changes
- Promotes atherothrombosis
- Increased oxidative stress
- Endothelial dysfunction
- Myocardial necrosis
- Apoptosis

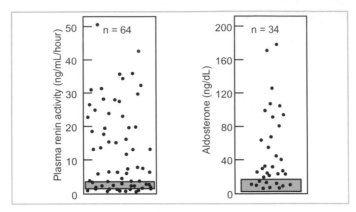

FIG. 2: In patients with systolic heart failure, plasma renin activity and aldosterone blood levels are increased.

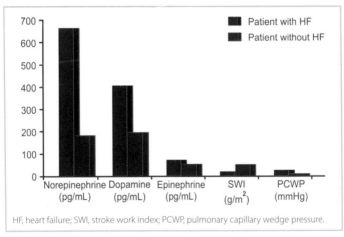

HF, heart failure; SWI, stroke work index; PCWP, pulmonary capillary wedge pressure.

FIG. 3: Mean values of circulating catecholamines and hemodynamic parameters in patients with or without heart failure.

(Fig. 4). Endothelins are also significantly elevated in patients with HFrEF. Endothelins are potent vasoconstrictors and produce adverse vascular and ventricular remodeling.

Angiotensin Inhibitors

A large number of clinical trials have documented the beneficial effects of angiotensin inhibitors in patients with HFrEF. Angiotensin I is formed from angiotensinogen in the liver by renin. Renin is primarily synthesized in the juxtaglomerular cells of kidney. The stimuli for the release of renin are reduced renal blood flow, hypotension, sodium depletion, diuresis and β-adrenergic stimulation. Angiotensin II is formed from angiotensin I by angiotensin-converting enzyme. Angiotensin II stimulates the angiotensin receptor subtypeI, the principal mechanism of the adverse cardiovascular effects of angiotensin. The synthesis of angiotensin II can be

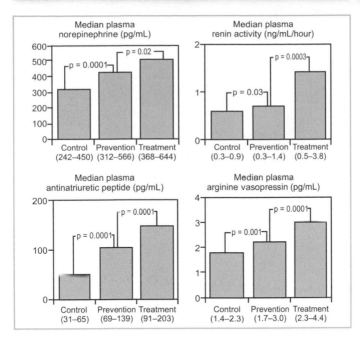

FIG. 4: Neurohormonal activation in patients with systolic heart failure is illustrated. Plasma norepinephrine, angiotensin and vasopressins are higher in patients with heart failure compared to controls. Neurohormonal activation is more pronounced in symptomatic than asymptomatic patients with systolic dysfunction.[10]

attenuated by inhibiting renin and angiotensin-converting enzymes. The adverse effects of angiotensin II can also be attenuated by blocking angiotensin II receptors. For treatment of HF, angiotensin-converting enzyme inhibitors (ACEIs) and angiotensin II receptor blockers (ARBs) have been investigated most extensively.

In the first placebo-controlled randomized clinical trial, the Cooperative North Scandinavian Enalapril Survival Study (CONSENSUS), enalapril was used.[11] Patients with severe HF were randomized to receive enalapril or placebo. The use of enalapril was associated with a substantial reduction in mortality and morbidity. The summary of 32 randomized trials with the use of various types of ACEIs is illustrated in Figure 5. The risk of total mortality decreased by 23% with the use of ACEIs. The risk of death or hospitalization for HF decreased by 35% and that of fatal myocardial infarction (MI) by 20%.[12] The exercise tolerance and symptoms also improved with the use of ACEIs.

Angiotensin II receptor blockers have also been used for treatment of patients with HFrEF. The agents that have been used are candesartan, losartan and valsartan. In the Candesartan in Heart failure Assessment of Reduction in Mortality and morbidity (CHARM) trial, the use of candesartan was associated with similar benefit in reduction in mortality

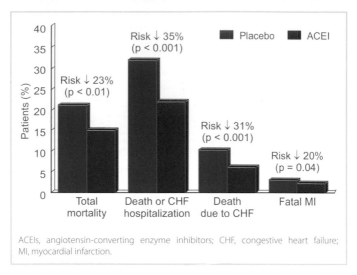

ACEIs, angiotensin-converting enzyme inhibitors; CHF, congestive heart failure; MI, myocardial infarction.

FIG. 5: The results of 32 randomized trials of angiotensin-converting enzyme inhibitors in patients with systolic heart failure are illustrated. There was a significant reduction in total and cardiovascular mortality. There was also reduction in death due to myocardial infarction.[12]

and morbidity to those of ACEIs.[13] In the losartan HF study (ELITE II), the effects of ARBs (losartan) were compared to those of the ACEIs (enalapril).[14] The beneficial effects of losartan and enalapril in decreasing mortality and morbidity in patients with HFrEF were similar.

The major side effect of ACEIs is cough, and it is related to increased bradykinin production. Angioedema, though occurs rarely with an approximate incidence of 1%, is a contraindication for the use of ACEIs. Significant hyperkalemia is also uncommon but is a contraindication for their use. Another contraindication for their use is pregnancy. Occasionally, skin rash and extreme bradycardia can develop, but these complications are extremely rare (Fig. 6). The dose of various ACEIs and ARBs used in HF are summarized in Table 7.

The 2013 American College of Cardiology Foundation (ACCF)/American Heart Association (AHA) Task Force on Practice Guidelines for Management of Heart Failure Recommendations for the Use of ACEI or ARBs[1]

Class I

ACEIs should be used in all patients with HFrEF (with or without symptoms) even if they have not experienced MI. (*Level of Evidence: A*)

An ARB should be used in stage C HFrEF patients and post-MI stage B HFrEF patients who are intolerant of ACEIs. (*Level of Evidence: A*)

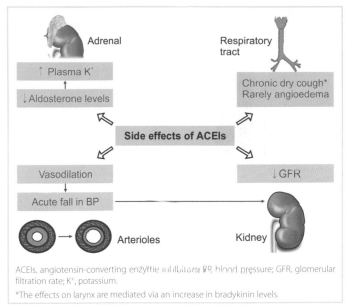

ACEIs, angiotensin-converting enzyme inhibitors; BP, blood pressure; GFR, glomerular filtration rate; K+, potassium.
*The effects on larynx are mediated via an increase in bradykinin levels.

FIG. 6: Side effects of angiotensin-converting enzyme inhibitors.

TABLE 7: Dose of various angiotensin-converting enzyme inhibitors and angiotensin II receptor blockers used in heart failure

Agents	Dose (mg)	Frequency
ACEIs		
Captopril	75–150	BD
Enalapril	10–40	BD
Fosinopril	10–40	OD
Lisinopril	10–40	OD
Quinapril	10–40	OD or BD
Ramipril	2.5–20	OD or BD
Trandolapril	1–4	OD
ARBs		
Losartan	25–50	BD
Valsartan	150–300	BD
Candesartan	4–16	OD

ACEIs, angiotensin-converting enzyme inhibitors; ARBs, angiotensin II receptor blockers.

Adrenergic Antagonists

In patients with HF, sympathoadrenergic systems are activated. The centrally mediated sympathetic nerve activity is increased. The circulating catecholamines are increased. There is also increased cardiac adrenergic activity. There is increased cardiac norepinephrine release, as evident from the higher norepinephrine concentration in the coronary sinus blood compared to that in arterial blood (Fig. 7). Increased cardiac

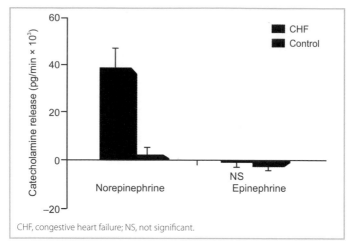

CHF, congestive heart failure; NS, not significant.

FIG. 7: Cardiac adrenergic activity in patients with systolic heart failure is illustrated. Cardiac catecholamine release is substantially increased in patients with systolic heart failure. Catecholamine release was calculated from the product of coronary sinus blood flow and the difference of the coronary sinus venous and arterial catecholamine concentrations.

adrenergic activity is associated with increased myocardial oxygen demand, calcium overload and myocardial ischemia. There is myocyte hypertrophy and myocyte necrosis and apoptosis.

Increased systemic sympathetic activity is associated with peripheral venous and arterial vasoconstriction. There is increased systemic vascular resistance, which is associated with impaired left ventricular systolic function. There is also adverse ventricular and vascular remodeling. Ventricular dilatation with increase in end-diastolic and end-systolic volumes along with reduction in EF occurs. There is also disruption of extracellular matrix with increased myocardial fibrosis.

The rationale of β-blocker therapy in HFrEF is to produce beneficial reverse ventricular remodeling, to relieve symptoms and to decrease mortality and morbidity. A number of β-adrenergic antagonists have been reported to produce beneficial effects in HFrEF. The three β-blockers that have been demonstrated to decrease mortality and morbidity of patients with HFrEF in large randomized clinical trials are carvedilol, slow release metoprolol and bisoprolol.

Carvedilol is a nonselective β-blocker and blocks both β1 and β2 receptors. It also possesses β-adrenergic antagonist property and has antioxidant effect. A number of clinical trials have been performed with the use of carvedilol in the management of HFrEF. In the Carvedilol Prospective Randomized Cumulative Survival (COPERNICUS) trial, 2,289 patients were randomized to receive either carvedilol or placebo.[15] The target dose of carvedilol was 25 mg twice a day. During a mean follow-up of 10.4 months, there was a 35%

reduction in the risk of mortality. In the USA carvedilol trial, 1,094 patients were randomized either to receive carvedilol or placebo. There was a 65% reduction in all-cause mortality with carvedilol therapy.[16]

In the Metoprolol CR/XL Randomized Intervention Trial in Congestive Heart Failure (MERITHF), 3,991 patients were randomized to receive either metoprolol XL or placebo.[17] During an average follow-up period of 12 months, there was a reduction of mortality by 34%. The target dose of metoprolol XL in this trial was 200 mg daily.

In the Cardiac Insufficiency Bisoprolol Study II (CIBIS-II), 2,647 patients were randomized to receive either bisoprolol or placebo.[18] There was a 34% reduction in the risk of total mortality, 44% reduction in the risk of sudden cardiac death and a 20% risk reduction in hospitalization for treatment of HF.

In the Study of Effects of Nebivolol Intervention on Outcomes and Rehospitalization in Seniors with Heart Failure (SENIORS) study, effect of nebivolol was evaluated in patients with HFrEF.[19] Nebivolol, a selective $\beta 1$ adrenergic antagonist with nitric oxide-mediated vasodilator property decreased the risk of composite endpoint of death or cardiovascular hospitalization.

The effects of carvedilol have been compared to those of short-acting immediate release metoprolol in the Carvedilol Or Metoprolol European Trial (COMET).[20] In this trial, 3,000 patients with moderately severe HF were randomized either to receive metoprolol tartrate or carvedilol. The target dose of carvedilol was 25 mg twice a day and that of metoprolol tartrate, 50 mg twice a day. With carvedilol, there was 17% greater reduction of mortality.

Bucindolol, a β-blocker similar to carvedilol was investigated and used in the β-blocker Evaluation Survival Trial (BEST).[21] In this trial, 2,708 NYHA class III or IV HF patients were randomized either to receive bucindolol or placebo. There was no survival benefit of bucindolol. Lack of bucindolol benefit may be related to its inverse agonist and intrinsic sympathomimetic activity.[22,23]

Centrally acting sympatholytic agents, such as moxonidine can produce adverse effects on cardiovascular mortality in patients with HF. In the Moxonidine in Congestive heart failure (MOXCON) trial, there was a higher mortality and morbidity in patients treated with moxonidine.[24] Thus, the adrenergic antagonists that are recommended for treatment of HFrEF at present are carvedilol, bisoprolol and long-acting slow-release metoprolol. The β-blockers should be instituted slowly. The initiating dose should be lower in patients with more severe HF. Particularly in relatively hypotensive patients, the lowest possible dose should be used initially. The initiating dose of carvedilol is usually 3.125 mg, metoprolol XL 12.5 mg and bisoprolol 2.5 mg in patients with HF and hypotension. In patients without hypotension, larger doses of β-blockers can be used as the initiating dose. The doses should be increased gradually till optimal dose or the maximal tolerated doses are attained. When larger doses are used initially, hypotension is likely to develop.

The usual complications of β-blockers are fatigue, impaired exercise tolerance and sometimes worsening symptoms of HF. It should be appreciated that these side effects occur initially and resolve within 6–8 weeks of treatment. Thus, the patients and the physicians should be encouraged to continue treatment.

The 2013 ACCF/AHA Task Force on Practice Guidelines for Management of Heart Failure Recommendations for the Use of β-blockers in HFrEF[1]

Class I

- Evidence based β-blockers should be used in all patients with stage C HFrEF unless contraindicated. (Level of Evidence: A)
- β-blockers should be used in all stage B HFrEF patients with a history of MI. (Level of Evidence: B)
- β-blockers should be used in all stage B HFrEF patients without a history of MI. (Level of Evidence: C)

Aldosterone Antagonists

In patients with HFrEF, aldosterone levels are elevated. Aldosterone promotes myocyte hypertrophy, increased collagen synthesis, myocardial fibrosis and adverse ventricular remodeling. It also promotes coronary atherosclerosis. There is decreased norepinephrine uptake. Renal adverse effects consist of glomerulosclerosis, tubulointerstitial fibrosis, sodium and water retention, and potassium and magnesium wasting. In the vasculature, it promotes atherosclerosis, endothelial and vascular smooth muscle cell hypertrophy and vasomotor dysfunction.

Aldosterone receptor antagonists, spironolactone and eplerenone, have the potential to produce beneficial left ventricular reverse remodeling, decrease in endsystolic and end-diastolic volumes with an increase in EF and also reduction in myocardial fibrosis.[25-28] In a substudy of the Eplerenone Post-acute Myocardial Infarction Heart Failure Efficacy and Survival Study (EPHESUS), serum levels of collagen biomarkers were measured and, after treatment with eplerenone, levels of aminoterminal peptide of types I and III procollagen were significantly lower at 6 months.[26]

In randomized clinical trials, aldosterone antagonists have been demonstrated to decrease mortality and morbidity in patients with HFrEF. In the Randomized Aldactone Evaluation Study (RALES), 1,663 patients with NYHA class III or IV HFrEF were randomized to receive either spironolactone (target dose 25 mg/day) or placebo.[29] After an average follow-up of 24 months, there was a 30% reduction in all-cause mortality. There was a reduction in the risk of sudden cardiac death as well as in HF death with spironolactone (Fig. 8).

The effects of eplerenone, a selective aldosterone antagonist, have also been evaluated both in post-acute MI patients and in patients with chronic HFrEF. In the EPHESUS, 6,642 postinfarction patients with LVEF of 40% or less were randomized within 3–14 days after infarction to receive either placebo or eplerenone (target dose 50 mg daily).[30] With the treatment of eplerenone, there was a 15% reduction in all-cause mortality, sudden cardiac death and hospitalizations for HF (Fig. 9). Treatment with eplerenone in postacute MI patients also decreases the mean length of hospital stay.[31]

The effects of eplerenone on mortality and morbidity of patients with NYHA class II chronic HFrEF were assessed in the placebo-controlled randomized trial, Eplerenone in Mild Patients Hospitalization and Survival Study in Heart Failure (EMPHASIS-HF).[32] In this trial, 2,737 patients more than 55 years with LVEF ≤35% were randomized either to receive eplerenone or placebo. Patients with an estimated glomerular filtration rate (GFR) of less than 30 mL/min/1.73 m^7 or serum

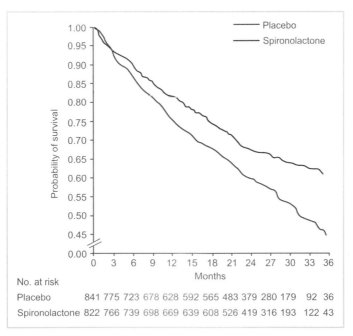

FIG. 8: The results of RALES trial in which aldosterone antagonist spironolactone, was used in patients with severe chronic systolic congestive heart failure.[29]

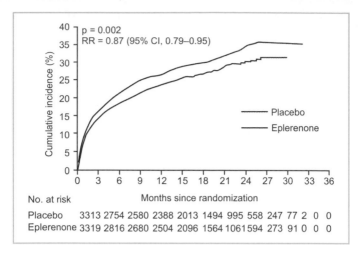

FIG. 9: The effects of aldosterone specific antagonist, eplerenone in post-acute myocardial infarction with reduced ejection fraction are illustrated. Eplerenone reduced the risks of mortality and development of heart failure.[30]

potassium ≥5.0 mmol/L were excluded. The inclusion criteria were: cardiac hospitalization within 6 months; BNP level more than 250 pg/mL, NT-proBNP more than 500 pg/mL (men), or more than 750 pg/mL (women); and QRS duration 130 ms or greater in patients with EF between 31% and 35%. The background treatment consisted of β-blockers and angiotensin inhibitors in the majority of patients in both groups. After a median of 21 months of follow-up, there was a significant reduction of primary composite endpoint of cardiovascular death or hospitalization for HF [hazard ratio (95% CI), 0.63 (0.54–0.74); P <0.001] and of all-cause mortality [hazard ratio (95% CI), 0.76 (0.62–0.93)]. There was also a significant reduction in the composite endpoint of all-cause, cardiac and HF hospitalizations. The number of patients needed to be treated was 51 to reduce one death/year during follow-up. The annual mortality rate in the placebo group was 7.1%.

The active metabolite of spironolactone is canrenone. The effect of canrenone on left ventricular remodeling was evaluated in a randomized placebo-controlled double-blind trial in patients with mild HFrEF, the antiremodeling effect of canrenone in patients with mild chronic HF (AREA IN-CHF) study.[33] In this trial, 467 patients in NYHA class II HF with LVEF ≤45% were randomized to receive canrenone or placebo. Almost all patients received angiotensin inhibitors and β-blockers before randomization. During follow-up of 12 months, there was no significant change in left ventricular end-diastolic volume with canrenone; however, the magnitude of LVEF was higher with canrenone than with placebo. There was a statistically insignificant trend toward reduction in all-cause mortality with canrenone (2.8% vs. 5.4%, P = 0.17).

However, there was a significant reduction of the composite of cardiac death or hospitalization with canrenone compared to placebo (8% vs. 15.1%, P = 0.02).

In a meta-analysis of 19 randomized clinical trials (14 studies of spironolactone, 3 studies of eplerenone and 3 studies of canrenone) on the effect of aldosterone antagonists in HFrEF, 10,807 patients were included for analysis.[34] There was 20% reduction in all-cause mortality and 3.1% increase in LVEF with aldosterone antagonists in patients with HFrEF.

The major side effects of aldosterone antagonists are hyperkalemia. In a meta-analysis of 19 randomized trials, incidence of serious hyperkalemia was 5.9% with the use of aldosterone antagonists.[34] In the EMPHASIS-HF trial, serum potassium concentration of more than 5.5 mmol/L occurred in 11.8% patients with eplerenone.[32] Serum potassium more than 6 mmol/L occurred in 2.5% of eplerenone-treated patients. In a nonrandomized cohort study, the incidence of serum potassium more than 6 mmol/L was 2.9%.[35] It should be appreciated that in randomized trials, the patients at a risk of hyperkalemia are excluded. Thus, the reported incidences in these trials are likely to be lower than what occurs in clinical practice.

There are several risk factors for hyperkalemia. Advanced age, diabetes, pre-existing renal dysfunction, hypovolemia and concomitant use of angiotensin inhibitors increase the risk of development of hyperkalemia. The use of nonsteroidal drugs, potassium supplements, potassium containing salt substitutes and concurrent use of other potassium sparing drugs may precipitate hyperkalemia. Whenever aldosterone antagonist therapy is initiated, careful monitoring of electrolytes, including serum potassium and renal function should be performed. Lack of adequate monitoring may be associated with severe unexpected hyperkalemia and increased mortality.[36]

Aldosterone antagonists should be initiated at low doses (spironolactone 6.25–12.5 mg and eplerenone 12.5 mg). Serum potassium and renal function should be monitored at 72 hours, at 1 and 2 weeks and then at 3 months or as required, based on the changes in clinical status.

Renal function impairment may occur but is uncommon. Severe hyponatremia is also an uncommon complication of these agents. Gynecomastia and breast enlargements are complications of spironolactone and do not occur with eplerenone. Spironolactone possesses antiandrogenic effects. It inhibits the effects of dihydrotestosterone at receptor sites. It also increases peripheral conversion of testosterone to estradiol.[37] The overall incidence of gynecomastia in the randomized trials is 2.8%.[34]

Drug Interactions

Spironolactone inhibits P-glycoprotein.[38] As digoxin is a substrate for P-glycoprotein, spironolactone can decrease renal clearance of digoxin and increase serum level of digoxin.[38]

The serum concentration of eplerenone is affected by the concomitant use of cytochrome P450 3A4 inhibitors as eplerenone is a substrate of cytochrome P450 3A4.[39] Drugs like ketoconazole can increase the serum level of eplerenone by 5-fold and should not be used concurrently. Erythromycin increases the serum level of eplerenone by 2–3 fold and the dose of eplerenone should be reduced when use of both drugs is necessary.

Contraindications

Aldosterone antagonists are contraindicated in patients with serum potassium more than 5.0 mEq/L or with serum creatinine more than 2.5 mg/dL.

The 2013 ACCF/AHA Task Force on Practice Guidelines for Management of Heart Failure Recommendations for the Use of Aldosterone Antagonists in HFrEF[1]

Class I

- Aldosterone antagonist is recommended for patients with NYHA classes II–IV HF with reduced LVEF of less than 35% while receiving standard therapy, including ACEI (or ARB) and β-blocker. (Level of Evidence: A)
- Following an acute MI, aldosterone antagonist is recommended in patients who have an LVEF of less than 40% and has clinical HF or history of diabetes mellitus. Patients should be on standard therapy, including ACEI (or ARB) and a β-blocker. (Level of Evidence: B)

Class III

Aldosterone antagonists are not recommended when creatinine is more than 2.5 mg/dL or creatinine clearance is less than 30 mL/min or serum potassium is more than 5 mmol/L or in conjunction with other potassium sparing diuretics. (Level of evidence: B)

Hydralazine and Nitrates

Hydralazine is an arteriolar dilator, and it dilates primarily the resistance vessels. The hemodynamic effects of hydralazine are characterized by a decrease in systemic vascular resistance associated with an increase in cardiac output. Frequently, mean arterial pressure and heart rate remain unchanged.[40] In patients with associated severe mitral regurgitation, hydralazine causes a greater increase in forward stroke volume because of reduction of systemic vascular resistance.[41] Hydralazine can produce sustained beneficial hemodynamic effects in patients with chronic HF during its long-term administration.[42]

Nitrates are predominantly venodilators. They also cause a modest increase in aortic compliance, which decreases left ventricular afterload. Because of venodilatation with nitrates, there is a decrease in venous return and a reduction in ventricular preload. There is a reduction in systemic (right atrial) and pulmonary venous (pulmonary capillary wedge) pressures with a little or no change in stroke volume and cardiac output. In patients with HF, there is also no reflex increase in heart rate.

The hemodynamic profile of patients with severe HFrEF is low cardiac output and increased right atrial and pulmonary capillary wedge pressures. Hydralazine increases cardiac output and nitrates decrease right atrial and pulmonary capillary wedge pressures. The hemodynamic advantage of combining hydralazine and nitrates in treating HFrEF is apparent.[43]

The effects of combination of hydralazine and nitrates have been assessed in a number of randomized clinical trials. In the Veteran Administration Heart Failure trial (VHeFT), 1,642 veterans with NYHA class II or III HF were randomized to receive either hydralazine and isosorbide dinitrate combination or prazosin (α-adrenergic blocking agent) or placebo.[44] There was no difference in mortality between prazosin and placebo. However, with hydralazine and isosorbide dinitrate combination therapy, there was a significant improvement in survival compared to placebo.

A large randomized trial (African-American Heart Failure Trial—AHeFT) was performed to assess the effects of combination of hydralazine and isosorbide dinitrate in the selfreported black patients with severe HFrEF.[45] In this trial, 1,050 patients in NYHA class III or IV HF were randomized to receive hydralazine and isosorbide dinitrate combination or placebo. The majority of patients received as background treatments, angiotensin inhibitors (87%) and β-blockers (74%). Only 39% were on spironolactone. The dose of hydralazine was 37.5–75 mg thrice a day and that of isosorbide dinitrate, 20–40 mg thrice a day. The trial was terminated prematurely, as there was a substantial survival benefit with hydralazine and isosorbide dinitrate combination therapy. The risk of all-cause mortality decreased by 43% and of first hospitalization by 39%.

It has been postulated that the beneficial effects of hydralazine and isosorbide dinitrate combination therapy are related to nitric oxide availability. Nitrates are nitric oxide donors, and it has been suggested that hydralazine decreases nitric oxide breakdown and enhances nitric oxide availability. However, some studies have suggested that hydralazine does not decrease nitric oxide resistance in chronic HF.[46]

Adverse Effects

The dose of hydralazine that is used for treatment of HFrEF rarely produces any significant adverse reactions. Occasionally, hypotension can occur. Lupus-like syndrome only occurs with larger doses. Skin rashes are rarely observed.

The complication of nitrates is headache at the initiation of treatment. Nitrate tolerance is decreased when used with hydralazine. Rarely, hypotension occurs with nitrates in HF.

The 2013 ACCF/AHA Task Force on Practice Guidelines for Management of Heart Failure Recommendations for the Use of Hydralazine and Nitrate in HFrEF[1]

Class I

A combination of hydralazine and nitrate is recommended to improve outcomes for patients self described as African-Americans with NYHA III-IV HFrEF on optimal therapy with ACEIs, β-blockers and diuretics (*Level of Evidence: A*).

Class IIA

A combination of hydralazine and nitrate is reasonable in patients with stage C HFrEF who cannot be given an ACEI or ARB because of drug intolerance, hypotension or renal insufficiency (*Level of Evidence: B*).

Calcium Channel Blockers

Both dihydropyridine and nondihydropyridine calcium channel blockers (CCBs) exert negative inotropic effects and they are contraindicated in patients with HFrEF. Although they exert peripheral and coronary vasodilatation, the beneficial effects due to vasodilatation have not been documented.

Amlodipine is a dihydropyridine CCB. The effect of amlodipine has been assessed in prospective randomized trials. In the Prospective Randomized Amlodipine Survival Evaluation (PRAISE) study, there was a trend for benefit in patients with nonischemic dilated cardiomyopathy, but the overall results were neutral.[47] Subsequent study has also demonstrated no beneficial effect of amlodipine in patients with nonischemic dilated cardiomyopathy. Thus, its use is not recommended except in patients with persistent hypertension despite adequate angiotensin inhibition and β-blocker therapy.

The 2013 ACCF/AHA Task Force on Practice Guidelines for Management of Heart Failure Recommendations for the Use of Calcium Channel Blocker in HFrEF[1]

Class III

Calcium channel blockers are not indicated as routine treatment for HF in stage C HFrEF patients. (Level of Evidence: A)

Diuretics

Diuretics are necessary to relieve congestive symptoms in patients with HFrEF (stages C and D). For long-term management, usually oral loop diuretics are used. The most frequently used loop diuretic is furosemide. However, ethacrynic acid, bumetanide and torsemide are also used but much less frequently than furosemide.

In an open-label randomized trial, 234 patients were randomized to receive either furosemide or torsemide.[48] The primary endpoint in this trial was the rate of hospital admissions. During the follow-up period of approximately 12 months, the hospital admission rate with torsemide was 17% and that with furosemide 32%.

Doses

The daily dose of furosemide is 20–240 mg, bumetanide 0.5–10 mg, ethacrynic acid 50–200 mg and torsemide 10–200 mg. However, in clinical practice the usual daily dose of furosemide is 40–80 mg, bumetanide 2–3 mg and torsemide 20–50 mg.

Complications

Aggressive diuretic therapy can produce several complications. Electrolyte imbalances, such as hypokalemia and hypomagnesemia are risk factors for life-threatening ventricular arrhythmias. Diuretic therapy can also produce hyponatremia, hyperuricemia and hyperglycemia. When large dose of furosemide is used, transient deafness may occur. Deterioration of renal function is common. Increased uric acid excretion and precipitation of gout may occur during diuretic therapy. Skin rash is also observed with loop diuretics.

Intravenous administration of furosemide can produce transient depression of left ventricular function with decreased cardiac output and increased pulmonary capillary wedge pressure. This hemodynamic deterioration results from transient increase in norepinephrine and vasopressin.[49]

The 2013 ACCF/AHA Task Force on Practice Guidelines for Management of Heart Failure Recommendations for the Use of Diuretics in HFrEF[1]

Class I

Diuretics are indicated in stage C HFrEF patients with fluid retention. (Level of Evidence: C)

Positive Inotropic Agents

The positive inotropic drugs, such as digoxin, catecholamines and cardiospecific phosphodiesterase inhibitors (PDEIs), are in general, not indicated in patients with stable chronic HFrEF.

Digoxin

Digoxin and other cardiac glycosides exert their positive inotropic effect by increasing intracellular calcium. It inhibits Na^+/K^+ adenosine triphosphatase (ATPase) and increases intracellular sodium. Sodium-calcium exchanger system is activated resulting in an increase in intracellular calcium.

Digitalis also exerts electrophysiologic effects both directly and by modulating autonomic nervous system. It decreases sinus rate and atrioventricular nodal conduction. Electrocardiogram shows sinus bradycardia and prolonged PR interval. Repolarization effects of digoxin are manifested by decreased T-wave amplitude and scooping of the ST segments.

Long-term oral digoxin therapy has been reported to improve hemodynamics and left ventricular function in patients with HFrEF.[50] There is an increase in left ventricular stroke work index along with a decrease in pulmonary capillary wedge pressure, indicating improvement in left ventricular function. Two randomized digoxin withdrawal studies have been performed. In the Prospective Randomized study of Ventricular failure and the efficacy of Digoxin (PROVED) study and in the Randomized Assessment of Digoxin in Inhibitors of AngiotensinConverting Enzyme (RADIANCE) study, the withdrawal of digoxin therapy was associated with a decrease in LVEF and deterioration in clinical status, functional capacity and exercise performance.[51,52] It should be appreciated that these studies were performed before the introduction of β-blocker therapy in HFrEF. In the randomized Digitalis Investigation Group (DIG) trial, long-term oral digoxin therapy was not associated with any improvement in survival in patients with chronic HFrEF.[53] In this trial, 6,800 patients with symptoms and signs of HF with LVEF of ≤45% were randomized either to receive digoxin or placebo. The median dose of digoxin used in this trial was 0.25 mg/day. Although digoxin did not decrease overall mortality, HF mortality tended to be lower. There was a statistically significant reduction in the composite endpoints of HF mortality or hospitalization for HF. However, toxicity was higher in digoxin treated patients compared to placebo (2% vs. 0.9%, p <0.001). Furthermore, in patients with digoxin blood level of 1.2 ng/mL or higher, there was increased mortality due to arrhythmia. Thus, if digoxin is used, the digoxin blood level should be kept below 1.2 ng/mL. It should be appreciated that the DIG trial was performed before β-blocker therapy was introduced. Presently, digoxin is used primarily in patients with atrial fibrillation to decrease ventricular response.[54]

The oral dose of digoxin is 0.0625–0.25 mg daily. In presence of renal failure, the dose should be decreased and administered less frequently. The usual maintenance dose of digoxin is 0.125–0.25 mg daily. The intravenous dose of digoxin is 0.25–1.0 mg, which should be given by slow infusion. Rapid bolus injection of digoxin is associated with coronary and mesenteric vasoconstriction.

The 2013 ACCF/AHA Task Force on Practice Guidelines for Management of Heart Failure Recommendations for the Use of Digoxin in HFrEF[1]

Class IIa

If there are no contraindications, digoxin can be beneficial in stage C HFrEF patients to decrease HF-related hospitalizations. (Level of Evidence: B)

The 2013 ACCF/AHA Task Force on Practice Guidelines for Management of Heart Failure Recommendations for the Use of Parenteral Positive Inotropic Drug in HFrEF[1]

Class III

Long-term use of a parenteral positive inotropic drug may be harmful and is not recommended for patients with stage C HFrEF, except as palliation for patients with end stage disease who cannot be stabilized with standard medical treatment. (Level of Evidence: C)

DRUG TREATMENT FOR ACUTE HEART FAILURE SYNDROMES

Diuretic Therapy

All patients with exacerbation of chronic HF with congestive symptoms require aggressive diuretic therapy. Most frequently, intravenous furosemide either by bolus or by infusion is used. The rationale for the use of intravenous diuretics is that, following oral administration, the absorption is slow and the critical serum level is obtained slowly.

Vasopressor and Inotropic Therapy

In hypotensive patients, the use of vasopressors and inotropic agents is necessary. The vasopressors that are commonly used are dopamine, norepinephrine, phenylephrine and vasopressin.

Dopamine can exert vasodilation, inotropic and vaso-constrictive effects, which are determined by the dose used. The low doses of dopamine (1–2 µg/kg/min) activate dopaminergic receptors 1 and 2 (DA1 and DA2). Activation of DA1 receptors produces renal and mesenteric vasodilatation. Activation of DA2 receptors decreases presynaptic reuptake of norepinephrine, which also promotes vasodilatation. With larger doses of dopamine (3–10 µg/kg/min), positive inotropic effects are observed. This is due to activation of β1 and β2 adrenergic receptors. There is an increase in cardiac output along with a modest increase in heart rate. With a further increase in the dose of dopamine, the vasopressor effects occur. The dose of dopamine that exerts vasopressor effects is usually higher than 10 μg/kg/min. Sometimes, very high doses exceeding 20 μg/kg/min are used to increase blood pressure. The higher doses of dopamine stimulate vascular α-receptors and cause an increase in systemic vascular resistance and arterial pressure. It should be appreciated that with an increase in systemic vascular resistance (left ventricular afterload), there might be a decrease in cardiac output. The higher doses of dopamine may also cause excessive tachycardia. Pulmonary capillary wedge and pulmonary artery pressure may also increase.[55]

Norepinephrine and phenylephrine are also used in hypotensive patients to increase blood pressure. Norepinephrine is predominantly an α-adrenergic agonist with a modest β-receptor agonist property. Phenylephrine is primarily an α-agonist. Both norepinephrine and phenylephrine increase systemic vascular resistance and blood pressure. However, cardiac output may decrease due to increased left ventricular afterload.

A synthetic catecholamine, dobutamine is predominantly a β1 adrenergic receptor agonist. It also stimulates β2 adrenergic receptors. The hemodynamic effects of dobutamine are characterized by a substantial increase in cardiac output, a reduction in systemic vascular resistance and a slight decrease in mean arterial pressure. There is only a slight increase in heart rate. The pulmonary capillary wedge and pulmonary artery pressure usually do not change significantly.

The phosphodiesterase 3 inhibitor, milrinone is an inodilator that is frequently used in patients with refractory HFrEF (stage D). It exerts a positive inotropic and vasodilator effect. The vasodilator effect is much more pronounced than its positive inotropic effect.[56] It increases cardiac output and decreases pulmonary capillary wedge and pulmonary artery pressures. There is a slight or no increase in heart rate; however, ventricular arrhythmias may be precipitated.

Inotropic drug therapy may be associated with myocyte necrosis, myocardial injury and worsening HF. It can be associated with a higher incidence of ventricular arrhythmias and increased mortality.

Vasodilator Therapy

In relatively hypertensive patients with acute HF syndromes, intravenous vasodilators, particularly sodium nitroprusside should be considered. Standard therapy with proven benefit should be instituted eventually.

DRUG TREATMENT OF HYPONATREMIA

Hyponatremia is defined as serum sodium level of less than 135 mEq/L and is observed in approximately 20–30% of patients with decompensated HFrEF. It is associated with increased mortality and morbidity. It can occur in hypovolemic, euvolemic, or hypervolemic patients. In congestive HF (CHF), it occurs most frequently in patients with volume overload.

Most patients with CHF who develop hyponatremia do not experience symptoms related to hyponatremia until the serum sodium level falls to 120 mEq/L or less. Signs and symptoms include nausea, vomiting, headache, confusion, lethargy and muscle spasms. With more severe hyponatremia, decreased consciousness, coma and seizures may occur. The neurologic complications of severe hyponatremia result from cerebral edema.

The mechanisms of hyponatremia are multifactorial. In CHF, hyponatremia results when water retention exceeds sodium retention. Decreased renal perfusion, activation of renin-angiotensin-aldosterone system and impaired natriuretic response cause sodium retention. Water retention results from excessive water reabsorption in proximal tubules and increased arginine vasopressin activation. Patients with CHF also develop excessive thirst due to stimulation of thirst center by angiotensin, which is elevated in HF. Excessive thirst is associated with increased intake of sodium-free water. In hyponatremic patients, total body water is greater than total body sodium.

Correction of Hyponatremia in Heart Failure

Fluid restriction to 1–2 L or less/day should be encouraged. However, most patients cannot adhere to fluid restriction because it is uncomfortable, and it induces thirst, which is associated with increased water intake.

Intravenous administration of isotonic or hypertonic saline with or without concomitant use of loop diuretics has been used to correct hyponatremia. However, in patients with HF, there is increased risk of volume overload and pulmonary congestion with intravenous saline infusion. Furthermore, rapid correction of hyponatremia can cause central pontine myelinolysis that is often fatal. It should also be appreciated that the use of loop diuretics can exacerbate hyponatremia due to activation of renin-angiotensin-aldosterone system. Thiazide diuretics and aldosterone antagonists also exacerbate hyponatremia. Diuretics can cause hypokalemia and hypomagnesemia, which can precipitate life-threatening arrhythmias.

Demeclocycline is a tetracycline antibiotic that has been used for treatment of hyponatremia. It inhibits effects of arginine vasopressin, and induces diabetes insipidus and enhances free water clearance. It can also produce nephrotoxicity.

Arginine vasopressin antagonists can also correct hyponatremia in patients with HF. There are three subtypes of arginine vasopressin receptors—V1a, V1b, and V2. Activation of V1a receptors causes vasoconstriction and cardiac myocyte hypertrophy. Stimulation of V1b receptors is associated with increased adrenocorticotropic hormone and β-endorphin release. The V2 receptors are primarily present in the principal cells of renal collecting duct and their stimulation causes renal free water reabsorption. The V2 receptors activate water channel aquaporin 2, which is associated with decreased water permeability, increased water retention, volume overload and hyponatremia. For correction of hyponatremia, V1a and V2 receptors antagonists are used. Tolvaptan, lixivaptan and conivaptan are the vasopressin antagonists that have been used for treatment of hyponatremia in HF.

Tolvaptan is a selective non-peptide V2 receptor antagonist. It is administered orally and it has a half-life of 6–8 hours. In the Acute and Chronic Therapeutic Impact of Vasopressin Antagonist in Congestive Heart Failure (ACTIV in CHF) trial, 319 patients with HFrEF with LVEF of less than 40% were randomized to receive 30, 60, or 90 mg/day of tolvaptan or placebo.[57] The patients receiving tolvaptan had a significant reduction in body weight, an improvement in dyspnea score and decrease in the length of hospital stay compared to placebo.

In the Efficacy of Vasopressin Antagonism in Heart Failure Outcome Study with Tolvaptan (EVEREST) trial, 4,133 patients were randomized to receive 30 mg/day of tolvaptan or placebo.[58] All patients were hospitalized, and were in NYHA class III or IV HF and had LVEF of less than 40%. The treatment was continued for 60 days. The mean follow-up period was 9.9 months. There was no significant difference in total mortality, cardiovascular mortality, or hospitalizations with tolvaptan treatment compared to placebo. However, there was an improvement in dyspnea scores, a decrease in body weight and peripheral edema. Serum sodium increased to a greater extent compared to placebo.

Lixivaptan is a nonpeptide and highly specific V2 receptor vasopressin antagonist. It is administered orally. In a randomized clinical trial, one dose of lixivaptan was found to increase urine volume and free water clearance.[59] There was also significant increase in serum sodium concentration.

Conivaptan is a nonpeptide and both V1a and V2 vasopressin receptor antagonist. It is administered intravenously. In a randomized trial, the effects of conivaptan were assessed in hyponatremic-hospitalized patients.[60] In this trial, 84 patients were randomized either to receive intravenous conivaptan (20 mg loading dose followed by 40 or 80 mg infusion for

96 hours) or placebo. There was a significant increase in serum sodium. In another randomized trial, the hemodynamic effects of conivaptan were determined in patients with advanced HFrEF who first underwent pulmonary artery catheterization.[61] In this trial, 142 patients with NYHA class III or IV HF were randomized to receive either a single dose of conivaptan or placebo. With conivaptan, there was a significant decrease in pulmonary capillary wedge and right atrial pressures. There was also significant increase in urine volume and free water clearance and decrease in urine osmolality.

The 2013 ACCF/AHA Task Force on Practice Guidelines for Management of Heart Failure Recommendations for the Use of Arginine Vasopressin Antagonists[1]

Class IIb

AV receptor selective or nonselective vasopressin antagonist therapy is reasonable in hospitalized HF patients who are hypervolemic and have persistent, severe and symptomatic (or at risk for symptoms) hyponatremia despite water restriction and guideline-directed medical therapy. (Level of Evidence: B)

MANAGEMENT OF HEART FAILURE WITH PRESERVED EJECTION FRACTION

The drug treatment of HFpEF is limited. The congestive symptoms are treated with diuretics and/or nitrates. However, there is no improvement in survival. In the Hong Kong Diastolic Heart Failure Study, the patients were randomized to receive diuretic alone, or diuretics and an ACEI, or diuretics and the ARB, irbesartan.[62] The hospital admission rates decreased and exercise performance improved in all three groups. There was, however, no survival benefit.

In a large randomized clinical trial, the efficacy of perindopril, an ACEI, was evaluated in elderly patients (≥70 years) with HFpEF.[63] In this trial, 850 patients were randomized to receive either perindopril or placebo. The primary endpoint was combined all-cause mortality and unexpected hospitalization for the treatment of HF. There was no significant reduction in the primary endpoints with perindopril compared to placebo.

In a number of randomized clinical trials, the efficacy of ARBs was assessed in the management of HFpEF. In the CHARM-Preserved trial, 3,023 patients were randomized to receive either candesartan or placebo.[64] The primary endpoint in this trial was cardiovascular death or hospitalization for HF. There was no significant benefit with candesartan treatment. In another randomized prospective clinical trial, 4,128 patients were randomized to receive irbesartan or placebo.[65] There was no difference in mortality or morbidity between irbesartan and placebo during the follow-up of over 4 years.

To assess the efficacy of aldosterone antagonists in the management of HFpEF, prospective randomized trials have been undertaken. In the Treatment of Preserved Cardiac Function Heart Failure with an Aldosterone Antagonist trial (TOPCAT), a large number of patients were randomized to receive either spironolactone or placebo.[66] There was no benefit in mortality or morbidity.

The β-blockers are useful to decrease heart rate and to improve ventricular filling. However, the effect of β-blockers on mortality and hospitalization in patients with HFpEF is not clearly established yet. In a meta-analysis of 15 observational studies and two randomized control trials involving a total of 27,099 patients with HFpEF, observational studies showed that β-blockers reduced all-cause mortality [RR (95% CI), 0.81 (0.72–0.90); P <0.001], but not HF hospitalization rates [RR (95% CI), 0.79 (0.57–1.10), P <0.001]. The two trials did not find a significant reduction in all-cause mortality with β-blocker therapy [RR (95% CI), 0.94 (0.67–1.32), P = 0.72] or HF hospitalization [RR (95% CI), 0.90 (0.54–1.49), P = 0.68].

Sildenafil, an orally active type 5 cyclic guanosine mono-phosphate (GMP)-specific PDEI, has been reported to improve clinical outcomes in patients with HFpEF and pulmonary hypertension.[67] In this study, 50 mg of sildenafil, thrice a day was used. Treatment with sildenafil was associated with a decrease in pulmonary artery pressure and pulmonary vascular resistance. There was also improvement in exercise tolerance. The sample size in this study was too small to assess any effect on mortality. A large multicenter, double-blind, placebo-controlled, parallel-group, randomized clinical trial, PhosphdiesteRasE-5 Inhibition to Improve CLinical Status and EXercise Capacity in Diastolic Heart Failure (RELAX) trial of 216 stable outpatients with HFpEF, EF ≥50%, elevated N-terminal BNP or elevated invasively measured filling pressures and reduced exercise capacity has been subsequently performed to determine the effect of the sildenafil compared with placebo on exercise capacity and clinical status in HFpEF.[68] Among patients with HFpEF, administration of sildenafil for 24 weeks, compared with placebo, did not result in significant improvement in exercise capacity or clinical status.

NEWER PHARMACOLOGIC AGENTS FOR TREATMENT OF HEART FAILURE

The newer drugs that are being developed for treatment of HF are not yet available for clinical use and are not approved by USFDA.

Heart Failure with Reduced Ejection Fraction

Inotropic Drugs

Calcium-sensitizing agents, such as levosimendan and pimobendan enhance the affinity of cardiac myosin filaments to calcium. They are also cardiac specific type III PDEI. The effect of levosimendan on human coronary hemodynamics has been evaluated. Levosimendan does not appear to increase myocardial oxygen consumption.[69] The use of levosimendan in patients with acute decompensated HF has been associated with increased incidence of atrial fibrillation and flutter, ventricular arrhythmias and hypotension and increased or no significant improvement in mortality.[70,71]

Cardiac myosin activator, omecamtiv mecarbil, increases contractility, directly affecting the sarcomere function. It does not change intracellular calcium metabolism. The inotropic effect is related to prolongation of ejection time. A clinical prospective, randomized, double-blind, clinical trial has reported that the positive inotropic effect of omecamtiv mecarbil is directly proportional to the magnitude of prolongation of left ventricular systolic ejection time.[72] Excessive prolongation of systolic ejection time may compromise diastolic filling time and induce myocardial ischemia.[73]

Istaroxime is an inotropic agent that inhibits Na^+/K^+ ATPase activity and stimulates the sarcoplasmic reticulum calcium ATPase activity. It increases contractility and enhances relaxation. In a phase II trial (Hemodynamic effects of Istaroxime in patients with worsening heart failure and Reduced LV Systolic Function—HORIZON-HF), 120 patients with HFrEF were randomized either to receive istaroxime or placebo. There was a reduction in pulmonary capillary wedge pressure and with the highest dose, there was also an increase in cardiac output.[74]

Vasodilators—Relaxin

Relaxin is a circulating peptide. It is a potent vasodilator. It is normally found in pregnant women. The vasodilatation is mediated by activation of nitric oxide synthase. The hemodynamic effects consist of decreased systemic vascular resistance and increased cardiac output. There is also a decrease in pulmonary capillary wedge pressure. In human, infusion of relaxin increases renal plasma flow without any change in GFR. Serelaxin is a recombinant human relaxin-2.

In a prospective phase IIb, PreRELAXA-HF study, 214 patients with acute HF with systolic blood pressure more than 125 mmHg were enrolled.[75] These patients also had mild-to-moderate renal impairment with estimated creatinine clearance of 30–75 mL/min/1.73 m^2. With the infusion of relaxin, there was an improvement in dyspnea score compared to placebo and there was a trend toward reduction of inhospital worsening HF, length of hospital stay and mortality at 60 days.

The RELAX-AHF, an international, double-blind, placebo-controlled trial, randomly-assigned 1161 patients hospitalized for acute HF to standard care and 48 hours intravenous infusions of placebo or serelaxin within 16 hours from presentation.[76] Serelaxin significantly improved dyspnea compared with placebo. It had no significant effect on cardiovascular death or readmission to hospital for HF or renal failure [hazard ratio (95% CI), 1·02 (0·74–1·41); P = 0·89] or days alive out of the hospital up to day 60, but was associated with significantly fewer deaths at day 180 [hazard ratio (95% CI), 0·63 (0·42–0·93); P = 0·019].

Sarcoplasmic Reticulum Calcium Adenosine Triphosphatase Activators

In HFrEF, calcium handling is abnormal. There is partial depletion of calcium in the sarcoplasmic reticulum. In animal models of HF, enhanced calcium uptake by the sarcoplasmic reticulum is associated with improved systolic and diastolic function, improved metabolic reserve and decreased mortality, and increased resistance for developing HF during prolonged pressure overload.[77]

A randomized clinical trial of gene therapy to increase sarcoplasmic reticular calcium has been performed. Thirty-four patients with NYHA class III or IV were randomized in Calcium Upregulation by Percutaneous Administration of Gene Therapy in Cardiac Disease (CUPID) study to receive gene therapy or placebo. Gene therapy to enhance sarcoplasmic reticular calcium was associated with symptomatic improvement, beneficial reverse remodeling and decreased natriuretic peptide levels.[78] Although these results are encouraging, large clinical trials will be required to establish the efficacy of such gene therapy for treatment of HF in clinical practice.

Ryanodine Receptor Stabilizers

In the myocyte, calcium release is mediated by activation of ryanodine receptor 2. Dysfunctional ryanodine receptor 2 may cause diastolic calcium leak and abnormal calcium handling in HF, which may cause cardiac dysfunction. There is increasing interest to develop drugs to prevent diastolic calcium leak and stabilize ryanodine receptors. A new class of drugs known as calcium release channel stabilizers (rycals) are being developed to prevent sarcoplasmic calcium leak which might be beneficial in treatment of HF.[79] It has been demonstrated that calcium/calmodulin-dependent kinase II (CaMKII) can mediate calcium leakage through ryanodine 2 receptors. It has been also reported that CaMKII is upregulated in HF and correlates with reduced EF. In endstage failing myocardium, both in animals and human, CaMKII inhibition reduces sarcoplasmic reticular calcium leak and enhances myocardial contractile function. Thus, CaMKII inhibitors may be useful in treatment of HFrEF.[80]

Neuregulins

The neuregulins are growth-promoting proteins. Neuregulin1 appears to exert a protective effect in HF.[81] The potential beneficial effects of neuregulin1 were evaluated in rats with coronary ligation models. Recombinant neuregulin1 was used, and there was an improvement in ventricular function and reverse ventricular remodeling. Early phase II studies have been performed with recombinant neuregulin1 in patients with HF, and a beneficial effect on cardiac function and structure was reported.[82] It increased cardiac output and produced vasodilation. It should be appreciated that there are potential adverse effects, including acceleration of tumor growth.

New Renin-Angiotensin-Aldosterone Blocking Agents

The effects of direct renin inhibitors, such as aliskiren in the management of HF have been investigated. In the Aliskiren Observation of heart Failure Treatment (ALOFT) trial, 302 patients with HF were randomized to receive aliskiren (150 mg/day) or placebo.[83] The patients were in NYHA classes II–IV, but majority of patients were in NYHA class II. With aliskiren treatment, there were a significant reduction in BNP as well as in adverse ventricular remodeling. However, there are potential adverse effects of adding aliskiren to ACEIs. Significant hyperkalemia may develop.

Neutral Endopeptidase Inhibitors

Neutral endopeptidase inhibitors prevent degradation of natriuretic peptides. Large randomized clinical trials have been performed to assess the efficacy of neutral endopeptidase inhibitors in the management of HFrEF. Omapatrilat was used in the Inhibition of Metallo Protease by BMS186716 in a Randomized Exercise and Symptoms (IMPRESS) study.[84] In this study, 573 patients were randomized to receive either 40 mg of omapatrilat or 20 mg of lisinopril every day. The patients were in NYHA classes II–IV and had EF less than 40%. During 24 weeks of treatment, there was no difference in the primary endpoint of exercise tolerance between the two groups. However, with omapatrilat, there was a significant reduction in the predefined composite endpoint of death, admission for HF, or discontinuation of HF treatment because of worsening symptoms. In a large phase III Omapatrilat Versus Enalapril Randomized Trial of Utility in Reducing Events (OVERTURE) study, 5,770 patients were randomized either to receive 40 mg of omapatrilat once a day or 10 mg of enalapril twice a day.[85] During follow-up of 14.5 months with omapatrilat, there was a small insignificant reduction in the composite endpoint of death or hospitalization for HF requiring intravenous treatment. Furthermore, increased incidence of angioedema occurred with omapatrilat. Thus, the omapatrilat studies have been discontinued.

Neprilysin inhibitor slows breakdown of natriuretic peptides. It has been combined with ARBs. A large double-blind randomized clinical trial (PARADIGM-HF) compared the combination therapy using the angiotensin receptor–neprilysin inhibitor LCZ696 (200 mg twice daily) with enalapril (10 mg twice daily) in 8,442 patients who had class II-IV HFrEF, in addition to recommended therapy.[86] After a median follow-up of 27 months, LCZ696 significantly reduced a composite of death from cardiovascular causes or hospitalization for HF [hazard ratio (95% CI), 0.80 (0.73–0.87); P <0.001], all-cause mortality [hazard ratio (95% CI), 0.84 (0.76–0.93); P <0.001], death from cardiovascular causes [hazard ratio (95% CI), 0.80 (0.71–0.89); P <0.001] and the risk of HF-related hospitalization (21% reduction, P <0.001) compared with enalapril. Hypotension and nonserious angioedema were more commonly seen in the LCZ696 group. Enalapril group had higher proportions of patients with renal impairment, hyperkalemia and cough. These beneficial results may prove to be a new paradigm shift in the treatment of patients with HF.

Aldosterone Blockade

Nonsteroidal mineralocorticoid blocking agents have been developed to assess their efficacy in treatment of hypertension and HF. These agents are undergoing clinical trials.

Aldosterone Synthase Inhibitors

The aldosterone synthase inhibitors have the potential to attenuate the deleterious effects of aldosterone on ventricular remodeling. In a rat model of failing ventricle, aldosterone synthase inhibitor has been reported to improve hemodynamics, left ventricular function, and to produce beneficial effects on ventricular remodeling.[87]

Selective Sinus Node Inhibitors

High resting heart rate is associated with adverse outcomes in patients with chronic HF. It has been hypothesized that heart rate reduction may improve clinical outcomes in patients with HF.

Ivabradine is a selective sinus node inhibitor.[88] It selectively blocks cardiac pacemaker cell f-channels from intracellular aspect and specifically inhibits I_f current. I_f current is the determinant of the spontaneous slow diastolic depolarization slope of the cardiac pacemaker cells. Thus, ivabradine reduces the heart rate without affecting other cardiac ionic currents.

A randomized, double-blind, placebo-controlled, parallel-group study (SHIFT trial) assessed the safety and efficacy of ivabradine in 6,558 patients with symptomatic HFrEF who had LVEF of 35% or lower, were in sinus rhythm with heart rate 70 beats per min or higher, were hospitalized for HF within the previous year, and were on stable background treatment including a β-blocker if tolerated.[89] Patients in the ivabradine group had a significant reduction in the composite primary endpoint of cardiovascular death or hospitalization for worsening HF [hazard ratio (95% CI), 0.82 (0.75–0.90), P <0.0001], hospitalization for worsening HF [hazard ratio (95% CI), 0.74 (0.66–0.83), P <0.0001] and HF-related deaths [hazard ratio (95% CI), 0.74 (0.58–0.94), P = 0.014] compared with the placebo after a median follow-up of 22.9 months. There was significantly higher proportion of symptomatic bradycardia (5% vs. 1%, P <0.0001) and visual side effects (3% vs. 1%, P <0.0001) in the ivabradine group than the placebo group. A small open label study of 10 consecutive patients with acute decompensated HFrEF with LVEF less than 40% and heart rates more than 70 beats per minute, and without other acute conditions or inotropic therapy showed that oral ivabradine safely reduced heart rate by mean of 16.3 beats per minute at discharge and lower heart rate at discharge was associated with better functional class (P = 0.033).[90]

Trimetazidine

Though the complete mechanisms of action are not known, trimetazidine exerts a cytoprotective effect via selective inhibition of the final enzyme in the β-oxidation pathway of free fatty acid, long-chain 3-ketoacyl coenzyme A thiolase.[91] It also increases pyruvate dehydrogenase activity. This restores the imbalance in glucose oxidation and glycolysis that occurs during ischemia. It is a direct inhibitor of cardiac fibrosis. It improves sarcolemmal mechanoresistance.

A systematic meta-analysis of 17 randomized controlled trials including 955 chronic HF patients found that trimetazidine significantly improved LVEF in patients with both ischemic and non-ischemic HF, reduced left ventricular end-systolic volume, improved NYHA class and increased exercise duration (P <0.01 for all) compared with placebo.[92] There was a greater reduction in all-cause mortality [RR (95% CI), 0.29 (0.17–0.49); P <0.00001] and cardiovascular events and hospitalization [RR (95% CI), 0.42 (0.30–0.58); P <0.00001] in the trimetazidine group than the placebo group. Another meta-analysis of 16 randomized controlled trials involving 884 patients with chronic HF also found that trimetazidine may reduce cardiac hospitalization and left ventricular remodeling, and improve clinical symptoms and cardiac function.[93] However, larger multicenter trials are necessary to confirm these beneficial findings.

Vitamin D Supplementation

Several observational and experimental studies have found an association between low levels of vitamin D and HF.[94] However, it is unclear whether low vitamin D levels result in progression of HF and whether vitamin D supplementation can prevent worsening of cardiac function. Interventional studies investigating the role of vitamin D supplementation have yielded conflicting results. A single-center, open-label, blinded endpoint randomized controlled trial of 101 stable chronic HF patients with reduced LVEF showed 6 weeks of daily 2,000 IU oral vitamin D3 decreased plasma renin activity and plasma renin concentration compared with the control.[95] A meta-analysis of 11 trials involving 50,252 individuals reported that calcium or vitamin D supplementation had no effect on major cardiovascular events [OR (95% CI), 1.03 (0.94–1.12); P = 0.54], MI (OR (95% CI), 1.08 (0.96–1.22); P = 0.21), or stroke [OR (95% CI), 1.01 (0.91–1.13); P = 0.80] in comparison to a placebo.[96]

Heart Failure with Preserved Ejection Fraction

Presently, there is no effective treatment available for the management of patients with HFpEF. Thus, there is increasing interest to develop newer treatment modalities for HFpEF. Advanced glycation end-products and collagen crosslinking modulators are being investigated.

To decrease myocardial stiffness, titin modulators are being developed. However, large clinical trials are lacking to assess the efficacy of such therapeutic approaches for management of HFpEF.

CONCLUSION

There has been a considerable advance in the understanding of pathophysiology and ventricular remodeling in both HFrEF and HFpEF. There have been advances in the management of HFrEF.

Recognition and management of acute decompensated HF have improved. However, the treatment of HFpEF has been disappointing. Furthermore, the drug treatment of HFrEF continues to improve with new advances in basic and clinic research. Thus, research should continue to develop new drugs for treatment of HF.

REFERENCES

1. Yancy CW, Jessup M, Bozkurt B, et al. 2013 ACCF/AHA guideline for the management of heart failure: a report of the American College of Cardiology Foundation/American Heart Association Task Force on Practice Guidelines. J Am Coll Cardiol. 2013;62:e147-239.

2. Lloyd-Jones DM, Larson MG, Leip EP, et al. Lifetime risk for developing congestive heart failure: the Framingham Heart Study. Circulation. 2002;106:3068-72.

3. McMurray JJ, Petrie MC, Murdoch DR, et al. Clinical epidemiology of heart failure: public and private health burden. Eur Heart J. 1998;19 Suppl P:P9-16.

4. Go AS, Mozaffarian D, Roger VL, et al. Heart disease and stroke statistics—2014 update: a report from the American Heart Association. Circulation. 2014;129:e28-292.

5. Heidenreich PA, Albert NM, Allen LA, et al. Forecasting the impact of heart failure in the United States: a policy statement from the American Heart Association. Circ Heart Fail. 2013;6:606-19.

6. Owan TE, Redfield MM. Epidemiology of diastolic heart failure. Prog Cardiovasc Dis. 2005;47:320-32.

7. Sweitzer NK, Lopatin M, Yancy CW, et al. Comparison of clinical features and outcomes of patients hospitalized with heart failure and normal ejection fraction (> or =55%) versus those with mildly reduced (40% to 55%) and moderately to severely reduced (<40%) fractions. Am J Cardiol. 2008;101:1151-6.

8. Kitzman DW, Gardin JM, Gottdiener JS, et al. Importance of heart failure with preserved systolic function in patients > or = 65 years of age. CHS Research Group. Cardiovascular Health Study. Am J Cardiol. 2001;87:413-9.

9. McKee PA, Castelli WP, McNamara PM, et al. The natural history of congestive heart failure: the Framingham study. N Engl J Med. 1971;285:1441-6.

10. Francis GS, Benedict C, Johnstone DE, et al. Comparison of neuroendocrine activation in patients with left ventricular dysfunction with and without congestive heart failure. A substudy of the Studies of Left Ventricular Dysfunction (SOLVD). Circulation. 1990;82:1724-9.

11. Effects of enalapril on mortality in severe congestive heart failure. Results of the Cooperative North Scandinavian Enalapril Survival Study (CONSENSUS). The CONSENSUS Trial Study Group. N Engl J Med. 1987;316:1429-35.

12. Garg R, Yusuf S, Bussmann W, et al. Overview of randomized trials of angiotensin-converting enzyme inhibitors on mortality and morbidity in patients with heart failure. JAMA. 1995;273:1450-6.

13. Granger CB, McMurray JJ, Yusuf S, et al. Effects of candesartan in patients with chronic heart failure and reduced left-ventricular systolic function intolerant to angiotensin-converting-enzyme inhibitors: the CHARM-Alternative trial. Lancet. 2003;362:772-6.

14. Pitt B, Poole-Wilson PA, Segal R, et al. Effect of losartan compared with captopril on mortality in patients with symptomatic heart failure: randomised trial--the Losartan Heart Failure Survival Study ELITE II. Lancet. 2000;355:1582-7.

15. Packer M, Coats AJ, Fowler MB, et al. Effect of carvedilol on survival in severe chronic heart failure. N Engl J Med. 2001;344:1651-8.

16. Packer M, Bristow MR, Cohn JN, et al. The effect of carvedilol on morbidity and mortality in patients with chronic heart failure. U.S. Carvedilol Heart Failure Study Group. N Engl J Med. 1996;334:1349-55.

17. Effect of metoprolol CR/XL in chronic heart failure: Metoprolol CR/XL Randomised Intervention Trial in Congestive Heart Failure (MERIT-HF). Lancet. 1999;353:2001-7.

18. The Cardiac Insufficiency Bisoprolol Study II (CIBIS-II): a randomised trial. Lancet. 1999;353:9-13.

19. Flather MD, Shibata MC, Coats AJ, et al. Randomized trial to determine the effect of nebivolol on mortality and cardiovascular hospital admission in elderly patients with heart failure (SENIORS). Eur Heart J. 2005;26:215-25.

20. Poole-Wilson PA, Swedberg K, Cleland JG, et al. Comparison of carvedilol and metoprolol on clinical outcomes in patients with chronic heart failure in the Carvedilol Or Metoprolol European Trial (COMET): randomised controlled trial. Lancet. 2003;362:7-13.

21. Beta-Blocker Evaluation of Survival Trial I. A trial of the beta-blocker bucindolol in patients with advanced chronic heart failure. N Engl J Med. 2001;344:1659-67.

22. Maack C, Cremers B, Flesch M, et al. Different intrinsic activities of bucindolol, carvedilol and metoprolol in human failing myocardium. Br J Pharmacol. 2000; 130:1131-9.

23. Andreka P, Aiyar N, Olson LC, et al. Bucindolol displays intrinsic sympathomimetic activity in human myocardium. Circulation. 2002;105:2429-34.

24. Cohn JN, Pfeffer MA, Rouleau J, et al. Adverse mortality effect of central sympathetic inhibition with sustained-release moxonidine in patients with heart failure (MOXCON). Eur J Heart Fail. 2003;5:659-67.

25. MacFadyen RJ, Barr CS, Struthers AD. Aldosterone blockade reduces vascular collagen turnover, improves heart rate variability and reduces early morning rise in heart rate in heart failure patients. Cardiovasc Res. 1997;35:30-4.

26. Iraqi W, Rossignol P, Angioi M, et al. Extracellular cardiac matrix biomarkers in patients with acute myocardial infarction complicated by left ventricular dysfunction and heart failure: insights from the Eplerenone Post-Acute Myocardial Infarction Heart Failure Efficacy and Survival Study (EPHESUS) study. Circulation. 2009;119:2471-9.

27. Tsutamoto T, Wada A, Maeda K, et al. Effect of spironolactone on plasma brain natriuretic peptide and left ventricular remodeling in patients with congestive heart failure. J Am Coll Cardiol. 2001;37:1228-33.

28. Udelson JE, Feldman AM, Greenberg B, et al. Randomized, double-blind, multicenter, placebo-controlled study evaluating the effect of aldosterone antagonism with eplerenone on ventricular remodeling in patients with mild-to-moderate heart failure and left ventricular systolic dysfunction. Circ Heart Fail. 2010;3:347-53.

29. Pitt B, Zannad F, Remme WJ, et al. The effect of spironolactone on morbidity and mortality in patients with severe heart failure. Randomized Aldactone Evaluation Study Investigators. N Engl J Med.1999;341:709-17.

30. Pitt B, Remme W, Zannad F, et al. Eplerenone, a selective aldosterone blocker, in patients with left ventricular dysfunction after myocardial infarction. N Engl J Med. 2003;348:1309-21.

31. Gheorghiade M, Khan S, Blair JE, et al. The effects of eplerenone on length of stay and total days of heart failure hospitalization after myocardial infarction in patients with left ventricular systolic dysfunction. Am Heart J. 2009;158:437-43.

32. Zannad F, McMurray JJ, Krum H, et al. Eplerenone in patients with systolic heart failure and mild symptoms. N Engl J Med. 2011;364:11-21.

33. Boccanelli A, Mureddu GF, Cacciatore G, et al. Anti-remodelling effect of canrenone in patients with mild chronic heart failure (AREA IN-CHF study): final results. Eur J Heart Fail. 2009;11:68-76.

34. Ezekowitz JA, McAlister FA. Aldosterone blockade and left ventricular dysfunction: a systematic review of randomized clinical trials. Eur Heart J. 2009;30:469-77.

35. Wei L, Struthers AD, Fahey T, et al. Spironolactone use and renal toxicity: population based longitudinal analysis. BMJ. 2010;340:c1768.

36. Shah KB, Rao K, Sawyer R, et al. The adequacy of laboratory monitoring in patients treated with spironolactone for congestive heart failure. J Am Coll Cardiol. 2005;46:845-9.

37. Rose LI, Underwood RH, Newmark SR, et al. Pathophysiology of spironolactone-induced gynecomastia. Ann Intern Med. 1977;87:398-403.

38. Kim RB. Drugs as P-glycoprotein substrates, inhibitors, and inducers. Drug Metab Rev. 2002;34:47-54.

39. Cook CS, Berry LM, Burton E. Prediction of in vivo drug interactions with eplerenone in man from in vitro metabolic inhibition data. Xenobiotica. 2004;34:215-28.

40. Chatterjee K, Parmley WW, Massie B, et al. Oral hydralazine therapy for chronic refractory heart failure. Circulation. 1976;54:879-83.

41. Greenberg BH, Massie BM, Brundage BH, et al. Beneficial effects of hydralazine in severe mitral regurgitation. Circulation. 1978;58:273-9.

42. Chatterjee K, Ports TA, Brundage BH, et al. Oral hydralazine in chronic heart failure: sustained beneficial hemodynamic effects. Ann Intern Med. 1980;92:600-4.

43. Massie B, Chatterjee K, Werner J, et al. Hemodynamic advantage of combined administration of hydralazine orally and nitrates nonparenterally in the vasodilator therapy of chronic heart failure. Am J Cardiol. 1977;40:794-801.

44. Cohn JN, Archibald DG, Ziesche S, et al. Effect of vasodilator therapy on mortality in chronic congestive heart failure. Results of a Veterans Administration Cooperative Study. N Engl J Med. 1986;314:1547-52.

45. Taylor AL, Ziesche S, Yancy C, et al. Combination of isosorbide dinitrate and hydralazine in blacks with heart failure. N Engl J Med. 2004;351:2049-57.

46. Chirkov YY, De Sciscio M, Sverdlov AL, et al. Hydralazine does not ameliorate nitric oxide resistance in chronic heart failure. Cardiovasc Drugs Ther. 2010;24:131-7.

47. Packer M, O'Connor CM, Ghali JK, et al. Effect of amlodipine on morbidity and mortality in severe chronic heart failure. Prospective Randomized Amlodipine Survival Evaluation Study Group. N Engl J Med. 1996;335:1107-14.

48. Murray MD, Deer MM, Ferguson JA, et al. Open-label randomized trial of torsemide compared with furosemide therapy for patients with heart failure. Am J Med. 2001;111:513-20.

49. Francis GS, Siegel RM, Goldsmith SR, et al. Acute vasoconstrictor response to intravenous furosemide in patients with chronic congestive heart failure. Activation of the neurohumoral axis. Ann Intern Med. 1985;103:1-6.

50. Arnold SB, Byrd RC, Meister W, et al. Long-term digitalis therapy improves left ventricular function in heart failure. N Engl J Med. 1980;303:1443-8.

51. Uretsky BF, Young JB, Shahidi FE, et al. Randomized study assessing the effect of digoxin withdrawal in patients with mild to moderate chronic congestive heart failure: results of the PROVED trial. PROVED Investigative Group. J Am Coll Cardiol. 1993;22:955-62.

52. Packer M, Gheorghiade M, Young JB, et al. Withdrawal of digoxin from patients with chronic heart failure treated with angiotensin-converting-enzyme inhibitors. RADIANCE Study. N Engl J Med. 1993;329:1-7.

53. Digitalis Investigation G. The effect of digoxin on mortality and morbidity in patients with heart failure. N Engl J Med. 1997;336:525-33.

54. Jorge E, Baptista R, Martins H, et al. Digoxin in advanced heart failure patients: a question of rhythm. Rev Port Cardiol (English Edition). 2013;32:303-10.

55. Leier CV, Heban PT, Huss P, et al. Comparative systemic and regional hemodynamic effects of dopamine and dobutamine in patients with cardiomyopathic heart failure. Circulation. 1978;58:466-75.

56. Baim DS, McDowell AV, Cherniles J, et al. Evaluation of a new bipyridine inotropic agent--milrinone--in patients with severe congestive heart failure. N Engl J Med. 1983;309:748-56.

57. Gheorghiade M, Gattis WA, O'Connor CM, et al. Effects of tolvaptan, a vasopressin antagonist, in patients hospitalized with worsening heart failure: a randomized controlled trial. JAMA. 2004;291:1963-71.

58. Konstam MA, Gheorghiade M, Burnett JC Jr, et al. Effects of oral tolvaptan in patients hospitalized for worsening heart failure: the EVEREST Outcome Trial. JAMA. 2007;297:1319-31.

59. Abraham WT, Shamshirsaz AA, McFann K, et al. Aquaretic effect of lixivaptan, an oral, non-peptide, selective V2 receptor vasopressin antagonist, in New York Heart Association functional class II and III chronic heart failure patients. J Am Coll Cardiol. 2006;47:1615-21.

60. Zeltser D, Rosansky S, van Rensburg H, et al. Assessment of the efficacy and safety of intravenous conivaptan in euvolemic and hypervolemic hyponatremia. Am J Nephrol. 2007;27:447-57.

61. Udelson JE, Smith WB, Hendrix GH, et al. Acute hemodynamic effects of conivaptan, a dual V(1A) and V(2) vasopressin receptor antagonist, in patients with advanced heart failure. Circulation. 2001;104:2417-23.

62. Yip GW, Wang M, Wang T, et al. The Hong Kong diastolic heart failure study: a randomised controlled trial of diuretics, irbesartan and ramipril on quality of life, exercise capacity, left ventricular global and regional function in heart failure with a normal ejection fraction. Heart. 2008;94:573-80.

63. Cleland JG, Tendera M, Adamus J, et al. The perindopril in elderly people with chronic heart failure (PEP-CHF) study. Eur Heart J. 2006;27:2338-45.

64. Yusuf S, Pfeffer MA, Swedberg K, et al. Effects of candesartan in patients with chronic heart failure and preserved left-ventricular ejection fraction: the CHARM-Preserved Trial. Lancet. 2003;362:777-81.

65. Massie BM, Carson PE, McMurray JJ, et al. Irbesartan in patients with heart failure and preserved ejection fraction. N Engl J Med. 2008;359:2456-67.

66. Dalzell JR, Pitt B, Pfeffer M, et al. Spironolactone for heart failure with preserved ejection fraction. N Engl J Med. 2014;371:179.

67. Guazzi M, Vicenzi M, Arena R, et al. Pulmonary hypertension in heart failure with preserved ejection fraction: a target of phosphodiesterase-5 inhibition in a 1-year study. Circulation. 2011;124:164-74.

68. Redfield MM, Chen HH, Borlaug BA, et al. Effect of phosphodiesterase-5 inhibition on exercise capacity and clinical status in heart failure with preserved ejection fraction: a randomized clinical trial. JAMA. 2013;309:1268-77.

69. Michaels AD, McKeown B, Kostal M, et al. Effects of intravenous levosimendan on human coronary vasomotor regulation, left ventricular wall stress, and myocardial oxygen uptake. Circulation. 2005;111:1504-9.

70. Cleland JG, Freemantle N, Coletta AP, et al. Clinical trials update from the American Heart Association: REPAIR AMI, ASTAMI, JELIS, MEGA, REVIVE II, SURVIVE, and PROACTIVE. Eur J Heart Fail. 2006;8:105-10.

71. Mebazaa A, Nieminen MS, Packer M, et al. Levosimendan vs dobutamine for patients with acute decompensated heart failure: the SURVIVE Randomized Trial. JAMA. 2007;297:1883-91.

72. Cleland JG, Teerlink JR, Senior R, et al. The effects of the cardiac myosin activator, omecamtiv mecarbil, on cardiac function in systolic heart failure: a double-blind, placebo-controlled, crossover, dose-ranging phase 2 trial. Lancet. 2011;378:676-83.

73. Teerlink JR, Clarke CP, Saikali KG, et al. Dose-dependent augmentation of cardiac systolic function with the selective cardiac myosin activator, omecamtiv mecarbil: a first-in-man study. Lancet. 2011;378:667-75.

74. Gheorghiade M, Blair JE, Filippatos GS, et al. Hemodynamic, echocardiographic, and neurohormonal effects of istaroxime, a novel intravenous inotropic and lusitropic agent: a randomized controlled trial in patients hospitalized with heart failure. J Am Coll Cardiol. 2008;51:2276-85.

75. Teerlink JR, Metra M, Felker GM, et al. Relaxin for the treatment of patients with acute heart failure (Pre-RELAX-AHF): a multicentre, randomised, placebo-controlled, parallel-group, dose-finding phase IIb study. Lancet. 2009;373:1429-39.

76. Teerlink JR, Cotter G, Davison BA, et al. Serelaxin, recombinant human relaxin-2, for treatment of acute heart failure (RELAX-AHF): a randomised, placebo-controlled trial. Lancet. 2013;381:29-39.

77. Kiriazis H, Kranias EG. Genetically engineered models with alterations in cardiac membrane calcium-handling proteins. Ann Rev Physiol. 2000;62:321-51.

78. Jessup M, Greenberg B, Mancini D, et al. Calcium Upregulation by Percutaneous Administration of Gene Therapy in Cardiac Disease (CUPID): a phase 2 trial of intracoronary gene therapy of sarcoplasmic reticulum Ca^{2+}-ATPase in patients with advanced heart failure. Circulation. 2011;124:304-13.

79. Andersson DC, Marks AR. Fixing ryanodine receptor Ca^{2+} leak–a novel therapeutic strategy for contractile failure in heart and skeletal muscle. Drug Discov Today Dis Mech. 2010;7:e151-7.

80. Bers DM. CaMKII inhibition in heart failure makes jump to human. Circ Res. 2010;107:1044-6.

81. Liu X, Gu X, Li Z, et al. Neuregulin-1/erbB-activation improves cardiac function and survival in models of ischemic, dilated, and viral cardiomyopathy. J Am Coll Cardiol. 2006;48:1438-47.

82. Gao R, Zhang J, Cheng L, et al. A Phase II, randomized, double-blind, multicenter, based on standard therapy, placebo-controlled study of the efficacy and safety of recombinant human neuregulin-1 in patients with chronic heart failure. J Am Coll Cardiol. 2010;55:1907-14.

83. McMurray JJ, Pitt B, Latini R, et al. Effects of the oral direct renin inhibitor aliskiren in patients with symptomatic heart failure. Circ Heart Fail. 2008;1:17-24.

84. Rouleau JL, Pfeffer MA, Stewart DJ, et al. Comparison of vasopeptidase inhibitor, omapatrilat, and lisinopril on exercise tolerance and morbidity in patients with heart failure: IMPRESS randomised trial. Lancet. 2000;356:615-20.

85. Packer M, Califf RM, Konstam MA, et al. Comparison of omapatrilat and enalapril in patients with chronic heart failure the Omapatrilat Versus Enalapril Randomized Trial of Utility in Reducing Events (OVERTURE). Circulation. 2002;106:920-6.

86. McMurray JJV, Packer M, Desai AS, et al. Angiotensin–neprilysin inhibition versus enalapril in heart failure. N Engl J Med. 2014;371:993-1004.

87. Mulder P, Mellin V, Favre J, et al. Aldosterone synthase inhibition improves cardiovascular function and structure in rats with heart failure: a comparison with spironolactone. Eur Heart J. 2008;29:2171-9.

88. DiFrancesco D, Camm JA. Heart rate lowering by specific and selective I(f) current inhibition with ivabradine: a new therapeutic perspective in cardiovascular disease. Drugs. 2004;64:1757-65.

89. Swedberg K, Komajda M, Böhm M, et al. Ivabradine and outcomes in chronic heart failure (SHIFT): a randomised placebo-controlled study. Lancet. 2010;376:875-85.

90. Sargento L, Satendra M, Longo S, et al. Heart rate reduction with ivabradine in patients with acute decompensated systolic heart failure. Am J Cardiovasc Drugs. 2014;14(3):229-35.

91. Chrusciel P, Rysz J, Banach M. Defining the role of trimetazidine in the treatment of cardiovascular disorders: some insights on its role in heart failure and peripheral artery disease. Drugs. 2014;74:971-80.

92. Gao D, Ning N, Niu X, et al. Trimetazidine: a meta-analysis of randomised controlled trials in heart failure. Heart. 2011;97(4):278-86.

93. Zhang L, Lu Y, Jiang H, et al. Additional use of trimetazidine in patients with chronic heart failure: a meta-analysis. J Am Coll Cardiol. 2012;59:913-22.

94. Dalbeni A, Delva P, Minuz P. Could vitamin D supplements be a new therapy for heart failure? Possible pathogenic mechanisms from data of intervention studies. Am J Cardiovasc Drugs. 2014;14:357-66.

95. Schroten NF, Ruifrok WPT, Kleijn L, et al. Short-term vitamin D3 supplementation lowers plasma renin activity in patients with stable chronic heart failure: An open-label, blinded end point, randomized prospective trial (VitD-CHF trial). Am Heart J. 2013;166:357-64.e2.

96. Mao PJ, Zhang C, Tang L, et al. Effect of calcium or vitamin D supplementation on vascular outcomes: A meta-analysis of randomized controlled trials.Int J Cardiol. 2013;169:106-11.

Drugs for Stable Angina

Kanu Chatterjee, Wassef Karrowni

INTRODUCTION

In the Oxford Dictionary, "angina pectoris" is defined as "strangulation in the chest". Angina is the most common manifestation of coronary artery disease (CAD). It is the presenting symptom in approximately 50% of patients with chronic ischemic heart disease.[1] It remains a very common symptom in patients with acute coronary syndromes even after revascularization.[2]

CHRONIC STABLE ANGINA

Incidence and Prognosis

It has been estimated that for every one patient admitted to the hospital for acute myocardial infarction, there are thirty patients with chronic stable angina.[1] Thus stable angina is a very common clinical condition. In the United States of America, approximately 400,000 new patients/year are diagnosed to have stable angina and it has been estimated that the incidence is likely to increase by 50% during the next three decades.[3] Presently, in the United States, between 6.5 and 16.5 million of patients have stable angina. The global incidence of stable angina remains unknown.

Stable angina is also associated with considerable mortality and morbidity. Chronic ischemic heart disease with silent or manifest myocardial ischemia has been reported to cause one of five deaths/year indicating that the prognosis of patients with chronic stable angina is not entirely benign. The one-year mortality of patients with chronic stable angina is approximately 4%.[4] The adverse prognostic factors are age older than 75 years, diabetes, left bundle branch block, and reduced left ventricular ejection fraction. The cost of management of stable angina is also considerable. Noninvasive and invasive tests that are performed to establish the diagnosis, to formulate therapies and determine prognosis are expensive procedures. Furthermore, treatment of comorbidities, such as diabetes and hypertension, are also expensive.

Pathophysiology

Angina is a manifestation of myocardial ischemia. Myocardial ischemia results from an imbalance between myocardial oxygen demand and oxygen supply. The determinants of myocardial oxygen demand and supply are summarized in Tables 1 and 2. The major determinants of myocardial oxygen demand are heart rate, left ventricular wall stress and contractility. The higher the heart rate, the greater is the myocardial oxygen demand. Enhanced contractility is also associated with increased myocardial oxygen demand. Left ventricular wall stress is directly proportional to its pressure and volume. An increase in left ventricular volume or pressure, left ventricular wall stress increases with a concomitant increase in myocardial oxygen demand. Increase in both systolic and diastolic wall stress is associated with increased myocardial oxygen requirement. Systolic wall stress is primarily determined by systemic arterial pressure (blood pressure). The higher the systolic blood pressure, the greater is the myocardial oxygen demand. The rationale for the use of antihypertensive drugs for treatment of angina is apparent. Left ventricular diastolic pressure and volume are the major determinants of diastolic wall stress. The higher the left ventricular diastolic pressure, the greater is the myocardial oxygen demand. Similarly, the larger the left ventricular diastolic volume, the greater is the myocardial oxygen demand. Pharmacologic agents that decrease left ventricular diastolic volume and/or pressure have the potential to decrease myocardial ischemia and relief angina.

The determinants of myocardial oxygen supply are summarized in Table 2.

Myocardial oxygen consumption is the product of coronary blood flow and myocardial oxygen extraction. The myocardial oxygen extraction is near maximum even at rest and does not vary significantly with changes in myocardial oxygen demand. Thus, myocardial oxygen supply is primarily determined by coronary blood flow.

TABLE 1: Major determinants of myocardial oxygen demand

- Heart rate
- Contractility
- Wall stress
  - Systolic blood pressure
  - Ventricular volume
  - Wall thickness

TABLE 2: Major determinants of oxygen supply in chronic stable angina

- Arterial oxygen content
- Coronary blood flow
  - Perfusion pressure
  - Perfusion time
  - Degree of coronary artery stenosis
  - Coronary vascular resistance
  - Coronary sinus venous pressure
  - Ventricular diastolic pressure
- Collateral blood flow

Coronary blood flow occurs predominantly during diastole. Aortic diastolic pressure is the perfusion pressure and remains the major determinant of coronary blood flow and left ventricular myocardial perfusion. Normally coronary blood flow remains relatively constant during changes in perfusion pressure due to autoregulation. Changes in coronary vascular resistance are the major regulatory mechanism of autoregulation. When aortic diastolic pressure decreases, coronary vascular resistance also decreases to maintain the coronary blood flow. When aortic diastolic pressure increases, coronary vascular resistance increases and coronary blood flow remains unchanged. In absence of autoregulation, however, coronary blood flow is proportional to perfusion pressure. During myocardial ischemia, coronary vascular bed is maximally dilated and autoregulation is absent. In presence of myocardial ischemia, coronary blood flow decreases with decreasing aortic diastolic pressure.

When there is stenosis of the epicardial coronary arteries, the perfusion pressure is the pressure distal to the stenosis. The poststenotic pressure is related to pressure gradient across the stenotic segment. More severe the stenosis, greater is the pressure drop distal to the stenosis, and lower is the perfusion pressure. It should be also appreciated that the autoregulatory reserve is reduced in presence of severe coronary artery stenosis. Autoregulatory reserve is defined as the capacity to maintain coronary blood flow by decreasing coronary vascular resistance. Although at rest, coronary blood flow may be maintained by autoregulation, autoregulatory reserve can be exhausted during exercise. When coronary vascular resistance becomes minimal and there is no further increase in coronary blood flow myocardial ischemia is precipitated. In patients with classic (Heberden's) angina, the mechanism of angina during exercise is not only due to increased myocardial oxygen demand but also due to reduced autoregulatory reserve (Fig. 1).

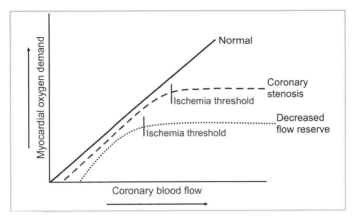

FIG. 1: Ishchemia threshold in stable angina.

Myocardial oxygen supply is also related to hemoglobin content and oxygen saturation of arterial blood. In presence of normal oxygen saturation, lower hemoglobin content is associated with decreased oxygen supply. However, there is a compensatory and obligatory increase in coronary blood flow resulting from decreased coronary vascular resistance.

Increased coronary sinus pressure increases coronary venous pressures and impairs myocardial perfusion. Left ventricular diastolic pressure is an important determinant of subendocardial blood flow. Higher the left ventricular diastolic pressure less is the subendocardial blood flow, which may be associated with subendocardial ischemia. The pharmacologic agents that decrease left ventricular diastolic pressure can decrease subendocardial ischemia and relief angina.

The magnitude of collateral blood flow to myocardial segments is an important determinant of maintaining perfusion to the myocardial segments supplied by the stenotic coronary arteries. At rest, collateral blood flow is frequently adequate to prevent myocardial ischemia. During increased myocardial oxygen demand as during exercise, collateral blood flow can be inadequate and is associated with myocardial ischemia and a greater risk of myocardial necrosis. An increase in collateral blood flow by angiogenesis has the potential to decrease myocardial ischemia and relief of angina.

SUBSETS OF STABLE ANGINA

A number of subsets of angina can be recognized clinically (Table 3). A careful history is usually sufficient to establish the diagnosis of these clinical subsets. However, it is often necessary to perform other investigations to determine the etiology and pathophysiologic mechanism of the clinical subsets. Noninvasive tests, such as stress tests and invasive tests including coronary angiography may be required to confirm

TABLE 3: Clinical subsets of stable angina

- Classic angina (Heberden's angina, effort angina)
  - Demand and supply ischemia
- Vasospastic angina (Prinzmetal angina)
  - Supply ischemia
- Mixed angina
  - Demand and supply ischemia
- Walk-through-angina
  - Supply ischemia
- Linked angina
  - Supply ischemia
- Syndrome "X"
  - Supply ischemia

the presence of and to establish the mechanism of myocardial ischemia. The pathophysiologic mechanisms of angina in these clinical subsets are also summarized in Table 3.

CLASSIC ANGINA (HEBERDEN'S ANGINA, EFFORT ANGINA)

Clinical Manifestations

The classic description of angina was first given by Dr William Heberden in 1768 when he gave his lecture in the Royal College of Physicians of London.[5] There has not been a better description of effort angina since then. In his presentation, he said, "those who are inflicted with it, are seized while they are walking, and more particularly after they walk soon after eating, with a painful and most disagreeable sensation in the breast, which seems as if it would take their life away, if it were to increase or to continue: the moment they stand still all this uneasiness vanishes."

The most common site of the chest discomfort is retrosternal; however, it can be located over epigastrium, left pectoral and interscapular regions. The predictive value of localization of the site of discomfort by the patient in the diagnosis of presence of CAD has been evaluated in a prospective, blinded study.[6] When the patient localizes the site of pain with a fist over the sternum, it is called "Levine sign". The "Levine sign" has been regarded diagnostic of angina for many years. Sometimes, the patient cannot localize the site of chest discomfort precisely and indicates the site of pain over left precordium by the hand. This is termed as "hand sign". If the patient can localize the site of the pain with fingertips, it is termed as "point sign". The "point sign" has a negative predictive value for angina and significant CAD over 97%. The positive predictive value of "Levine sign" and "hand sign" is approximately 50%. Thus, these classical clinical signs cannot be used to diagnose the presence of obstructive CAD.

The radiation of pain may occur to left or right arm or to both arms. Radiation to lower jaw is very suggestive of angina. Radiation to lower extremities on the other hand is extremely unlikely to be due to angina.

The character of pain is more often pressure or heaviness rather than pain. It can be squeezing or like indigestion. It is usually "deep and dull" and not "sharp and superficial". The duration of chest discomfort is usually a few minutes. If the duration is very brief like a "fraction of a second" or very prolonged like hours, it is unlikely to be angina. The chest discomfort is usually relieved with sublingual nitroglycerin in 1–3 minutes. If the relief is instantaneous with sublingual nitroglycerin, it is unlikely to be angina.

For establishing the diagnosis of myocardial ischemia, stress electrocardiography, or stress myocardial perfusion imaging is frequently performed. For the diagnosis of presence or absence of obstructive CAD, invasive coronary arteriography or noninvasive contrast computed coronary angiography is necessary.

Management

There are two major therapeutic goals for management of stable angina: (1) to reduce the risks of myocardial infarction and death and (2) to relieve angina/angina equivalent and to decrease myocardial ischemia. Revascularization therapy, whether surgical or percutaneous, plays an important role in chronic stable angina patients. Table 4 summarizes the current indications for revascularization in chronic stable angina.

Pharmacologic Management to Reduce the Risks of Future Adverse Cardiovascular Events

There are a number of drugs that have been demonstrated to reduce the risks of adverse cardiovascular complications in patients with stable angina.

TABLE 4: Indications for revascularization therapy in chronic stable angina

- Left main coronary artery disease
- Major three vessel coronary artery disease
- Two vessel disease with proximal LAD involvement
- Large area of myocardium at risk
- Persistent symptoms despite adequate medical therapy
- Symptomatic patients refusing anti-anginal drugs therapy

LAD, left anterior descending.

Antiplatelet Drugs

Aspirin is most frequently used antiplatelet drug in patients with atherosclerotic CAD. Aspirin inhibits synthesis of platelet thromboxane–A2 by irreversible acetylation of the enzyme cyclooxygenase. It is an effective antithrombotic agent and decreases the risk of myocardial infarction. In studies involving more than 3,000 patients with stable angina, there was an average 33% reduction of adverse cardiovascular events with the aspirin.[3,7,8] In asymptomatic patients, 325 mg of aspirin given on alternate days has been reported to decrease the incidence of myocardial infarction.[9] The use of low dose (75 mg) of aspirin decreases the risk of myocardial infarction and sudden cardiac death by approximately 32% in patients with stable angina.[10]

Aspirin should be used in all patients with stable angina in absence of contraindications. It should be used for primary prevention of cardiovascular complications in patients with risk factors for CAD, such as diabetes, hypertension, obesity, hyperlipidemia and smoking. The use of aspirin is indicated for secondary prevention of adverse cardiovascular events in all patients with documented coronary artery disease with or without previous myocardial infarction and with or without manifest myocardial ischemia.

The usual dose of aspirin is 75–325 mg both for primary and secondary prevention of cardiovascular events. In Europe, 75 mg strength is available. In the USA, 81 mg (baby aspirin) strength is available. Both lower and higher doses of aspirin produce similar cardiovascular beneficial effects. However, the risks of complications are higher with larger doses. The 81 mg strength tablet is more expensive than the 325 mg strength.

The most common side effect of aspirin is gastric intolerance and symptoms of indigestion. Frank gastric and duodenal ulcers are less common. However, gastric erosion can occur. Hepatotoxicity, exacerbation of asthma, skin rashes and renal toxicity are also uncommon complications of aspirin.

The gastrointestinal blood loss is the most serious complication of long-term use of aspirin. The fecal blood loss is dose-related. In patients who develop anemia, appropriate investigations for gastrointestinal blood loss including endoscopy should be undertaken. After treatment of gastritis or gastric erosions, lower dose of aspirin can be reinstituted and given every other day or even twice weekly. Long-term use of aspirin is contraindicated in patients with severe asthma.

The American College of Cardiology (ACC)/American Heart Association (AHA) guidelines recommend the use of aspirin in all patients with stable angina in absence of absolute contraindication (*Class I, Level of Evidence A*).

Clopidogrel

Clopidogrel exerts its antithrombotic effect by reducing platelet aggregation by inhibiting adenosine diphosphate pathway (ADP). Clopidogrel is a thienopyridine derivative and it irreversibly blocks platelet surface ADP receptors affecting ADP-dependent activation of glycoprotein IIb-IIIa complex. It does not affect prostaglandin metabolism.

In a randomized clinical trial, clopidogrel was compared in patients at risk of adverse cardiovascular events. It was reported that clopidogrel was slightly better than aspirin in reducing the adverse cardiovascular events.[11]

Clopidogrel is not used routinely in patients with stable angina except when coronary artery stents are used. It is used for 4–6 weeks when bare metal stents are used and for at least 1 year when drug-eluting stents are used.

The dose of clopidogrel for its long-term use is 75–81 mg daily orally. The duration of antiplatelet effect is 7–10 days. Clopidogrel is well tolerated and the side effects are uncommon. The skin rash has been observed infrequently. Neutropenia and thrombocytopenic purpura are very rare complications of clopidogrel.

Aspirin and clopidogrel resistance has been observed and its reported incidence varies between 5% and 75%. This wide variation in their incidence is partly due to the various definitions used for resistance. Various methods have been also developed and approved by FDA to detect and treat aspirin and clopidogrel resistance.

ACC/AHA guidelines recommend use of clopidogrel in patients with stable angina when aspirin is absolutely contraindicated (*Class IIa, Level of Evidence: B*).

Dipyridamole

Dipyridamole is an antiplatelet agent and it exerts its antiplatelet function by inhibiting adenosine uptake and cyclic guanosine monophosphate diesterase activity. It also possesses vasodilating property. It is seldom used as an antiplatelet agent for the management of patients with atherosclerotic cardiovascular diseases. In cardiology, dipyridamole is primarily used as a pharmacologic stress agent for nuclear perfusion myocardial imaging test. Occasionally, it is used in combination with warfarin for prevention of thromboembolic complications in patients with prosthetic mechanical valves.

ACC/AHA guidelines recommend against use of dipyridamole in patients with stable angina. (*Class III, Level of Evidence: B*).

Cilostazol

Cilostazol is a phosphodiesterase inhibitor. It inhibits platelet aggregation and also has vasodilating effect. It is primarily used for treatment of intermittent claudication.

Warfarin

The potential beneficial effect of low-intensity anticoagulation with warfarin has been investigated in asymptomatic patients with risk factors of atherosclerosis. It has been suggested that it can be beneficial in selected patients with stable angina. However, presently it is not clear whether anticoagulation therapy with warfarin alone without aspirin, is any better than aspirin alone.[3]

ACC/AHA guidelines recommend use of long-term low-intensity anticoagulation with warfarin along with aspirin in selected patients with stable angina. (*Class IIb, Level of Evidence: B*).

Lipid-lowering Agents

All patients with established coronary artery disease or with high-risk for coronary artery disease should be treated with 3-hydroxy-3-methylglutaryl coenzyme A (HMG CoA) reductase inhibitors (statins) in absence of contraindication.

In Scandinavian Simvastatin Survival Study (4S), 4,444 patients with dyslipidemia and coronary artery disease were randomized either to receive placebo or simvastatin. During a follow-up period of 5.4 years, treatment with simvastatin was associated with a 26% reduction in new onset or worsening angina and a 37% reduction for the need of revascularization.[12] There was also a significant reduction in the risks of fatal and nonfatal myocardial infarction.[12] In the Cholesterol and Recurrent Events (CARE) study, statin therapy with pravastatin was associated with a 37% reduction in the relative risks of fatal myocardial infarction in patients with documented coronary artery disease.[13] In the Atorvastatin Versus Revascularization Treatment (AVERT) trial, patients with stable angina associated with coronary artery disease were randomized to receive 80 mg of atorvastatin or percutaneous coronary intervention with or without stent implantation. Atorvastatin treatment was associated with a statistically significant lower risk of the primary composite endpoint defined as one of the outcomes: Death from cardiac causes, nonfatal myocardial infarction, cerebrovascular accident, coronary artery bypass graft surgery (CABGS), angioplasty, resuscitation after cardiac arrest and worsening angina requiring hospitalization. Studies comparing the effects of intensive versus moderate lipid-lowering strategies on the extent of myocardial ischemia in patients with stable coronary artery disease have been performed.[14,15] There was a significant reduction in myocardial ischemia with both intensive and moderate lipid-lowering therapy.[14,15]

In the Double-Blind Atorvastatin Amlodipine (DUAAL) trial, the anti-ischemic effect of atorvastatin was compared to that of a calcium channel blocker amlodipine. After 24 weeks of treatment, both treatment modalities caused similar reduction of myocardial ischemia detected by stress testing or by ambulatory electrocardiography.[16]

In the Vascular Basis for the Treatment of Myocardial Ischemia Study, intensive or moderate antilipid treatment strategies were compared in patients with dyslipidemia and stable coronary heart disease.[15] During 12 months of treatment, both treatment strategies reduced the incidence and duration of myocardial ischemia detected by stress testing or ambulatory electrocardiography.

In the Study Assessing Goals in the Elderly (SAGE) trial, the effect of intensive (atorvastatin 80 mg daily) was compared to moderate (pravastatin 40 mg daily) statin therapy in 900 elderly patients with coronary heart disease.[17] After 1 year of treatment, both strategies were associated with a 37% reduction of total duration of myocardial ischemia during ambulatory electrocardiography. Intensive lipid-lowering therapy with atorvastatin was associated with a 77% risk reduction in total mortality.

In the Clinical Outcome Utilizing Revascularization and Aggressive Drug Evaluation (COURAGE) trial, patients with chronic stable angina were randomized to receive medical therapy or revascularization.[18] Medical therapy included statin therapy. In this trial, medical therapy was as effective as percutaneous coronary artery intervention in reducing the future adverse coronary events and myocardial ischemia.

The results of these clinical trials suggest that statins should be used in patients with chronic stable angina in absence of absolute contraindication.

ACC/AHA guidelines recommend use of lipid lowering-therapy in patients with documented or suspected CAD and LDL cholesterol more than 130 mg/dL with a target LDL less than 100 mg/dL (Class I, Level of Evidence A).

The presently available statins for clinical use are simvastatin, lovastatin, atorvastatin, rosuvastatin, pravastatin and fluvastatin. Statins should be taken in the evening after dinner as cholesterol synthesis occurs predominantly at night.

Lovastatin and simvastatin are pro-drugs. Atorvastatin, rosuvastatin and fluvastatin are active as they are administered. Gastrointestinal absorption of statins is 40–70% except that of fluvastatin, which is fully absorbed. The half-lives of most of the statins are between 1 and 3 hours except atorvastatin (14 hours) and rosuvastatin (19 hours).

The mechanism of action of statins is primarily due to inhibition of HMG-CoA reductase inhibition. They increase the hepatic high-affinity low-density lipoprotein receptors (LDL). There is increased scavenging of the circulating LDL cholesterols. This is the primary mechanism for the reduction of LDL levels with statins.

The major adverse effects of statin therapy are elevation of serum aminotransferase activity. If the liver function abnormalities continue, statins should be discontinued. Skeletal muscleache is rather common however, marked myositis and rhabdomyolysis are rare. The metabolism of lovastatin, simvastatin and atorvastatin involves primarily CYP3A4 and that of fluvastatin and rosuvastatin CYP2C9. Pravastatin is metabolized by the different mechanisms including sulfation. In patients who cannot tolerate simvastatin or atorvastatin, pravastatin may be used.

The drug interactions of statins with macrolide antibiotics, cyclosporine, ketoconazole, HIV protease inhibitors and fibrates have been observed. Concomitant use of verapamil or amiodarone and statin increase the risk of myopathy.

For monitoring the adverse effects of statin therapy, periodic assessment of liver function and measurement of creatinine kinase (CK) is recommended.

The dose of simvastatin is 5–80 mg daily. Recently FDA has recommended not to use 80 mg dose of simvastatin because of the increased risk of rhabdomyolysis.

The dose of lovastatin is 10–40 mg, atorvastatin 10–80 mg, rosuvastatin 10–40 mg and that of pravastatin 10–80 mg daily.

Angiotensin-inhibiting Drugs

Angiotensin inhibition therapy has the potential to reduce the adverse cardiovascular events in patients with stable angina. The use of an angiotensin-converting enzyme inhibitor ramipril, in a high-risk population, such as with history of coronary artery disease, stroke, peripheral vascular disease, diabetes, hypertension, hyperlipidemia and without overt manifestation of myocardial ischemia is associated with a substantial reduction of adverse cardiovascular events.[19] Perindopril, another angiotensin-converting enzyme inhibitor was associated with decreased risk of adverse cardiovascular complications in patients with ischemic heart disease.[20] In postmyocardial infarction patients with decreased left ventricular ejection fraction, angiotensin-converting enzyme inhibitor captopril has been shown to decrease the risk of mortality and morbidity.[21] There are, however, studies which have reported lack of benefit of routine angiotensin-converting enzyme inhibitor treatment in patients with low-risk patients with stable coronary artery disease.[22] In the PEACE trial, trandolapril, another angiotensin-converting enzyme inhibitor was used in patients with chronic ischemic heart disease. The patients in this randomized trial, the risk factors were treated as well. The majority of patients were treated with statins and also had revascularization therapy.[23] In this trial, the event rate of adverse cardiovascular events was lower in the placebo-treated group than in the trandolapril-treated group. Based on the result of PEACE trial, ACC/AHA guideline committee recommends against use of angiotensin-converting enzyme inhibitors in the low-risk patients.[24] However, even in the low-risk patients with elevated biomarkers of cardiovascular stress, such as of midregional pro-atrial natriuretic peptide, midregional pro-adrenomedullin, C-terminal pro-endothelin–I and copeptin, use of trandolapril was associated with decreased risk of cardiovascular death and heart failure.[25] It should be also appreciated that in the majority of the randomized studies, it was observed that angiotensin inhibition therapy is beneficial and thus should be used in patients with documented coronary artery disease in absence of absolute contraindication.[22]

ACC/AHA guidelines recommend that angiotensin-converting enzyme inhibitors should be used in all patients with coronary artery disease and diabetes and/or left ventricular systolic dysfunction (*Class I, Level of Evidence A*). It should be also used in patients with coronary artery disease without diabetes or other vascular disease (*Class IIa, Level of Evidence B*).

Beta-adrenergic Receptor Antagonists (Beta-blockers)

It has been amply demonstrated that β-blockers improve left ventricular systolic function and decrease mortality and morbidity of patients with reduced left ventricular ejection fraction.[26] However, there is limited data available to assess the effect of β-blocker therapy on mortality and morbidity of patients with stable angina without previous myocardial infarction and with preserved left ventricular systolic function. In the atenolol silent ischemia study, asymptomatic or minimally symptomatic patients were randomized to receive either atenolol or placebo.[27] Treatment with atenolol was associated with a significant lower risk of the primary combined endpoint (death, resuscitation from ventricular tachycardia/fibrillation, nonfatal myocardial infarction, hospitalization for unstable angina, aggravation of angina requiring known antianginal therapy or need for myocardial revascularization during the follow-up period of 1 year). There was, however, no difference between atenolol or placebo treatments in the individual hard endpoints such as death and nonfatal myocardial infarction.

ACC/AHA guidelines recommend use of β-blockers in patients with stable angina if not contraindicated to reduce the risks of future adverse cardiovascular events (*Class I, Level of Evidence B*).[3]

Other Therapies to Decrease the Risks of Adverse Cardiovascular Events

Folate therapy should be considered when homocysteine levels are elevated. The treatment of depression is also recommended.

Adequate control of hypertension and diabetes is essential. Cessation of smoking is highly recommended. Weight loss should be encouraged in overweight patients. Sedentary lifestyle should be discouraged and regular aerobic exercise should be encouraged. The therapies to decrease the risks of adverse cardiovascular events are summarized in Table 5.

Drugs to Relieve Angina and Myocardial Ischemia in Patients with Stable Angina (Table 6)[28-30]

Beta-adrenergic Receptor Antagonists (Beta-blockers)

Three types of β-adrenergic receptors, β-1, β-2, and β-3 have been recognized. Beta-1 receptors are present in cardiac

TABLE 5: Therapies to decrease the risks of adverse cardiovascular events in patients with stable angina

- Antiplatelet drugs
- Lipid-lowering agents
- Angiotensin-inhibiting drugs
- Beta-blockers
- Adequate control of hypertension
- Adequate control of diabetes
- Folate therapy if homocysteine level is elevated
- Treatment of depression
- Cessation of smoking
- Weight loss in overweight patients
- Regular exercise

TABLE 6: Drugs to relieve angina and myocardial ischemia

- Beta-adrenergic receptor antagonists (β-blockers)
- Nitroglycerin and nitrates
- Calcium channel blocking agents
- Late sodium current blocking agent—Ranolazine
- Nicorandil
- Trimetazidine
- I_f current inhibition—Ivabradine
- Vasopeptidase inhibition—Omapatrilat
- Rho-kinase inhibition—Fasudil

I_f, funny current.

myocytes, sinoatrial and atrioventricular nodal cells. Activation of β-1 receptors is associated with increased contractility and heart rate and enhanced atrioventricular nodal conduction.

Beta-2 receptors are present in cardiac myocytes but are more abundant in bronchial and peripheral vascular smooth muscle cells. Activation of β-2 receptors causes bronchodilatation and peripheral vasodilatation. There is a small increase in myocardial contractility.

Beta-3 receptors are present in the heart and in adipose tissue. Activation of β-3 receptors reduces contractility.[28]

Beta-blockers in general inhibit β-1 and β-2 adrenergic receptors. Inhibition of β-1 receptors is associated with a decrease in heart rate and contractility, which decrease myocardial oxygen demand. Activation of β-2 receptors causes vasodilatation and decreases systemic vascular resistance. Beta-2 receptors stimulation is also associated with coronary vasodilatation and increased coronary blood flow. Thus, with the use of β-blockers, potential exists for the decrease in coronary blood flow with inhibition of β-2 receptors due to increase in coronary vascular resistance. The clinical relevance of this effect of β-blockers on coronary hemodynamics remains uncertain.

Beta-blockers can be selective or nonselective. Some β-blockers also possess intrinsic sympathomimetic property (ISA). Beta-blockers with ISA have partial agonist property and exert stimulation of adrenoreceptors at rest. Thus, resting heart rate and contractility are not diminished. However, exercise-induced increase in heart rate and contractility is inhibited.

Selective β-blockers inhibit β-1 receptors which are present predominantly in the cardiac myocytes. Selective β-blockers decrease heart rate and contractility. They cause less bronchoconstriction and less peripheral vasodilation than the nonselective β-blockers, which inhibit both β-1 and β-2 receptors. There are β-blockers, which also inhibit α-adrenergic receptors and have direct vasodilating properties.

The major mechanism by which β-blockers relief angina and myocardial ischemia is by reduction of myocardial oxygen demand. However, with a reduction in heart rate, myocardial perfusion time increases with improved myocardial perfusion.

It should be appreciated that with a marked reduction in heart rate, left ventricular end-diastolic volume increases which also increases myocardial oxygen demand. Thus, the beneficial effect of β-blockers may be partially offset. Concomitant use of nitrates, which decrease left ventricular end-diastolic volume, may be more effective for relief of myocardial ischemia.

TABLE 7: Beta-adrenergic blocking agents in stable angina

Agent	Selectivity	Partial agonist activity (ISA)	Half-life (hours)	Dose (mg/day)
Atenolol	β1	No	6–9	25–100
Acebutolol	β1	Yes	3–4	1200
Bisoprolol	β1	No	9–12	10
Carvedilol	None	No	7–10	50
Metoprolol	β1	No	3–4	200
Nadolol	None	No	14–24	160
Propranolol	None	No	3.5–6	180
Timolol	None	No	4–5	20

ISA, intrinsic sympathomimetic activity.

The selective and nonselective β-blockers decrease frequency and severity of episodes of angina and increase exercise tolerance in patients with stable angina have been reported in several studies.[1,3,18-20] Nonselective β-blockers with α-blocking property, carvedilol has been also reported to be effective in the treatment of stable angina.[31-33] Carvedilol (25–50 mg twice daily) appears to be as effective as nifedipine (20 mg twice daily), verapamil (120 mg twice daily) or immediate release metoprolol (100 mg twice daily) in reducing the frequency of angina and in improving exercise duration.[31-33] Beta-blockers with ISA are not generally recommended for treatment of angina. The pharmacokinetics of β-blockers is summarized in Table 7.

ACC/AHA guidelines recommendations for the use of β-blockers in stable angina:

Beta-blockers should be used as initial therapy in absence of contraindications in patients with prior myocardial infarction (*Class I, Level of Evidence: A*)

Beta-blockers should be used as initial therapy in absence of contraindications in patients without prior myocardial infarction (*Class I, Level of Evidence: B*)

Nitroglycerin and Nitrates

Nitroglycerin was introduced for treatment of angina by William Murrell in 1879.[34] It has been used since then for treatment of all subsets of angina. Presently, it is used not only for stable angina but also for acute coronary syndrome.

Mechanism of Action

Nitroglycerin and nitrates cause dilatation of veins and arteries by relaxation of vascular smooth muscle cells. Relaxation of vascular smooth muscle cells is mediated by generation of nitric oxide and sulfhydryl-nitrosothiols. Nitroglycerin and nitrates are first metabolized to 1,2-glyceryl dinitrate and nitrite and then to nitric oxide and sulfhydryl-nitrosothiols.

Effects on Systemic and Coronary Hemodynamics

Nitroglycerin and nitrates are predominantly venodilators and cause dilatation primarily of larger capacitance veins and the venules are least affected. Venodilation is associated with decreased systemic venous return, which decreases ventricular volumes.

Dilatation of arterial system with nitroglycerin is much less pronounced. It causes minimal or no dilatation of the smaller arteries such as of the intramyocardial coronary arteries. Nitrates also have minimal effects on arterioles. However, nitroglycerin and nitrates decrease stiffness of the larger arteries, such as of aorta and cause dilatation of the larger arteries including aorta. Decreased aortic stiffness (increased compliance) is associated with a modest decrease in systolic blood pressure. Nitrates also cause dilatation of the epicardial coronary arteries. In the atherosclerotic coronary artery disease, nitroglycerin dilates not only the nonstenotic segments but also the atherosclerotic stenotic epicardial coronary artery segments. The epicardial coronary artery vasodilatory effects are associated with an increase in coronary blood flow. Dilatation of the smooth muscles of the epicardial coronary arteries relieves coronary artery spasm—the principal mechanism for relief of vasospastic angina. An improvement in endothelial function has been proposed to be a mechanism of epicardial coronary artery dilatation.

The systemic hemodynamic effects of nitroglycerin are characterized by a decrease in right atrial and pulmonary capillary wedge pressures. There is usually no change in cardiac output. There is a reduction in right and left ventricular diastolic volumes and pressures. As there is also a decrease in arterial pressure, both systolic and diastolic wall stress is decreased, which is associated with decreased myocardial oxygen demand. If there is a marked reduction in ventricular volumes, stroke volume and arterial pressure may decrease and syncope may occur (nitroglycerin syncope). A fall in arterial pressure is associated with a reflex increase in heart rate and contractility. It should be appreciated that nitroglycerin does not possess any direct positive inotropic effect.

Usually with a fall in blood pressure with nitroglycerin, there is a reflex increase in heart rate. In some patients if there is a marked decrease in left ventricular volume associated with a reflex increase in contractility, ventricular vagal afferent "C" fibers can be stimulated and may cause cardioinhibitory and vasodepressor responses resulting in bradycardia and hypotension (paradoxical response of nitroglycerin).

Mechanism of Relief of Angina and Myocardial Ischemia

The principal mechanism of relief of myocardial ischemia by nitroglycerin and nitrates is by reduction of myocardial oxygen demand. The decrease in ventricular volumes and arterial pressure is associated with a reduction in wall stress, which decreases myocardial oxygen demand. Decreased left ventricular diastolic volume and pressure can also increase subendocardial blood flow and decrease subendocardial ischemia. A reduction of subendocardial ischemia may be contributory for relief of angina.

It should be appreciated that the reflex increase in heart rate and contractility in response to fall in blood pressure may decrease the beneficial effects of nitroglycerin. The concurrent use of β-blockers can minimize these potential adverse effects of nitroglycerin. For maintenance treatment of stable angina, combination of nitrates and β-blockers are frequently employed.

Nitroglycerin and Nitrate Preparations

The nitroglycerin and nitrate preparations that are used for treatment of angina are summarized in Table 8.

Sublingual, buccal or spray preparations of nitroglycerin are used for the immediate relief of angina. For maintenance therapy, isosorbide dinitrate or mononitrate is used. Short-acting nitrates can be used before physical exercise is undertaken. The dose and duration of action of nitroglycerin and nitrates are summarized in Table 8.

The most common side effect of nitroglycerin and nitrates is headache. Dizziness and presyncope may also occur. Frank syncope is a rare complication. Nitrate tolerance may develop during its prolonged use. A nitrate-free interval of 10–12 hours is recommended to decrease the incidence of nitrate tolerance.[35]

ACC/AHA guidelines recommendation for the use of nitroglycerin and nitrates in stable angina:

Sublingual nitroglycerin or nitroglycerin spray for the immediate relief of angina (*Class I, Level of Evidence: C*).

TABLE 8: Dose and duration of action of nitroglycerin and nitrates

Nitroglycerin and nitrates	Dose	Duration of action
Nitroglycerin (SL, buccal)	0.15–1.2 mg/PRN	10–30 minutes
Nitroglycerin patch	10–25 mg/24 hours	8–10 hours
Isosorbide dinitrate	10–60 mg/4–6 hours	4–6 hours
Isosorbide mononitrate	30–120 mg/24 hours	6–10 hours

SL, sublingual; PRN, pro-re nata (as the circumstance arises).

Long-acting nitrates with or without calcium channel blockers as initial therapy when β-blockers are contraindicated (*Class I, Level of Evidence: B*).

Long-acting nitrates with or without calcium channel blockers in combination with β-blockers when initial treatment with β-blockers is not successful (*Class I, Level of Evidence: B*).

Long-acting nitrates with or without calcium channel blockers as a substitute for β-blockers if initial treatment with β-blockers leads to unacceptable side effects (*Class I, Level of Evidence: C*).

Calcium Channel Blockers[3]

Mechanism of Action

Calcium channel blocking agents decrease transmembrane flux of calcium via the calcium channels. Three types of voltage-dependent calcium channels are recognized: L type, T type and N type. The L type channels have large conductance. The T type exerts transient duration of opening of calcium channel. The N type has primarily neuronal distribution.

For treatment of angina, most frequently L-type calcium channel blockers are used. The major mechanism of action of L-type calcium channel blockers is by inhibition of calcium influx into myocytes as well as into vascular smooth muscle cells. Reduced calcium influx into myocytes causes decrease in contractility, which decreases myocardial oxygen demand. Nondihydropyridine heart rate regulating calcium channel blockers, such as verapamil, and diltiazem, exert inhibitory effect on sinus node cells, which is associated with decreased sinus rate. In addition, verapamil and diltiazem slow atrioventricular nodal conduction which is associated with decreased ventricular rate. Decreased sinus rate and ventricular rate are also associated with decreased myocardial oxygen demand.

Reduced calcium influx into vascular smooth muscle cells causes vasodilatation of the systemic and coronary arteries. Systemic vasodilation is associated with decreased systemic vascular resistance and arterial pressure which decrease myocardial oxygen demand. Coronary vasodilatation decreases coronary vascular resistance and increases coronary blood flow. Calcium channel blockers dilate both epicardial conductance vessels and myocardial resistance vessels.

The major mechanism of relief of angina and myocardial ischemia with calcium channel blockers is by reduction of myocardial oxygen demand. However, increased coronary blood flow may be contributory. Dilatation of the epicardial coronary arteries is the principal mechanism of the beneficial effect of calcium channel blockers in patients with vasospastic angina.

Dilatation of the myocardial resistance vessels, although is associated with increased coronary blood flow, there is potential for diversion of coronary blood flow from the ischemic myocardium to nonischemic myocardium which may enhance ischemia in the ischemic myocardial segments (Steel phenomenon).

With dihydropyridine calcium channel blockers, there is a reflex increase in heart rate, which increases myocardial oxygen demand, partially offsetting their beneficial effects. Concomitant use of β-blockers, however, prevents tachycardia.

Slow-release and long-acting dihydropyridines are effective for treatment of stable angina. Similarly, heart rate regulating nondihydropyridine calcium channel blockers are effective for maintenance therapy of stable angina. Although both dihydropyridine and nondihydropyridine calcium channel blockers relieve angina and improve exercise tolerance, they do not improve angina threshold.[33]

The T type calcium channel blocker mibefradil also exerts negative inotropic effect and decreases myocardial oxygen demand. It has been withdrawn from clinical use because of adverse drug interaction.

Calcium channel blockers that are used for treatment of angina are summarized in Table 9. Their duration of action and pharmacokinetics are also summarized.

The adverse effects of calcium channel blockers are primarily related to their pharmacologic properties.

Hypotension can occur with the use of any of the calcium channel blockers. However, it is more pronounced with dihydropyridines such as nifedipine. All calcium channel

TABLE 9: Calcium channel blocking agents that can be used for treatment of stable angina

Agent	Half-life	Dose
Amlodipine	30–50 hours	5–10 mg/day
Nifedipine	4–5 hours	20–40 mg TD
Diltiazem	3–4 hours	30–80 mg QD
Diltiazem slow release	Long	120–320 mg/day
Verapamil	6 hours	80–160 mg TD
Verapamil slow release	Long	120–480 mg/day
Felodipine	11–16 hours	5–10 mg/day
Isradipine	8 hours	2.5–10 mg BD
Nicardipine	2–4 hours	20–40 mg TD
Nimodipine	1–2 hours	40 mg every 4 hours
Nisoldipine	6–12 hours	20–40 mg OD
Nitrendipine	5–12 hours	20 mg OD or BD

OD, once a day; BD, twice a day; TD, thrice a day; QD, four times a day.

blockers exert negative inotropic effect and can exacerbate or cause worsening of systolic heart failure.

Lower extremity edema is complication of all types of calcium channel blockers during their long-term use. The severity of edema is dose-dependent—larger the dose of calcium channel blockers used, worse is the lower extremity edema. The calcium channel blockers-induced edema is usually diuretics resistant. It should be appreciated that the mechanism of edema caused by the calcium channel blockers remains unexplained.

Constipation, often severe can occur with the use of any type of the calcium channel blockers. This is related to decreased calcium influx to the vascular smooth cells of the intestine, which is associated with decreased intestinal motility.

Calcium channel blockers can cause arrhythmia. Dihydropyridines cause reflex tachycardia due to activation of adrenergic system. Dihydropyridines do not alter sinus node discharge rate or atrioventricular conduction. Thus, they do not cause sinus node dysfunction or atrioventricular block.

Nondihydropyridine calcium channel blockers, such as diltiazem or verapamil can cause sinus bradycardia and atrioventricular block. They decrease sinus node discharge rate and slow atrioventricular conduction. Sinus bradycardia and atrioventricular block with diltiazem or verapamil are accentuated with concomitant use of digoxin or amiodarone, which also exerts similar pharmacologic effects on sinus node function and atrioventricular conduction. Calcium channel blockers also alter digoxin clearance and digitalis toxicity may occur with the concomitant use of the calcium channel blockers and digoxin.

ACC/AHA guidelines recommendations for the use of calcium channel blockers for management of stable angina:

Heart rate regulating calcium channel blockers as initial therapy when β-blockers are contraindicated (*Class I Level of Evidence B*).

Heart rate regulating calcium channel antagonist and/or long-acting nitrates in combination with β-blockers when initial treatment with β-blockers is not successful (*Class I, Level of Evidence B*).

Heart rate regulating calcium channel antagonists as substitute for β-blockers if initial treatment with β-blockers leads to unacceptable side effects (*Class I Level of Evidence C*).

Ranolazine

Ranolazine is an antianginal drug, which does not either decrease myocardial oxygen demand or increase coronary blood flow. It has been proposed that it decreases myocardial ischemia by inhibiting late sodium inward current (Fig. 2).

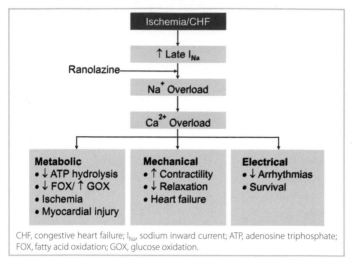

CHF, congestive heart failure; I_{Na}, sodium inward current; ATP, adenosine triphosphate; FOX, fatty acid oxidation; GOX, glucose oxidation.

FIG. 2: Potential role of ranolazine in modifying pathophysiology of angina.

The late sodium current channels are upregulated during ischemia and heart failure. Activation of these channels causes increased sodium influx into myocytes. Increased intracellular sodium increases intracellular calcium by activating sodium-calcium exchange mechanism. Myocardial calcium overload causes metabolic, functional and electrical dysfunction.[36,37]

Myocardial metabolic dysfunction is characterized by increased adenosine triphosphate (ATP) hydrolysis, increased free fatty acid oxidation and decreased glucose oxidation. This metabolic dysfunction is associated with myocardial injury, myocyte necrosis and apoptosis.

Myocardial mechanical dysfunction is manifested by decreased contractility and impaired relaxation. Impaired relaxation is associated with increased left ventricular end-diastolic pressure. Myocardial calcium overload may also cause subendocardial ischemia and myocardial necrosis.

Calcium overload-induced electrical dysfunction causes ventricular and atrial arrhythmias. There is increased frequency of ventricular premature beats and nonsustained ventricular tachycardia. There is increased risk of arrhythmogenic mortality.

Ranolazine has been demonstrated to attenuate these adverse effects of calcium overload. It improves myocardial metabolic, mechanical and electrical function. In the Metabolic Efficiency with Ranolazine for Less Ischemia in Non-ST-Elevation Acute Coronary Syndrome–Thrombolysis in Myocardial Infarction 36 (MERLIN-TIMI 36) trial, 6,560 patients were randomized to receive either placebo or ranolazine. Treatment with ranolazine was associated with a significant reduction in the incidence of ventricular premature beats and nonsustained ventricular tachycardia. There was also a significant reduction of recurrent episodes of myocardial ischemia.

Ranolazine inhibits inward sodium influx and decreases calcium overload. Ranolazine has the potential to ameliorate the deleterious effects of calcium overload.

Decreased metabolic dysfunction is associated with reduced myocardial injury. Experimental studies suggest that ranolazine can decrease myocardial injury.

Ranolazine improves left ventricular compliance and decreases left ventricular end-diastolic pressure. It can also reduce subendocardial ischemia.

The antiarrythmic effects of ranolazine are characterized by the reduction of frequency of premature ventricular complexes and ventricular tachycardia.

The potential beneficial antianginal effects of ranolazine have been studied in a number of placebo-controlled studies. In the Monotherapy Assessment of Ranolazine In Stable Angina (MARISA) trial, ranolazine compared to placebo improved exercise tolerance, increased time to ST-segment depression during treadmill exercise test.[38] It also improves exercise tolerance with a background treatment with β-blockers and calcium channel blockers.[39]

Ranolazine is extensively metabolized, approximately 70% through the cytochrome P450 3A4 pathway. Ranolazine is the major bioactive compound. The maximum dose of ranolazine should be reduced when it is used with the drugs that also inhibit cytochrome P450 3A4 pathway such as verapamil and diltiazem.

Contraindications for the Use of Ranolazine

Ranolazine is contraindicated in patients receiving ketoconazole, which is a strong inhibitor of cytochrome P450 34A pathway. It is also contraindicated in patients with severe hepatic insufficiency or cirrhosis.

Concomitant doses of statins that inhibit P450 cytochrome pathway should be reduced. Thus, the doses of lovastatin and simvastatin should be reduced. The dose of simvastatin should not exceed 20 mg daily and the dose of ranolazine should also be reduced.

Side Effects of Ranolazine

The side effects of ranolazine are relatively minor. The dizziness and nausea can occur at the initiation of the treatment with ranolazine. Dose-related asthenia and constipation occur in 3–10%. Although electrocardiogram can reveal prolongation of QT interval, ventricular arrhythmias resulting from prolongation from QT does not occur. Indeed, ranolazine exerts protective effect against ventricular arrhythmia.

ACC/AHA guidelines recommendations for use of ranolazine in chronic stable angina:

Refractory angina (*Class IIa: Level of Evidence A*).

There are evolving new mechanistic approaches to address myocardial ischemia, which are summarized in Table 10 and discussed below. In addition, there are several current non-pharmacologic antianginal strategies that are summarized in Table 11.

Trimetazidine

Normally free fatty acid oxidation is the principal metabolic source for myocardial energy utilization. In presence of hypoxia, glucose oxidation is preferable to free fatty acid oxidation as there is more generation of ATP for maintaining myocyte and myocardial metabolic function. The agents that inhibit oxidation of free fatty acids have the potential to enhance oxygen supply and relief ischemia and angina.

Trimetazidine is a partial inhibitor of oxidation of free fatty acids and has been demonstrated to be effective for treatment of stable angina. In a number of randomized clinical trials, it has been shown to relieve frequency of angina and improve exercise tolerance.[40-42] In a randomized clinical trial, effects of

TABLE 10: New mechanistic approaches to myocardial ischemia

Mechanism	Therapy
Rho-kinase inhibition	Fasudil
Metabolic modulation	Trimetazidine
Preconditioning	Nicorandil
Sinus node inhibition	Ivabradine
Adenosine triphosphate potassium channel opener	Nicorandil
Nitric-oxide donor	Molsidomine
Increased calcitonin generalated peptide release	Capsaicin

TABLE 11: Current non-pharmacologic antianginal strategies

- Exercise training
- Enhanced external counterpulsation (EECP)
  - ↑ Endothelial function
  - Promotes coronary collateral formation
  - ↓ Peripheral vascular resistance
  - ↑ Ventricular function
  - Placebo effect
- Transmyocardial revascularization
  - Sympathetic denervation
  - Angiogenesis
- Spinal cord stimulation (SCS)
  - ↓ Neurotransmission of painful stimuli
  - ↑ Release of endogenous opiates
  - Redistributes myocardial blood flow to ischemic areas

trimetazidine were assessed on the frequency of myocardial ischemia, in patients with noninsulin-dependent diabetes. The frequency of ischemia was assessed by ambulatory electrocardiography. The use of trimetazidine was associated with a significant reduction in the frequency of ischemia.[43] Trimetazidine is usually used in combination with other antianginal drugs.

Side Effects

Myalgia, nausea, vomiting and fatigue are the reported side effects.

Contraindications

Trimetazidine is well tolerated; there are no absolute contraindications.

European Society of Cardiology (ESC) guidelines recommendations: *Class IIb, Level of Evidence B*.

Nicorandil

Nicorandil is similar to nitroglycerin in their pharmacodynamic effects. It also produces similar hemodynamic effects.

Nicorandil enhances production of nitric oxide but also activates ATP sensitive inward—rectifier potassium channels. The hemodynamic effects are characterized by a significant reduction of right atrial and pulmonary capillary wedge pressures with a modest increase in cardiac output. There is little or no change in heart rate or contractility. There is reduction of left ventricular preload and afterload.[44-46] The net effects are reduction of myocardial oxygen demand, which is the principal mechanism for relief of angina and ischemia.

In the Impact of Nicorandil in Angina (IONA) trial,[44] over 5,000 patients with stable angina were randomized to receive either nicorandil or placebo. The results of this study reported a significant reduction in the composite endpoint of death from coronary heart disease, nonfatal myocardial infarction and hospital readmission for cardiac chest pain during a follow-up of about 18 months. The predominant beneficial effect was related to the reduction in hospital admission rates for chest pain but not reduction in death or nonfatal myocardial infarction. It is also of interest that the beneficial effects of nicorandil were not observed in women, may be related to a smaller number of women enrolled in the study.

The report of a meta-analysis of 20 studies indicated no advantage of nicorandil in reduction in the frequency of angina attacks or in the time to ST-segment changes during exercise tests.[46]

Dose and Side Effects

The usual dose of nicorandil is 10–20 mg twice daily. The major side effect is development of tolerance as like nitrate tolerance.

The ESC guidelines recommendations for the use of nicorandil:

Class I, Level of Evidence C, for patients with intolerance or contraindications to β-adrenergic receptor or calcium channel blockers.

Class IIa, Level of Evidence C, for patients who have been unsuccessfully treated with two antianginal drugs.

Ivabradine

Ivabradine is a selective inhibitor of the funny (If) current.[47,48] The If current is an inward potassium current and it is activated by hyperpolarization of the myocytes. The myocytes of the sinoatrial nodal cells possess the If current channels and they are absent in the atrioventricular nodal cells. Inhibition of If currents is associated with a reduction in sinus rate and a prolonged sinus node recovery time. The complete blockade of If currents by ivabradine is associated with a 30–40% reduction of sinus rate. It has no effect on atrioventricular conduction and thus it does not decrease ventricular response in patients with atrial fibrillation. The magnitude of reduction in heart rate by ivabradine depends on the resting heart rate. The faster the resting heart rate, greater is the magnitude of reduction of heart rate by ivabradine. The QT interval is prolonged by ivabradine; however, corrected QT interval for heart rate is only slightly prolonged.

It should be appreciated that the If current inhibitor ivabradine does not exert negative inotropic effects like β-adrenergic antagonists.

In a randomized clinical trial, ivabradine has been reported to decrease the frequency of angina, nitroglycerin consumption and to increase exercise duration and the time to ST-segment depression during treadmill exercise test.[49-53] In the Morbidity-Mortality Evaluation of the If Inhibitor Ivabradine in Patients with Coronary Disease and Left Ventricular Dysfunction (BEAUTIFUL) trial, [54] almost 11,000 patients with left ventricular ejection fraction of less than 40% were randomized to receive either ivabradine or placebo. The majority of patients received β-blockers as background therapy. During the follow-up of approximately 2 years, there was no change in cardiovascular mortality with ivabradine. However, there was a significant reduction in the rate of hospital admission for myocardial infarction or heart failure. In the BEAUTIFUL trial, about 14% of patients had stable angina at baseline. In patients with resting heart rate of

70 beats/min or higher, there was almost 60% reduction in the need of revascularization.

Dose and Side Effects

The usual dose is 5.0–7.5 mg twice daily. In elderly patients, a lower dose is recommended. Blurred vision or sharp flashes in the eyes are the most common side effects. The retina and brain cells have If channel isoforms. Other side effects are headache, dizziness and symptomatic bradycardia.

Contraindications

Ivabradine is metabolized through the cytochrome P450 3A4 hepatic pathway. It is contraindicated in patients receiving inhibitors of this metabolic pathway. It is also contraindicated in patients with moderate-to-severe hepatic insufficiency.

Rho-kinase Inhibitors

Rho-kinase is a guanosine triphosphate (GTP) binding protein, which is involved in signaling pathway for intracellular calcium handling. It promotes intracellular calcium entry and increases vascular tone. In coronary circulation, it enhances coronary vasoconstriction. Rho-kinase inhibitors decrease coronary vascular resistance and increase coronary blood flow. This is the principal mechanism for relief of myocardial ischemia and angina by Rho-kinase inhibitors.

In a randomized, double-blind placebo-controlled trial, the efficacy of a Rho-kinase inhibitor, fasudil was compared to that of placebo.[55] Fasudil was reported to increase the time to ST-segment depression during treadmill exercise test.

Allopurinol

Allopurinol is a xanthine oxidase inhibitor and has been reported to be of benefit in patients with stable angina. In a randomized placebo-controlled study, allopurinol in a dose of 300 mg daily was reported to improve exercise tolerance and to increase the time to ST-segment depression during treadmill exercise tests.[56] The precise mechanism of the beneficial effect of allopurinol remains unknown.

Vasopeptidase Inhibitors

These agents inhibit both bradykinin and angiotensin formation by inhibiting angiotensin-converting enzyme. They have the potential to decrease coronary vascular resistance, increase coronary blood flow and decrease myocardial oxygen demand concurrently. These agents, therefore, have the potential to be of benefit in management of chronic stable angina. The risk of angioedema prohibits their use.

Angiogenesis

To promote development of new blood vessels to the ischemic myocardial segments potentially can be of benefit in relieving ischemia and angina. Vascular endothelial growth factors and fibroblast growth factors as angiogenic factors and have been studied. However, the results remain inconclusive.

Intracoronary infusion of stem cells and angiogenic agents to the ischemic myocardium to improve angiogenesis has been also attempted. The results remain inconclusive.

VASOSPASTIC ANGINA

Vasospastic angina (Prinzmetal angina) results from focal spasm of the epicardial coronary arteries. Coronary vasodilators, such as nitrates and calcium channel blocking agents are the appropriate pharmacologic agents.

MIXED ANGINA

The clinical features of mixed angina are the variable angina threshold. The patients can exercise on occasions more without developing angina, on other occasions angina develops at a much lower level of exercise. The mechanism appears to be due to increase in myocardial oxygen demand and concurrent increase in coronary vascular resistance. The pharmacologic agents that decrease myocardial oxygen demand and cause coronary vasodilatation are appropriate.

LINKED ANGINA

In these patients, there is a reflex increase in coronary vascular resistance and centrally mediated decrease in coronary blood flow. The activation of the afferent receptors which are located in the gastroesophageal junction occurs during acid reflux and produce reduction of coronary blood flow. The H2 blockers appear to be appropriate treatment.

WALK-THROUGH-ANGINA

In these patients, angina develops at the beginning of exercise. The angina is relieved even when patients continue to the same level of exercise. The mechanism appears to be due to increase in coronary vascular resistance and decrease in coronary blood flow at the beginning of exercise. During continued exercise, metabolically related coronary vascular resistance declines with a concomitant increase in coronary blood flow. The pharmacologic agents with coronary vasodilating properties are appropriate.

SYNDROME "X"

In this syndrome, during exercise, angina with evidence of myocardial ischemia develops in absence of significant atherosclerotic obstructive coronary artery disease. Inadequate coronary vasodilatory reserve appears to be the principal mechanism. The pharmacologic agents with coronary vasodilatory property are appropriate.

CONCLUSION

Chronic stable angina is a common clinical manifestation of ischemic heart disease. It usually results from disproportionate increase in myocardial oxygen demand. However, a concomitant reduction in autoregulatory reserve decreases angina threshold.

The effective pharmacologic treatment consists of agents that decrease myocardial oxygen demand. In certain clinical subsets, however, the pharmacologic agents that increase coronary blood flow concurrently may be useful.

The newer pharmacologic agents have some beneficial roles but only in selected patients. Reperfusion therapy should be reserved only for patients with refractory angina.

REFERENCES

1. Deedwania PC, Carbajal EV, Bobba VR. Trials and tribulations associated with angina and traditional theraputic approaches. Clin Cardiol. 2007;30(Suppl I) 116-24.
2. Holubkov R, Lasky WK, Haviland A, et al. Angina 1 year after percutaneous coronary interventions: a report from the NHLBI Dynamic registry. Am Heart J. 2002;144:826-33.
3. Gibbon RJ, Abrams J, Chatterjee K, et al. ACC/AHA 2002 guidelines update for the management of patients with stable angina—a summary article: A report of the American College of Cardiology/American Heart Association Task Force on Practice Guidelines (Committee to Update the 1999 Guidelines for the Management of Patients with Chronic Stable Angina). Circulation. 2003;107:149-58.
4. Gitt AK, et al. Circulation. 2004;110:III-626.
5. Heberden W. Some account of disorders of the breast. Med Trans. 1772;2:59.
6. Marcus GM, Cohen J, Varosy P, et al. The utility of gestures in patients with chest discomfort. AM J Med. 2007;120:83-9.
7. Ridker PM, Manson JE, Gaziano JM, et al. Low-dose aspirin for chronic stable angina. A randomized, placebo-controlled clinical trial. Ann Intern Med. 1991;114:835-9.
8. Collaborative overview of randomized trials of antiplatelet therapy—I: Prevention of death, myocardial infarction and stroke by prolonged antiplatelet in various categories of patients. Antiplatelet Trialists' Collaboration. BMJ. 1995;308:81-106.
9. Final report on the aspirin component of the ongoing Physicians' Health Study. Steering Committee of the Physicians' Health Study Research Group. N Engl J Med. 1989;321:129-35.
10. Juul-Moller S, Edvardsson N, Jahnmatz B, et al. Double-blind trial of aspirin in primary prevention of myocardial infarction in patients with stable chronic angina pectoris. The Swedish Angina Pectoris Trial (SAPAT) Group. Lancet. 1992;340:1421-5.

11. CAPRIE Steering Committee. A randomized , blinded, trial of clopidogrel versus aspirin in patients at risk of ischemic events (CAPRIE). Lancet. 1996;348: 1329-39.

12. Randomized trial of cholesterol lowering in 4,444 patients with coronary heart disease–the Scandinavian Simvastatin Survival Study (4S). Lancet. 1994;344: 1383-9.

13. Cholesterol and Recurrent Events Trial Investigators (CARE). The effect of pravastatin on coronary events after myocardial infarction in patients with average cholesterol levels. N Engl J Med. 1996;335:1001-9.

14. Deedwania PC. Study Assessing Goals in the Elderly steering committee and investigators. Effect of aggressive versus moderate lipid-lowering therapy on myocardial ischemia: the rational, design, and baseline characteristics of the Study Assessing Goals in the Elderly (SAGE). Am Heart J. 2004;148:1053-9.

15. Stone PH, Lloyd-Jones DM, Vascular Basis Study Group, et al. Effect of intensive lipid lowering, with or without antioxidant vitamins compared with moderate lipid lowering on myocardial ischemia in patients with stable coronary artery disease: the Vascular Basis for the Treatment of Myocardial Ischemia Study. Circulation. 2005;111:1747-55.

16. Deanfield JE, Sellier P, Thaulow E, et al. Potent anti-ischemic effects of statins in chronic stable angina :incremental benefit beyond lipid lowering? Eur Heart J. 2010;31: 2650-9.

17. Deedwania P, Stone PH, Bairey Merz CN, et al. Effects of intensive versus moderate lipid-lowering therapy on myocardial ischemia in older patients with coronary heart disease: results of the Study Accessing Goals in the Elderly (SAGE). Circulation. 2007;115:700-7.

18. Boden WE, O'Rourke RA, Teo KK, et al. Optimal medical therapy with or without PCI for stable coronary disease. N Engl J Med. 2007;356:1503-16.

19. The Heart Outcomes Prevention Evaluation Study Investigators. Effects of an angiotensin-converting-enzyme inhibitor, ramipril on cardiovascular in high-risk patients. N Engl J Med. 2000;342:145-53.

20. The European trial on reduction of cardiac events with perindopril in stable coronary artery disease investigators. Efficacy of perindopril in reduction of cardiovascular events among patients with stable coronary artery disease: randomized, double-blind, placebo-controlled, multicenter trial (the EUROPA study). Lancet. 2003;362:782-8.

21. Pfeffer MA, Braunwald E, Moye LA, et al. Effect of captopril on mortality and morbidity in patients with left ventricular dysfunction after myocardial infarction: results of the survival and ventricular enlargement Trial. The SAVE Investigators. N Engl J Med. 1992;327:669-77.

22. Al-Mallah MH, Theyjeh IM, Abdel-Latif AA, et al. Angiotensin-converting enzyme inhibitors in coronary artery disease and preserved left ventricular systolic function: a systematic review and meta-analysis of randomized controlled trials. J Am Coll Cardiol. 2006;47:1576-83.

23. Braunwald E, Domanski MJ, PEACE Trial Investigators, et al. Angiotensin-converting-enzyme inhibition in stable coronary artery disease. N Engl J Med. 2004;351:2058-68.

24. Fraker TD Jr, Flin SD, Gibbons RJ, et al.2007 Chronic angina focused update of the ACC/AHA 2002 guidelines for the management of patients with chronic stable angina : a report of the American College of Cardiology/American Heart Association Task Force on Practice Guidelines Writing Group to develop the focused update of the 2002 guidelines for the management of patients with chronic stable angina. Circulation. 2007;116:2762-72.

25. Sabatine MS, Morrow DA, de Lemos JA, et al. Evaluation of multiple biomarkers of cardiovascular stress for risk prediction and guiding medical therapy in patients with stable coronary disease. Circulation. 2012;125:233-40.

26. Chatterjee K, De Marco T, McGlothlin D. Remodeling in systolic heart failure—effects of neurohormonal modulators: basis for current pharmacotherapy. Cardiology Today. 2005;9:270-7.

27. Pepine CJ, Cohn PF, Deedwania PC, et al. The Atenolol Silent Ischemia Study (ASIST). Effects of treatment on outcome in mildly symptomatic patients with ischemia during daily life. Circulation. 1994;90:762-8.

28. Abrams J. Clinical practice. Chronic stable angina. N Engl J Med. 2005;352:2524-33.

29. Abrams J, Thadani U. Therapy of stable angina pectoris: the uncomplicated patient. Circulation. 2005;112: e255-9.

30. Reiter MJ. Cardiovascular drug class specificity: beta-blockers. Prog Cardiovasc Dis. 2004;47:11-33.

31. Weiss R, Ferry D, Pickering E, et al. Effectiveness of three different doses of carvedilol for exertional angina. Carvedilol-Angina Study Group. Am J Cardiol. 1998;82:927-31.

32. van der Does R, Hauf-Zachariou U, Pfarr E, et al. Comparison of safety and efficacy of carvedilol and metoprolol in stable angina pectoris. Am J Cardiol. 1999;83:643-9.

33. Hauf-Zachariou U, Blackwood RA, Gunawardena KA, et al. Carvedilol versus verapamil in chronic stable angina: a multicenter trial. Eur J Clin Pharmacol. 1997;52:95-100.

34. Murrell W. Nitro-glycerine as a remedy for angina pectoris. Lancet. 1879;1:80-1.

35. Gumbrielle T, Freedman SB, Fogarty L, et al. Efficacy, safety and nitrate-free interval to prevent tolerance to transdermal nitroglycerin in effort angina. Eur Heart J. 1992;13:671-8.

36. Antzelovitch C, Belardinelli L, Zygmunt AC, et al. Electrophysiological effects of ranolazine, a novel antianginal agent with antiarrythmic properties. Circulation. 2004;110:904-10.

37. Maklelski JC, Valdivia CR. Ranolazine and late cardiac sodium current—a therapeutic target for angina, arrhythmia and more? Br J Pharmacol. 2006;148:4-6.

38. Chaitman BR, Skettino SL, Parker JO, et al. Antiischemic effects and long term survival during ranolazine monotherapy in patients with chronic severe angina. J Am Coll Cardiol. 2004;43:1375-82.

39. Chaitman BR, Pepine CJ, Parker JO, et al. Effects of ranolazine with atenolol, amlodipine, or diltiazom on exercise tolerance and angina frequency in patients with severe chronic angina. JAMA. 2004;291:309-16.

40. Ciapponi A, Pizzarro R, Harrison J. Trimetazidine for stable angina. Cochrane Database Syst Rev. 2005;4:CD003614.

41. Ribeiro LW, Ribeiro JP, Stein R, et al. Trimetazidine added to combined hemodynamic antianginal therapy in patients with type 2 diabetes: a randomized crossover trial. Am Heart J. 2007;154:78.e1-7.

42. MacInnes A, Fairman DA, Binding P, et al. The antianginal agent trimetazidine does not exert its functional benefit via inhibition of mitochondrial long-chain 3-ketoacyl coenzyme A thiolase. Circ Res. 2003;93(3):,e26-e32.

43. Marazzi G, Wajngarten M, Vitale C, et al. Effect of fatty acid inhibition on silent and symptomatic myocardial ischemia in diabetic patients with coronary artery disease. Int J Cardiol. 2007;120:79-84.

44. IONA Study Group. Effect of nicorandil on coronary events in patients with stable angina: the Impact of Nicorandil in Angina (IONA) randomized trial. Lancet. 2002;359:1269-75.

45. Simpson D, Wellington K. Nicorandil: a new of its use in the management of stable angina pectoris, including high-risk patients. Drugs. 2004;64:1941-55.

46. Hanai Y, Mita M, Hishinuma S, et al. Systematic review on the short-term efficacy and safety of nicorandil for stable angina pectoris in comparison with those Beta-blockers, nitrates and calcium antagonists. Yakugaku Zasshi. 2010;130:1549-63.

47. DiFrancesco D. The role of the funny current in pacemaker activity. Circ Res. 2010;106:434-46.

48. Bauruscotti M, Barbuti A, Bucchi A. The cardiac pacemaker current. J Mol Cell Cardiol. 2010;48:55-64.

49. Fernandez SF, Tandar A, Boden WE. Emerging medical treatment for angina pectoris. Expert Opin Emerg Drugs. 2010;15:283-98.

50. TardifJC, Ponikowski P, Kahan T, et al. Efficacy of the If current inhibitor ivabradin in patients with chronic stable angina receiving beta-blocker therapy: a 4-month, randomized, placebo-controlled trial. Eur Heart J. 2009;30:540-8.

51. Borer JS, Fox K, Jaillon P, et al. Antianginal and antiischemic effects of ivabradine, an If inhibitor, in stable angina: a randomized, double-blind, multicentered, placebo-controlled trial. Circulation. 2003;107:817-23.

52. Tardif JC, Ford I, Tendera M, et al. Efficacy of ivabradine, a new selective If inhibitor, compared with atenolol in patients with chronic stable angina. Eur Heart J. 2005;26:2529-36.

53. Tendera M, Borer JS, Tardif JC. Efficacy of If inhibition with ivabradine in different subpopulations with stable angina pectoris. Cardiology. 2009;114:116-25.

54. Fox K, Ford I, Steg PG, et al. Ivabradin for patients with stable coronary artery disease and left ventricular systolic dysfunction (BEAUTIFUL): a randomized double-blind ,placebo-controlled trial. Lancet. 2008;372:807-16.

55. Chaitman BR, Sano J. Novel therapeutic approaches to treating chronic angina in the setting of chronic ischemic heart disease. Clin Cardiol. 2007;30(Suppl 1):125-30.

56. Norman A, Ang DS, Ogston S, et al. Effect of high-dose allopurinol on exercise in patients with chronic stable angina: a randomized, placebo controlled crossover trial. Lancet. 2010;375:2161-7.

Drugs for Pulmonary Hypertension

Ravinder Kumar, Sif Hansdottir

INTRODUCTION

The pulmonary vasculature under normal conditions is a low pressure and low-resistance system. Pulmonary hypertension (PH) is a hemodynamic state characterized by elevated pressure in the pulmonary vascular bed. The pressure in the pulmonary artery is considered elevated when the resting mean pulmonary arterial pressure (mPAP) is above or equal to 25 mmHg, measured during right heart catheterization (RHC). Many clinical conditions can lead to PH and an extensive evaluation focused on elucidating underlying etiology is the key to successful management. This chapter provides an overview of the classification of PH and reviews in detail the therapies currently available for the management of pulmonary arterial hypertension (PAH). Since the publication of the first edition of this book, several new drugs have been approved by the US Food and Drug Administration (US FDA) and added to the armamentarium of medical therapy available to treat PAH.

NOMENCLATURE AND CLASSIFICATION

Clinically, the World Health Organization (WHO) classifies PH into five major categories on the basis of pathological, physiological and therapeutic characteristics (Table 1).[1] Recent modifications and updates in the classification, proposed during the 5th World Symposium held in 2013 in Nice, have been incorporated in this chapter. The nomenclature can be quite confusing and is worth reviewing. The term PH encompasses all WHO categories. WHO group 1 PAH includes idiopathic PAH (iPAH), hereditary PAH (hPAH) and PH associated with several clinical conditions. The clinical conditions are detailed in Table 1 and have similar pathophysiology and treatment response as iPAH. Idiopathic PAH was previously referred to as "primary PH", but this term has been abandoned. WHO group 2 PH is PH owing to elevated left heart pressures that result from

TABLE 1: Updated WHO classification of pulmonary hypertension[1]

1. Pulmonary arterial hypertension
    1.1 Idiopathic PAH (previously primary pulmonary hypertension)
    1.2 Heritable PAH
        1.2.1 Bone morphogenic protein receptor type 2 (BMPR2)
        1.2.2 Activin receptor-like kinase type 1 (ALK1), endoglin, caveolin-1, SMAD9
        1.2.3 Unknown
    1.3 Drug and toxin induced
    1.4 Associated with:
        1.4.1 Connective tissue disease
        1.4.2 Human immunodeficiency virus (HIV) infection
        1.4.3 Portal hypertension
        1.4.4 Congenital heart disease
        1.4.5 Schistosomiasis

1'. Pulmonary veno-occlusive disease and/or pulmonary capillary hemangiomatosis

1''. Persistent pulmonary hypertension of the newborn (PPHN)

2. Pulmonary hypertension due to left heart disease
    2.1 Left ventricular systolic dysfunction
    2.2 Left ventricular diastolic dysfunction
    2.3 Valvular disease
    2.4 Congenital/acquired left heart inflow/outflow tract obstruction and congenital cardiomyopathies

3. Pulmonary hypertension due to lung diseases and/or hypoxia
    3.1 Chronic obstructive pulmonary disease
    3.2 Interstitial lung disease
    3.3 Other pulmonary diseases with mixed restrictive and obstructive pattern
    3.4 Sleep disordered breathing
    3.5 Alveolar hypoventilation disorders
    3.6 Chronic exposure to high altitude
    3.7 Developmental lung diseases

4. Chronic thromboembolic pulmonary hypertension (CTEPH)

5. Pulmonary hypertension with unclear multifactorial mechanism
    5.1 Hematological disorders: chronic hemolytic anemia, myeloproliferative disorders, splenectomy
    5.2 Systemic disorders: sarcoidosis, pulmonary histiocytosis, lymphangioleiomyomatosis
    5.3 Metabolic disorders: glycogen storage disease, Gaucher disease, thyroid disorders
    5.4 Others: tumoral obstruction, fibrosing mediastinitis, chronic renal failure, segmental PH

either left-sided valvular disease or heart failure. This group is also referred to as pulmonary venous hypertension (PVH) or postcapillary PH. The other two major categories of PH are WHO group 3 PH due to lung disease or sleep-disordered breathing and WHO group 4 PH from chronic thrombotic and/or embolic disease. Lastly, WHO group 5 PH consists of various miscellaneous conditions that have been found to be risk factors for PH, but the pathophysiology is unclear.

The hemodynamic classification of PH has two major components—mPAP and left heart pressures. The 5th World Symposium recommends that mPAP above or equal to 25 mmHg at rest by RHC should be considered elevated.[2] Based on left heart pressures, i.e., left atrial pressure as estimated by pulmonary artery wedge pressure (PAWP) or the more directly measured left ventricular end-diastolic pressure (LVEDP), PH can be further categorized as precapillary (PAWP or LVEDP ≤15 mmHg) and postcapillary (PAWP or LVEDP >15 mmHg). WHO group 1 PAH, WHO group 3 PH due to lung disease and/or hypoxia, WHO group 4 chronic thromboembolic PH (CTEPH) and WHO group 5 PH with unclear or multifactorial mechanism all result in precapillary PH and cannot be distinguished based on hemodynamics alone. Patients with PAH are characterized by precapillary PH with mPAP above or equal to 25 mmHg, PAWP below or equal to 15 mmHg and elevated pulmonary vascular resistance (PVR) more than 3 Wood units.

WHO Group 1 Pulmonary Arterial Hypertension

World Health Oraganization group 1 PAH has been the focus of intense research over the last 20 years and major advances have been made in the understanding of pathophysiology and treatment of this condition. The clinical conditions that fall into this category (Table 1) have been found to have similar pathology, clinical presentation, hemodynamics and response to treatment. The exact prevalence of PAH is unclear but ranges between 15 and 50 cases per million in Western countries.[3,4] PAH is a progressive and often fatal disease and the pathophysiology is characterized by vasoconstriction, excessive cellular proliferation, inflammation and in situ thrombosis. Patients with PAH have an imbalance between endothelial production of vasodilatory and antiproliferative agents like nitric oxide and prostacyclin, and vasoconstrictive and proliferative substances like endothelin-1. The outcome is obstructive remodeling of the pulmonary vessels and an increase in pulmonary arterial pressure (PAP) and PVR. The progressive increase in PVR ultimately leads to right ventricular (RV) hypertrophy and dilatation and, eventually, RV failure.

Better understanding of the pathophysiology of PAH has resulted in the availability of multiple medical treatment options that target one of three pathways, i.e., the prostacyclin, nitric oxide or endothelin pathways (Fig. 1). Prior to 1995, there was no specific treatment for PAH, and patients were treated empirically with calcium-channel blockers (CCBs), digoxin, diuretics and anticoagulation. The first PAH-specific treatment, epoprostenol, was approved by the US FDA in 1995. Since then, the number of US FDA-approved therapeutic options has increased steadily with 12 PAH-specific therapies available at the end of the year of 2014 (Fig. 2).

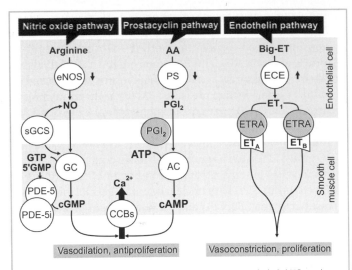

AA, arachidonic acid; ET, endothelin; NO, nitric oxide; eNOS, endothelial NO synthase; sGCS, soluble guanylate cyclase stimulator; PS, prostacyclin synthase; ECE, endothelin-converting enzyme; PGI$_2$, production of prostaglandin I$_2$; ETRA, endothelin receptor antagonist; GTP, guanylate triphosphate; ATP, adenosine triphosphate; GC, guanylate cyclase; AC, adenylate cyclase; PDE-5i, phosphodiesterase 5 inhibitor; CCB, calcium channel blocker; cAMP, cyclic adenosine monophosphate; cGMP, cyclic guanylate monophosphate.

FIG. 1: Three mechanistic pathways disturbed in patients with PAH. The short, thick, black arrows depict aberrations observed in these pathways in patients with PAH. The points at which drug treatment affects these mechanistic processes are shown in pink circles.

Left, the NO pathway. NO is created in endothelial cells by type III (i.e., endothelial) eNOS, which in pulmonary arterial smooth muscle cells (PASMCs) induces GC to convert GTP to cGMP. Riociguat, a direct stimulator of soluble guanylate cyclase enhances production of cGMP. cGMP is a second messenger that constitutively maintains PASMC relaxation and inhibition of PASMC proliferation by ultimately reducing inward flux of calcium ions (Ca^{2+}). Cyclic GMP is removed by the PDE-5 enzyme to yield the inactive product 5'GMP. Patients with PAH have reduced expression and activity of eNOS.

Middle, the prostacyclin pathway. The production of PGI$_2$ is catalyzed by PS in endothelial cells. In PASMCs, PGI$_2$ stimulates AC, thus increasing production of cAMP from ATP. cAMP is a second messenger that constitutively maintains PASMC relaxation and inhibition of PASMC proliferation. Patients with PAH have reduced expression and activity of PS.

Right, the ET pathway. Big-(i.e., pro-) ET is converted in endothelial cells to ET$_1$ (a 21-amino acid peptide) by endothelin-converting enzyme (ECE). ET$_1$ binds to PASMC ET$_A$ and ET$_B$ receptors, ultimately leading to PASMC contraction, proliferation, and hypertrophy. Endothelin-1 also binds to endothelial cell ET$_B$ receptors (not illustrated). Patients with PAH have increased expression and activity of ECE.

TREATMENT

This chapter focuses on the treatment of WHO group 1 PAH, starting with general treatment measures, followed by supportive therapies and the role of CCBs and lastly disease-specific therapies. These therapeutic options are generally not applicable to non-WHO group 1 PH.

Before 1995	CCBs, anticoagulation, digitalis, diuretics
1995	Epoprostenol (intravenous)
2001	Bosentan
2002	Treprostinil (subcutaneous)
2004	Treprostinil (intravenous) and iloprost (inhaled)
2005	Sildenafil
2007	Ambrisentan
2009	Tadalafil and treprostinil (inhaled)
2013	Treprostinil (oral), Macitentan, Riociguat

CCBs, calcium channel blockers.

FIG. 2: Timeline of USFDA approval of pulmonary arterial hypertension specific therapies.

Goals of Treatment in Pulmonary Arterial Hypertension

With advances in our understanding of the pathophysiology of PH and availability of increasing number of therapeutic options there has been a shift in therapeutic goals from short-term functional changes to improvements in long-term outcomes. Variables used in clinical practice to determine response to therapy and prognosis include improvement in functional class to I or II, normal or near normal RV size and function based on echocardiographic or magnetic resonance imaging (MRI) evaluation, normalization of right atrial pressure (RAP) (<8 mmHg) and CI (>2.5–3.9L/minute/m^2), 6-minute walk distance (MWD) more than 380–440 m, peak oxygen uptake (VO$_2$) more than 15 mL/minute/kg and normal B-type natriuretic peptide level.[5]

General Treatment Measures

Diet

Limiting fluid and sodium intake (<2.4 g/day) is advised and is particularly important in patients with symptomatic right heart failure for managing the volume status.

Rehabilitation and Exercise Training

Results from three randomized controlled trials suggest that supervised exercise training improves functional capacity, quality of life and functional class.[6-8] Exercise training programs should be implemented by centers experienced in management of patients with PAH.

Immunizations

Routine immunizations against influenza and pneumococcal pneumonia are advised.

Pregnancy

According to current guidelines, pregnancy should be avoided or terminated as early as possible in women with PAH. The hemodynamic fluctuations during pregnancy, labor, delivery and the postpartum period are potentially devastating. In fact, maternal mortality rate as high as 30–50% has been observed in some series.[9] It is important to discuss effective birth control with women of childbearing age. Use of estrogen-containing contraceptives may increase the risk of venous thromboembolism, but preparations with a lower dose can be used with concurrent warfarin anticoagulation. Use of barrier methods or surgical sterilization can also be used as alternatives.

Supportive Therapies for Pulmonary Arterial Hypertension

Supportive therapies are treatments that are directed at the consequences of PAH. Supportive therapies have only been studied in retrospective and/or nonrandomized trials. Recommendations regarding their use are thus based on expert opinion.[10]

Oxygen

Oxygen supplementation is recommended to maintain arterial blood oxygen pressure above or equal to 60 mmHg to avoid hypoxia-mediated pulmonary vasoconstriction. Patients with hypoxemia should be evaluated for pulmonary embolism and right-to-left shunt. Exposure to high altitudes may worsen hypoxia and result in hypoxic pulmonary vasoconstriction. Similarly, some patients may require oxygen during air travel. Although there is no data from controlled trials, it is recommended that if the patient's pre-flight oxygen saturation as determined by pulse oximetry is less than 92%, he or she should receive supplemental oxygen.[11]

Anticoagulation

The pathologic evidence of in situ thrombosis and abnormal platelet function provides a rationale for anticoagulation in patients with PAH.[12] Anticoagulants have been studied in three noncontrolled observational series in patients with mainly iPAH.[13-15] An improvement in survival with warfarin anticoagulation has been observed. Anticoagulation is recommended in patients with iPAH and those with advanced disease requiring intravenous therapy (International Randomized Ratio goal of 1.5–2.5).[10] The role of newer anticoagulants, such as thrombin and factor Xa inhibitors, has not been studied in PAH.

Diuretics

Diuretics are used to manage RV volume overload, which manifests as elevated jugular venous pressure, lower extremity edema and abdominal distention. Loop diuretics including furosemide, bumetanide and torsemide are frequently used in clinical practice. Goals of therapy are to reduce the central venous pressure and eliminate renal and hepatic congestion without causing hypotension. Aldosterone antagonists, such as spironolactone can be used in patients to help conserve K^+ and may also have beneficial effects on RV remodeling. Renal function and electrolytes should be closely monitored in patients receiving diuretics.

Digoxin

Digoxin is sometimes used in patients with RV failure and low cardiac output or in patients with atrial arrhythmias. One study demonstrated that giving intravenous digoxin to iPAH patients produced a modest increase in cardiac output and a reduction in circulating norepinephrine levels after 2 hours. Longer-term data are not available.[16] There is a narrow therapeutic window and the goal serum digoxin level, as with any other heart failure patient being treated with digoxin, is 0.5–0.8 ng/mL. Levels should be closely monitored in elderly and patients with renal dysfunction.

Calcium-Channel Blockers

Acute vasodilator testing and the use of CCBs in PAH have mainly been studied in patients with iPAH. The rationale for vasodilator testing in diagnostic evaluation of PAH is based on two factors: (1) acute vasodilator responsiveness identifies patients with a better prognosis and (2) responders are more likely to have a sustained response to oral CCBs than nonresponders and can be treated with these less expensive drugs.[17] Acute vasodilator testing should be done only in referral centers and preferably using inhaled nitric oxide (iNO); although, intravenous epoprostenol or intravenous adenosine may be used as an alternative. A positive response is defined as a decrease in mPAP by at least 10 mmHg to an absolute level of mPAP below 40 mmHg without a decrease in cardiac output.

Calcium-channel blockers have been used in iPAH since 1992 when a study demonstrated 95%, 5-year survival in patients who exhibited an acute vasodilator response.[13] The typical agents used in PAH are dihydropyridines, including amlodipine or nifedipine, or the non-dihydropyridine diltiazem. The choice of CCB is based upon the patient's heart rate with relative bradycardia favoring the dihydropyridines and tachycardia favoring diltiazem. Verapamil is not used because of its potential negative inotropic effects. If a patient who meets the definition of an acute responder does not improve to WHO functional class I or II on CCB, the patient should no longer be considered a responder, and alternative or additional PAH-specific therapy should be instituted. Only approximately 8% of iPAH will continue to respond to CCB therapy over the following year.[17] In order to achieve the maximum benefit, patients generally need high doses of CCBs that are higher than those conventionally used to treat systemic hypertension, 20–30 mg/day of amlodipine, 180–240 mg/day of nifedipine and 720–960 mg/day of diltiazem.

Acute vasoreactivity testing is recommended in patients with idiopathic pulmonary PAH to identify patients that are likely to favorably respond to long-term treatment with high doses of CCBs.[10] Vasoreactivity testing is not recommended in non-WHO group 1 PH. Lastly, testing should be done with caution in patients with concomitant left ventricular disease as pulmonary edema has been reported in patients with stable left-sided heart failure.

Pulmonary Arterial Hypertension—Approved Drugs

Prior to 1995, there was no specific treatment for PAH. Extensive research over the last two decades has resulted in the development of several new treatment options. Currently, there are four classes of PAH approved drugs: (1) prostacyclin analogues, (2) endothelin receptor antagonists (ERAs), (3) phosphodiesterase-5 inhibitors (PDE-5is) and (4) soluble guanylate cyclase stimulators. Historically, approval of drug therapies in PAH has been largely supported by data from relatively small, randomized, placebo-controlled studies of 12–16 weeks duration demonstrating modest improvements in functional class, exercise capacity and hemodynamics. However, several more recent studies have been designed to prospectively assess long-term morbidity and mortality. Evidence supporting survival benefits of current PAH therapies is mostly surmised from observational post *hoc* analyses, referencing historical control data and meta-analysis. It should be noted that PAH-specific therapies have mainly been evaluated in patients with iPAH, hPAH, PAH associated with connective tissue disease (CTD) and in patients with PAH from anorexigen use. Extrapolation of findings to other PAH subgroups should be done with caution and this data does not apply to other categories of PH (Table 2).

Prostacyclins or Its Analogues

Prostacyclins are generated through the breakdown of arachidonic acid using prostacyclin synthase, an enzyme that is reduced in PAH patients (Fig. 1). The arachidonic acid

TABLE 2: Disease-specific therapies for pulmonary arterial hypertension

Drug	Dose	Side effects	Comments
Prostacyclin analogues			
Epoprostenol (IV)	Started at low dose of 1–2 ng/kg/min and increased by 1–2 ng/kg/minute weekly or biweekly, as tolerated to an optimal dose of 20–45 ng/kg/minute	Headache, flushing, jaw pain, nausea, diarrhea, hypotension, dizziness, thrombocytopenia, leg pain cough (inhaled) and site pain (subcutaneous	Interruption of IV therapy can cause life-threatening worsening of pulmonary hypertension
Treprostinil (SC, IV, inhaled and oral)	Treprostinil (SC and IV) started at low dose of 1–2 ng/kg/minute and increased to 20–80 ng/kg/minute		Bolus of IV therapy can cause severe side effects, in particular hypotension
	Treprostinil (inhaled) 3–9 breaths 4 times daily while awake		Line infections and thrombosis can occur in patients with indwelling catheters
	Treprostinil oral is started at a dose of 0.25 mg every 12 hours, increased every 3–4 days by 0.25–0.5 mg BID to a maximum dose of 21 mg every 12 hours		
Iloprost (inhaled)	Iloprost (inhaled), every 2 hours 6–9 times a day		
Endothelin receptor antagonists			
Bosentan	Started at 62.5 mg BID and titrated to 125 mg BID after 4 weeks	Peripheral edema, liver toxicity, anemia, teratogenicity, reduced hormonal contraceptive efficacy, reduced sperm count, and drug-drug interactions with strong inducers or inhibitors of CYP450 enzymes	Monthly LFTs with bosentan (US FDA recently removed the monthly monitoring requirement for ambrisentan)
Ambrisentan	Ambrisentan is started at a dose of 5 mg daily and is up titrated to 10 mg daily		Monthly pregnancy test for women of childbearing potential
Macitentan	Macitentan is started at 10 mg daily		

(continued)

Table 2 (*continued*)

Drug	Dose	Side effects	Comments
Phosphodiesterase-5 inhibitors			
Sildenafil	USFDA approved dose—20 mg TID	Headache, dizziness, nausea, priapism, epistaxis, hearing loss, AION and optic atrophy	Nitrates contraindicated due to potential life-threatening hypotension
Tadalafil	USFDA approved dose—40 mg daily		
Soluble guanylate cyclase stimulator			
Riociguat	USFDA approved initial dose is 1 mg TID. Consider 0.5 mg TID if patient becomes hypotensive. If systolic BP >95 mmHg and no symptoms of hypotension, up-titrate dose by 0.5 mg PO TID with dose increase no sooner than 2 weeks apart to highest tolerated dose (not to exceed 2.5 mg PO TID)	Nausea, vomiting, diarrhea, dyspepsia, gastritis, constipation, dizziness, headache, hypotension, anemia, serious bleeding, hemoptysis	Contraindicated in combination with PDE-5is because of hypotension

AION, anterior ischemic optic neuropathy; BID, twice a day; LFT, liver function test; TID, three times a day; PDE-5i, phosphodiesterase-5-inhibitors.

metabolism is shifted toward production of thromboxane (a vasoconstrictor and promoter of platelet aggregation), which contributes to the pathogenesis of PAH. The vasodilator and antiproliferative effects of prostacyclin I_2 are mediated through the production of cyclic adenosine monophosphate (cAMP) (Fig. 3).[18] Prostacyclin and its analogues also inhibit platelet aggregation.

Prostacyclins are US FDA approved for use in patients with PAH. Their use has been associated with reduced survival in patients with systolic heart failure (WHO group 2 PH) and increased pulmonary shunt flow and hypoxemia in patients with lung disease (WHO group 3 PH).[19-21]

There are three approved prostacyclins and four different modes of delivery:

1. Intravenous epoprostenol
2. Intravenous treprostinil, subcutaneous treprostinil, inhaled treprostinil, oral treprostinil
3. Inhaled iloprost.

The choice of prostacyclin and the route of administration are determined by a combination of severity of illness and patient factors. Severity of illness is based mainly on WHO functional class, but other risk factors should also be taken into consideration (Table 3). Patient factors include patient's preference of route, social support, manual dexterity and

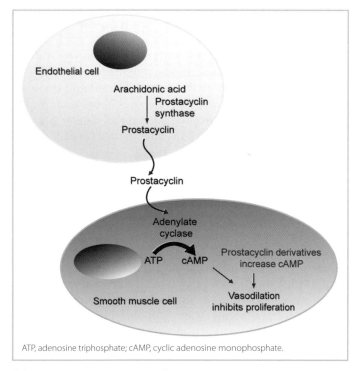

ATP, adenosine triphosphate; cAMP, cyclic adenosine monophosphate.

FIG. 3: Prostacyclins: Mechanism of action in pulmonary arterial hypertension.

TABLE 3: Determinants of prognosis in pulmonary arterial hypertension

Determinants of risk	Lower	Higher
Clinical evidence of RV failure	No	Yes
Progression	Gradual	Rapid
WHO class	II and III	IV
6-MWD	Longer (>400 m)	Shorter (<300 m)
CPET	Peak VO_2 >10.4 mL/kg/minute	Peak VO_2 <10.4 mL/kg/min
BNP	Minimally elevated	Significantly elevated
Echocardiographic findings	Minimal RV dysfunction	Pericardial effusion and significant RV dysfunction
Hemodynamics	RAP <10 mmHg CI >2.5 L/minute/m²	RAP >20 mmHg CI <2.0 L/minute/m²

6-MWD, 6-minute walk distance; BNP, B-type natriuretic peptide; CPET, cardiopulmonary exercise testing; RAP, right atrial pressure; RV, right ventricular; CI, confidence interval.

distance of the patient from a hospital with staff trained in their management.

Epoprostenol

Epoprostenol has a very short half-life of 3–6 minutes and is administered as a continuous intravenous infusion through a central venous catheter.

Epoprostenol was found to be beneficial in three unblinded randomized controlled trial in patients with iPAH[22,23] and in those with PAH associated with scleroderma spectrum of diseases.[24] Epoprostenol improves symptoms, exercise capacity and hemodynamics in both clinical conditions. Up until recently it was the only treatment shown to improve survival in iPAH.[23] Macitentan, as discussed later in this chapter, has also been shown to improve morbidity and mortality in patient with PAH (composite endpoint).[25]

Epoprostenol is US FDA-approved therapy for PAH. It is unstable at room temperature and needs to be maintained on ice after reconstitution. In 2010, a room temperature stable form of epoprostenol was approved for usage in PAH. Epoprostenol is started at a low dose of 1–2 ng/kg/minute and increased slowly by 1–2 ng/kg/minute weekly or biweekly, depending on tolerability and side effects to an optimal dose of 20–45 ng/kg/minute. A more rapid up-titration can be done under close monitoring in an intensive care unit. Because epoprostenol has a very short half-life, interruption of the infusion can result in rebound worsening of PH, which can be life-threatening. Likewise, inadvertent bolus administration can lead to life-threatening systemic vasodilation and hypotension.

Treprostinil

Treprostinil is a more stable prostanoid with an elimination half-life of about 4.5 hours. Treprostinil was initially studied as a subcutaneous infusion but is now also available as an intravenous infusion and as an inhaled formulation.

The following studies led to US FDA approval of various delivery forms of treprostinil. In a 12-week, double-blind, placebo-controlled, multicentre trial of 470 patients with functional classes II, III or IV PAH, subcutaneous treprostinil resulted in a modest but statistically significant median increase of 16 m of the 6-MWD, which was dose-related.[26,27] The TRUST trial (Treprostinil for Untreated Symptomatic PAH Trial) was a 12-week placebo-controlled study of intravenous treprostinil in 44 patients with New York Heart Association (NYHA) class III symptoms due to iPAH and hPAH. Six-MWD improved by a placebo corrected median of 83 m in patients treated with treprostinil (p = 0.0008).[28] Treprostinil patients also had a reduction in Borg scale of dyspnea by a median of 2 units (p = 0.02) and improved NYHA functional class by a median of class 1 (p = 0.051). The TRIUMPH trial (inhaled TReprostinil sodiUM in Patients with severe Pulmonary arterial Hypertension) showed that inhaled treprostinil improved exercise capacity, N-terminal pro-brain natriuretic peptide (NT-proBNP) and quality of life in PAH patients on background therapy with either bosentan or sildenafil.[29] Lastly, oral treprostinil at peak dose improved 6-MWD by 26 m in a randomized controlled trial of patients with de novo PAH not on any background therapy.[30]

The US FDA approved subcutaneous treprostinil in 2002 for use in functional classes II, III and IV PAH and intravenous treprostinil in 2004 for patients who do not tolerate the subcutaneous infusion. Inhaled treprostinil was approved by US FDA in 2009. Oral treprostinil was approved by US FDA in 2013.

Treprostinil (subcutaneous and intravenous) is started at a low dose of 1–2 ng/kg/minute and is increased gradually to a dose of 20–80 ng/kg/minute. If a rapid up-titration is needed, it should be done with close monitoring of the hemodynamic status. Inhaled treprostinil is administered via an ultrasonic nebulizer and the total dose is administered in less than a minute with 3–9 breaths four times a day. Oral treprostinil is started at a dose of 0.25 mg every 12 hours, increased every 3–4 days by 0.25–0.5 mg BID to a maximum dose of 21 mg every 12 hours.

Iloprost

Iloprost is a synthetic analogue of prostacyclin PGI_2. In the AIR trial (Aerosolized Randomized Iloprost Study) inhaled iloprost was compared to placebo inhalation in patients with PAH and CTEPH. The study showed improvement in exercise capacity, symptoms, PVR and clinical events.[31]

The US FDA approved inhaled iloprost in 2004 for functional class III and IV PAH. Iloprost is administered via the hand-held portable I-neb Adaptive Aerosol Delivery System every 2 hours while the patient is awake for a total of 6–9 treatments daily. The device also contains a computer microchip, which can be analyzed with software that provides useful information, such as patient compliance and treatment times.

Selexipag

Selexipag is an oral, selective prostacyclin receptor agonist. A large multicenter, double-blind, placebo-controlled, phase III study (GRIPHON) to demonstrate the efficacy and safety of selexipag was completed in 2014. This study is the largest study that has been completed in PAH and enrolled 1,156 patients. This was an event-driven study and the primary endpoint was time to first clinical worsening. Patients were treated for up to 4.3 years with selexipag 200–1600 µg or placebo twice a day. The results of this study have not been published but based on information provided by the company selexipag decreased the morbidity/mortality by 39% compared to placebo (p <0.0001). Selexipag has been submitted to the US FDA for approval for treatment of PAH.

Prostacyclin Side Effects

Common side effects of prostacyclin and prostacyclin analogues include headache, flushing, jaw pain, nausea, diarrhea, hypotension, dizziness and leg pain. Patients with intravenous catheters are at risk of infection and thrombosis as well as interruption of therapy. When given as a subcutaneous infusion (treprostinil), approximately 85% of patients experience infusion pain and/or infusion site reactions, which can be mitigated by rotating the infusion site. However, 5–23% of patients discontinue the subcutaneous infusion due to this complication. The inhaled agents are commonly associated with cough.

Endothelin Receptor Antagonists

Endothelin-1 is a vasoconstrictor and smooth muscle mitogen that may contribute to the development of PAH. The actions of endothelin-1 are mediated via two endothelin receptors, ET-A and ET-B (Fig. 1). Although activation of ET-A leads to vasoconstriction and ET-B tends to lead to vasodilatation and release of antiproliferative factors, selective versus nonselective blockade of receptors does not appear to affect clinical outcome (Fig. 4).

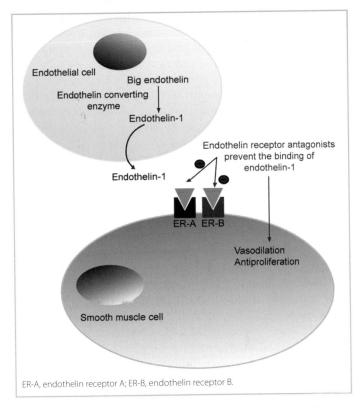

ER-A, endothelin receptor A; ER-B, endothelin receptor B.

FIG. 4: Endothelin receptor antagonists: Mechanism of action in pulmonary arterial hypertension.

Like prostacyclins, ERAs are only approved for use in WHO group 1 PAH. Benefits of therapy have not been shown in other types of PH and inappropriate use may result in harm. In patients with chronic left heart failure and PVH (WHO group 2), bosentan did not improve hemodynamic parameters. More patients, however, stopped therapy due to adverse effects including worsening of heart failure and death.[32] Similarly, studies on patients with WHO group 3 PH due to lung disease have not found ERAs to be beneficial and some have shown a decrease in exercise capacity and worsening of hypoxemia.[33,34]

Bosentan

Bosentan is a dual endothelin receptor antagonist. Five randomized controlled trials [Study-351, BREATH (Bosentan Randomized trial of Endothelin Antagonist Therapy)-1, BREATH-2, BREATH-5 and EARLY (Endothelin Antagonist Trial in Mildly symptomatic pulmonary arterial hypertension patients)] showed improvement in exercise capacity, functional class, hemodynamic parameters, echocardiographic and Doppler variables, and time to clinical worsening.[35-39]

Most studies on PAH-specific therapies have been performed on patients with advanced functional class (III or IV). In the EARLY study, bosentan therapy was evaluated in mildly symptomatic (WHO functional II) PAH. Patients were randomized to receive bosentan or placebo for 26 weeks. There was a significant improvement in PVR, but not in 6-MWD. There was a significant improvement in time to clinical worsening.[38] In patients with Eisenmenger syndrome, bosentan reduced PVR index, decreased mPAP and increased exercise capacity.

Bosentan was the first oral agent approved by the US FDA in 2001. The recommended starting dose is 62.5 mg twice a day with up-titration to 125 mg twice a day after 4 weeks.

Ambrisentan

Ambrisentan is a relatively selective endothelin-A receptor antagonist. The efficacy of ambrisentan was evaluated in a pilot study[40] and two large randomized controlled trials [AIRES (Ambrisentan in Pulmonary Arterial Hypertension, Randomized, double-blind, placebo-controlled, multicentre, Efficacy Study)-1 and AIRES-2).[41] Subjects who received ambrisentan had improvement in symptoms, exercise capacity, hemodynamics and time to clinical worsening when compared to placebo.

Use of ambrisentan has been studied in a small cohort of patients with portopulmonary hypertension (POPH). In this small study, 13 patients with POPH were given ambrisentan. The investigators found that ambrisentan decreased mPAP and PVR but no change in liver function tests (LFTs).[42]

The US FDA approved ambrisentan for use in PAH in 2007. It is given orally and the recommended starting dose is 5 mg daily, and it can be up-titrated to 10 mg daily.

Macitentan

Macitentan is a dual ERA that was developed by modifying the structure of bosentan to increase safety and efficacy. Macitentan is characterized by sustained receptor binding and enhanced tissue penetration. In the event-driven SERAPHIN (Study with an Endothelin Receptor Antagonist in Pulmonary Arterial Hypertension to Improve Clinical Outcome), Macitentan significantly reduced morbidity and mortality among patients with PAH and also increased exercise capacity. The primary endpoint of this study was the time from the initiation of treatment to the first occurrence of a composite endpoint of death, atrial septostomy, lung transplantation, initiation of treatment with intravenous or subcutaneous prostanoids or worsening of PAH. The benefits were observed regardless of whether the patient was receiving therapy for PAH.[25]

Macitentan was approved by US FDA in 2013 for treatment of PAH to delay disease progression. It is started at a dose of 10 mg/day.

Side Effects of Endothelin Receptor Antagonists

Side effects of the ERAs include peripheral edema, potential for liver toxicity, anemia, teratogenicity and drug-drug interactions with strong inducers or inhibitors of cytochrome P450 enzymes.

Bosentan leads to dose-related increases in liver transaminases in 10–15% patients,[36,43] For this reason, the US FDA mandates that LFTs be monitored monthly in all patients on bosentan. Monthly LFTs are not required in patients on ambrisentan and macitentan but periodic liver function testing is still recommended as part of the routine management of all patients with PAH, who may develop right heart failure and associated liver dysfunction.

Lower extremity edema can develop in up to 28% of patients treated with ambrisentan but may be less frequent with bosentan.[36,41] Although the etiology of edema has not been established, it is likely related to fluid retention rather than peripheral vasodilation. The side effect can usually be anticipated and controlled with diuretic adjustment without the need for drug discontinuation in most patients. It may be better to avoid initiating these therapies in patients with acutely decompensated right heart failure until the congestion has been adequately treated.

Nitric Oxide Pathway

The vasodilatory effects of nitric oxide depend upon its ability to augment and sustain cyclic guanosine monophosphate (cGMP) content in vascular smooth muscle. Nitric oxide activates guanylate cyclase, which increases cGMP production. This cGMP in turn causes vasorelaxation, but the effects are short-lived, as cGMP undergoes rapid degradation to GMP, and this is mediated by PDEs. PDE-5 hydrolyzes cAMP and cGMP, limiting their intracellular signaling (Fig. 1). Two classes of PAH-approved drugs affect the NO pathway, phosphodiesterase-5 inhibitors and soluble guanylate cyclase stimulators.

Sildenafil and tadalafil are PDE-5is and enhance the effects of vasodilating (and perhaps antiproliferative) cyclic nucleotides (Fig. 5). Like prostacyclins and ERAs, PDE-5is are currently only approved for use in PAH. Several small studies have looked at the role of PDE-5is in the treatment of WHO group 2 PH secondary to congestive heart failure.[44-46] These studies indicate that PDE-5is may improve exercise capacity in patients with PH due to heart failure, but further studies are needed. PDE-5is have also been studied in patients

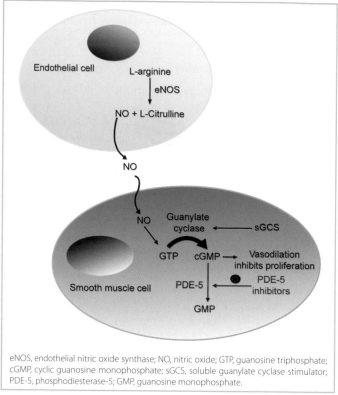

eNOS, endothelial nitric oxide synthase; NO, nitric oxide; GTP, guanosine triphosphate; cGMP, cyclic guanosine monophosphate; sGCS, soluble guanylate cyclase stimulator; PDE-5, phosphodiesterase-5; GMP, guanosine monophosphate.

FIG. 5: Phosphodiesterase-5 inhibitors: Mechanism of action in pulmonary arterial hypertension.

with WHO group 3 PH due to lung disease. A small study of patients with chronic obstructive lung disease found that sildenafil acutely improved hemodynamics but inhibited hypoxic vasoconstriction resulting in impairment of arterial oxygenation.[47] A study of 180 patients with idiopathic pulmonary fibrosis found no improvement in 6-MWD after 12 weeks of sildenafil therapy.[48] At this time, there is no clear role for PDE-5is in the setting of PH due to lung disease.

Sildenafil

Sildenafil was the first PDE-5i that was approved for use in patients with PAH. It has a short half-life of 3–4 hours and needs to be administered three times a day. Sildenafil is mostly used orally but is also available intravenously.

In the landmark SUPER-1 (Sildenafil Use in Pulmonary Arterial Hypertension) study, sildenafil improved 6-MWD in patients with PAH.[49] Sildenafil reduced the mPAP and improved functional class. The incidence of clinical worsening did not differ significantly between the patients treated with sildenafil versus placebo.

The US FDA approved sildenafil in patients with PAH in 2005 and the recommended dose is 20 mg orally three times a day.

Tadalafil

Tadalafil is a longer acting PDE-5i with a half-life of 17.5 hours and can be dosed once a day. Tadalafil at a dose of 40 mg/day, in the PHIRST trial (Pulmonary Arterial Hypertension and Response to Tadalafil) significantly improved 6-MWD and time to clinical worsening. There was no difference in change in functional class or Borg dyspnea score between tadalafil and placebo.[50]

The US FDA approved tadalafil for use in patients with PAH in 2009, and the recommended dose is 40 mg/day.

Side Effects of Phosphodiesterase-5 Inhibitors

Side effects of PDE-5is include headache, dizziness, nausea, epistaxis and priapism. There have been rare reports of patients treated with PDE-5is developing anterior ischemic optic neuropathy and optic atrophy, but causal association has not been clearly defined. Patients who develop visual changes while taking these medications should seek medical attention and discontinue use in the event of sudden vision loss. Hearing loss has been reported, but causality and mechanism remain unclear.

Use of nitrates is contraindicated in patients on PDE-5is because of the potential for life-threatening hypotension. Patients on PDE-5is should be advised to avoid all nitrates, including nitroglycerin and isosorbide mononitrate and isosorbide dinitrate. In patients who develop acute coronary syndrome, nitrates can be administered with close hemodynamic monitoring, 24 hours after the last dose of sildenafil and 48 hours after the last dose of tadalafil. Caution should be exercised when using α-blockers with PDE-5is because of the potential for orthostatic hypotension.

Riociguat (Soluble Guanylate Cyclase Stimulator)

Riociguat is a direct stimulator of the soluble guanylate cyclase independent of NO availability. It enhances the production of cGMP and is potentially effective also in conditions in which endogenous NO is depleted. In the PATENT (Pulmonary Arterial Hypertension Soluble Guanylate Cyclase-Stimulator Trial)-1 riociguat showed favorable results on exercise capacity, hemodynamics, WHO functional class and time to clinical worsening in PAH patients.[51]

Riociguat was approved by US FDA for PAH in 2013. The initial dose is 1 mg TID. Consider 0.5 mg TID if patient becomes hypotensive. If systolic BP is above 95 mmHg and no symptoms of hypotension, up-titrate dose by 0.5 mg PO TID with dose increase no sooner than 2 weeks apart to highest tolerated dose (not to exceed 2.5 mg PO TID).

The adverse effects of riociguat include nausea, vomiting, diarrhea, dyspepsia, gastritis, constipation, dizziness, headache, hypotension, anemia, serious bleeding and hemoptysis.

The combination of riociguate and PDE-5is is contraindicated because of hypotension.

Combination of Currently Approved Disease-specific Therapies for Pulmonary Arterial Hypertension

The management of PAH has been extensively studied over the last two decades, resulting in the development of many new treatment options. However, many questions remain; for example, is one drug therapy better than another, should more than one therapy be started simultaneously upon diagnosis, should a second drug be added later in the course of the disease, and if so, when. Given the availability of medications that target different pathologic processes, combination therapy is an attractive theoretical option. The fact that PAH is an orphan disease makes it difficult to conduct studies that have enough power to answer questions like this. However, several small studies have been performed on combination therapies, and more studies are underway. A recent meta-analysis on six randomized controlled trials showed that combination therapy reduced the risk of clinical worsening, increased 6-MWD and reduced mPAP, RAP and PVR.[52]

The approaches to institute combination therapy may be sequential or initial (upfront). Sequential combination therapy is the most widely utilized strategy. Drugs are added to monotherapy if there is inadequate clinical response or clinical deterioration. The PACES trial (Pulmonary Arterial Hypertension Combination Study of Epoprostenol and Sildenafil) studied the effects of the addition of sildenafil or placebo in PAH patients who remained symptomatic while on stable dose of intravenous epoprostenol for at least 3 months. Patients treated with sildenafil experienced a placebo-adjusted improvement in 6-MWD at 16 weeks, as well as improvement in mPAP, cardiac output and time to clinical worsening.[53] The TRIUMPH-1 study showed improvement in 6-MWD when inhaled treprostinil was added to either bosentan or sildenafil.[29] The COMPASS-1 study (The Effects of Combination of Bosentan and Sildenafil vs. Sildenafil Monotherapy on Morbidity and Mortality in Symptomatic Patients with Pulmonary Arterial Hypertension) investigated the acute pharmacodynamic effects of addition of sildenafil to bosentan in patients with PAH. Mean PVR was significantly reduced from baseline to 60 minutes following sildenafil administration. The reduction in PVR following sildenafil was comparable to that resulting from iNO.[54] Sequential combination therapy has been allocated a grade of recommendation I and level of evidence A in PAH patients with inadequate clinical response to initial monotherapy. Initial combination therapy has been allocated a grade of recommendation IIb and level of evidence C in WHO-FC IV PAH patients in case of nonavailability of IV prostanoids. The experience on randomized controlled trials with upfront combination therapy is limited to the small BREATH-2 study, which failed to demonstrate any significant difference between patients treated initially with the combination epoprostenol and bosentan as compared to epoprostenol alone.[37] In a more recent study, 23 treatment naïve PAH patients were treated with initial combination of epoprostenol and bosentan and compared with matched historical control group treated with epoprostenol. There was a statistically significant decrease in PVR in the initial combination therapy group but this hemodynamic benefit did not translate into statistically significant difference in survival, or in transplant-free survival.[55] The results of the AMBITION (A randomized, Multicenter Study of First-Line Ambrisentan and Tadalafil Combination Therapy in Subjects with Pulmonary Arterial Hypertension) were recently presented at the European Respiratory Society International Congress 2014 in Munich, Germany. This study compared first-line monotherapy with tadalafil, monotherapy with ambrisentan and combination therapy with tadalafil and ambrisentan in de novo WHO-FC II and III PAH patients. Combination therapy reduced the risk of clinical failure compared to pooled ambrisentan and tadalafil monotherapy arms. This was mainly driven by reduction in hospitalization. There was also significant decrease in NT-proBNP and improvement in 6-MWD.

Invasive Therapies

Lung and Combined Heart and Lung Transplantation

None of the current medical therapies for PAH are curative. Patients who have continued progression of the disease on medical therapies and patients with advanced disease (WHO-FCs III–IV) should be referred to a center that specializes in lung transplantation. Delayed referral in combination with the length of the waiting time, due to the shortage of organ donors, may increase the mortality on the waiting list and clinical severity at the time of transplantation. Patients who undergo lung transplantation for PAH have higher perioperative mortality, reflecting the hemodynamic severity of the disease;

however, the long-term post-transplant outcomes among those who survive the first year are similar to lung transplant recipients with other indications. The survival post-transplant is 52–75% at 5 years and 45–66% at 10 years.[56-58] The etiology of PAH may help the decision making because the prognosis varies according to the underlying condition. PAH associated with CTD has a worse prognosis than iPAH even when treated with prostanoids, while patients with PAH associated with congenital heart disease have a better survival. The worst prognosis is seen in patients with pulmonary veno-occlusive disease and pulmonary capillary hemangiomatosis because of the lack of effective medical treatments and these patients should be listed for transplantation at diagnosis.

Atrial Septostomy

As the right heart function worsens in response to ongoing severe PAH, patients experience progressive dyspnea, ascites, lower extremity edema and may have presyncope or syncope. Atrial septostomy creates a right-to-left interatrial shunt, decreasing RV filling pressure and improving RV function and LV filling. While the created shunt decreases systemic arterial oxygen saturation, it is anticipated that improved cardiac output will result in overall augmentation of systemic oxygen delivery.

The procedure can be performed either surgically or in the cardiac catheterization laboratory with balloon septostomy. A percutaneous approach is preferred in most patients because of the very high risk of surgery. The procedure can be considered for patients with recurrent syncope despite optimization of medical therapies as a bridge to lung transplantation or palliation in patients who are not transplant candidates. The procedure-related mortality is high (around 16%). Several recommendations have been made to minimize the risk. Atrial septostomy should be performed in centers with experience in its use and management of potential complications. A mean RAP above 20 mmHg, PVR index more than 55 Wood units/m^2 and a predicted 1-year survival less than 40% are significant predictors of a procedure-related death. Before cardiac catheterization, patients should have systemic oxygen saturation more than 90% in room air and optimized cardiac function.

Pulmonary Thromboendarterectomy

Patients with suspected PAH should undergo evaluation for WHO-group 4 PH, i.e., CTEPH. The screening tool of choice for CTEPH is a ventilation perfusion scan. If indicative of CTEPH, a pulmonary angiogram should be performed. Patients are considered to be candidate for pulmonary thrombo-endarterectomy (PTE) if they have surgically accessible disease and present acceptable surgical risk. The goal of PTE is to remove sufficient material from the pulmonary arteries to substantially lower PVR and improve cardiac output. This complex and life-saving procedure is best performed at high volume centers.

Patients who have no surgical targets and thus have inoperable CTEPH and patients who have persistent PH after PTE have been shown to benefit from the guanylate cyclase stimulator riociguat. The CHEST (Chronic Thromboembolic Pulmonary Hypertension Soluble Guanylate Cyclase-Stimulator Trial)-1 trial showed that riociguat improved exercise capacity and PVR in this group of patients.[59]

Riociguat was approved by the US FDA in 2013 for use in patients with CTEPH. For dosing and side effects see section on guanylate cyclase stimulators.

PROGNOSIS

Pulmonary arterial hypertension is a progressive disease, and the overall prognosis is poor. Estimated median survival of patients with iPAH before available therapy was 2.8 years after diagnosis.[60] With the advent of new therapies over the last two decades, however, contemporary survival and quality of life of patients with PAH have improved substantially compared with prior survival estimates.[60-62] A meta-analysis of all the randomized, controlled trials performed from 1990 to 2008 demonstrated a reduction in mortality of 43%. Number of patients to be treated to prevent one death was 61.6 and 16.2 deaths were prevented in each 1,000 patients treated.[63] Predictors of a poor outcome include clinical evidence of RV failure, rapid progression of disease and advanced functional class, poor exercise capacity as measured by 6-MWD or cardiopulmonary exercise test, elevated brain natriuretic peptide, RV dysfunction or pericardial effusion by echocardiogram and high RA pressure, high PVR and low cardiac index by RHC (Table 3). Information from two large present-day registries of patients with PAH gives us the opportunity to better understand the prognosis of PAH, its determinants and outcomes in the current treatment era. These registries are the French National Registry and the REVEAL Registry (the Registry to Evaluate Early and Long-Term PAH Disease Management). French National Registry enrolled 354 consecutive idiopathic, heritable and anorexigen-associated patients from October 2002 to October 2003. The 1-year, 2-year and 3-year survival rates per this registry are 82.9%, 67.1% and 58.2%, respectively. Univariate analysis suggested that the factors associated with better prognosis were female sex, functional class I or II symptoms, greater 6-MWD, lower RAP and higher cardiac output. The multivariate analysis reduced this list to three independent factors, namely, sex, 6-MWD and cardiac output at diagnosis.[61,64] The REVEAL Registry analyzed 2,716 patients with PAH and found 1-year survival to be 91% from the date of enrollment and the 1-year and 3-year survival rates from the time of PAH diagnosis of 87.7% and 72.1%, respectively. Sex, functional class, 6-MWD, origin of PAH, age, PVR, RAP, renal insufficiency, resting systolic blood pressure and heart rate, BNP, presence of a pericardial effusion and diffusing capacity of the lung for carbon monoxide were predictive of outcome.[65]

TREATMENT ALGORITHM AND EVALUATING RESPONSE TO THERAPY

There is emerging evidence that earlier initiation of therapy when patients are mildly symptomatic improves functional and clinical status. The decision to initiate vasodilator therapy and the specific agents used depend on the patients' WHO-FC, risk profile and preference. PAH patients with symptoms that result in slight limitation of physical activity (WHO-FC II) should be started on oral agents, either ERAs or PDE-5is. Patients that are unable to carry out any physical activity without symptoms (WHO functional class IV) need more aggressive therapy and prostacyclin therapy should be considered. The guidelines propose a wide range of treatment options for patients who are asymptomatic at rest but have marked limitation of physical activity (WHO-FC III). Patients with WHO-FC III symptoms and poor prognostic factors should be considered for prostacyclin therapy, while patients with good prognostic profile can be started on oral therapy.

Close follow-up is crucial in all patients started on PAH-specific therapy. Stable patients on oral therapy can be followed every 4–6 months. Patients with more advanced and/or progressive symptoms, right heart failure and patients on intravenous therapy need to be seen at least every 3 months. With each clinic visit, WHO-FC, BNP/NT-proBNP and exercise capacity (6-MWD or graded treadmill) is checked to help determine response to therapy. A repeat echocardiogram is done at least 6 months after commencing PAH-specific therapy. The timing of repeat RHC varies between PH centers. RHC should be considered in patients with progressive symptoms in spite of therapy, prior to addition of a new PAH specific agent, and many experts routinely repeat RHC after 1 year on therapy, particularly in patients on prostacyclin therapy (Fig. 6).

Patients who have inadequate clinical response on monotherapy, i.e., symptoms progress or do not improve

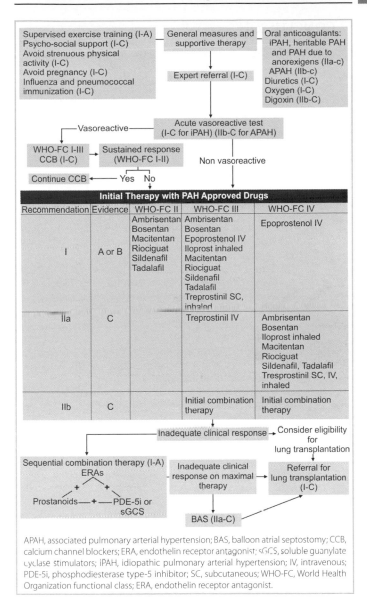

FIG. 6: Evidence-based treatment algorithm for the management of pulmonary arterial hypertension. Drugs within the same grade of evidence are listed in alphabetical order and not order of preference.[10]

to WHO-FC I or II may benefit from switching PAH-specific agents or from a combination of agents. As discussed above, combining PAH-specific therapies that affect different pathways make therapeutic sense and are currently under intense investigation. Lastly, invasive therapies like lung transplantation or atrial septostomy may be an option for patients who have progressive symptoms in spite of optimization of medical therapies.

CONCLUSION

Over the last two decades, remarkable progress has been made in the understanding of the pathophysiology and pathogenesis of PAH. Improvement in knowledge has resulted in many new treatment options. PAH has evolved from a rare, untreatable and fatal entity to that of an effectively managed disease with improvement in quality of life and survival. There is still much to learn and accomplish in managing this complex disease.

REFERENCES

1. Simonneau G, Gatzoulis MA, Adatia I, et al. Updated clinical classification of pulmonary hypertension. J Am Coll Cardiol. 2013;62(25 Suppl):D34-41.
2. Hoeper MM, Bogaard HJ, Condliffe R, et al. Definitions and diagnosis of pulmonary hypertension. J Am Coll Cardiol. 2013;62(25 Suppl):D42-50.
3. Humbert M, Sitbon O, Chaouat A, et al. Pulmonary arterial hypertension in France: results from a national registry. Am J Respir Crit Care Med. 2006;173(9):1023-30.
4. Peacock AJ, Murphy NF, McMurray JJ, et al. An epidemiological study of pulmonary arterial hypertension. Eur Respir J. 2007;30(1):104-9.
5. McLaughlin VV, Gaine SP, Howard LS, et al. Treatment goals of pulmonary hypertension. J Am Coll Cardiol. 2013;62:D73-81.
6. Mereles D, Ehlken N, Kreuscher S, et al. Exercise and respiratory training improve exercise capacity and quality of life in patients with severe chronic pulmonary hypertension. Circulation. 2006;114(14):1482-9.
7. Weinstein AA, Chin LM, Keyser RE, et al. Effect of aerobic exercise training on fatigue and physical activity in patients with pulmonary arterial hypertension. Respir Med. 2013;107(5):778-84.
8. Chan L, Chin LM, Kennedy M, et al. Benefits of intensive treadmill exercise training on cardiorespiratory function and quality of life in patients with pulmonary hypertension. Chest. 2013;143(2):333-43.
9. Weiss BM, Zemp L, Seifert B, et al. Outcome of pulmonary vascular disease in pregnancy: a systematic overview from 1978 through 1996. J Am Coll Cardiol. 1998;31(7):1650-7.
10. Galie N, Corris PA, Frost A, et al. Updated treatment algorithm of pulmonary arterial hypertension. J Am Coll Cardiol. 2013;62(25 Suppl):D60-72.
11. Mohr LC. Hypoxia during air travel in adults with pulmonary disease. Am J Med Sci. 2008;335(1):71-9.
12. Johnson SR, Mehta S, Granton JT. Anticoagulation in pulmonary arterial hypertension: a qualitative systematic review. Eur Respir J. 2006;28(5):999-1004.
13. Rich S, Kaufmann E, Levy PS. The effect of high doses of calcium-channel blockers on survival in primary pulmonary hypertension. N Engl J Med. 1992;327(2):76-81.
14. Fuster V, Steele PM, Edwards WD, et al. Primary pulmonary hypertension: natural history and the importance of thrombosis. Circulation. 1984;70(4):580-7.
15. Frank H, Mlczoch J, Huber K, et al. The effect of anticoagulant therapy in primary and anorectic drug-induced pulmonary hypertension. Chest. 1997;112(3):714-21.
16. Rich S, Seidlitz M, Dodin E, et al. The short-term effects of digoxin in patients with right ventricular dysfunction from pulmonary hypertension. Chest. 1998;114(3):787-92.
17. Sitbon O, Humbert M, Jais X, et al. Long-term response to calcium channel blockers in idiopathic pulmonary arterial hypertension. Circulation. 2005;111(23):3105-11.
18. Humbert M, Sitbon O, Simonneau G. Treatment of pulmonary arterial hypertension. N Engl J Med. 2004;351(14):1425-36.
19. Califf RM, Adams KF, McKenna WJ, et al. A randomized controlled trial of epoprostenol therapy for severe congestive heart failure: The Flolan International Randomized Survival Trial (FIRST). Am Heart J. 1997;134(1):44-54.

20. Olschewski H, Ghofrani HA, Walmrath D, et al. Inhaled prostacyclin and iloprost in severe pulmonary hypertension secondary to lung fibrosis. Am J Respir Crit Care Med. 1999;160(2):600-7.

21. Ghofrani HA, Wiedemann R, Rose F, et al. Sildenafil for treatment of lung fibrosis and pulmonary hypertension: a randomised controlled trial. Lancet. 2002;360(9337):895-900.

22. Rubin LJ, Mendoza J, Hood M, et al. Treatment of primary pulmonary hypertension with continuous intravenous prostacyclin (epoprostenol). Results of a randomized trial. Ann Intern Med. 1990;112(7):485-91.

23. Barst RJ, Rubin LJ, The Primary Pulmonary Hypertension Study Group, et al. A comparison of continuous intravenous epoprostenol (prostacyclin) with conventional therapy for primary pulmonary hypertension. N Engl J Med. 1996;334(5):296-302.

24. Badesch DB, Tapson VF, McGoon MD, et al. Continuous intravenous epoprostenol for pulmonary hypertension due to the scleroderma spectrum of disease. A randomized, controlled trial. Ann Intern Med. 2000;132(6):425-34.

25. Pulido T, Adzerikho I, Channick RN, et al. Macitentan and morbidity and mortality in pulmonary arterial hypertension. N Engl J Med. 2013;369(9):809-18.

26. Laliberte K, Arneson C, Jeffs R, et al. Pharmacokinetics and steady-state bioequivalence of treprostinil sodium (Remodulin) administered by the intravenous and subcutaneous route to normal volunteers. J Cardiovasc Pharmacol. 2004;44(2):209-14.

27. Simonneau G, Barst RJ, Galie N, et al. Continuous subcutaneous infusion of treprostinil, a prostacyclin analogue, in patients with pulmonary arterial hypertension: a double-blind, randomized, placebo-controlled trial. Am J Respir Crit Care Med. 2002;165(6):800-4.

28. Hiremath J, Thanikachalam S, Parikh K, et al. Exercise improvement and plasma biomarker changes with intravenous treprostinil therapy for pulmonary arterial hypertension: a placebo-controlled trial. J Heart Lung Transplant: the official publication of the International Society for Heart Transplantation. 2010;29(2):137-49.

29. McLaughlin VV, Benza RL, Rubin LJ, et al. Addition of inhaled treprostinil to oral therapy for pulmonary arterial hypertension: a randomized controlled clinical trial. J Am Coll Cardiol. 2010;55(18):1915-22.

30. Jing ZC, Parikh K, Pulido T, et al. Efficacy and safety of oral treprostinil monotherapy for the treatment of pulmonary arterial hypertension: a randomized, controlled trial. Circulation. 2013;127(5):624-33.

31. Olschewski H, Simonneau G, Galie N, et al. Inhaled iloprost for severe pulmonary hypertension. N Engl J Med. 2002;347(5):322-9.

32. Kaluski E, Cotter G, Leitman M, et al. Clinical and hemodynamic effects of bosentan dose optimization in symptomatic heart failure patients with severe systolic dysfunction, associated with secondary pulmonary hypertension—a multi-center randomized study. Cardiology. 2008;109(4):273-80.

33. Stolz D, Rasch H, Linka A, et al. A randomised, controlled trial of bosentan in severe COPD. Eur Respir J. 2008;32(3):619-28.

34. King TE Jr, Brown KK, Raghu G, et al. BUILD-3: a randomized, controlled trial of bosentan in idiopathic pulmonary fibrosis. Am J Respir Crit Care Med. 2011;184(1):92-9.

35. Channick RN, Simonneau G, Sitbon O, et al. Effects of the dual endothelin-receptor antagonist bosentan in patients with pulmonary hypertension: a randomised placebo-controlled study. Lancet. 2001;358(9288):1119-23.

36. Rubin LJ, Badesch DB, Barst RJ, et al. Bosentan therapy for pulmonary arterial hypertension. N Engl J Med. 2002;346(12):896-903.

37. Humbert M, Barst RJ, Robbins IM, et al. Combination of bosentan with epoprostenol in pulmonary arterial hypertension: BREATHE-2. Eur Respir J. 2004;24(3):353-9.

38. Galie N, Rubin L, Hoeper M, et al. Treatment of patients with mildly symptomatic pulmonary arterial hypertension with bosentan (EARLY study): a double-blind, randomised controlled trial. Lancet. 2008;371(9630):2093-100.

39. Galie N, Beghetti M, Gatzoulis MA, et al. Bosentan therapy in patients with Eisenmenger syndrome: a multicenter, double-blind, randomized, placebo-controlled study. Circulation. 2006;114(1):48-54.

40. Galie N, Badesch D, Oudiz R, et al. Ambrisentan therapy for pulmonary arterial hypertension. J Am Coll Cardiol. 2005;46(3):529-35.

41. Galie N, Olschewski H, Oudiz RJ, et al. Ambrisentan for the treatment of pulmonary arterial hypertension: results of the ambrisentan in pulmonary arterial hypertension, randomized, double-blind, placebo-controlled, multicenter, efficacy (ARIES) study 1 and 2. Circulation. 2008;117(23):3010-9.

42. Cartin-Ceba R, Swanson K, Iyer V, et al. Safety and efficacy of ambrisentan for the treatment of portopulmonary hypertension. Chest. 2011;139(1):109-14.

43. McLaughlin VV, Sitbon O, Badesch DB, et al. Survival with first-line bosentan in patients with primary pulmonary hypertension. Eur Respir J. 2005;25(2):244-9.

44. Guazzi M, Samaja M, Arena R, et al. Long-term use of sildenafil in the therapeutic management of heart failure. J Am Coll Cardiol. 2007;50(22):2136-44.

45. Guazzi M, Vicenzi M, Arena R, et al. Pulmonary hypertension in heart failure with preserved ejection fraction: a target of phosphodiesterase-5 inhibition in a 1-year study. Circulation. 2011;124(2):164-74.

46. Lewis GD, Shah R, Shahzad K, et al. Sildenafil improves exercise capacity and quality of life in patients with systolic heart failure and secondary pulmonary hypertension. Circulation. 2007;116(14):1555-62.

47. Blanco I, Gimeno E, Munoz PA, et al. Hemodynamic and gas exchange effects of sildenafil in patients with chronic obstructive pulmonary disease and pulmonary hypertension. Am J Respir Crit Care Med. 2010;181(3):270-8.

48. Zisman DA, Schwarz M, Anstrom KJ, et al. A controlled trial of sildenafil in advanced idiopathic pulmonary fibrosis. N Engl J Med. 2010;363(7):620-8.

49. Galie N, Ghofrani HA, Torbicki A, et al. Sildenafil citrate therapy for pulmonary arterial hypertension. N Engl J Med. 2005;353(20):2148-57.

50. Galie N, Brundage BH, Ghofrani HA, et al. Tadalafil therapy for pulmonary arterial hypertension. Circulation. 2009;119(22):2894-903.

51. Ghofrani HA, Galie N, Grimminger F, et al. Riociguat for the treatment of pulmonary arterial hypertension. N Engl J Med. 2013;369(4):330-40.

52. Galie N, Palazzini M, Manes A. Pulmonary arterial hypertension: from the kingdom of the near-dead to multiple clinical trial meta-analyses. Eur Heart J. 2010;31(17):2080-6.

53. Simonneau G, Rubin LJ, Galie N, et al. Addition of sildenafil to long-term intravenous epoprostenol therapy in patients with pulmonary arterial hypertension: a randomized trial. Ann Inter Med. 2008;149(8):521-30.

54. Gruenig E, Michelakis E, Vachiery JL, et al. Acute hemodynamic effects of single-dose sildenafil when added to established bosentan therapy in patients with pulmonary arterial hypertension: results of the COMPASS-1 study. J Clin Pharmacol. 2009;49(11):1343-52.

55. Kemp K, Savale L, O'Callaghan DS, et al. Usefulness of first-line combination therapy with epoprostenol and bosentan in pulmonary arterial hypertension: an observational study. J Heart Lung Transplant. 2012;31(2):150-8.

56. Toyoda Y, Thacker J, Santos R, et al. Long-term outcome of lung and heart-lung transplantation for idiopathic pulmonary arterial hypertension. Ann Thorac Surg. 2008;86(4):1116-22.

57. Fadel E, Mercier O, Mussot S, et al. Long-term outcome of double-lung and heart-lung transplantation for pulmonary hypertension: a comparative retrospective study of 219 patients. Eur J Cardiothorac Surg. 2010;38(3):277-84.

58. de Perrot M, Granton JT, McRae K, et al. Outcome of patients with pulmonary arterial hypertension referred for lung transplantation: a 14-year single-center experience. J Thorac Cardiovasc Surg. 2012;143(4):910-8.

59. Ghofrani HA, D'Armini AM, Grimminger F, et al. Riociguat for the treatment of chronic thromboembolic pulmonary hypertension. N Engl J Med. 2013;369(4):319-29.

60. D'Alonzo GE, Barst RJ, Ayres SM, et al. Survival in patients with primary pulmonary hypertension. Results from a national prospective registry. Ann Inter Med. 1991;115(5):343-9.

61. Humbert M, Sitbon O, Yaici A, et al. Survival in incident and prevalent cohorts of patients with pulmonary arterial hypertension. Eur Respir J. 2010;36(3):549-55.

62. Thenappan T, Shah SJ, Rich S, et al. Survival in pulmonary arterial hypertension: a reappraisal of the NIH risk stratification equation. Eur Respir J. 2010;35(5):1079-87.

63. Galie N, Manes A, Negro L, et al. A meta-analysis of randomized controlled trials in pulmonary arterial hypertension. Eur Heart J. 2009;30(4):394-403.

64. Humbert M, Sitbon O, Chaouat A, et al. Survival in patients with idiopathic, familial, and anorexigen-associated pulmonary arterial hypertension in the modern management era. Circulation. 2010;122(2):156-63.

65. Benza RL, Miller DP, Gomberg-Maitland M, et al. Predicting survival in pulmonary arterial hypertension: insights from the Registry to Evaluate Early and Long-Term Pulmonary Arterial Hypertension Disease Management (REVEAL). Circulation. 2010;122(2):164-72.

Cardiac Drugs in Pregnancy and Lactation

Wassef Karrowni, Kanu Chatterjee

INTRODUCTION

Cardiovascular diseases (CVD) complicate 0.2–4% of all pregnancies in western industrialized countries.[1] In addition, the risk of CVD in pregnancy is expected to increase due to increasing age at first pregnancy and increasing prevalence of cardiovascular risk factors.[2] Since only few medications have specifically been tested for safety and efficacy during pregnancy and lactation, physicians caring for pregnant women have very little information to help them decide whether the potential benefits to the mother outweigh the risks to the fetus.[3] It should be appreciated, however, that current methods to assess teratogenicity consist mainly of pregnancy registries and case-control surveillance studies with very few randomized controlled trials available.

Several factors have to be taken into consideration when prescribing a drug to a pregnant or breastfeeding woman. These factors include, but are not limited to, gestational age of the embryo or fetus, route of drug administration, whether the drug crosses the placenta or is excreted in breast milk and the necessary effective dose of the drug.[4] Awareness of the unique physiologic changes of pregnancy (increase in cardiac output and glomerular filtration rate, increase in body fat and decrease in plasma albumin concentration) that affect the pharmacokinetics of medications used by pregnant women is of critical importance in deciding the dosage and frequency of administration and monitoring. A major concern is the potential harm to the fetus or nursing infant, but equally important is the assessment of the potential harm to the mother that withholding a drug can cause.[4] Thus, in these situations, when prescribing a drug, the decision comes down to "Does the benefit of the drug outweigh its risks?"

It is of paramount importance to start by identifying cardiovascular drugs of known teratogenic effects. Drugs that irreversibly alter growth, structure or function of the developing embryo or fetus are classified as teratogens. Commonly used cardiovascular drugs that are classified as teratogens include inhibitors of the renin-angiotensin system, warfarin and 3-hydroxy-3-methylglutaryl-coenzyme A (CoA) reductase inhibitors (Table 1).

To help guide physicians, the US Food and Drug Administration (USFDA) has developed categories of risk of medication used during pregnancy (Table 2). Categories A and B generally are considered safe in humans. Category C medications have not been definitively shown to be harmful to human fetuses, but reasons exist to be cautious when prescribing them. Category D drugs are those with evidence of human fetal risk based on well-controlled human studies. Finally, category X drugs are very high risk to the human fetus and should never be used in pregnancy.

TABLE 1: Cardiovascular drugs with teratogenic effects

Drug	Teratogenic effects
Inhibitors of the renin-angiotensin system	Renal or tubular dysplasia, prolonged renal failure in neonates, ossification disorders of skull, oligohydramnios, growth retardation, lung hypoplasia, contractures, large joints, anemia and intrauterine fetal death
Warfarin	Fetal hemorrhage, skeletal and central nervous system defects, Dandy-Walker syndrome*
3-hydroxy-3-methylglutaryl-CoA reductase inhibitors (statins)	Skeletal malformations

*A congenital brain malformation involving the cerebellum and the fluid filled spaces around it.
CoA, coenzyme A.

TABLE 2: USFDA pregnancy risk category for medications

USFDA category	Definition
A	No risk in controlled human studies
B	No risk in controlled animal studies; or animal studies have shown an adverse effect, but adequate and well-controlled studies in pregnant women have failed to demonstrate a risk to the fetus
C	Small risk in controlled animal studies; or no animal studies have been conducted and there are no adequate and well-controlled studies in pregnant women
D	Strong evidence of risk to the human fetus, but the benefits from use in pregnant women may be acceptable, despite the risk
X	Never to be used in pregnancy; very high risk to the human fetus

HYPERTENSIVE DISEASE IN PREGNANCY AND LACTATION

Hypertensive disorders are the most frequent cardiovascular complications during pregnancy, complicating up to 15% of pregnancies and accounting for about a quarter of all antenatal admissions.[5] Hypertension in pregnancy is not a single entity but comprises and is generally classified into four different entities, including preexisting hypertension and gestational hypertension (develops after 20 weeks of gestation).[6] It remains a major cause of maternal, fetal, and neonatal morbidity and mortality. These women are at higher risk for severe complications, such as abruptio placentae, cerebrovascular accident, organ failure and disseminated intravascular coagulation, and the fetus is at risk for intrauterine growth retardation, prematurity and intrauterine death.[2]

Antihypertensive therapy for mild-to-moderate hypertension in pregnancy [defined as systolic blood pressure (SBP) of 140–169 mmHg and diastolic blood pressure (DBP) of 90–109 mmHg] does not seem to decrease the incidence of preeclampsia nor affect maternal or perinatal outcomes.[7] Thus, avoidance of drug therapy is suggested in mild hypertension where nonpharmacological therapies may suffice.[8] Chronic antihypertensive therapy can be stopped during pregnancy under close observation and resumed, if necessary. Alternatively, a woman whose arterial pressure was well controlled by antihypertensives before pregnancy may continue with the same agents [except for angiotensin-converting enzymes inhibitors (ACEIs), angiotensin receptor blockers (ARBs) and direct renin inhibitors, which are contraindicated]. On the other hand, drug treatment of severe hypertension (SBP ≥160–170 mmHg or DBP ≥110 mmHg) in pregnancy is beneficial and is required.

The different antihypertensive medications and their potential usage in pregnancy are listed in Table 3. The drug of choice for long-term treatment of hypertension during pregnancy is methyldopa (centrally acting agent leading to a reduction in the sympathetic outflow).[9] Multiple other agents could also be used, such as the α-/β-blocker labetalol, β-adrenoceptor antagonists (metoprolol and propranolol) and calcium channel blockers (nifedipine). Diuretics may decrease blood flow in the placenta and should be avoided for treatment of hypertension.[2] In hypertensive crises, the drug of choice is sodium nitroprusside, given as an intravenous infusion at 0.25–5.0 μg/kg/min.[2] In the case of preeclampsia associated with pulmonary edema, intravenous nitroglycerin infusion (20–200 μg/min) is the drug of choice.[2] Labetalol can also be administered in intravenous form and used for treatment of severe hypertension. Intravenous hydralazine use is associated

TABLE 3: Drugs commonly used to treat hypertension in pregnancy and lactation

Drug	USFDA category	Route of administration	Placental permeability	Reported adverse effects
Methyldopa	B	Oral	Yes	Mild neonatal hypotension
Labetalol	C	Oral/intravenous	Yes	Intrauterine growth retardation (second and third trimesters), neonatal bradycardia and hypotension (used near term)
Nifedipine	C	Oral	Yes	Tocolytic; potential synergism with magnesium sulfate may induce maternal hypotension and fetal hypoxia
Metoprolol	C	Oral/intravenous	Yes	Bradycardia and hypoglycemia in fetus
Propranolol	C	Oral	Yes	Bradycardia and hypoglycemia in fetus
Nitroglycerin	B	Intravenous	Unknown	Bradycardia, tocolytic
Hydralazine	C	Oral	Yes	Maternal lupus-like symptoms; fetal tachyarrhythmias. Intravenous use is associated with more perinatal adverse effects and is avoided
Hydrochlorothiazide	B	Oral	Yes	Oligohydramnios

with more perinatal adverse effects than other drugs and is no longer the drug of choice.[2] All antihypertensive agents taken by the nursing mothers are excreted into breast milk; however, most are present at very low concentrations and are considered compatible with breastfeeding. The exceptions are propranolol and nifedipine, whose concentrations in breast milk are similar to those in maternal plasma.[2]

ACUTE CORONARY SYNDROME AND STABLE CORONARY ARTERY DISEASE IN PREGNANCY AND LACTATION

Coronary artery disease (CAD) management during pregnancy has been an increasingly encountered challenge by the physicians because of the increasing maternal age. Acute coronary syndrome (ACS) is rare during pregnancy, but it has devastating consequences with maternal mortality of 5–10%.[2] The spectrum of causes of ACS during pregnancy is different from the general population. Spontaneous coronary artery dissection makes a substantial proportion and is mostly reported around delivery or in the early postpartum period.[10] Thus, coronary angiography with the possibility of coronary intervention (PCI) is the preferred first-line therapy for patients presenting with ST-elevation myocardial infarction.[2] PCI in pregnancy can be considered relatively safe, taking into account the minimal risk of radiation exposure to the fetus, especially during the period of organogenesis. On the other hand, thrombolytic therapy should be reserved for life-threatening ACS with no access to PCI.[11] Coronary artery bypass surgery can be performed during pregnancy and the maternal mortality equals mortality in nonpregnant cardiac surgery. However, the fetal mortality risk is still high with an incidence of 20%.[12] Drug therapy during pregnancy for patients with ACS is summarized in Table 4.

The management of patients with stable CAD aims to reduce the progression of atherosclerosis and prevent anginal symptoms. The classes of medications used include antiplatelet agents, lipid-lowering agents and antianginal drugs (Table 5). In pregnant patients with CAD, aspirin in low doses (<150 mg/day) should be used and is considered safe.[15,16] On the other hand, higher doses are associated with fetal and maternal hemorrhage, premature closure of the ductus arteriosus and fetal congenital abnormalities. It is well established that reduction in low-density lipoprotein is associated with decrease in the risk of coronary heart disease and all-cause mortality. Statins are the first-line therapy for dyslipidemias in the general population, but are contraindicated in pregnancy. They are labeled USFDA category X for possible teratogenic effects (mainly skeletal defects observed in animal studies).[17]

TABLE 4: Drug therapy in pregnancy and acute coronary syndrome

Drug	USFDA category	Maternal considerations	Fetal considerations	Breastfeeding	Comments
Thrombolytics					
Streptokinase Recombinant plasminogen activators	C	Hemorrhage risk ~8% (mostly from the genital tract)[13]	Do not cross the placenta in animals (unknown in human) Causes subplacental bleeding Fetal loss 6%[14] Preterm delivery 6%[14]	No data on excretion into human milk	Relatively contraindicated Reserved for life-threatening ACS with no access to PCI
Antithrombotics					
Unfractionated heparin Low-molecular-weight heparin	B	Regular monitoring of therapeutic levels is needed	Does not cross the placenta	Compatible	Because of scarce data, fondaparinux should not be used in pregnancy Bivalirudin is not recommended during pregnancy due to lack of safety data
Antiplatelet agents					
Low-dose aspirin (<150 mg/day)	B	Large trials demonstrated relative safety during pregnancy	Crosses human placenta	Well tolerated	Higher doses have teratogenic effects Avoid breastfeeding with high dose
Clopidogrel	C	During pregnancy use only when strictly needed (e.g., after stenting) and for the shortest duration possible (ESC) Bare metal stents should be the first choice if percutaneous coronary intervention is needed	Unknown	Unknown	The use of glycoprotein of IIb/IIIa inhibitors, prasugrel, and ticagrelor is not recommended during pregnancy given the absence of safety data

TABLE 5: Drug therapy in pregnancy and stable coronary artery disease

Drugs	USFDA category	Maternal considerations	Fetal considerations	Excretion in milk	Comments
Antiplatelet agents					
Low-dose aspirin (<150 mg/day)	B	Large trials demonstrated relative safety during pregnancy	Crosses human placenta	Well tolerated	Higher doses are associated with teratogenic effects Avoid breastfeeding if using high dose
Antianginal drugs					
Nitrates (Isosorbide dinitrate)	B	Maternal hypotension should be avoided (subsequent fetal hypoperfusion)	Unknown if crosses human placenta	Unknown	Bradycardia; isosorbide mononitrate class C
Calcium channel blockers	C	—	Crosses the placenta	Yes	Diltiazem has teratogenic effects in animals (should not be used)
β-blockers	C	—	Risk of mildly lower birth weight, bradycardia and hypoglycemia in fetus	—	Avoid atenolol (USFDA category D)
Lipid-lowering drugs					
Statins	X	Should be started in the postpartum period	Crosses human placenta	Unknown	Causes congenital anomalies
Fenofibrate	C	—	Crosses human placenta	Yes	No adequate human data available
Gemfibrozil	C	—	Crosses human placenta	Unknown	No adequate human data available
Colestipol, cholestyramine	C	—	Unknown	Transfer to breast milk lowering neonatal fat soluble vitamins (e.g., vitamin K)	May predispose to neonatal cerebral bleeding
Ezetimibe	C	—	Unknown	Unknown	Limited data available

The treatment of angina pectoris in pregnancy follows the same general principles, which include decreasing the myocardial oxygen demand and improving coronary perfusion. β-blockers decrease oxygen demand by slowing down the heart rate. In general, β-blockers are relatively safe with the exception of atenolol (USFDA category X). However, caution should be used as severe bradycardia can lead to uteroplacental hypoperfusion. The use of β-blockers is associated with a mildly lower birth weight, bradycardia and hypoglycemia in fetus. On the other hand, atenolol use should be avoided as it has been associated with hypospadias (first trimester) and birth defects, low birth weight, bradycardia and hypoglycemia in fetus (second and third trimesters).[2]

The antianginal effect of nitrates and calcium channel blockers is via vasodilatation. This results in decreased cardiac workload (decreased afterload from peripheral vasodilation) and improved coronary perfusion (coronary vasodilatation). Similar to β-blockers, caution has to be practiced with high doses, which may cause maternal hypotension and subsequent fetal hypoperfusion. Nifedipine appears to be safe and is frequently used during pregnancy for the treatment of hypertension. On the other hand, diltiazem should not be used, as it has teratogenic effects (skeletal abnormalities) in animals, and there is no information about its use in human pregnancy.[18] Diltiazem is also excreted in milk in concentration similar to that in maternal plasma and should be avoided during breastfeeding.

CARDIOMYOPATHIES AND HEART FAILURE IN PREGNANCY AND LACTATION

Cardiomyopathies are rare but serious disease during pregnancy with peripartum cardiomyopathy (PPCM) representing the most common cause of severe complications.[2,19] PPCM is defined as an idiopathic cardiomyopathy that presents with heart failure secondary to left ventricular (LV) systolic dysfunction toward the end of pregnancy or in the months after delivery, in the absence of any other cause of heart failure.[20] When diagnosed during pregnancy, the majority of patients present in third trimester, with a few patients presenting in the second trimester.[21]

In general, the medical management of pregnant or lactating patient with cardiomyopathy should follow the standard drug therapy for acute and chronic heart failure, except that drug therapy may need to be altered because of potential detrimental effects on the fetus or the lactating infant.[22] The drugs commonly used for the management of patients with cardiomyopathy during pregnancy or lactation are summarized in Table 6. It is important to note that ACEIs

TABLE 6: Drugs commonly used in the management of heart failure patients during pregnancy

Drug	USFDA category	Route of administration	Placental permeability	Reported adverse effects
Inotropy				
Dopamine	C	Intravenous	—	Increased uterine resistance; animal studies demonstrated decrease in newborn survival rate and potential for cataract formation
Dobutamine	B	Intravenous	—	No evidence of harm to the fetus
Milrinone	C	Intravenous	Yes	No teratogenicity in animal studies
Digoxin	C	Intravenous/oral	Yes	Serum levels unreliable
Preload reduction				
Furosemide	C	Intravenous/oral	Yes	Oligohydramnios
Hydrochlorothiazide	B	Oral	Yes	Oligohydramnios
Afterload reduction				
Nitrates	B	Intravenous/oral	Unknown	Bradycardia, tocolytic
Nitroprusside	C	Intravenous	—	Prolonged use associated with thiocyanate toxicity
Hydralazine	C	Oral	Yes	Maternal lupus-like symptoms; fetal tachyarrhythmias. Intravenous use is associated with more perinatal adverse effects and is avoided
β-blockers				
Metoprolol	C	Intravenous/oral	Yes	Bradycardia and hypoglycemia in fetus
Bisoprolol	C	Oral	Yes	Bradycardia and hypoglycemia in fetus

despite being hallmark for therapy of patients with heart failure, given their effect on ventricular remodeling, are teratogenic in pregnancy and, therefore, should be strictly avoided.[23] Few data are available regarding ARBs in pregnancy, but are also contraindicated in pregnancy because their actions are similar to that of ACEIs.[24] Thus, during pregnancy, the combination of organic nitrates and hydralazine should be used as a substitute for ACEIs or ARBs; and in the acute setting, intravenous nitroglycerin is considered first line for afterload reduction.[22] The ACEIs considered compatible with breastfeeding are benazepril, captopril and enalapril.[2,25] Currently, there is no data describing the use of other ACEIs or ARBs during human lactation.[8]

The use of aldosterone antagonists should be avoided during pregnancy.[26] Spironolactone (USFDA category D) can be associated with antiandrogenic effects in first trimester. However, it is considered compatible with breastfeeding.[25] Data for eplerenone are lacking, otherwise, most other drugs used for the management of heart failure are compatible with breastfeeding.[22] In addition, a recent study reported that the rate of recovery of LV function was significantly higher in lactating women.[27] Thus, clinically stable women with PPCM should not be discouraged from breastfeeding their infants.[22]

ARRHYTHMIA IN PREGNANCY AND LACTATION

Arrhythmias are divided into two categories—bradyarrhythmias and tachyarrhythmias. During pregnancy, there is an increased incidence of maternal cardiac arrhythmias explained in part by the metabolic, hormonal and hemodynamic changes.[28] In addition, there are increased numbers of women with congenital cardiac malformations reaching reproductive age with the advances in cardiac surgery, and these patients are known to be more prone to cardiac arrhythmias.[29]

The most common maternal arrhythmias during pregnancy are simple ventricular and atrial ectopy (reported in 50-60% of pregnant women).[30] Bradyarrhythmias are rare during pregnancy and usually have a favorable outcome in the absence of underlying heart disease.[2] Characteristic arrhythmia in the fetus are supraventricular tachycardia (SVT) and atrial flutter.[31] In these cases, the mother is simply the conduit for transplacental administration of the drug.

The major concern regarding the use of antiarrhythmic drugs during pregnancy is their potential adverse effects on the fetus, and all antiarrhythmic drugs should be regarded as potentially toxic to the fetus (Tables 7 and 8).[2] The smallest recommended dose should be used initially and the patient should be monitored regularly with measurement of serum drug levels

TABLE 7: Drugs commonly used for treatment of supraventricular tachyarrhythmias during pregnancy and lactation

Drug	Drug class*	USFDA category	Placental permeability	Breastfeeding considerations	Reported adverse effects
Adenosine	—	C	No	Compatible	No fetal adverse effects reported
Metoprolol	II	C	Yes	Compatible	Bradycardia and hypoglycemia in fetus
Digoxin	—	C	Yes	Compatible	Serum levels unreliable
Diltiazem	IV	C	No	Compatible	Increased risk of birth defects
Verapamil	IV	C	Yes	Compatible	Maternal hypotension, fetal bradycardia and heart block
Sotalol	III	B	Yes	Compatible	Bradycardia and hypoglycemia in fetus
Flecainide	Ic	C	Yes	Compatible	Safe in structurally normal hearts
Propafenone	Ic	C	Yes	Unknown	Limited experience
Amiodarone	III	D	Yes	Avoid	Fetal hypothyroidism, hyperthyroidism, goiter, bradycardia, growth retardation, premature birth

*Vaughan-Williams classification of antiarrhythmic drugs.

TABLE 8: Drugs commonly used for treatment of ventricular tachyarrhythmias during pregnancy and lactation

Drug	Drug class*	USFDA category	Placental permeability	Breastfeeding considerations	Reported adverse effects
Metoprolol	II	C	Yes	Compatible	Bradycardia and hypoglycemia in fetus
Verapamil	IV	C	Yes	Compatible	Maternal hypotension, fetal bradycardia and heart block
Sotalol	III	B	Yes	Compatible	Bradycardia and hypoglycemia in fetus; Torsade de pointes
Procainamide	Ia	C	Yes	Compatible but long-term therapy should be avoided	Lupus-like syndrome with long-term use, Torsade de pointes
Flecainide	Ic	C	Yes	Compatible	Safe in structurally normal hearts
Propafenone	Ic	C	Yes	Unknown	Limited experience
Amiodarone	III	D	Yes	Avoid	Fetal hypothyroidism, hyperthyroidism, goiter, bradycardia, growth retardation, premature birth

*Vaughan-Williams classification of antiarrhythmic drugs.

(when available) along with reassessment for continued need for medication.[31] In the setting of minimally symptomatic simple arrhythmias (such as, premature ventricular or atrial beats), no treatment is necessary. On the other hand, patients with SVT (atrioventricular nodal reentry tachycardia, atrioventricular reentry tachycardia, atrial fibrillation, atrial flutter, etc.) and severe symptoms or hemodynamic compromise need medical intervention. Serious ventricular arrhythmias (ventricular tachycardia or fibrillation) are rare during pregnancy but are life-threatening, so prompt treatment is needed.

Patients with SVT and hemodynamic instability require immediate electrical cardioversion (which seems to be safe in all stages of pregnancy).[2] Intravenous adenosine is safe to terminate SVTs in the hemodynamically stable patient, if the vagal maneuver fails, and in the absence of preexcitation (class I: conditions for which there is evidence and/or general agreement that a given procedure is useful and effective). Intravenous metoprolol or propranolol can also be considered for the same purpose (class IIa: weight of evidence/opinion is in favor of usefulness/efficacy). Alternatively, intravenous verapamil can be used (class IIb: usefulness/efficacy is less well established by evidence/opinion).[2] For long-term management, β-blockers (metoprolol or propranolol) and digoxin are drugs of first choice (class I). If these fail, oral sotalol or flecainide should be considered (IIa) and oral propafenone or procainamide may be considered as the last option if other suggested agents fail and before amiodarone is used (IIb). It is important to note that atenolol should not be used for any arrhythmia (USFDA risk category D) because of its known adverse effects on fetal growth. Amiodarone is also fetotoxic and should not be used unless other options fail. There is limited experience with dronedarone (a new antiarrhythmic drug) and should not be used during pregnancy.

Immediate electrical cardioversion is recommended for patients with sustained ventricular tachycardia (VT) and hemodynamic instability (class I). In stable patients with sustained VT, it is also desirable to restore normal sinus rhythm in a timely fashion.[2] This can be achieved via electrical cardioversion, antitachycardia pacing or antiarrhythmic drugs.[2] Intravenous sotalol (in the absence of prolonged QT interval) or procainamide should be considered in monomorphic VT (IIa; conditions for which there is conflicting evidence and/or a divergence of opinion about the usefulness/efficacy of a procedure and the weight of evidence favors usefulness/efficacy). The use of intravenous amiodarone should be reserved for patients with sustained monomorphic VT that is hemodynamically unstable, refractory to conversion or recurrent despite other agents (IIa).[2] Oral metoprolol, propranolol or verapamil is recommended for long-term management of idiopathic sustained VT (class I). If these drugs fail, oral sotalol, flecainide or propafenone should be considered (IIa). For long-term management of the congenital long QT syndrome, β-blocking agents are recommended during pregnancy and also postpartum (class I).[2] Mexiletine has been used during pregnancy without maternal or fetal complications

VENOUS THROMBOEMBOLISM AND THROMBOPROPHYLAXIS IN PREGNANCY AND LACTATION

In addition to venous thromboembolism (VTE) that occurs in increased frequency during pregnancy and postpartum period and represents a significant cause of morbidity and mortality, there are multiple other conditions, which need antithrombotic therapy during pregnancy and lactation. The increased thromboembolic risk in atrial fibrillation is assessed with the CHADS2 [C: congestive heart failure (or LV systolic dysfunction); H: hypertension: blood pressure consistently above 140/90 mmHg (or treated hypertension on medication); A: age ≥75 years; D: diabetes; S: prior stroke or transient ischemic attack] score or the CHA2DS2VASC [C: congestive heart failure (or LV systolic dysfunction); H: hypertension: blood pressure consistently above 140/90 mmHg (or treated hypertension on medication); A: age ≥75 years; D: diabetes; S: prior stroke or transient ischemic attack, or thromboembolism; V: vascular disease; A: age 65–74 years; SC: sex category] score, and thromboprophylaxis is recommended in high-risk pregnant patients.[2] Thromboprophylaxis is also advisable in PPCM patients from the time of the diagnosis until LV function recovers [LV ejection fraction (LVEF) >35%], because of the high incidence of thromboembolism (particularly during pregnancy and the first 6–8 weeks of postpartum).[22] Patients with mechanical valves carry the risk of valve thrombosis, which is increased during pregnancy. Thus, anticoagulation therapy (Table 9) in these women is recommended to prevent the occurrence of valve thrombosis and its lethal consequences for both mother and fetus.[2]

The choice of the anticoagulant is made according to the condition being treated and the stage of pregnancy. Low-molecular-weight heparin (LMWH) has become the drug of choice for the treatment of VTE (pulmonary embolism or deep vein thrombosis) in pregnancy. Because of more risk of thrombocytopenia, osteoporosis and less convenient dosing when compared with LMWH, unfractionated heparin is favored only in special situations like in patients with renal failure and in the acute treatment of massive pulmonary embolism.[2] On the other hand, multiple studies have shown that heparin

used and short-acting drugs are preferred. Finally, patients should always be informed about the risks and benefits of each medical therapy and should be involved in the decision-making process.

REFERENCES

1. Weiss BM, von Segesser LK, Alon E, et al. Outcome of cardiovascular surgery and pregnancy: a systematic review of the period 1984-1996. Am J Obstet Gynecol. 1998;179(6 Pt 1):1643-53.
2. European Society of Gynecology; Association for European Paediatric Cardiology; German Society for Gender Medicine, et al. ESC guidelines on the management of cardiovascular diseases during pregnancy: the Task Force on the Management of Cardiovascular Diseases during Pregnancy of the European Society of Cardiology (ESC). Eur Heart J. 2011;32(24):3147-97.
3. Koren G, Pastuszak A, Ito S. Drugs in pregnancy. N Engl J Med. 1998;338(16):1128-37.
4. Buhimschi CS, Weiner CP. Medications in pregnancy and lactation: part 1. Teratology. Obstet Gynecol. 2009;113(1):166-88.
5. James PR, Nelson-Piercy C. Management of hypertension before, during, and after pregnancy. Heart. 2004;90(12):1499-504.
6. Helewa ME, Burrows RF, Smith J, et al. Report of the Canadian Hypertension Society Consensus Conference: 1. Definitions, evaluation and classification of hypertensive disorders in pregnancy. CMAJ. 1997;157(6):715-25.
7. Abalos E, Duley L, Steyn DW, et al. Antihypertensive drug therapy for mild to moderate hypertension during pregnancy. Cochrane Database Syst Rev. 2007;(1):CD002252.
8. Ghanem FA, Movahed A. Use of antihypertensive drugs during pregnancy and lactation. Cardiovasc Ther. 2008;26(1):38-49.
9. Cockburn J, Moar VA, Ounsted M, et al. Final report of study on hypertension during pregnancy: the effects of specific treatment on the growth and development of the children. Lancet. 1982;1(8273):647-9.
10. Roth A, Elkayam U. Acute myocardial infarction associated with pregnancy. J Am Coll Cardiol. 2008;52(3):171-80.
11. Leonhardt G, Gaul C, Nietsch HH, et al. Thrombolytic therapy in pregnancy. J Thromb Thrombolysis. 2006;21(3):271-6.
12. Arnoni RT, Arnoni AS, Bonini RC, et al. Risk factors associated with cardiac surgery during pregnancy. Ann Thorac Surg. 2003;76(5):1605-8.
13. Turrentine MA, Braems G, Ramirez MM. Use of thrombolytics for the treatment of thromboembolic disease during pregnancy. Obstet Gynecol Surv. 1995;50(7):534-41.
14. Ahearn GS, Hadjiliadis D, Govert JA, et al. Massive pulmonary embolism during pregnancy successfully treated with recombinant tissue plasminogen activator: a case report and review of treatment options. Arch Intern Med. 2002;162(11):1221-7.
15. CLASP: a randomised trial of low-dose aspirin for the prevention and treatment of pre-eclampsia among 9364 pregnant women. CLASP (Collaborative Low-dose Aspirin Study in Pregnancy) Collaborative Group. Lancet. 1994;343(8898):619-29.
16. Roberts JM, Catov JM. Aspirin for pre-eclampsia: compelling data on benefit and risk. Lancet. 2007;369(9575):1765-6.
17. Pollack PS, Shields KE, Burnett DM, et al. Pregnancy outcomes after maternal exposure to simvastatin and lovastatin. Birth Defects Res A Clin Mol Teratol. 2005;73(11):888-96.
18. Tan HL, Lie KI. Treatment of tachyarrhythmias during pregnancy and lactation. Eur Heart J. 2001;22(6):458-64.
19. Pearson GD, Veille JC, Rahimtoola S, et al. Peripartum cardiomyopathy: National Heart, Lung, and Blood Institute and Office of Rare Diseases (National Institutes of Health) workshop recommendations and review. JAMA. 2000;283(9):1183-8.

20. Sliwa K, Hilfiker-Kleiner D, Petrie MC, et al. Current state of knowledge on aetiology, diagnosis, management, and therapy of peripartum cardiomyopathy: a position statement from the Heart Failure Association of the European Society of Cardiology Working Group on peripartum cardiomyopathy. Eur J Heart Fail. 2010;12(8):767-78.

21. Elkayam U, Akhter MW, Singh H, et al. Pregnancy-associated cardiomyopathy: clinical characteristics and a comparison between early and late presentation. Circulation. 2005;111(16):2050-5.

22. Elkayam U. Clinical characteristics of peripartum cardiomyopathy in the United States: diagnosis, prognosis, and management. J Am Coll Cardiol. 2011;58(7): 659-70.

23. Alwan S, Polifka JE, Friedman JM. Angiotensin II receptor antagonist treatment during pregnancy. Birth Defects Res A Clin Mol Teratol. 2005;73(2):123-30.

24. Siu SC, Sermer M, Colman JM, et al. Prospective multicenter study of pregnancy outcomes in women with heart disease. Circulation. 2001;104(5):515-21.

25. American Academy of Pediatrics Committee on Drugs. Transfer of drugs and other chemicals into human milk. Pediatrics. 2001;108(3):776-89.

26. Mirshahi M, Ayani E, Nicolas C, et al. The blockade of mineralocorticoid hormone signaling provokes dramatic teratogenesis in cultured rat embryos. Int J Toxicol. 2002;21(3):191-9.

27. Safirstein JG, Ro AS, Grandhi S, et al. Predictors of left ventricular recovery in a cohort of peripartum cardiomyopathy patients recruited via the internet. Int J Cardiol. 2012;154(1):27-31.

28. Widerhorn J, Widerhorn AL, Rahimtoola SH, et al. WPW syndrome during pregnancy: increased incidence of supraventricular arrhythmias. Am Heart J. 1992;123(3):796-8.

29. Perloff JK. Pregnancy and congenital heart disease. J Am Coll Cardiol. 1991;18(2):340-2.

30. Shotan A, Ostrzega E, Mehra A, et al. Incidence of arrhythmias in normal pregnancy and relation to palpitations, dizziness, and syncope. Am J Cardiol. 1997;79(8):1061-4.

31. Joglar JA, Page RL. Antiarrhythmic drugs in pregnancy. Curr Opin Cardiol. 2001;16(1):40-5.

32. Salazar E, Izaguirre R, Verdejo J, et al. Failure of adjusted doses of subcutaneous heparin to prevent thromboembolic phenomena in pregnant patients with mechanical cardiac valve prostheses. J Am Coll Cardiol. 1996;27(7):1698-703.

33. Vitale N, De Feo M, De Santo LS, et al. Dose-dependent fetal complications of warfarin in pregnant women with mechanical heart valves. J Am Coll Cardiol. 1999;33(6):1637-41.

34. European Heart Rhythm Association; European Association for Cardio-Thoracic Surgery; Camm AJ, et al. Guidelines for the management of atrial fibrillation: the Task Force for the Management of Atrial Fibrillation of the European Society of Cardiology (ESC). Europace. 2010;12(10):1360-420.

Future Directions: Role of Genetics in Drug Therapy

Eric J Topol

INTRODUCTION

There has been considerable progress in the genomics of cardiovascular drug interactions, but unfortunately little of this has yet been incorporated into clinical care. Let me divide the advances that have been made into two major categories—common genomic variants, which means those occurring in more than 5% of the population, and rare variants.

COMMON VARIANTS

The genome-wide association studies, which used micro-arrays with approximately 1 million single nucleotide variants, identified many important pharmacogenomic sequence variants for drugs such as statins, clopidogrel and warfarin. At Vanderbilt University, 10,000 patients were screened for the CYP2C19 common variants that affect clopidogrel efficacy, the myopathy side effects of statins (SCOLB1 variant) and sequence variants in the genes affecting warfarin dosing (VKORC1 and CYP2C9). A significant minority of patients carried at least one of the high-risk variants for these commonly used cardiovascular drugs (Fig. 1).[1]

However, such well-established sequence variants are not assessed in most patients due to practical considerations including cost, turnaround time and the gap in knowledge base for the majority of practicing cardiologists. These issues need to be addressed in the future with point-of-care rapid genotyping at low cost and educational initiatives to bring physicians up to speed on the utility of using pharmacogenomics in routine patient care.

There has been, in general, fixation on the individual's DNA for pharmacogenomics. But a discovery that the gut micro-biome can harbor bacteria that make drugs ineffective, such as digoxin, has broadened the basis of DNA-drug interactions.[2]

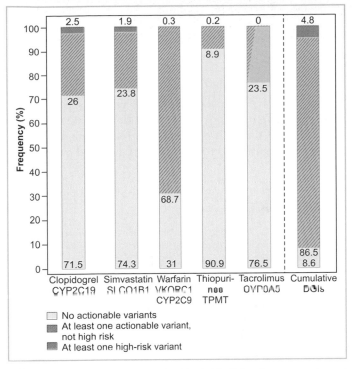

FIG. 1: In 10,000 patients screened at Vanderbilt University, commonly used medications were associated with a substantial number who had actionable variants.[1]

Much more gut microbiome sequencing will be necessary to understand the implications on other commonly used cardiovascular medications.

RARE VARIANTS

By sequencing, two genes, both affecting lipids, have been shown to mark protective effects. PCSK9 loss-of-function mutations lead to very low low-density lipoprotein (LDL) levels in the blood, and afford substantial protection against coronary disease. Similarly, loss-of-function mutations in the gene APOC3, which lead to low triglycerides, also provide approximately 40% reduction in ischemic heart disease. Because both these gene mutations are rare (<1% of the population), they required sequencing to be discovered. As a result, both have led to new drug development. The PCSK9 trials have moved far along to Phase 3 and have to date achieved very marked LDL lowering without significant side effects.[3] The drugs are monoclonal antibodies, which require at least once monthly subcutaneous injection.

For simulating loss-of-function of APOC3,[4] an antisense drug is being tested. It substantially lowers triglyceride levels but, like PCSK9, it remains to be seen whether major reductions in adverse cardiovascular outcomes will be achieved. Undoubtedly, in the era of sequencing that has now reached the $1,000 per whole genome level of cost, many more important low frequency and rare sequence variants will be discovered. New drug classes will be developed, but always there will be the question as to whether administering a drug later in life, with potential off-target effects, will be comparable with a mutation in nature that endows the individual from the time of conception. Nevertheless, this represents an exciting path for the future of cardiovascular drugs based on genomic guidance.

REFERENCES

1. Van Driest SL, Shi Y, Bowton EA, et al. Clinically actionable genotypes among 10,000 patients with preemptive pharmacogenomic testing. Clin Pharmacol Ther. 2014;95(4):423-31.

2. Haiser HJ, Gootenberg DB, Chatman K, et al. Predicting and manipulating cardiac drug inactivation by the human gut bacterium Eggerthella lenta. Science. 2013;341(6143):295-8.

3. Blom DJ, Hala T, Bolognese M, et al. A 52-week placebo-controlled trial of evolocumab in hyperlipidemia. N Engl J Med. 2014;370:1809-19.

4. Jorgensen AB, Frikke-Schmidt R, Nordestgaard BG, et al. Loss-of-function mutations in APOC3 and risk of ischemic vascular disease. N Engl J Med. 2014;371(1):32-41.

Index

Page numbers followed by *f* refer to figure and *t* refer to table.